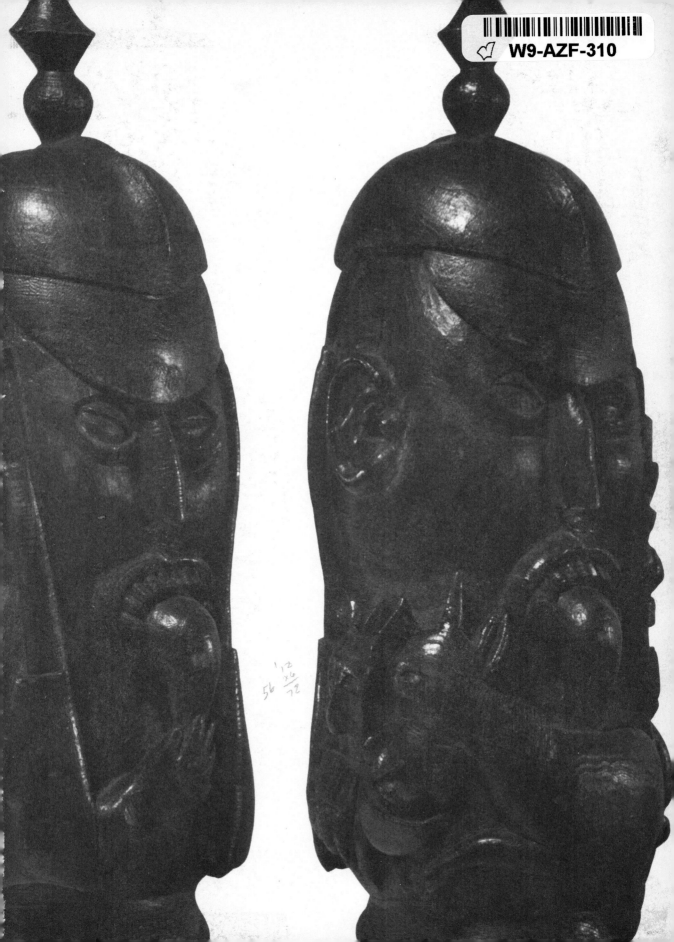

EPHRAIM ROSEN

Late Professor of Psychology
University of Minnesota

RONALD E. FOX

Associate Professor of Psychology
Ohio State University

IAN GREGORY

Professor and Chairman
Department of Psychiatry
Ohio State University

abnormal psychology

SECOND EDITION

1972 —— W. B. SAUNDERS COMPANY — Philadelphia · London · Toronto

W. B. Saunders Company: West Washington Square
Philadelphia, Pa.   19105

12 Dyott Street
London, WC1A   1DB

1835 Yonge Street
Toronto 7, Canada

Abnormal Psychology

ISBN 0-7216-7696-0

Print No.:   9   8   7   6   5   4   3   2   1

To our wives

MARGARET FOX

and

JEAN GREGORY

It is a thing of no great difficulty to raise objections against another man's
oration—nay, it is a very easy matter; but to produce a better in its place
is a work extremely troublesome.
Plutarch, *Of Hearing*

PREFACE

Any comprehensive view of man's behavior must be based on information from a variety of disciplines that include genetics, physiology, biochemistry, psychology, sociology and anthropology. Because of the tremendous advances being made in each field of study, however, scholars have tended to become isolated by specialization. Even in such closely related disciplines as psychology, psychoanalysis and psychiatry, students are frequently unaware of each other's literature and viewpoints, and may therefore be unable to communicate effectively. This is not the first textbook of abnormal psychology to be written jointly by psychologists and a psychiatrist, but we believe it is unique in its attempt to integrate psychoanalytic theory, experimental psychology and practical clinical experience with research in the various biological and social sciences.

This book begins with an introduction to the general principles of abnormal psychology, and then proceeds to an application of these principles to the analysis of each of the main syndromes of abnormal behavior. The chapters are structured in terms of definition and description, development and dynamics, causation and treatment. This method of analyzing abnormal behavior has provided a logical basis for the presentation of the subject matter as a whole. Within this systematic framework we are concerned with such questions as: What is abnormality? What abnormal behavior is associated with a given diagnosis? What are the characteristic dynamics or modes of adaptation? What is the developmental history? What causal factors probably initiated or perpetuated this abnormal behavior? What approaches to treatment have been adopted?

The desire to simplify information for the undergraduate student sometimes leads to a glossing over of conflicting findings or interpretations, and the presentation of a one-sided or reductionistic point of view. This book, however, is intended for serious students, and there has been no attempt to avoid any aspect of the subject because of difficulty or controversy. We have not avoided discussion of methodological issues, presentation of contradictory evidence, or use of statistics and tables. We have taken great pains, however, to explain every new concept clearly and to use whatever forms of illustration seemed desirable for clarification, including a large number of case histories which are discussed in some detail. The latter are not restricted to any particular age group or socioeconomic status, but include a representative selection of cases seen in private offices, public clinics, general hospitals and various institutions restricted to psychiatric patients.

In preparing this second edition, our aim was to update the material so that it would reflect current knowledge and practice. Thus, most of the chapters have been modified and some have been rewritten entirely. The current upsurge of interest in learning theory and humanistic-existential approaches is reflected in a

presentation of these alternatives to psychoanalysis in discussions of both
definition and treatment. The theoretical discussion throughout has been
changed to reflect a more ego-analytic and eclectically dynamic bias. This
change should be particularly noticeable in the chapters in which abnormality,
development and treatment are defined. New material has been added on the
effects of drugs on abnormality and the relationship between pornography and
sexual deviation. The chapters on biological and hereditary determinants of
behavior have been condensed and combined into a single chapter since the
original material seemed overly detailed for an undergraduate text. The chapters
on treatment and diagnosis have been rewritten and moved near the end of the
book, following the presentation of the major syndromes. There is a new chapter
on the community mental health movement and the resulting changes in our
ideas about intervention.

Professor Rosen died shortly before the publication of the first edition.
However, in a real sense his contribution is still evident even after the major
revision.

We wish to express our appreciation to the various authors and publishers who
kindly consented to our reproducing tables, figures and other material. In particular we wish to thank Herrn Dr. Joseph Neugebauer, Vize-Direktor of Sandoz A.C.
in Basel, Switzerland. Dr. Neugebauer was instrumental in obtaining the prints
used in the end-plates and for chapter-opening illustrations. All these pictures
are works of art created by persons suffering from emotional problems and are
part of a series distributed by Sandoz in Europe. Their use here is not intended
to demonstrate anything about the nature of emotional disturbance other than
the fact that some such persons have artistic talent. We appreciate the patient
work of Jackie Gundling in translating some materials which were available
only in the French language. A final thanks goes to Miss Lena Ross whose
services as a librarian made much of our work infinitely easier.

RONALD E. FOX

IAN GREGORY

Description of front end sheets. Wood carvings produced by Karl Brendel, a European stone mason and artist who left a large legacy of sculpture. In his late teens and early twenties he had several convictions for assault and battery, resisting authority and procuring. At age 35, he was hospitalized with a diagnosis of schizophrenia with the symptoms of delusions of grandeur and persecution, hallucinations, confused speech and aggressive outbursts. He had repeated hospitalizations over the next six years. During one of these periods he began modeling obscene figures with chewed bread crumbs and later turned to a voluminous outpouring of wood sculpture such as shown here.

Description of back end sheets. The home of Karl Junker, a German architect, painter, and sculptor who suffered from a para-noid schizophrenic psychosis. Junker worked on his home con-tinuously for over 30 years, designing both the interior and exterior, as well as all the furniture. Disappointments in love and failure to obtain desired artistic acclaim led him to live an increasingly secluded life. Gradually, his behavior grew more and more peculiar. He would not leave the house during the day, and he worked far into the night for months on end, carving, decorating and elaborately ornamenting every piece of wood in the house. In his later years, he allowed no one to approach him except a neighbor who fur-nished him the necessities of life. He was often observed to stand in his garden at night declaiming in a loud voice. He once dis-closed that he knew the most secret thoughts of the pope, was not called "Junker" for nothing, and was working on a new style "which would perhaps be understood in a hundred years."

CONTENTS

1 INTRODUCTION: THE NATURE AND SCOPE OF ABNORMAL
   PSYCHOLOGY 3

2 THE HISTORICAL BACKGROUND OF ABNORMAL PSYCHOLOGY 17

3 MODERN CLASSIFICATION OF ABNORMALITY 35

4 DEVELOPMENT OF THE NORMAL PERSONALITY............................. 51

5 THE NATURE OF CAUSATION... 71

6 HEREDITARY AND BIOLOGICAL DETERMINANTS........................... 77

7 PSYCHOLOGICAL DETERMINANTS.. 101

8 SOCIOCULTURAL DETERMINANTS 127

9 PSYCHONEUROTIC DISORDERS... 147

10 PSYCHOPHYSIOLOGIC DISORDERS 169

11 AFFECTIVE DISORDERS 191

12 SCHIZOPHRENIA... 213

13 PARANOID STATES 245

14 DELINQUENCY, CRIME AND ANTISOCIAL PERSONALITY 255

15   SEXUAL DEVIATION.. 273

16   ALCOHOLISM AND DRUG ADDICTION... 301

17   BRAIN SYNDROMES... 325

18   MENTAL SUBNORMALITY... 355

19   DISORDERS OF CHILDHOOD 383

20   EVALUATION.. 413

21   TREATMENT... 429

22   MODERN TRENDS IN TREATMENT: COMMUNITY MENTAL HEALTH............ 465

      GLOSSARY... 473

      SELECTED REFERENCES 481

      NAME INDEX... 501

      SUBJECT INDEX... 509

LIGHTLY

abnormal psychology

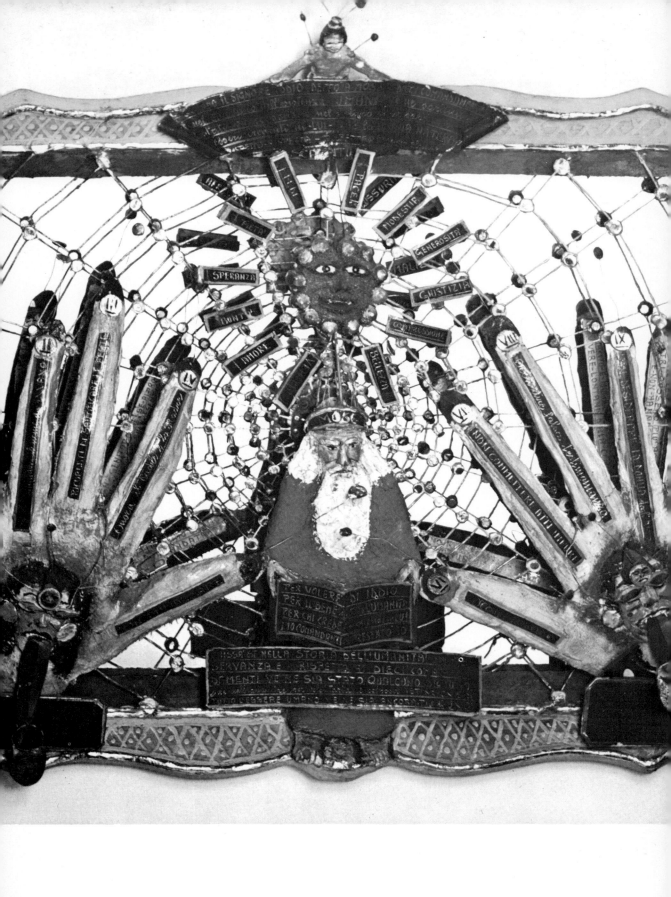

Mental disease appears greatly to tax the attention of good observers
because it presents itself to us as a mixture of incoherence and confusion.

Philippe Pinel, Introduction to *Medical-Philosophic Treatise on Mania,* 1801

1

INTRODUCTION: THE NATURE AND SCOPE OF ABNORMAL PSYCHOLOGY

Since recorded history began man has been continuously preoccupied with that most fascinating object of study—man himself. Quite simply, we amaze ourselves. How people behave, how they think, how they feel and how they perceive are of interest to all of us in helping to understand ourselves and others. Of particular interest have been those unusual experiences which by their very uniqueness command our attention. Nightmares, dreams, bizarre actions, frightful feelings, hallucinations and the like have been observed and recorded throughout all of history. The black moods of King Saul, the bizarre behavior of Nero and the "animal fits" of Nebuchadnezzar are just a few of the ancient and well-known examples.

Why do people have nightmares? How can a person feel such despair that he kills himself without apparent reason? What happens to a person so that he imagines himself to be Napoleon even though he "knows" that Napoleon died long ago? Many persons come to the study of abnormal psychology because of such questions. Certainly the answers to these questions are encompassed by abnormal psychology but the field is a very broad one.

Abnormal psychology is the application of the methods, concepts, principles and findings of general psychology—primarily, the psychology of perception, learning and development, and social psychology—to deviant behaviors and experiences. Abnormal psychology is an attempt to understand and explain the abnormal in the framework of the normal and general. This definition is incomplete, in that it does not specify what is meant by "normal," "abnormal" or "deviant." The criteria for judging that a behavior or experience is abnormal are discussed later in the chapter.

In this chapter the nature of abnormal psychology is explored as follows: First, some examples of abnormal behaviors and experiences are described and analyzed. Immediately following, the question of how and why such phenomena are judged abnormal is discussed. The next section illustrates the usefulness and also the difficulties of applying the concepts of general psychology to abnormal behavior. Since biology and sociology, as well as general psychology, are rich sources for the understanding of abnormal phenomena, the following two sections illustrate the application of biological

3

and sociocultural concepts to abnormal behavior. Finally, the discussion then focuses on a philosophical problem posed by the fact that abnormal psychology is concerned with both psychological and biological phenomena. This is the classic problem of the relation of mind to body.

EXAMPLES OF DEVIANT BEHAVIOR AND EXPERIENCE

Let us look at three examples as an introduction to the data and concepts of abnormal psychology.

Case 1. A 35-year-old man had been working as a salesman for a large corporation for several years. His progress was satisfactory to his company, his family and himself. He was promoted to the position of sales manager and began his new work with great optimism, confidence and eagerness. He received excellent cooperation from his associates. But within a couple of months it became clear that something was wrong. He had always been accurate in numerical computation but now he began to make errors. He sometimes addressed people in an offensive manner. He began to sleep badly, smiled much less than formerly and often seemed irritable, upset and depressed. Occasionally he expressed the feeling that he could not handle the job and that he must be stupid or incompetent. Then he decided that his only problem was that some of his colleagues were against him and were sabotaging him. In previous years he drank liquor on social occasions only, but now he began to drink more often, frequently when alone.

Analysis. Our definition of abnormal psychology referred to the two realms of behavior and experience. Abnormalities of both are present in the unhappy sales manager. A number of his difficulties are purely behavioral and can be observed objectively, and some can even be quantified numerically. His increasing inefficiency, difficulty in sleeping (insomnia), change in facial expression, increased frequency of aggressive language and increased consumption of alcohol are all observable phenomena. But his feelings of depression, wavering self-confidence and belief that others were undermining him are not directly observable; they are subjective experiences that have to be inferred from behavior. An important part of abnormal psychology is concerned with such experiences. A disturbed individual's self-concept, feelings of inferiority, unexpressed hostility and guilt feelings are as important as his overt speech

and motor behavior. For the sake of convenience, however, the term "behavior" is often used to stand for both behavior and experience.

The sales manager's difficulties also illustrate the fact that deviant phenomena vary in seriousness and degree of irrationality. His unfounded conviction that he was being persecuted constitutes a delusion. Most people would agree that a delusion is more serious than such difficulties as insomnia or irritability. Each of these is a *symptom,* that is, a manifestation of an illness or emotional disturbance.

Symptoms almost never come singly but occur in clusters called *syndromes.* For example, one of the syndromes of psychological disturbance, involutional melancholia, includes such symptoms as feelings of guilt, agitated restlessness, anxiety and fears, delusional ideas and suicidal impulses. Another syndrome, compulsive personality, consists of symptoms that exaggerate common personality traits, particularly excessive orderliness, obstinacy and stinginess. A given syndrome is more severe in some cases than in others; there are mild and severe compulsives, and mild and severe melancholics.

Symptoms may be grouped into several categories. The sales manager's numerical errors and delusion of persecution are deviations of intelligence and thought. His depression is a deviation of affect, mood or feeling. His anxiety, increased use of alcohol, aggressiveness and loss of confidence indicate disordered motivation. Two other categories of symptoms are frequent: symptoms of disordered sensation and perception, and of verbal and motor behavior. These will all be encountered in later discussions of the different syndromes.

Case 2. A staff sergeant in World War II adjusted well to noncombat duties during the first two years of his army service. In his third year he was in combat for months on end and developed symptoms in one leg that appeared to be due to sciatica. (Sciatica is pain in those regions of the thigh and leg that are innervated by the sciatic nerve.) He began to have nightmares in which he tried to escape from pursuing monsters. During the day, he manifested a number of physiological signs of anxiety: excessive sweating, shaking, muscular weakness and facial pallor. The sciatic symptoms soon disappeared, but he became completely paralyzed in both legs. Medical examination revealed no physical basis for this symptom and it was concluded that its origin was emotional. He was discharged from the armed services and in time the paralysis vanished almost completely. However, new behavior difficulties soon appeared. He began to beat his wife and children brutally and to get into fist fights with casual acquaintances. He was jailed three times and fired from 15 successive jobs. Finally, when he experienced a strong impulse to "punch a bus in the nose," he realized that he needed help and voluntarily committed himself to a hospital.

Analysis. To understand this case it is necessary to explore the complex concept of *anxiety.* The patient manifested anxious *responses* such as sweating and shaking. But anxiety is a drive as well as a type of response, and as such it motivated much of the patient's behavior. For example, his leg paralysis was an unconscious, involuntary, defensive attempt to avoid being overwhelmed by anxious feelings. So long as he could not move he could not be sent into combat. On a conscious level he did not fear combat at all and in fact rather gloried in it, but in order to understand his behavior we can assume that he was unconsciously afraid. That is to say, he behaved in a manner indicative of fear without being aware of the implications of his behavior. His nightmares support the assumption, for they are indicative of anxiety as the term is commonly used. The case thus illustrates the fact that explanations of abnormal phenomena involve unconscious as well as conscious processes.

Although the paralysis was ameliorated when he was discharged from the army, the patient's unconscious anxiety persisted, driving him to aggressive behavior toward his family, comparative strangers and even inanimate objects. The immediate cause of the fear (combat) was gone but his anxiety had persisted or become chronic. Anxiety is evidenced in so many ways, is an important component of so many disorders, and can persist for so long a time that it may be considered one of the central concepts of modern abnormal psychology.

Case 3. A 55-year-old woman with no prior history of difficulties began to deteriorate mentally. Fairly simple intellectual problems became impossible for her to solve, particularly if they involved abstract ideas or generalizations. She became disoriented: she did not know where she was, the month of the year or the identity of people with whom she had talked many times. Her memory became vague, especially for recent events. Frequently she would make silly, pointless statements and repeat meaningless phrases over and over. She liked being with people and was interested in the happenings around her, yet her emotional responses lacked richness, variation and subtlety to the extent that she seemed childlike. In time her speech became incoherent and she developed such muscular difficulties as partial paralyses and convulsions.

Analysis. Behavior of this sort is characteristic of patients with a severe brain disorder. The case just cited is an example of *Alzheimer's disease,* a progressive, widespread deterioration of the cerebral cortex that severely impairs intellectual functioning.

In the first two cases no medical factors operated causally (except for an attack of sciatica preceding the sergeant's leg paralysis). In the present case the patient's symptoms can be understood only as a consequence of medical causes. Psychological abnormality may result from emotional, non-medical, so-called "functional" causes; or mainly from medical, so-called "organic" causes; or both.

WHAT IS ABNORMALITY?

Everyone knows what abnormality is. It is those behaviors or thought processes which are commonly agreed to be bizarre, unusual or odd. People who hear voices or think they are Christ or are subject to uncontrollable fits of violence or depression seem to be obviously emotionally disturbed. Abnormality is for many persons merely a polite synonym for craziness, lunacy or madness.

Yet, the cases cited demonstrate that abnormality embraces many different and complicated phenomena. These may be objective or subjective; may be relatively severe or mild; and may occur as difficulties of intellectual functioning, as disordered affect and mood, as disturbed motivation, or as disturbances of perceptual, motor, or verbal behavior. The phenomena of abnormality often require analysis at both conscious and unconscious levels. Finally, they may or may not involve organic difficulties.

Those persons in the above cases seem to be obviously disturbed people. Yet it must be mentioned that we are able to benefit from hindsight and a listing of all symptoms which each person manifested over a period of time. On a day to day basis such persons may not appear to be emotionally disturbed or abnormal. In fact, these cases were chosen for illustrative purposes and are not representative of the typical person who presents himself for psychological help. Many persons who come to psychological clinics for counseling or psychotherapy do not appear seriously disturbed and often outwardly resemble the so-called "man on the street." In addition, as we shall see repeatedly in this book, there are very few symptoms of abnormality which have not been experienced at one time or another by the bulk of the persons in the general population. At what point is a person being abnormal rather than evidencing one of the many strange but common quirks of human behavior? For purposes of scientific study, of experimentation, and of diagnosis, such distinctions are critical. Even though we all "know" what abnormality is in its more obvious, extreme forms, a precise definition which covers all behaviors, in any person in every situation has proved to be extremely difficult to devise.

In the following sections several of the most frequently used criteria of normality and abnormality are presented and critically evaluated.

Normal is Average: The Statistical Definition

A common-sense approach to the problem of definition has been to label normal those behaviors or traits which are frequent, typical or commonly occur in most persons. The term abnormal is then applied to any forms of behavior (including thoughts and feelings) which are infrequent, atypical or very rare in the experience of most persons. This view received particular impetus several decades ago when psychologists discovered that many traits which are measureable can be arranged into a frequency distribution so that most scores cluster around the mean or average.

Intelligence tests for example can be constructed in such a way that most persons will score in the average range. Very bright persons will score higher than average while dull persons will score lower. Figure 1–1 shows the theoretical distribution of scores on a standard intelligence test for a large representative sample of the adult population in the United States. The distribution of scores conforms to the statistical principle of the bell-shaped curve, in which most scores fall in the middle range and fewer scores occur with increasing distance from the average. As can be seen in the figure, 82. 2 per cent of all persons tested obtain scores between 80 and 120 on this test, and 95.6 per cent fall between the scores of 70 and 130. Thus, depending on how broad a range of scores one is willing to define as average, every person scoring above or below the defined range can be labeled abnormal with respect to intellectual functioning.

This type of statistical perspective is widely used in biology and medicine. One can have too high or too low a white blood cell count; his body temperature can be too high or too low.

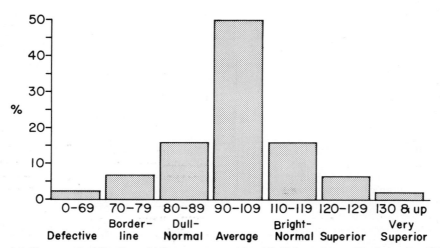

Figure 1–1. *Intelligence classification of I.Q. scores, age 16 to 75. (Adapted from Wechsler, D., 1958. The Measurement of Adult Intelligence. Baltimore, The Williams & Wilkins Co.)*

Only the middle range is considered normal.

In psychology, the statistical approach is similarly used. One can be too emotionally responsive or not responsive enough. A student can be so anxious that his performance on exams is disrupted or show so little anxiety that he has no motivation to study. It is the middle range of scores and associated attitudes which is considered normal; all else is abnormal.

The only prerequisites for a statistical definition of abnormality with respect to any measurable trait are the selection of two points on the distribution of scores for the population under study and the stipulation that scores between these cut-off points be termed normal while those outside the points be termed abnormal. For instance, we can select the 10th and 90th percentiles in a distribution showing the amount of alcohol consumed per person per year. Any person who consumes more or less alcohol than 90 per cent of the general population would be considered abnormal with respect to alcohol consumption. The abnormal may thus be equated with a strictly quantitative departure from the statistical average.

The statistical criterion of abnormality has a strong appeal for the psychologist who is eager to put abnormal psychology on a firmly scientific basis. But a rigid application of the criterion involves us in several difficulties.

1. The Problem of Arbitrary Divisions. The placement of the cutting points that divide a frequency distribution into normal and abnormal regions is arbitrary. An I.Q. of 80 will be termed abnormal if 90 is chosen as a cutting point but not if 70 is chosen. If 70 is chosen, a person who scores 69 is abnormal, even though he is not really different from the person who scores 70. People do not fall into the two simple classes of bright and dull; they are *more or less* bright (or dull).

The same consideration holds for any other trait so that there is little justification for the selection of any point whatsoever to effect a rigid division of behavior or subjective experience into the two classes of normal and abnormal. Analysis of the statistical criterion of abnormality thus leads to the important conclusion that there is a gradual continuum from the normal to the abnormal instead of a sharp separation between the two. The abnormal is usually an exaggeration of the normal.

The concept of a normal-abnormal continuum provides a logical basis for the generalization to abnormal phenomena of principles drawn from studies of normal individuals, as called for by our definition of abnormal psychology. In addition, the idea of a normal-abnormal continuum leads to attitudes of sympathy and acceptance toward the emotionally disturbed and mentally ill. The realization that a patient has much in common with us, no matter how disorganized and irrational his behavior may seem at first blush, may motivate efforts to understand and help him. One sees something of the patient in oneself and something of oneself in the patient.

2. The Problem of Combining Scores. Sometimes it is desirable to characterize as more or less deviant an entire syndrome or even a person, rather than a single trait or behavior. To do this statistically it is necessary to combine several measures into a total score. Suppose, for example, that an individual is troubled by hallucinations, physiological signs of anxiety and gaps in memory. Suppose further that each of these symptoms could be expressed as a score. If we tried to combine the three scores we would not know how much weight to give each, for we do not know the relative importance of each symptom in every syndrome. Weighting symptoms equally would ignore the fact that they vary in importance. Since the typical syndrome includes far more than three symptoms, it becomes quite impossible to derive a meaningful abnormality score for a syndrome or a person.

3. The Problem of Different Dimensions. The problem of weighting symptoms is complicated by the fact that there may be more than one fundamental way of being abnormal. The distinction between *neurosis* and *psychosis* illustrates this point. In neurotic disturbances, the individual suffers from internal conflicts, anxiety and an inability to integrate his drives with his moral standards and inhibitions. He attempts to defend himself against anxiety and fails, but he is rational and he perceives the outer world fairly accurately. The psychotic individual, on the other hand, either because of brain malfunctioning or emotional conflict, tends to misinterpret reality, may fail to communicate meaningfully with other people and is often lost in disorganized and irrational thought processes. A popular joke embodies the difference between the two: the psychotic thinks two and two make five; the neurotic knows perfectly well that two and two make four but it makes him nervous.

The implication of this distinction between neurosis and psychosis is that the dimension or continuum of normal-neurotic may be quite different from the dimension of normal-psychotic. There may be two independent axes of abnormality. In general, we tend to think of psychosis as more severe than neurosis because of the psychotic's defective relation to reality, yet we cannot say that a psychotic is *merely* more abnormal than a neurotic. Psychosis is not neurosis-plus. Although a neurotic patient sometimes becomes psychotic at a later time, more often he remains neurotic. Similarly, the psychotic seldom changes into a neurotic. Furthermore, there are relatively mild psychotics who are able to function more effectively in day-to-day living than some severe neurotics.

4. The Problem of Unequal Extremes. One more difficulty is our reluctance to term both extremes of a distribution abnormal unless somehow we can distinguish between them. Statistically, the genius is as abnormal as the mentally retarded individual; almost complete freedom from conflicts is as abnormal as being ridden by conflicts; and an extremely accurate perception of reality is as rare and abnormal as a marked distortion of reality. But there is a world of difference between the abnormally disturbed and the abnormally supernormal or between the dullard and the genius: one end of the continuum is considered undesirable and the other desirable. Strictly statistical criteria cannot by themselves dictate judgments of desirability and un-desirability. They must be supplemented by nonstatistical considerations if we are to be consistent with the universal assumption that health is better than sickness.

Normalcy is Personal Comfort

A second approach equates normalcy with the personal comfort felt by the individual. If he is depressed, unhappy, upset or troubled by inability to control his thoughts he is abnormal. If he is relatively untroubled and indifferent to his inner state and to the impression he makes on others, or if he manifests a state of well-being and euphoria, he is normal no matter how deviant his behavior appears to observers.

There is intuitive appeal to such an approach. Abnormal psychology has no "emotional thermometer" which can reliably detect when a person is disturbed. Its measures are still crude and in need of greater precision. In the absence of universally accepted, external criteria, a person's subjective state seems as good as any other. If a person feels good, how is anyone else to "prove" that he is disturbed.

The difficulties with the personal discomfort criterion stem from the fact that a disturbed person's complaints, moods, feelings and fears, although important, are an incomplete part of the picture.

1. The Problem of Subjective vs. Objective Symptoms. The discomfort criterion omits all consideration of behavior deviations that are not accompanied by subjective distress. A patient in the manic phase of the psychotic disorder termed manic-depressive reaction is likely to report that he feels fine, that his daily life is full of things that interest him and that he is sitting on top of the world. Yet he could be considered abnormal since he does not function efficiently in intellectual tasks, he is physically overactive, his speech may be hard to follow and he may hear nonexistent voices. In such a case the personal comfort and sense of well-being is itself considered to be a symptom of abnormality.

2. The Problem of Individual Reactions to Discomfort. The discomfort criterion omits the important matter of how an individual adjusts to his own feeling states. Two equally depressed persons may behave very dif-ferently: one resists his depressive feelings and struggles to carry on his daily activities while the other submits as if it were futile to expend energy on any activity whatever. Most of us would regard the second individual as far more ill than the first. A criterion of abnormality that does not distinguish between such diametrically different adjustments to felt discomfort is inadequate.

3. The Problem of Social Consequences. A final inadequacy of the discomfort criterion is its failure to consider the effect of deviant behavior on other people. To return to the thumbnail description of mania, it can be seen that a drop in intellectual efficiency may create difficulties for one's coworkers; confused speech puzzles and may upset people; and physical overactivity in a few cases leads to assaultive behavior. So important, in fact, are the social aspects of abnormality that it has been suggested that they alone are sufficient to define abnormality.

Normalcy is Social Conformity

From birth on, the individual lives in a social framework. Society expects him to conform to its standards with certain permitted exceptions. He is rewarded if he conforms and punished if he does not. The criterion of social nonconformity emerges from these considerations: an individual is deemed abnormal to the degree that he fails to conform to social standards and expectations.

Basically, this criterion is statistical since it defines degree of abnormality by degree of nonconformity. The criterion has several major difficulties.

1. The Problem of Criminality. It is often important to distinguish crime from psychological abnormality. Many criminals are disturbed psychologically—they are particularly likely to belong to a category known as sociopathic personality—but some criminals seem psychologically normal despite the fact that they are nonconformists. Crime is a legal, not a psychological, concept. The criminal violates the legal code of society; most disturbed individuals do not violate it or else violate it only as a secondary consequence of psychological disturbance (for example, bodily assault due to delusions). If a careful distinction is not made between criminal and psychological nonconformity there is a danger of incorrectly labeling all criminals as mentally ill, or—even worse—of labeling all mentally ill persons as criminals and thus countering the humanitarian attitude toward mental illness.

2. The Problem of Cultural Relativity. What constitutes conformity in one culture may constitute nonconformity in another. A few examples drawn from the field of cultural anthropology will illustrate the point.

If a member of a New Guinea tribe, the Kwoma, is frustrated by anyone but a relative he is expected to respond with strong verbal and physical aggression, even to the point of killing the individual who has frustrated him. Such behavior is unacceptable in our culture.

Among the Hopi Indians of the Southwest, on the other hand, both competitiveness and aggression are suppressed to a degree that would seem abnormal to most of us. Hopis show so strong a reluctance to outshine or

disapprove of others that in our culture their behavior would undoubtedly be labeled, "abnormally passive"; conversely, our tendency to compete in work and play and to respond aggressively when we feel threatened would constitute social nonconformity in Hopi society. The Hopis also display an intense fear of supernatural forces that would be labeled "anxiety reaction" in our culture.

One need not go outside our own culture to demonstrate variation in cultural expectancies and behavior. Within a single complex culture there are different subcultures: for example, it has been shown repeatedly that members of different classes in our culture respond differently in their thinking, emotional reactions and speech. One consequence of this diversity is that diagnoses depend in part on the background and class-conditioned values of the diagnostician. If he shares upper or middle-class values, the speech and thinking patterns of a lower-class patient may appear strange to him and he may be readier to diagnose such a patient as psychotic than one from his own class whose patterns of speech and thought are familiar.

3. The Problem of Undesirable Social Standards. A danger of the conformity criterion is that it may lead to the assumption that society is always right and the nonconforming individual always at fault. This assumption ignores the fact that cultures vary in their adequacy; cultural change is sometimes more desirable than conformity. The social nonconformity criterion of abnormality has at times been misused to argue for blind conformity to an undesirable status quo.

Related to the preceding problem is the danger of ignoring the fact that progress in human affairs has almost always been brought about by the efforts of innovators who took new paths in art, science and other domains. It is a mistake to assume that every nonconformist is a genius, but it is equally fallacious to assume that all innovators are merely abnormal. One recent and familiar example may be taken from the Civil Rights Movement in the United States where many persons refused to obey laws which in effect perpetrated racial discrimination. Their "criminal behavior" resulted in fairer laws and therefore scarcely could serve as an index of abnormality.

4. The Problem of the Conforming Neurotic. Most neurotics conform to social expectations more closely than do psychotics, so that the nonconformity criterion is not as readily applicable to neurosis as to psychosis. In fact,

change or acceptance

some neurotics are marked by a rigid overconformity.

Society maintains jails for the criminally nonconforming and hospitals for the psychiatrically nonconforming. Because of their nonconformity, psychotics are hospitalized far more often than neurotics; the criterion of social nonconformity, despite all its problems and difficulties, is usually the actual basis of a family, medical or legal decision to hospitalize a disturbed individual. The outwardly conforming, unhappy neurotic constitutes a fairly small percentage of involuntarily hospitalized patients. In addition to the three fundamental criteria just explored, several others have received increased emphasis in the last two decades. Offer and Sabshin (1966) present an excellent discussion of the concept of normality and abnormality.

OTHER APPROACHES TO THE DEFINITION OF ABNORMALITY

Normality is an Ideal   *NEVER REACHED*

In this approach normality is conceived of as a harmonious, optional blending of the diverse elements of the mental and emotional functions. A normal person then becomes a perfectly functioning, ideal organizer, an occurrence which exists only in theory or at least occurs quite infrequently.

This approach stems from Sigmund Freud's conception of normality as an ideal fiction, with everyone being neurotic to some extent. More modern theorists, such as Carl Rogers, Abraham Maslow and Charlotte Buhler, place less emphasis on the universality of neurosis but still talk of normalcy as a seldom realized ideal. They speak of the "fully functioning person" (Rogers, 1959) or the "self actualized" individual (Maslow, 1954), although relatively few persons ever become fully functioning or completely self-actualized.

Emphasizing the positive aspects of personality functioning tends to remove abnormal behavior from the realm of the unusual or different and calls attention instead to the positive ideals to which man has always aspired. However, the difficulty with an ideal is that few ever attain it, and from a pragmatic viewpoint, to say that people differ only in the degree to which they achieve the ideal brings us full circle. How do we measure the extent of normalcy? How do we recognize an abnormal person when we see one?

Normality is a Process

This view asserts that normality is a process: the end result of interacting systems that change over time. It asserts that healthy people strive to live up to their potentialities, to develop toward greater psychological maturity and to be able to cope effectively with stress. Inability to do these things or participate in the process is defined as abnormality.

The criterion often clashes with both the nonconformity and the personal discomfort criteria, because the individual who strives and achieves need not be a conformist and may often be tense and uncomfortable. Another limitation is that the choice of behaviors defining health as positive striving is equivalent to the ethical judgment that people *ought* to strive. Very different traits—for example, ability to relax or intensity of sensuous enjoyment—could just as well be chosen as the criterion of health.

Is an Absolute Criterion of Abnormality Possible?

The logical conclusion of the preceding analysis is that no criterion of abnormality is free of weaknesses. No index has so far been proposed that will unfailingly separate normal from abnormal behavior under any and all circumstances. Furthermore, it is doubtful that such an index is possible.

In cases of sufficiently severe disturbance, any of the fundamental criteria is likely to classify the individual as abnormal. Typically the very disturbed individual is statistically different from his fellows; most often he is subjectively upset and unhappy; and frequently he does not conform to all the standards of his social group. The absence of a universal, mostly foolproof criterion is important for borderline and questionable cases. For the most part we may explore abnormal behavior even though an absolute definition of the term is a current impossibility. After all, we all "know" what abnormality is!

A Note on Terminology

A number of different terms are widely used to designate the general class of "abnormal behavior." Many of the terms—for example, behavior deviation, psychological deviation, behavior disturbance and psychological disturbance—may be used synonymously, but others differ in emphases and shades of meaning. "Mental illness," "mental disorder" and "insanity"—the last a legal rather than a psychological term—may be used to refer to psychosis but not neurosis. "Emotional disturbance" and "emotional disorder" are terms with more than one meaning. In one sense, they are used to refer to neurosis rather than psychosis; in another sense, they are intended to refer to the emotional component of all psychological disturbances, including the psychoses.

"Behavior pathology" and "psychopathology" are terms that need careful examination. Since pathology is the study of disease, behavior pathology or psychopathology should mean the study of those aspects of behavior disturbance attributable to medical disease. But a broad analogy can be made between the processes present in physical disease and in psychological disorder so that the terms behavior pathology and psychopathology are often used to refer to all behavior deviations, whether or not they are due to organic disease. The expression "psychiatric disorder" also has two meanings. A psychiatrist is by definition a medical doctor; psychiatric disorders therefore may mean disorders with a known medical, organic basis. But since the psychiatrist may also diagnose and treat nonorganic behavior disturbances, psychiatric disorders may mean abnormal behavior in general.

The terms "behavior disorders" and "conduct disorders" are sometimes restricted to a special sub-type of behavior that is neither neurotic nor psychotic but marked by a particular kind of impulsive, antisocial behavior pattern.

ABNORMAL PSYCHOLOGY AND GENERAL PSYCHOLOGY

In the rest of this book the concepts of general psychology are applied to abnormal behavior again and again. As an introduction, we shall illustrate the manner in which some of the concepts and principles taken from the psychology of perception, learning, development and social psychology are useful to us.

The general principle of *perceptual selectivity* states that drives influence the choice of stimuli to which the individual pays attention or perceives, and also just what he perceives in the stimuli. It is known from several experiments, for example McClelland and Atkinson (1948), that hungry individuals are more likely than others to perceive ambiguous stimuli as food objects. A frightened person is apt to misperceive neutral objects as frightening; for example, he may perceive a neutral face as threatening. Thirst produces mirages. Sexual deprivation alters the perception of the attractiveness of others.

This principle is of great importance in explaining hallucinations, that is, visual, tactile, auditory or other perceptions that have no basis in reality. (Hallucinations are symptomatic of many psychotic disturbances.) The principle of perceptual selectivity is relevant to hallucinations because the perceptions of psychotic individuals are strongly affected by the drives of anxiety, guilt or fear of failure. Just as a hungry man misidentifies a neutral stimulus as an item of food, so the pressures of guilt and anxiety lead a hallucinating patient to the limit of misperception: he creates completely unreal perceptions that are congruent with his drives. Just as fear may make a normal person misperceive a face as threatening, so anxiety may make a psychotic hear threatening voices when there are no real voices at all.

The psychology of learning yields many concepts and principles of great value to abnormal psychology. An example is the concept of *stimulus generalization* and its relation to drive level. As implied in the previous example, disturbed persons tend to have strong, unsatisfied drives; since the anxiety of schizophrenic patients is particularly intense, their drive level should be especially high. An important hypothesis from the field of learning is that the higher this level of drive, the greater is the tendency to stimulus generalization, i.e., the tendency to respond in a particular way to stimuli other than the stimulus to which the response was initially learned. Applying this hypothesis to schizophrenics, neurotics and normals, the schizophrenic group would be expected to show the greatest degree of stimulus generalization. Knopf and Fager (1961) tested this deduction by an experimental procedure in which subjects were presented with several lamps and instructed to push a switch when the appropriate lamp was lighted; the experimental situation was so arranged that only one lamp was the appropriate one. Stimulus generalization in this situation meant pushing the switch in response to any of the other lamps being lit. Schizophrenics responded to the incorrect stimuli more often than neurotics or normals, thus confirming the prediction. More than a clever and well designed experiment is involved here, for the learning concepts that help explain the experimental results can be extended to the everyday behavior of schizophrenics and other psychotics. One feature of such behavior is disorganization, a failure to respond coherently and meaningfully to the succession of stimuli constantly impinging on the organism. It may well be that this disorganization consists partly of errors of stimulus generalization; the psychotic's thoughts, emotions and motor responses may not "fit" reality because his high drive level makes it impossible for him to discriminate accurately between stimulus situations that are real and stimulus situations that exist only in his fantasies. He responds to the former as if they were the latter, and vice versa.

Developmental concepts are particularly important for abnormal psychology because many disturbances of behavior develop over time; psychopathological development may be regarded as a special case of normal development. For example, a cornerstone of the psychoanalytic theory constructed and formulated by Sigmund Freud (1943) is the idea of *developmental, psychosexual stages*. This concept is embedded in hypotheses that assert that every individual normally passes through a series of predictable sexual stages and that emotional disorder may be conceived as a *fixation* (failure to progress to the next stage) or *regression* (return) to a formerly pleasurable psychosexual stage. These hypotheses are developed later in some detail; for the moment, the point is that the concepts of developmental stages, fixation, and regression bind developmental and abnormal psychology together closely.

Finally, an example of the application of a social-psychological concept to behavioral deviations is the concept of *role-taking*. Paraphrasing Cameron and Cameron (1951), a social role may be defined as an organized and interrelated set of attitudes and responses prescribed by the social environment. The behaviors appropriate to a mother constitute a social role; so do the behaviors appropriate to a 10-year-old boy, a skilled mechanic, a concert musician, and so forth.

Role-taking, the expression in day-to-day existence, fantasy and play of the behaviors that constitute a social role, is difficult for many disturbed persons. Whether because of biological defects, unfortunate childhood experiences or cultural deprivations, they cannot carry through the behaviors appropriate to their capacities or positions and they cannot put themselves in the place of another person in fantasy. They find it hard to imagine or to anticipate someone else's responses. Much of the social awkwardness, difficulty in communication and peculiar thinking of psychotic individuals may stem from these difficulties in role-taking.

Some Difficulties in the Application of General Concepts to Abnormal Psychology

The attempt to apply general psychological principles to the data and problems of abnormal psychology is not uniformly successful; one reason is that our current knowledge and understanding of normal behavior are very incomplete.

A consequence of the gaps in our knowledge is that very often a choice among incompatible concepts and principles is possible. In the field of learning, for example, there are several theories that disagree on such issues as how many fundamental types of learning there are, the place of reward and punishment in learning and the relation of learning to motivation and perception. Similarly, there is lack of agreement among psychologists as to the basic nature of perception, social-psychological processes and development. For example, Freud's theory of sexual stages is not subscribed to unanimously and his hypotheses that developmental stages are basically sexual and universal, and that emotional difficulty is best conceptualized as a regression, have been widely challenged.

Given this lack of unanimity, the wisest course is to be judiciously eclectic and apply a variety of different concepts and points of view to the phenomena of abnormal psychology. The alternative approach is to subscribe to one of the contending theories of general psychology and make use of it alone, rigidly excluding all other concepts and principles. However, no general theory so far constructed seems sufficiently sound and comprehensive enough to warrant the adoption of this alternative.

ABNORMAL PSYCHOLOGY AND BIOLOGY

A human being before all else is a biological organism. Biological structure and function set limits to an individual's behavior and are at the root of many behavioral disturbances. For example, it has been observed that Huntington's chorea, a psychotic disorder caused by a pathological process in the brain, occurs in approximately half of all offspring of a parent with the disorder. The remaining offspring are free of Huntington's chorea and do not transmit it to their own children. This pattern is explained completely by the biological concept of inheritance through a single dominant gene.

The importance of biological considerations in abnormal psychology can also be illustrated by considering *psychophysiologic disorders*. These include certain cases of asthma, peptic ulcer, high blood pressure and other disorders that stem from continuous and exaggerated physiological accompaniments of various emotional states. The physiological activity eventually leads to pathological changes in the structure or functioning of some organ of the body. To understand such disorders one must be familiar with the physiological accompaniments of emotion and with the role of the autonomic nervous system in both emotional expression and the functioning of those organs in which psychophysiologic symptoms occur.

In general, the disorders we shall be concerned with may be divided into two major groups. One group—for which the most helpful explanations are psychological—includes the neuroses, most psychoses, and special disturbances of the personality. The second group—for which explanations are wholly or largely biological—includes disturbances due to brain damage, endocrine gland malfunction or autonomic overactivity. But even for the first group biology is not irrelevant, for every organism has a certain heredity and constitution. Nor are general psychological principles wholly irrelevant to the second group, for the organism with structural damage or physiological malfunctioning also perceives, learns, develops and interacts socially. Sometimes it is best to pay more attention to the psychological basis of abnormalities and sometimes to the biological basis; it is never wise to ignore either completely. We are, in short, psychological, sociological, biological organisms; neither more nor less.

ABNORMAL PSYCHOLOGY AND SOCIOCULTURAL VARIABLES

The position of an individual in the social structure affects the likelihood of his becoming emotionally disturbed or mentally ill, the partic-

ular kind of disturbance or illness he manifests and even the kind of treatment to which he responds favorably. Let us illustrate each of these points.

Hollingshead and Redlich (1958) made a pioneering study of the relations between social class and mental illness. They divided the residents of a New England city into five social classes and found that the rate of occurrence of many disorders varied systematically from class to class. Schizophrenia, for example, was most prevalent in the two lowest classes. Hollingshead and Redlich speculated that the probability of schizophrenic breakdown increases if the individual has had a "loveless infancy," that is, deprivation of affection in infancy. It is possible that children in the lower socioeconomic classes receive insufficient love and affection due to the necessity for mothers to work and the frequency of broken homes. We can thus interrelate a sociocultural variable (class membership) to a fact of abnormal psychology (the probability of occurrence of schizophrenia) through a link provided by the concept of deprivation of affection.

The same study provided evidence that the prevalence of neurosis in different classes does not follow the pattern of schizophrenia. Neurotic patients in treatment were concentrated at the upper-class levels, indicating that the effect of sociocultural factors is different for different behavioral deviations.

Another example of the importance of sociocultural factors in abnormality is contained in a study by Singer and Opler (1961). They investigated the nature of the symptoms manifested by two groups of schizophrenic patients in the United States, one of Irish and the other of Italian extraction, and found that the Irish patients tended to evidence a greater degree of fantasy and the Italian patients a greater degree of impulsive, overtly aggressive behavior. The differences between the patients seem to correspond to differences between the cultures of the two parent national groups.

ABNORMAL PSYCHOLOGY AND THE MIND-BODY PROBLEM

A popular but erroneous conception of the nature of abnormal psychology arises from the use of the terms "mental illness" and "mental disorder." It is tempting to believe that the fact that some mental illnesses have organic causes demonstrates that the body affects the mind.

For psychophysiologic disorders the reverse is sometimes maintained: the mind affects the body and makes it ill. Both assertions—that abnormal phenomena demonstrate the effect of body on mind or vice versa—are based on the belief that abnormal psychology deals with two kinds of "stuff," mind and matter, the first intangible, elusive and shadowy, and the second tangible and concrete.

In actual fact, abnormal psychology, like general psychology, deals exclusively with events and processes that are tangible and real. Some of these are best observed or measured by biological methods and others by psychological methods; the events and processes are just as real when observed by psychological as by biological methods. Biological procedures are used to measure pulse rate, blood pressure, changes in the electrical rhythm of the brain or the amount of damage in the brain cells. Psychological procedures such as personality tests, interviews or examination of written documents are used to observe or measure verbal or motor behavior. From the latter observations, such

psychological variables as fantasies, fears, guilt feelings, irritability, unconscious hostility, disorganized thinking and perceptual disturbances may be inferred in the same way that a material but invisible disease process in the tissues may be inferred from x-ray pictures. Furthermore, biological processes, e.g., brain degeneration, typically are accompanied by behavioral changes, and behavioral changes are accompanied by nervous system activity. An individual is fundamentally a unitary organism. The word "psychological" does not mean nonmaterial; it merely denotes a special set of techniques for observing the organism, the particular behaviors observed by these techniques and the inferences about the organism made from the behaviors.

In the next chapter, the history of abnormal psychology is traced in order to locate current theory and practice in their long-range context. If the matrix from which abnormal psychology has developed is understood, its present status will be better appreciated.

2
THE HISTORICAL BACKGROUND OF ABNORMAL PSYCHOLOGY

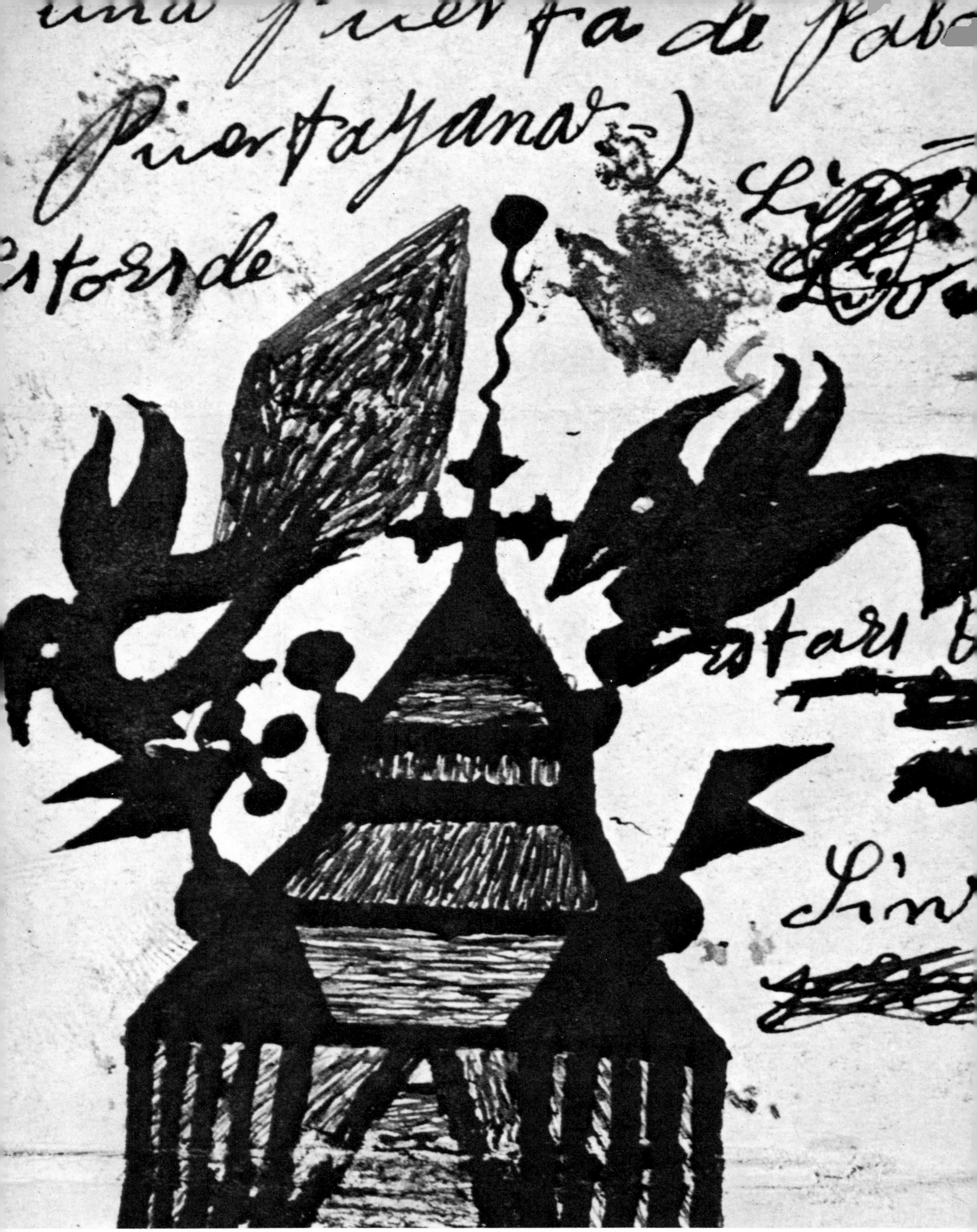

The scientific approach to medical psychology to a very great extent depends on and varies with man's attitude toward himself and the outside world. This attitude has never been fully objective.

Gregory Zilboorg, *A History of Medical Psychology*

THE HISTORICAL BACKGROUND OF ABNORMAL PSYCHOLOGY

ORGANIC – a pathological (diagnosis & treatment, disease) condition arising from a physio. deficiency. MEDICAL

FUNCTIONAL – emotional, non-medical, no organic cause.

The madman, the crazy person, the man possessed by evil spirits, the lunatic, or, in modern parlance, the emotionally disturbed person, has always been a part of the total human experience. Explanations of the causes of such behavior and treatments based on these explanations have been available at least since the Stone Age. As customs change, as science advances, and as civilization becomes more complex, attitudes toward emotional disorders change. The relative humaneness or cruelty of treatment of the insane has often mirrored, as we shall see, the overall humaneness and respect for the individual of the society at large.

The evolution of the understanding and treatment of the emotionally disturbed has culminated in present-day abnormal psychology. Three major trends run through this fascinating historical evolution. First, there has been a trend toward *empiricism,* the view that knowledge must be based on experience rather than speculation. As observations have accumulated, faith in empiricism has grown. In recent years a special type of empiricism has come to the fore with the development of experimental psychopathology, the use of experimental laboratory methods to investigate psychopathological problems.

Second, *naturalism* has replaced magic and supernaturalism in the explanation of abnormality. Two types of natural causes can be distinguished: organic causes, first emphasized by physicians in ancient Greece, and functional psychological causes, not given much attention until the latter part of the nineteenth century.

The third trend has been toward *humanitarianism.* Sympathy for the mentally ill person has grown; asylums have replaced jails and hospitals have replaced asylums. Barbaric punishments and tortures have decreased and, although many mental hospitals still fall far short of ideal conditions, rational management of patients has greatly increased.

These broad trends are interdependent. A humanitarian attitude toward a troubled person is furthered by observing him understandingly, because understanding reduces one's own anxiety and reduced anxiety permits sympathy. In turn, a sympathetic attitude furthers the empirical approach since unsympathetic hostility to the mentally ill erects a barrier that blocks accurate observation. A naturalistic theory of causation grows out of empiricism and leads to rational and humane treatment. Non-naturalistic theories have usually been accompanied by unbridled speculation and have often been used to justify harshness and cruelty.

The three trends have not followed an unbroken line through history. Some knowledge has been lost over long periods and regressions to primitive beliefs and attitudes have occurred. Fortunately, recovery from these regressions has also taken place.

THE PRIMITIVE ERA

Early man made no distinction between physical and mental disease. All disease, like life itself, was explained by the action of the spirits who were believed to animate natural forces, objects, animals and men.

There were two kinds of spirits: good spirits, the gift of the gods, and evil spirits or demons, the punishment of the gods for men's transgressions. Demonology—the term for these beliefs—was the prevailing theory of disease in the Stone Age and among the Hebrews, Egyptians, early Greeks and Chinese.

In time, demonology became associated with mental more than physical disorders. The physically sick person is usually in pain; he knows he is ill and he requests help. Although he was often feared in primitive societies, because disease can spread and weaken a tribe, he must also have been pitied, for we know that attempts were made to help him by the administration of herbs and other physical measures. The mentally ill person, on the other hand, typically has no insight into his disturbance and does not ask for help, yet acts strangely. Primitive man must have been very frightened by mental illness and his fears bred fantastic explanations. It was obvious to him that only an extraordinary agent such as a demon could lead to extraordinary behavior.

The theory of demonology has elements of the supernatural and the magical: supernatural in that the gods, working through spirits, interfere with the orderly progression of natural events, and magical in that an individual possessed by demons—a witch—may use the power of the demons to wreak evil on others. A belief gradually arose that possession by demons could be voluntary. The afflicted person and the demon could make a compact to give the witch magical powers in exchange for the demon's right to possess the witch's body and soul.

Archeological evidence from the Stone Age, the Bible and various other documents of antiquity indicates that mental disorder was explained by demonology. Stone Age skulls have been found that show evidence of an operation called trephining, in which a circle of bone was chipped from the skull, and there is little doubt that the purpose of trephining was to make an orifice through which the demons inhabiting the brain of the possessed individual could escape (see Figures 2–1 and 2–2). Some trephined patients apparently survived, as evidenced by signs of later bone change at the edges of the circle. Perhaps the operation actually helped a few persons who happened to have excessive pressure inside the skull. If so, this is the earliest instance of a theme frequently repeated later: a method of treatment that is effective for a reason quite different from the one propounded by its supporters. Thus electroshock treatment has helped many patients in the twentieth century although the

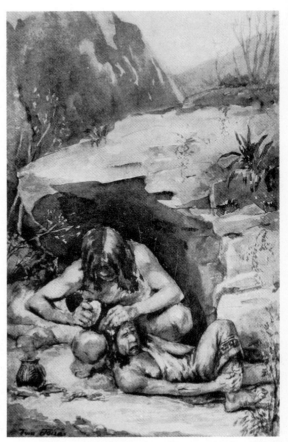

Figure 2–1. *Prehistoric trephining operation. (Bettman Archive.)*

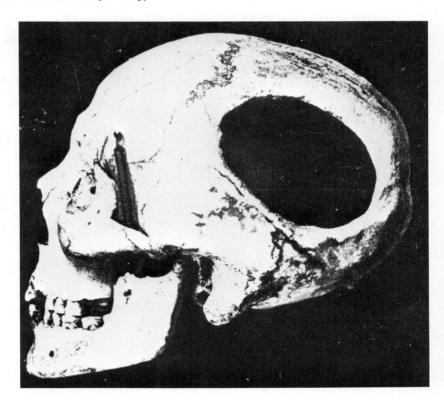

Figure 2–2. *Trephined Neolithic skull found at Nogent-les-Vierges. (Bettman Archive.)*

reason postulated by the inventors for its effectiveness is not tenable.

The Bible has many passages of interest to historians of abnormal psychology. Supernatural causation is expressed in the words, "The Lord shall smite thee with madness, and blindness, and astonishment of heart" (Deuteronomy 28:28). Saul, in the eleventh century B.C., was punished for disobedience by an evil spirit sent forth from God; he became manic, stripped off his clothes and tried to kill his son. David escaped from his enemies by feigning madness, for they believed that his symptoms were a mark of divine favor and should be met with reverence. Well into classical Greek times the disorder of epilepsy was referred to as the "sacred disease"; it was a sign that the gods wished to honor one. Nebuchadnezzar, the king of Babylon, under the delusion that he was a wild beast, ate grass. Christ exorcised the devils out of a man into the Gadarene swine.

Broadly speaking, the assumed cause of a disorder dictated the nature of its treatment. If the spirits were good, their possessor was honored; if they were evil, then either the gods had to be placated and coaxed to withdraw the demons, or the demons had to be exorcised, that is, forced to leave the body. Exorcism varied from

relatively mild to extremely severe and cruel procedures. Mild exorcism involved prayer and incantation. Centuries after the primitive era ended, in the medieval period, these practices were combined with other mild measures: the possessed individual touched relics, loud noises were made and malodorous substances were thrust under his nose to frighten and offend the demons and a priest stamped on crude pictures of the demons. Severe exorcism used flogging, starvation, torture and execution both as a punishment and as a favor to the transgressor: for his own sake, the evil demons inhabiting him had to be driven out at any cost. The statement, "Thou shalt not suffer a witch to live" (Exodus 22:18), constituted the ultimate rationale for the witchburning of the Middle Ages. Leviticus adds, "A man also or woman that hath a familiar spirit or that is a wizard, shall surely be put to death: they shall stone them with stones: their blood shall be upon them" (Leviticus 20:27).

The extreme hostility of these pronouncements must have stemmed from a fear of mental illness and also from a projection of unacceptable impulses onto the mentally ill. A powerful unconscious mechanism of defense consists of disowning the anxiety-provoking aspects of oneself by attributing them to others and then attacking them, thus bolstering a belief in one's moral worth. Unacceptable sexual and aggressive impulses, in particular, are projected in this fashion; the mentally ill are very convenient scapegoats and have often borne the brunt of others' projections of perverse and sadistic tendencies.

The mythology of early Greece is replete with references to mental illness caused by supernatural forces. Orestes saw furies that his sister Electra could not see. Ajax was visited with madness, slew a flock of sheep he believed to be his enemies and committed suicide. The daughters of Proetus, king of Argos, opposed the worship of the gods and were punished by the delusion that they were beasts.

Within this framework arose a new Greek institution, a kind of temple presided over by men who combined priestly and medical functions. These physician-priests, the *Aesculapiadae,* treated patients who made pilgrimages to the temples by religious ceremonies, interpretation of patients' dreams and administration of herbs chosen according to the nature of the dreams. A faint note of empiricism and naturalism enters the picture with the observation of dreams, even if they were then misinterpreted, and with the use of herbs for mental as well as physical disorders. The temples of the Aesculapiadae were the precursors of hospitals for the sick.

THE GREEK AND ROMAN EMERGENCE FROM PRIMITIVISM

The six hundred years between approximately 400 B.C. and 200 A.D. witnessed great advances in the observation, understanding and treatment of mental illness. First in Greece and then in Rome men struggled to emerge from the superstitions of earlier periods. In part they failed, for they could not free themselves completely from bias and from anxiety about psychopathology; nevertheless, their achievements were notable.

The period opens with its greatest figure, Hippocrates (c. 460–377 B.C.), the "Father of Medicine" and the true author of the empirical and naturalistic approaches to behavior disorders. Hippocrates approached mental disorders with few preconceived notions. He observed and reported the symptoms of depression or melancholia, psychosis after childbirth, neurotic phobia, and delirium. Hippocrates described each disorder in terms of its course and outcome and thus began the tradition of recording the progression of a psychiatric illness

to its final stage. He challenged the belief in a supernatural etiology. Writing about epilepsy, Hippocrates asserted:

It thus appears to me to be in no way more divine, nor more sacred than other diseases, but has a natural cause from which it originates. . . . If you cut open the head, you will find the brain humid, full of sweat, and smelling badly. And in this way you may see that it is not a god which injures the body, but disease.

The idea of anatomical causation in this quotation was new and important, regardless of the inaccuracy of Hippocrates' description of the epileptic's brain.

Hippocrates is credited with a number of conceptions and observations which have extended well into modern times. He observed that when a physical illness occurs during a mental illness, temporary mental improvement is likely. Modern motivation theories explain this phenomenon in terms of the priority of the drive for self-preservation, when threatened by physical illness, over the motives perpetuating the mental illness. Another observation foreshadowed Freud: Hippocrates asserted that dreams embody desires free from interference by the reality of the waking state. He gave the name to hysteria which was recognized as a neurosis in the late nineteenth century. Hippocrates believed that hysteria was a physical disorder which occurred only in women and which was attributable to a wandering of the uterus from its normal location (*hystera* is the Greek word for uterus). This theory was widely held for over 2000 years.

Hippocrates' theory of causation was simple: mental disorders were caused solely by brain disease, brain injury or an excessive amount of a bodily substance called a *humor.* Four humors —black bile, blood, yellow bile and phlegm— were postulated. Each corresponded to one of the four "elements"—earth, air, fire, and water— which were believed to be the fundamental components of the universe. An excess of a particular humor was held responsible for a particular type of personality or temperament, e.g., too much black bile led to a melancholic, depressed temperament (see Table 2–1). If the excess was great enough, the individual manifested more than an eccentric personality trait: he was emotionally disturbed and ill.

This fantastic humoral theory, elaborated over the next several centuries until it comprised nine different temperaments, had profound consequences. It began the tradition of classifica-

TABLE 2–1. The Humoral Theory of Temperament and Pathology
(as developed from Hippocrates to Galen)

Cosmic Elements	Humors Corresponding to the Elements		Temperament Resulting from Excess of One Humor
Earth	Black bile		Melancholic
Air	Blood	*excess of blood* →	Sanguine; optimistic
Fire	Yellow bile		Choleric; angry and anxious
Water	Phlegm		Phlegmatic; apathetic

tion of personality into types. It implied that personality distortions and emotional disorders were quantitative exaggerations of normality. And it tied abnormalities to an anatomical and physiological basis.

Plato (427–347 B.C.), Hippocrates' pupil, espoused a doctrine in which mind was the only true reality and matter a secondary substance that imperfectly copied the mental and ideal. This philosophical ideal had little patience for the material or the body. Plato distinguished between a rational soul and an irrational soul. The irrational soul was the source of anger and love, fear and hope, and pain and pleasure, and it became ill if the union between it and the rational soul was severed. Mental illness was therefore the absence of rationality and therapy should therefore consist of philosophical persuasion back to rationality. Plato made some telling clinical observations, such as the following description of the hypochondriac:

> [They] . . . are always doctoring and increasing and complicating their disorders and always fancying that they will be cured by any nostrum which anybody advises them to try . . . and the charming thing is that they deem him their worst enemy who tells them the truth.

The next great figure, Asclepiades, a Roman of about 50 B.C., was the first to distinguish clearly acute deliria due to fevers from chronic, long-standing mental disorders; illusions in which an actual stimulus is misperceived from hallucinations in which no stimulus exists to warrant the individual's perceptions; and apathetic states from excited, agitated states. Equally as important as these empirical contributions was his humanitarianism. He advocated soothing the excited patients rather than terrorizing them. He invented a swaying bed and many types of special baths that had sedative effects. He urged the use of music as a therapy. At this time the mentally ill were customarily kept in dark cells; Asclepiades protested against this practice and also against treating patients by bleeding them. Implicit in his program was the assumption that a mental disorder can be either improved or exacerbated by psychological treatment.

As a result of Asclepiades' work, persons who were neither philosophers nor physicians became concerned about mental illness. For example, the historian and biographer Plutarch (46–120 A.D.) wrote a description of depression that is both compassionate and clinically sound by modern standards:

> When a man is depressed, every little evil is magnified by the scaring spectres of his anxiety. He looks on himself as a man whom the gods hate and pursue with their anger. . . . He dares not employ any means of averting or of remedying the evil. . . . "Leave me," says the wretched man, "me the impious, the accursed, hated of the gods, to suffer my punishment. . . ." Asleep or awake he is haunted alike by the spectres of his anxiety. Awake he makes no use of his reason; and asleep he enjoys no respite from his alarms. . . . Nowhere can he find an escape from his imaginary terrors.

FAR-OUT

Soranus (second century A.D.) picked up the humanitarian theme of Asclepiades. In Soranus' time, alcohol was often prescribed to treat mental illness; quite reasonably he asked how intoxication could be expected to dispel mental states that themselves frequently resembled an intoxicated state of confusion and irrationality. He drew up a code for the rational management of patients:

> Maniacs must be placed in a moderately lighted room, which is of moderate temperature and where the tranquillity is not disturbed by noise. . . . Much tact and discretion should be employed in directing attention to their faults; sometimes misbehavior should be overlooked or met with indulgence. . . . The greatest precautions must be taken to avoid shock [in using physical restraints], for the careless application of restraining bands increases or even produces fury instead of appeasing it.

The last major figure of the Classical Age was Galen (130–200 A.D.). Through dissection and experiment he searched for anatomical bases of function and pathology. He regarded the central nervous system as the center for sensation, mobility and mental functions. Mental disorders were defined as disorders of the brain. He elaborated the humoral theory of body types and temperamental characteristics. Galen's influence dominated general medicine until approximately 1750 A.D. but his approach to mental disorders was soon submerged in the revived and expanded demonology of the medieval period.

THE MEDIEVAL REGRESSION

In the medieval period the return to primitivism in psychopathology began earlier, took deeper hold, and lasted longer—until the eighteenth century—than in any other domain of human affairs. Abnormal behavior was divorced from rationality, reassociated with the supernatural and magical (as many purely physical ills also were), and delivered to the clergy for treatment. The medieval mind did not doubt that evil magic, promoted by innumerable demons, flourished on every side. Salvation was considered the only valid goal of mankind and earthly concerns were depreciated; a naturalistic approach to the mind was unthinkable. By 429 A.D. the demonological point of view had developed sufficiently for magic to be officially condemned by the Church as equivalent to heresy.

For the next thousand years demonological theory was elaborated and refined. Certain symptoms, such as pigmented spots and areas of skin anesthesia (loss of tactile sensitivity, a classic sign of hysterical neurosis), where infallible signs of demonic possession. Late in the medieval period when the Inquisition took over the task of hunting down the possessed, special assistants known as prickers identified insensitive areas by pricking suspected witches in various bodily parts. If shouting a Biblical passage into the ear of a patient having convulsions produced a response, the illness was undoubtedly demonic, because the holy text had frightened the demon; if there was no response the illness was natural.

Therapy in the medieval period at first consisted of prayer, incantation, touching of relics and fantastic prescriptions that caricatured

naturalism. Thus an illness might be treated by obtaining organs removed from a dog and a toad, pulverizing them, mixing the powder in ale and giving the patient the liquid to drink when the moon was in a waning phase. Sick and frightened people are often suggestible; it is not surprising that patients believed in such treatment and were seemingly helped by it. An incantation of the tenth century illustrates the result of wedding supernaturalism to Hippocrates' theory of hysteria: for the treatment of a hysterical young woman referred to as N., the less extraordinary part of the incantation pronounced over her was (Zilboorg and Henry, 1941, pp. 131, 132):

. . . I conjure thee, O womb, in the name of the Holy Trinity, to come back to the place from which thou shouldst neither move nor turn away, without further molestation, and to return, without anger, to the place where the Lord has put thee originally. . . . I conjure thee not to harm that maid of God, N., not to occupy her head, throat, neck, chest, ears, teeth, eyes, nostrils, shoulder blades, arms, hands, heart, stomach, spleen, kidneys, back, sides, joints, navel, intestines, bladder, thighs, shins, heels, nails, but to lie down quietly in the place where God chose for thee, so that this maid of God, N., be restored to health.

Because mentally ill persons aroused great fear, they were often disavowed by their families. They roamed the countryside, looking less and less human as time passed, until their appearance seemed to justify the very superstition and anxiety originally responsible for their desperate condition.

From the fifth century on, an extraordinary social pathology appeared in many guises. For example, a phenomenon occurred called the dancing mania or St. Vitus' dance in which someone would suddenly leap up and run in great excitement to the market place where he might be joined by the entire population of the town. They danced wildly, tore off their clothes, beat each other, rolled on the ground, drank, sang and talked unceasingly. It is reasonable to suppose that this psychopathological social pattern was a temporary and violent release from the dangers and uncertainties of life in medieval times. The prevalence of belief in demonology is not surprising in such a social context.

As the medieval period continued, mental disease was more and more equated with sin, primarily sexual. Invisible devils called *incubi* had sexual intercourse with women, and others called *succubi* seduced men. Demons were responsible for sexual impotence, sterility and abortions, as well as for hatred, jealousy, physical disease and loss of reason. In 1494, two Dominican friars named Johann Sprenger and Heinrich Kraemer were authorized by the Pope to investigate and root out witchcraft, believed to be on the increase. They wrote a learned and scholarly book entitled *Malleus Maleficarum—"Witches' Hammer"*—that immediately became the official manual for the diagnosis and treatment of witches. For two and one-half centuries it was used to apprehend, try, torture, convict and execute witches, almost all of whom would now be recognized as obviously mentally ill. A few quotations from the *Malleus* reveal the temper of the age:

   . . . True faith teaches us that certain angels fell from heaven and are now devils, and we are bound to acknowledge that by their very nature they can do many wonderful things which we cannot do. And those who try to induce others to perform such evil wonders are called witches. And because infidelity in a person who has been baptized is technically called heresy, therefore such persons are plainly heretics.

   . . . The devil has extraordinary power over the minds of those who have given themselves up to him, so that what they do in pure imagination, they believe they have actually and really done in the body.

The latter passage has implications that may not be immediately obvious: not even a delusion ("pure imagination") excused one from being treated as a witch, because a delusion itself resulted from a compact with the devil. The patient's statements were taken either as factual truth or as equivalent to it. Zilboorg remarks:

It is as if today we listened to a person afflicted with a paranoid schizophrenia and heard him say that detectives were after him, that he had killed a good man, and that he heard voices coming to him by radio waves from the next building, and we then set out to look for the transmitter and at the same time instituted proceedings charging the patient with murder in the first degree.

"All witchcraft," says the *Malleus* "comes from carnal lust, which is in women insatiable. . . . Wherefore for the sake of fulfilling their lusts they consort even with devils." It has been estimated that about 50 women were condemned and burned for every man. For her trial after torture the female witch was stripped of her clothes, her marks of torture exposed, her hair shaven so no devils could hide in it and she was led into court backward so that her evil eye might not bewitch the judges. The degradation and hatred of women were rationalized as a struggle against sin; burning a witch was

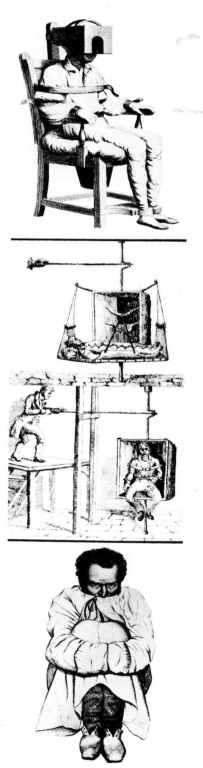

Figure 2–3. *Early methods of treating emotional disorders. (Reproduced by permission from Psychiatry and Social Science Review, Vol. 4, 1970.)*

rationalized as an act of mercy that freed her from the devil's clutches.

Another interesting practice common in the fourteenth and fifteenth centuries was to relinquish the insane to a boatman who would often deposit them in another city. As the practice increased it became difficult to unload the madmen on an unsuspecting city, with the result that many unfortunates were permanently bound to a "ship of fools" sailing from port to port. A popular pastime of the period was to go to the docks to watch the antics of the fools during the loading or unloading of a foreign ship (Foucault, 1965).

THE EMERGENCE FROM DEMONOLOGY IN THE RENAISSANCE

Although the last witch was executed in Switzerland as late as 1782, beginning in the Renaissance of the sixteenth century a few men protested against the *Malleus,* much as the Greek and Roman pioneers had argued against primitive barbarism. The sixteenth-century essayist Montaigne talked to witches and decided they were more demented than guilty. His contemporary, Juan Luis Vives, a deeply religious Spanish scholar, argued for compassion toward the mentally ill and for the desirability of understanding their feelings and emotions. This stress on empathy and understanding of the individual patient was a new and very modern note in the history of psychopathology.

Johann Weyer (1515–1588) was the major voice of reason raised in opposition to the *Malleus.* He was the first physician in history whose central interest was mental illness and he claimed that most witches were innocent, sick people. "I show that those illnesses the origin of which is attributed to witches come from natural causes," he wrote. The whole structure of the *Malleus* was grandiose nonsense to him. Symptoms such as skin anesthesia were signs of suggestibility, not possession. His descriptions of patients show a calm matter-of-factness, free of the emotional language of the *Malleus,* that has served as a model ever since. For example, he wrote:

I knew a melancholic who insisted that someone smelled of sulphur and tar. . . . He also said that his private parts were tormented with so much inflammation and stench that he was painfully afraid that they would rot and die away, yet these parts were found healthy. I could cite here an infinite number of ex-

amples in which you could see the senses involved in many ways, by humors and melancholic vapors [Weyer partially returned to the tradition of Galen] which affect the basis from which all these monstrous fantasies spring.

Men like Weyer made up a tiny minority, however. More representative of the age was James I of England, who in 1665 wrote and published a book to refute *The Discovery of Witchcraft,* by Reginald Scot, a scholarly attack on demonology (see Fig. 2–4). Not until 1700 was demonology definitely on the wane; half a century later it was all but dead.

THE MODERN ERA

The modern era may be divided into two periods. First, up to roughly 1900, but continuing beyond it, the *organic* point of view was dominant. Second, beginning about 1880, the height of the organic period, and continuing into the present there has been an increasing emphasis on the *psychological* sources of behavior disturbances. Both periods have their roots in earlier eras. The viewpoints and findings of both periods will be summarized here and elaborated in the ensuing chapters.

The Organic Period

The basis for the organic emphasis was the great advance in knowledge of human anatomy and physiology that began in the sixteenth century. This knowledge combined with a complete reaction against demonology to become the foundation for an empirical and naturalistic approach to the understanding of abnormal behavior.

The climactic figures of the organic period were Wilhelm Griesinger (1817–1868) and Emil Kraepelin (1856–1926). They were preceded by many scientists and physicians who had suggested that emotional disorder could result from exhaustion of the nervous system, peculiarities of brain shape or size, brain tissue destruction, heredity, childbirth, menopause or other organic factors. Griesinger, a German psychiatrist, systematized these accumulated organic observations and hypotheses in *Mental Pathology and Therapeutics* (1845). The thesis of this book was that all mental disorders were somatic diseases whose locus was the brain. Psychological causes for mental disorder did not exist. In one

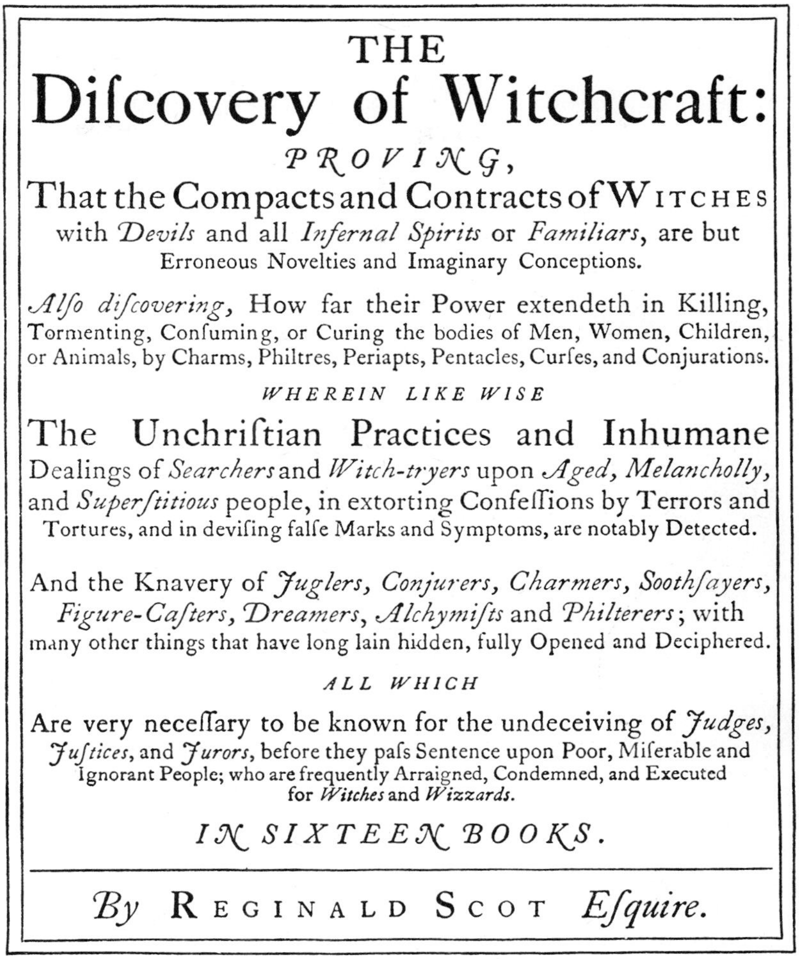

70
84
88
————
172
70
242
200
300
-172
28
20
3⌐242

Figure 2–4. Title page of Reginald Scot's Discovery of Witchcraft, edition of 1665.

THE
Discovery of Witchcraft:
PROVING,
That the Compacts and Contracts of Witches
with *Devils* and all *Infernal Spirits* or *Familiars*, are but
Erroneous Novelties and Imaginary Conceptions.

Also discovering, How far their Power extendeth in Killing,
Tormenting, Consuming, or Curing the bodies of Men, Women, Children,
or Animals, by Charms, Philtres, Periapts, Pentacles, Curses, and Conjurations.

WHEREIN LIKE WISE
The Unchristian Practices and Inhumane
Dealings of *Searchers* and *Witch-tryers* upon *Aged, Melancholly,*
and *Superstitious* people, in extorting Confessions by Terrors and
Tortures, and in devising false Marks and Symptoms, are notably Detected.

And the Knavery of *Juglers, Conjurers, Charmers, Soothsayers,*
Figure-Casters, Dreamers, Alchymists and *Philterers*; with
many other things that have long lain hidden, fully Opened and Deciphered.

ALL WHICH
Are very necessary to be known for the undeceiving of *Judges,*
Justices, and *Jurors,* before they pass Sentence upon Poor, Miserable and
Ignorant People; who are frequently Arraigned, Condemned, and Executed
for *Witches* and *Wizzards.*

IN SIXTEEN BOOKS.

By REGINALD SCOT *Esquire.*

sense, even mental disorders did not exist because mental symptoms were no more than indices of brain disease. Since the facts to back up these contentions were largely absent, the organic point of view depended on what has often been called a "brain mythology." But in time, organicism succeeded in explaining a number of mental disorders. By 1913 organic factors had been established as the primary determinants of alcoholic psychoses, paresis (conclusively proved in 1913 to be due to a syphilitic infection of the brain), senile psychoses, psychosis with cerebral arteriosclerosis (a disorder associated with hardening of the arteries in the brain) and many other behavior disturbances.

Kraepelin elaborated Griesinger's point of view into a systematic classification of diseases. His fundamental assumption was that the out-come of mental disease is predetermined. Patients either naturally recover, as often happens, for example, in manic-depression, or they naturally deteriorate, as Kraepelin mistakenly believed to be inevitable in schizophrenia. The course and outcome of a disease define it; the patient's feelings, thoughts, motives and anxieties are incidental and irrelevant. It is important to know that his hallucinations are auditory rather than visual, for the occurrence of auditory hallucinations argues for a schizophrenic diagnosis; but just what the hallucinated voices say is of no consequence.

Kraepelin's nosology defined and distinguished the important disorders of manic-depressive psychosis, a cyclic series of elations and depressions often accompanied by normal intervals between attacks, and dementia praecox, a psychosis that often begins in ado-

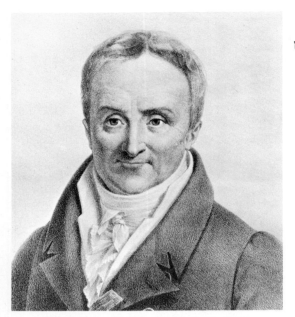

Figure 2–5. *Philippe Pinel (1745–1826).*

organic basis: it was intended to rearrange the brain and return it to a normal state.

Philippe Pinel (1745–1826), a French psychiatrist, broke through this atmosphere by obtaining governmental permission in 1793 to remove the chains from the patients in La Bicêtre hospital in Paris. To the surprise of the Parisian citizens most of the released patients were docile instead of violently assaultive. Pinel had had precursors in the trend to humanitarianism, from Asclepiades to the inhabitants of the town of Gheel in Belgium: In the fifteenth century a custom began of making pilgrimages to seek cures for mental illness at a shrine in Gheel. Many pilgrims stayed on in the homes of the inhabitants and there is still a colony of several thousand patients who live and work there and freely mix with the townfolk.

Pinel's achievement was paralleled by William Tuke, a wealthy English Quaker. In 1796 he established a retreat for the mentally ill at his estate and demonstrated that giving them freedom was both safe and beneficial. In the United States Dorothea Dix (1802–1887) spent four decades arousing the country to the brutal condition of patients in jails and county almshouses. As a result of her efforts, more than 30 state hospitals were founded.

Advances in organic treatment approaches were particularly notable in the 1930's with the development of insulin shock and electroshock

lescence. For these and for all other mental disorders Kraepelin gave an exhaustive description of symptoms based on the cumulative case histories of thousands of patients. He attributed all disorders to biological factors. Although this approach was quite narrow, his classification itself was so comprehensive and backed by so many descriptive facts that with minor revisions it has remained the standard system of psychiatric classification.

While medicine and abnormal psychology made great diagnostic strides, despite overemphasis on organic factors, treatment lagged far behind. Benjamin Rush (1745–1813), the first American psychiatrist and a signer of the Declaration of Independence, was at one with Celsus in advocating emetics, purgatives and bloodletting. Johann Reil (1759–1813), a relatively enlightened German psychiatrist, advocated "noninjurious torture." In a typical asylum such as Bethlem Hospital in London, patients were chained in cold cells, undernourished, encouraged to attack each other by sadistic jailers and exhibited to visitors for a small admission fee. The word "bedlam" is a corruption of the name of this hospital. Treatment included immersing the patient completely in water until he almost drowned and twirling him on a special stool until he became unconscious. The latter procedure had a mythological

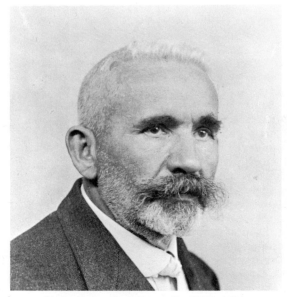

Figure 2–6. *Emil Kraepelin (1856–1926).*

therapy. These treatments utilized insulin or electricity to induce convulsion in patients suffering from various emotional ailments. While the original theories on which the treatments were based were soon disproved, both continued to be widely used until the mid 1950's. Electroshock therapy is still used with good effect in the treatment of severe and intractable depressions. The use of brain surgery or lobotomy also obtained prominence as a treatment during the 1930's. In one of the popular versions, the surgeon cuts the connective tissues between the frontal lobes and the rest of the brain. While this resulted in greater periods of calm in previously violent and unmanageable patients, there often resulted untoward and irreversible side effects.

Ataractic, mood-influencing drugs were introduced in the 1950's and had an immediate effect on the treatment of emotional disorders. Tranquilizers, mood elevators, mood depressors, and general muscle relaxants in various combinations were introduced. By rendering patients more acceptable to other forms of persuasion, such as psychotherapy, it was now possible to avoid hospitalizing increasing numbers of patients. The effect of these drugs can scarcely be minimized. Had the rate of hospitalization for mental disorders increased as expected before the advent of the ataractic drugs, more than 700,000 Americans would have been in mental hospitals in 1967. Instead the figure

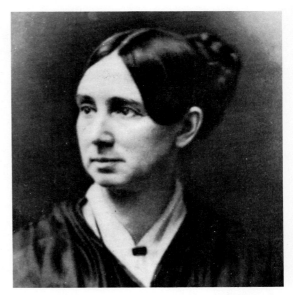

Figure 2–8. Dorothea Lynde Dix (1802–1887).

for 1967 was 426,000. Drugs cannot be credited with all of the reduction but they have played a significant role.

The Psychological Period

About 1880 there began a swing away from the rigidity of the completely organic point of view and toward the flexibility of an organic-psychological combination. This movement was precipitated by the realization that the explanation offered by the organic approach for the neuroses, the personality disorders and such psychoses as dementia praecox rested on hypothetical and unproved lesions of the brain. Although countless hours were spent examining cross sections of the brain tissue of deceased neurotics, no difference from normal brains was ever found. A second precipitating factor was the observation that many patients recovered despite the fact that the irreversibility of brain tissue destruction could be expected to lead to irreversible psychological consequences. The discrepancy might be explained by assuming that undamaged areas of the brain eventually take over the impaired functions of the destroyed brain cells, or by assuming that psychological difficulties can be caused by chemical disturbances in the brain without tissue destruction. But no empirical basis for such speculations existed in the nineteenth century.

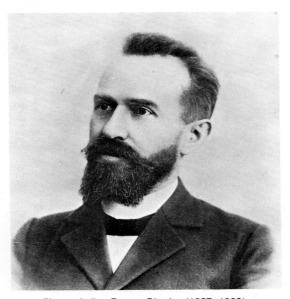

Figure 2–7. Eugen Bleuler (1857–1939).

The psychological revolution was in part an outgrowth of the tradition of humanitarianism and also of the discovery of hypnosis. Pinel's work implied that mental patients were human beings like everyone else; unshackling them inevitably led to interest in their psychology. The development of hypnosis started in Vienna with Franz Anton Mesmer (1733–1815). He announced the discovery of "animal magnetism," a hypothetical magnetic fluid that he claimed was present throughout the universe and was particularly concentrated in people. Mesmer believed that illness was due to a lack of equilibrium in this fluid and that he could reestablish the necessary balance by the induction of magnetic forces. He went to Paris where he built a kind of tub, called a *baquet,* which had vertical iron rods to be grasped by the patients. Mesmer stroked his patients and also waved a magnetic wand to coax the fluid into them from the rods, thus restoring the necessary equilibrium. When subjected to this procedure, many patients showed strange effects such as laughing, crying, "convulsions" and fainting. Animal magnetism was soon exposed by a committee of scientists (which included Benjamin Franklin) as nonexistent and the effects of mesmerism, as it came to be known, were attributed to imagination. In the latter half of the 1800's several British and French physicians continued to study the "trance state" which Mesmer had discovered. The phenomenon was given the name hypnosis (after the Greek word *hypnos,* for sleep) by the British physician James Braid (1795–1860). The study of hypnosis proved to be a crucial phase in the eventual discovery of the psychological bases for abnormal behavior.

Jean Martin Charcot (1825–1893), a French psychiatrist and neurologist sometimes referred to as the father of modern neurology, used hypnotism to make an extensive investigation into the nature of the neuroses, especially hysteria, at the Salpêtrière hospital in Paris. He mistakenly believed that only hysterics were hypnotizable and that the phenomena observed in hypnotized hysterics—trance-like states, muscular rigidity, anesthesias, hallucinatory perceptions and reflex changes—were caused by brain defects; hypnosis merely revealed the fundamental organic defects of the hysteric. It did not occur to Charcot that most people can be hypnotized and that the hypnotic procedure itself was responsible for the phenomena he observed. As we understand it today, certain hysteric symptoms may be

precipitated by a hypnotist's (or inquisitor's) questions, because hysterics tend to be suggestible.

At the time Charcot was working in Paris, two physicians in Nancy, Liébault (1823–1904) and Bernheim (1840–1919), began to use hypnotism to treat neurotics. They hypothesized that both hypnosis and hysteria were states of heightened suggestibility. Hypnosis was induced through suggestions imparted by others while hysteria seemed to be induced by auto- or self-suggestion. Hypnosis could produce hysteric-like symptoms in normals and could be used to treat and remove the symptoms of a true hysteric. The School of Nancy, as it is called, thus brought about the convergence of a number of important trends: true psychotherapy was finally born and with it came a shift in interest from organic to emotional determinants; it was recognized that neurotics and normals are similar and that the understanding of neurotics therefore can be furthered by studying normals; finally, the linkage of hysteria to the measurable variable of suggestibility, which can be studied in the laboratory, meant that an experimental foundation for abnormal psychology became possible.

Pierre Janet (1859–1947) described hysterical symptoms comprehensively and constructed a theory of hypnosis that combined the approaches of both Charcot and the Nancy school. Suggestibility, an important factor in Janet's theory of hysteria, was itself due to the hysteric's tendency to *dissociation,* a breakdown of the normal integration and association of psychological processes. Janet theorized that dissociation occurred because of hereditary or constitutional defects, so that hysteria was ultimately organic. Whether or not this hypothesis is correct, the concept of dissociation is important and comes very close to Freud's basic concept of *repression.* Janet also differentiated and described some neurotic states other than hysteria and he thus laid much of the basis for our current classification of the neuroses.

There were two gaps in Janet's approach. First, he did not undertake to interrelate motives and early experiences to the development of neurotic symptoms; second, he offered no rationale to explain the selective occurrence in a particular patient of a few particular symptoms, out of all those that might occur. It remained for Sigmund Freud (1856–1939) to fill these gaps. Freud had studied under Charcot and had familiarized himself with Bernheim's achievements. In Vienna, Freud collaborated with

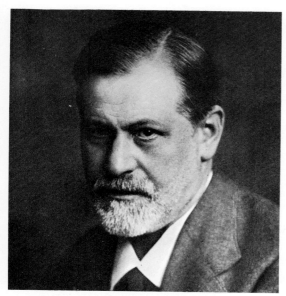

Figure 2–9. Sigmund Freud (1856–1939).

the physician Josef Breuer in exploring the latter's method for the treatment of hysterics by encouraging them to talk freely under hypnosis of the circumstances that had led to the onset of symptoms. Breuer and Freud's patients reported past events with an emotional outburst that was a cathartic release of previously pent-up affect; hence this variant of hypnotic treatment was called catharsis. In 1895, Breuer and Freud's *Studies on Hysteria* formulated a preliminary version of a theory of hysteria which became the basis of a general theory of all of the psychoneuroses.

While there were many modifications as Freud continued to develop his psychoanalytic theory over the next four decades, several important insights were evident in the initial publication (Strupp, 1967):

1. A relationship was established between hysterical symptoms and hypnosis.
2. The hysterical symptoms were often tied to painful feelings and memories of which the patient was unaware or could not express except under hypnosis (that is, there are *unconscious* thoughts that can influence the patient's mental life).
3. The original painful feelings are excluded from awareness (repressed).
4. The patient develops ways of thinking or perceiving which serve to ensure that the unpleasant feelings remain out of awareness (that is, the patient erects *defenses* against certain aspects of his own awareness).
5. An *intrapsychic* conflict develops in which the patient struggles to forget something which, by being extremely painful, begs to be remembered.
6. Denied proper expression, the feeling can be distorted or converted (thus the term conversion hysteria) into physical symptoms. At this point the patient thus both expresses his pain and "forgets" the original painful event.
7. This process can be reversed under hypnosis through having the patient recall the original painful feelings. The expression of the feelings often resulted in at least a temporary diminution of the physical symptoms.
8. The patient's relationship to the doctor was important to the success of the treatment.

Freud soon rejected hypnosis in favor of *free association,* in which the patient is required to say whatever comes to his mind without concern for logic or propriety. His patients' associations provided the empirical basis for his development of psychoanalytic theory over the next 40 years.

Three different aspects of psychoanalysis may be distinguished. It is a method of psychotherapy, a theory of abnormality, and a general theory of personality extrapolated and modified from the theory of neurosis.

Psychoanalytic therapy aims at insight and at better control over behavior. This is achieved via slow and careful analysis of the patient's free associations and dreams through which his unconscious childhood attitudes are revealed. As the patient comes to understand and accept this repressed material and its effect on current emotional events, he assumes greater voluntary control over behavior that previously had been at the mercy of his unconscious impulses.

The psychoanalytic theories of neurosis and general personality brought about an intellectual revolution. Psychoanalysis asserts that many of the crucial determinants of action, feeling and thinking are unconscious—a concept which is a challenge to man's narcissistic pride. Historians have remarked that the self concept of modern man has suffered three shattering intellectual blows: the Copernican revolution pushed aside his dwelling place from the center of the universe; the Darwinian revolution demoted him from his nonanimal status; and the Freudian revolution challenged the conviction that if he is an animal, at least he is a rational one.

Freudian or psychoanalytic theory sees man in a state of conflict in which he constantly seeks to balance opposing needs or demands within himself. In addition to the reality demands of the world dictated by reason, judgment, perception, intelligent planning and the like (a group of processes labeled *ego*), man is faced with both the unconscious demands of his biological, largely sexual, drives which constantly seek expression (*id* is the term used to refer to the biological drives), and with the largely unconscious moral prohibitions (*superego*) acquired in childhood which are specifically aimed at blocking impulse expression. Man's task, then, is to reconcile impulses and inhibitions with reality. The neurotic fails in this reconciliation, and his particular symptoms symbolize the conflicts in living which he has failed to resolve.

Psychoanalysis, as therapy and as theory, rapidly gained in acceptance during World War I (1914–1918). The stress of war precipitated neurotic breakdowns, particularly of a hysterical type, in hundreds of thousands of soldiers. It seemed to many observers that Freudian theory explained the unexpected mass breakdowns better than any competing theory. Psychoanalysis has had an increasing influence on the study and treatment of abnormal behavior ever since, especially in the United States. Although widely criticized because of its lack of attention to certain critical aspects of human experience, psychoanalysis still stands as the most comprehensive theory of personality and neurosis yet developed.

Various modifications of psychoanalytic theory have been proposed and elaborated. Carl Jung, Alfred Adler, Karen Horney and Harry Stack Sullivan have been particularly prominent in psychoanalytic revisions. Jung expanded Freud's concept of the *libido,* the energy of psychosexual impulses, to include all of the individual's "life force," of which sexuality is but one component. Adler suggested that the drive for power and superiority is a more fundamental motivation than Freud's sexual strivings. Karen Horney has theorized that basic anxiety and repressed hostility are the primary sources of personality difficulty. Sullivan has emphasized the social and interpersonal nature of neurosis and its origins. It is apparent that the major modifications of Freud have re-jected, in one way or another, his hypothesis that man's ultimate motives are sexual.

In addition to the development from hypnosis and suggestibility to Freudian theory and its modifications, a number of other important modern trends have appeared. Clifford Beers published *A Mind That Found Itself* (1908), in which he recounted the horrors of his own hospitalization for mental illness. As a result of Beers' exposé, the mental hygiene movement was founded in 1909. It has focused on community attempts to support mental hospitals and raise their standards of treatment, on prevention of mental disorders and on establishing clinics for disturbed children.

Another development in modern abnormal psychology was the discovery of the *experimental neurosis* in 1914 in the laboratory of the Russian physiologist and Nobel prize winner, Ivan Pavlov (1849–1936). Pavlov had established that if a dog was repeatedly presented with an auditory or visual stimulus (such as a bell or a circle) immediately prior to eating, he soon learned, or was conditioned, to salivate immediately upon presentation of the bell or circle alone. Furthermore, a conditioned response, such as salivation, would soon appear or be *generalized* to other stimuli such as the experimental room and other auditory or visual cues. Eventually the animal would learn to salivate or respond only to those sounds or sights which had been paired with food. Quite accidentally it

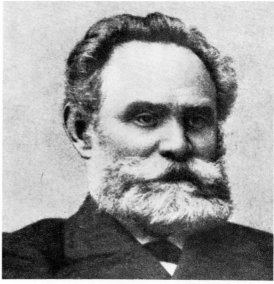

Figure 2–10. *Ivan Petrovich Pavlov (1849–1936).*

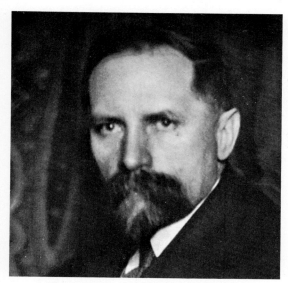

Figure 2–11. *Adolf Meyer (1866–1950).*

was discovered that animals forced to make more and more difficult discriminations (such as salivate to a circle and not to an almost circular ellipse) became noisy, violent, and often lost the ability to make discriminations which had been previously mastered. In a sense, they acted "neurotic" or abnormal. These unusual behaviors were found to generalize to persons and objects present during the original difficult learning situation. Although primitive by modern standards, Pavlov's early experiments established an important beginning for controlled laboratory studies of psychopathology. For the first time it was established that certain abnormal behaviors could be produced at will through specified procedures and that these behaviors are subject to the principles of learning, such as conditioning and stimulus generalization.

A quite different tendency in recent years has been the emphasis on the psychosomatic, holistic or organismic point of view, that is, the insistence that neither organic nor psychological factors should be ignored in behavioral disturbance. This approach stems particularly from Adolf Meyer (1866–1950), an outstanding figure in recent American psychiatry who popularized the need for the study of the patient and his personality in all relevant aspects, instead of concentrating on symptoms only. World War II strengthened this point of view because many of the war breakdowns were psychophysiologic. The organismic approach is needed to understand both the organic and emotional aspects of a psychophysiologic disorder.

THE IMPLICATIONS OF HISTORY FOR ABNORMAL PSYCHOLOGY

In addition to the uneven, interrupted march toward empiricism, naturalism and humanitarianism, a number of other trends and relationships can be observed in the historical events we have sketched. An awareness of these trends and relationships is helpful in evaluating the present status of abnormal psychology and attempting to anticipate its future:

The roots of treatment for emotional disorders are ancient as revealed by the evidence of trephining. All societies have had some kind of policy to cope with mental and physical disease, even when the two were not distinguished from each other.

Errors and superstitious practices may be traced to antiquity but so may some scientific practices. Trephining was the crude forerunner of brain surgery; Asclepiades' advocacy of music as therapy in 50 B.C. foreshadowed the widespread use of music in mental hospitals today; some of today's ideas and practices will be improved tomorrow.

Different areas of psychopathology have developed at different rates. By the first century A.D. several psychotic conditions had been adequately described and differentiated from each other but it was not until the nineteenth century that a similar stage was reached for the neurotic disorders.

The historical progressions and retrogressions of abnormal psychology are related to progress and decline in the general level of society; consequently the prevailing attitudes to mental illness seem to be a fair index of the social, political and cultural levels of the age. The mentally ill are the most vulnerable of all minorities, for they cannot adjust to the demands made on them and they do not understand why they cannot adjust. In a period of social turmoil or decline they become convenient scapegoats.

The history of psychopathology provides no firm guarantee against a future recurrence of cruelty or speculation unchecked by evidence. Undoubtedly another regression in social, political and cultural areas would be accompanied by a deterioration in attitudes toward abnormal behavior.

Several eras have ignored their immediate predecessors and elaborated on the tradition of temporally distant epochs. The Middle Ages ignored the Greco-Roman period and returned to pre-classical primitivism. The nineteenth century organicists skipped over the Dark Ages and revived the approach of the Greeks and Romans. The post-1880 emphasis on psychological sources of disorder swung away from the immediately preceding organic achievements. Current advances in genetics, endocrinology and brain physiology may possibly culminate in a revival of the pre-Freudian organic tradition.

The descriptions of disturbance in the literature of antiquity are dramatic and they stress wildly irrational behavior; minor difficulties seem to have been ignored. It may be inferred that standards have changed and that our own age is more sensitive than were past eras to signs of minor disturbance. But it is also true that the early descriptions fit many present-day cases. It follows that some forms of mental illness have been quite constant over the ages, although others have not (e.g., the dancing mania has disappeared). In different contemporary cultures one finds a considerable similarity in types of disturbance but not complete identity. Mental disorder largely transcends time and culture.

Throughout the organic subperiod of the nineteenth century, scientists felt that historical justification was needed for their theories and procedures. They sought a basis in the authority of Galen, Hippocrates and others. Today the attempt to justify a position by quoting a historical authority—for example, Freud—still exists, but the trend to empiricism has weakened this tendency. Empiricism means appeal to evidence, not to authority. The history of psychopathology thus culminates in a certain freedom from that very history.

ABNORMAL PSYCHOLOGY TODAY

The following are some major features of present-day abnormal psychology; each is an outgrowth of the past. The importance of each feature is apparent in many places in the rest of this book.

Differences of opinion abound in abnormal psychology but there is agreement that the test of a belief should be empirical and if possible experimental. With time, empirical research may be expected to lead to greater agreement on the causes and treatment of abnormal behavior.

Psychoanalysis is moving toward a rap-

prochement with the traditional psychology of learning, perception and so forth. The two developed independently of each other, the first from therapeutic work with neurotic patients and the second from laboratory investigations. However, traditional academic psychology has now incorporated a number of psychoanalytic concepts such as the defense mechanisms and, at the same time, psychoanalysis is becoming increasingly interested in the ego functions that have always been the concern of traditional psychology. E. H. Erikson (1950), H. Hartmann (1958) and E. Kris (1951) are among the analysts in the forefront of this trend.

Both intrapersonal and interpersonal factors are important in contemporary abnormal psychology. It is standard practice to investigate the processes within the individual and also outside him.

Assessment of disturbance is based largely on intelligence, aptitude, interest and personality tests developed in recent decades. The clinical psychologist, among other functions, specializes in administration and interpretation of tests and in research on tests. A good deal of effort is expended toward test improvement.

New methods of treating a group of patients simultaneously, combinations of hypnotic and nonhypnotic techniques, special methods for treating children and many other types of psychotherapy have multiplied and are in wide use. No single type of psychotherapy is the standard.

A new type of organicism based on careful experimentation may be arising. Improved techniques of physiological investigation have stimulated a host of recent studies of biological factors in mental disorders. It is not yet possible to predict the ultimate outcome of these studies.

In a number of communities, mental hospitals have been moving in two directions, both of which are logical developments of the humanitarian trend. The open hospital, an institution without locked doors, has been tried and found feasible. Second, a movement has begun away from the rural, often isolated, state hospital designed for large numbers of exclusively mental patients to small psychiatric divisions in ordinary, urban, general-medical hospitals. This trend obviously implies that a mental patient is not a special kind of organism to be segregated.

The organismic point of view is often implemented by the team approach. A group of experts—for example, a psychiatrist (an M.D. with postgraduate training in the medical specialty of psychiatry), a clinical psychologist (a Ph.D. in psychology who works with disturbed persons), and a psychiatric social worker (an M.S.W. trained to help patients, their families and other persons with whom patients interact)—together evaluate a patient or a family and plan treatment.

Mental health specialists have taken root in new environments, e.g., schools, colleges, churches and military organizations. Some industrial companies have hired staff psychologists and psychiatrists to help employees with emotional problems. More than in any period in the past, present-day society recognizes the value of a scientific and professional approach to psychological disorders.

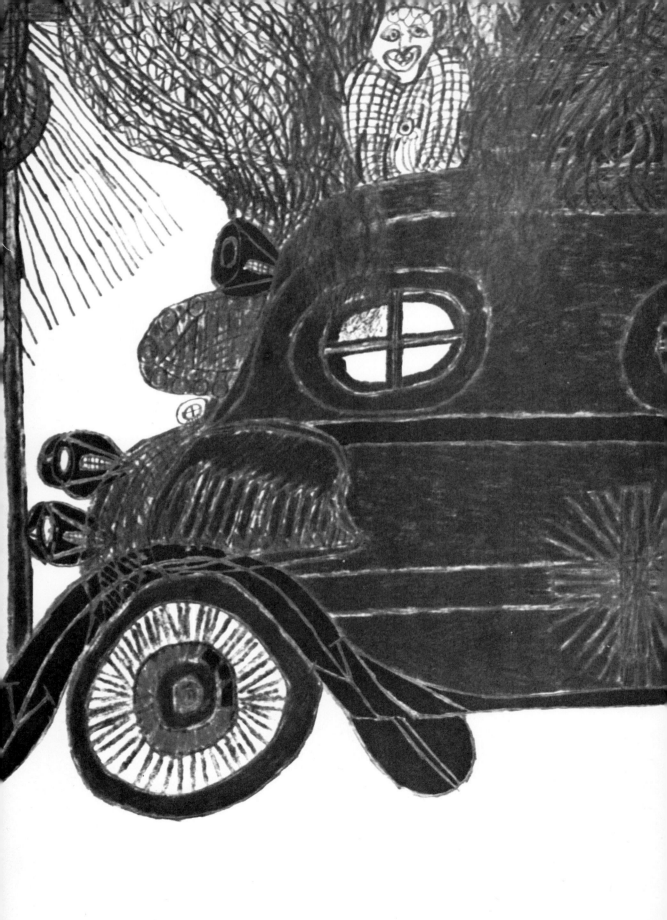

> "When I use a word," Humpty Dumpty said in rather a scornful tone, "it means just what I choose it to mean—neither more nor less."
>
> Lewis Carroll, *Through the Looking-Glass and What Alice Found There*

MODERN CLASSIFICATION OF ABNORMALITY

An emotionally disturbed woman, aged 42, was hospitalized for observation and treatment. She was unkempt, had dark circles under her eyes and appeared tired, fearful and tense. She avoided looking at anyone directly but glanced about rapidly or stared fixedly into the distance. Although she seemed to be above average in intelligence, she asked, after a routine blood test, "Are they going to take my memory away as well as my blood?" She was unable to report past events consistently. In talking about her family she sometimes said she had two brothers and sometimes one.

She rarely smiled and her voice indicated little emotion. However, she reported having had two abortions and as she talked of these incidents her manner revealed a deep sense of guilt.

For some years she had wandered from city to city living with different relatives. In an unemotional tone she said that she had let everyone down, was worthless and was "under investigation" for her misdeeds. She heard people calling her derogatory names. She believed someone was trying to steal the key to her apartment. She heard "spooks outside the door" who influenced her thoughts and actions.

She repeatedly stated that married people were very lucky; she herself had been divorced. She complained that she was bored, had no one to talk to and no one understood her. On the hospital ward she sometimes cried, sometimes sat in a stuporous fashion and sometimes busied herself with various routine activities. She considered herself to be well. If she had ever been ill, she said, she had gotten over it.

Obviously, this patient was emotionally disturbed and in need of help. To prescribe the proper treatment and make other decisions affecting her life, it was first necessary to diagnose the disorder from which she suffered. On the basis of a diagnosis it might be decided that she should be treated by psychotherapy, drugs, electroconvulsive therapy or some combination of these or other methods. Since the rate of recovery varies for different disorders, a diagnosis could be used as a basis for predicting the probability that she would recover and deciding whether to tell her family to expect improvement. Patients with some disorders often attempt suicide; a diagnosis would dictate whether she should be watched with special care.

The diagnosis in this case was paranoid schizophrenia. From her history and diagnosis it was then possible to predict: that the disorder had taken years to develop, that many different causes might have contributed to it, that the risk of suicide was slight, that the probability of improvement with treatment was well over 50 per cent, that improvement might be slow and treatment by ataractic drugs was indicated, *TRANQ.* preferably with concomitant psychotherapy.

A meaningful diagnosis can be made only if diagnosticians agree on a system of classification, that is, an organized summary of the syndromes into which diverse symptoms fall. Symptoms can be either subjective or objective manifestations of a disorder. Subjective symptoms are complaints such as tiredness, depression or fear. Objective symptoms are usually revealed in observable behavior such as faulty memory or inappropriate emotional reactions.

For convenience in presentation, psychological symptoms may be classified into five categories: disorders of sensation and perception, of intelligence and thought, of affect, of motivation, and of verbal and motor behavior. These categories are for discussion purposes only and should not be confused with *syndromes.* A syndrome refers to one of many commonly observed clusters of symptoms which may fall into several of the above categories. The paranoid schizophrenic patient just described displayed symptoms from all five of the categories.

In this chapter the major psychological symptoms are categorized and defined. Physiological symptoms as well as minor and infrequent psychological symptoms are omitted. Following the survey of symptoms, the major diagnostic syndromes are summarized and the reliability of the standard system of classification is discussed.

Three introductory points should be clarified. First, the categorization of symptoms is an abstraction from reality. A living organism simultaneously perceives, thinks, feels and acts, in a holistic pattern. It is artificial to break this organismic pattern into separate categories except for didactic purposes. Second, any single symptom may occur in many quite different psychological disorders, just as the symptom of fever may occur in many physical diseases. Consequently, a symptom is usually not important in itself but as a constituent with other symptoms of a syndrome. Third, the present chapter is primarily descriptive. The important problems of the dynamics and origins of symptoms and syndromes are reserved for discussion in later chapters.

THE SYMPTOMS OF ABNORMAL BEHAVIOR

Disordered Sensation and Perception

The brain receives nerve impulses from the specialized sense organs of the body, translates these impulses into sensations and integrates the sensations into perceptions of objects. In consequence, objects are perceived as oriented in space, visible, audible, painful, hot, cold, smooth, rough, or with particular odors or tastes. A sensation may be disturbed in several ways: it may be absent, present but decreased in intensity, increased in intensity, or distorted.

All disorders of sensation may result either from bodily diseases or emotional factors. Thus, in the neurosis called conversion reaction or conversion hysteria the patient may be completely unable to see, or have somewhat reduced vision, or complain that things are too bright and intense, or have distorted vision (as in double vision). A physical examination of the hysterical patient, however, reveals no causal organic process to account for these symptoms. To take another example, hysterics sometimes manifest glove anesthesia (an area of anesthesia on the hand and wrist that can be covered by a glove); since the anatomical distribution of nerve fibers does not conform to a glove pattern, the symptom has no neural basis. Disturbances in any other sense modality may also be manifested by conversion hysterics or by patients with various other syndromes. Schizophrenics, for example, often complain of peculiar and unpleasant bodily sensations, unpleasant odors and annoying sounds.

Turning from sensation to perception, a distinction should be made between two common perceptual symptoms, illusions and hallucinations. An *illusion* is a misinterpretation of external and real stimuli. A *hallucination* is a perception completely unwarranted by external stimuli. Illusions are mistaken perceptions; hallucinations are false perceptions without any basis in reality.

Both illusions and hallucinations may involve any of the senses: visual, auditory, olfactory, gustatory, tactile and others. Some visual illusions regarding the size and shape of objects are normal and universal, e.g., the familiar Müller-Lyer illusion (Fig. 3–1), but patients experience many illusions of various types and sometimes of considerable intensity that are

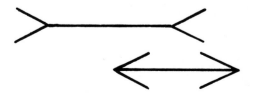

Figure 3–1. The Müller-Lyer illusion. The horizontal lines appear unequal because of the diagonal lines.

rare in normals. A delirious patient may misinterpret the shadows in the corner of his room as a crouching dog and a schizophrenic may misinterpret a friendly utterance as a threat.

Visual hallucinations occur in normal individuals in the form of dreams and occasionally in the hypnagogic state (the intermediate stage between waking and sleeping). Visual hallucinations in the waking state are common in brain disorders. Nonvisual hallucinations are rare in normals but common and vivid in many psychiatric syndromes. A schizophrenic may hear voices laughing at him, insulting him obscenely, warning him about the evil intentions of others or commanding him to perform various actions. For example, one patient heard a voice repeating "Kill Mary! Kill Mary!" (His daughter's name was Mary.) Such hallucinated commands are perfectly real to the person experiencing them. He may or may not attempt to carry out the command but he is certain that he hears it.

Another perceptual symptom, *clouding of consciousness,* consists of a state of confusion in which the individual's perceptions lack clarity. In clouding of consciousness, the individual apparently is not sufficiently attentive to his surroundings, either because he is so preoccupied by emotional turmoil that external reality cannot impress itself on him sharply, or because of brain damage.

Disordered Intelligence and Thought

The normal individual has, by definition, a normal intellectual level. Intellectual abnormality may take any of several major forms: low intellectual capacity, deterioration of intellectual ability later in life, intellectual functioning markedly below ability, or distorted memory and thinking, with or without intellectual deterioration.

Low intellectual capacity is usually defined as an intelligence quotient or I.Q. score of 70 or less, which is two or more standard deviations below the mean of the general population, and is variously termed *intellectual subnormality, mental deficiency, mental retardation* or *amentia.* It is marked by a limited capacity to comprehend or master new material, by memory deficits, and by difficulties in forming discriminations, making judgments and solving problems. At the lower ranges, below an I.Q. of 50, physical abnormalities frequently accompany the intellectual defect.

A deterioration in intellectual ability may

occur at any age but is more typical of older persons. Frequently the decline is attributable to one of a number of brain disorders. The intellectually impaired individual who formerly could solve algebraic problems may become unable to add simple numbers correctly. He finds it very difficult to compare two objects, for example, a fish and a bird, and decide how they are similar and how different. His memory for events of the same day, such as the breakfast menu or the past hour's activities, may be fuzzy and unreliable.

The brain is the basis of intelligent behavior and it is not surprising that intelligence should decline in brain disorders. Whether basic intellectual ability also declines in functional disorders such as schizophrenia is a matter of controversy, for the measurement of a schizophrenic's I.Q. is unreliable due to difficulty of motivating him to cooperate fully while being tested.

A marked disparity between an individual's intellectual ability and the effective use of that ability typically results from emotional difficulty. Almost no one makes full use of all his intellectual capabilities, but some individuals expend so much energy struggling with internal emotional problems that the energy available for other activities is greatly reduced and an unusually wide gap opens between potentiality and effectiveness. This pattern is often seen in unproductive neurotics who worry, ruminate or daydream excessively.

Distortions of memory take the form of a pathological loss of the ability to recall. Many individuals with emotional problems complain of a poor memory and yet appear to function reasonably well on various recall tests. In such cases it seems more precise to speak of a lack of confidence in the ability to remember rather than a real memory loss. In some organic brain syndromes or rare functional disorders, such as psychoneurotic dissociative reactions, there may be total lack of recall or amnesia. Typically the amnesia occurs after a precipitating event such as head injury or severe emotional shock. The individual may be unable to recall events preceding the precipitating shock (retrograde amnesia), or unable to recall events following the shock (anterograde amnesia), or both. Such lost memories are usually accompanied by *disorientation,* the inability to identify time, place or persons accurately, and by perplexity and confusion. There may also be a concomitant clouding of consciousness. Sometimes a patient manifests a complete distortion of memory called *confabulation* in which he fills amnesic gaps with imaginary experiences. If a confabulating hospital patient is asked to recount the events of his day he may state with complete conviction that he has been in a distant city and describe his adventures there in detail.

Amnesia accompanied by physical flight from the immediate environment is a *fugue.* The individual in a fugue state assumes a new identity and name; he may start life anew by adopting a new vocation and acquiring a new family.

Distortions of the *sequence, manner and content of thinking* are particularly important symptoms of many organic disorders and functional psychoses. These distortions diminish intellectual effectiveness even more than neurotic inefficiency does. A distorted belief that is completely out of tune with reality, e.g., an individual's delusion that he has an exalted Messianic mission or that he has invented a machine that can make people immortal, is obviously incompatible with effective day-by-day use of intellect.

The sequence of thought may be disturbed in several ways. *Flight of ideas* consists of a series of rapid jumps from one idea to another. The ideas may be connected only by an irrelevant memory or a similarity of word sounds (called a clang association) and they may be interrupted by a distracting environmental stimulus. Thus a patient may refer to a friend named Mr. Queen and then proceed, "The Queen of England's picture was in the newspaper this morning. I used to deliver newspapers. What's the news?—there's a scratch on my nose." Flight of ideas occurs most often in mania and schizophrenia. In mania it is usually possible to follow the sequence of associations but in some cases of schizophrenia the patient's thinking may be too fragmented to be comprehensible.

An opposite symptom is *retardation of ideas* in which the patient's thinking is slowed and laborious. This symptom is characteristic of depression. Somewhat similar to retardation is *blocking* in which there is a sudden stoppage of the sequence of thought. Blocking is usually felt to be unpleasant by the individual. Although it is fairly common in schizophrenia, its prototype occurs in normals, especially under emotional stress. In *impoverished ideation,* the patient produces only a few ideas which may recur over and over in a stereotyped fashion. Such poverty of ideas is common in mental deficiency, organic brain syndromes and

schizophrenia. Finally, *circumstantiality* is the term for a sequence of thoughts and spoken words in which trivial details are unnecessarily and explicitly elaborated. For example, a schizophrenic patient who was asked whether prior to hospitalization he had been living alone or had shared his apartment took over 40 minutes to answer the question. He detailed to an absurd degree the layout and furnishings of the apartment, the reasons why it might or might not have been desirable to have a roommate, the step-by-step changes from his initial preference for sharing the apartment to a later preference for solitude, and so forth.

Among the distortions of the *manner* of thinking, an important symptom is *concrete thinking,* the inability to generalize or to think abstractly. It may be found in intellectual subnormality or any variety of impaired intellectual functioning. *Autistic thinking* (also known as dereistic, magical or prelogical thinking) consists of highly subjective reasoning peculiar to the individual. It is insufficiently controlled by reality and is often guided by fantasy gratification of drives. Autistic thinking is particularly prominent in schizophrenia. The difference between concrete and autistic thinking may be illustrated by schizophrenic patients' interpretations of simple proverbs. One such patient responded to the request, "Tell me what 'a stitch in time saves nine' means" with the concrete interpretation, "If you had a tear in your clothing and sewed it up right away, you'd be saving time." Two other patients interpreted the proverb autistically: "If I would take one stitch ahead of time, I would know nine times better how to do another stitch," and, "I could do something and it would help everyone else."

Distortions of the *content* of thinking are extremely common in neuroses and are invariably found in one or another form in psychoses. An *obsession* is the persistent intrusion into consciousness of an unwanted and unpleasant thought or impulse. An irrational and obsessive fear, not warranted by an actual danger, is known as a *phobia.* Obsessions and phobias are the major symptoms of certain neuroses (obsessive-compulsive reaction and phobic reaction) but they also occur in many psychoses. A large number of words have been derived from Greek roots to designate different varieties of phobia (e.g., acrophobia for excessive fear of heights, agoraphobia for open spaces, claustrophobia for closed places, and even phobophobia for excessive and irrational fear of phobias). The names are much less commonly used than in former generations for they add nothing to the understanding of phobic phenomena.

The most dramatic and striking distortions of the content of thinking are *delusions*. A delusion may be defined as a false belief inconsistent with the individual's own knowledge and experience. It is maintained in the face of contrary objective evidence and logical argument and it is not shared by the individual's cultural group. Delusions are found in various types of psychosis and are typically accompanied by disordered perceptions (illusions or hallucinations), autistic thinking and disorders of affect, and often also by impaired memory. Hallucinations, in particular, are closely integrated with delusions: a hallucinated voice addressing insults to a psychotic individual corroborates his delusional belief that he is being persecuted; conversely, his conviction of persecution explains the insults.

One of the commonly known types of delusion is the delusion of grandeur. Under such a delusion the individual has an unrealistic and exaggerated belief in his own achievements or attributes. It is characteristically associated with an exaggerated feeling of physical and emotional well-being found in mania and also in various psychoses with paranoid features. A patient with an extreme form of grandiose delusion may believe that he is a famous historical or contemporary figure: Jesus, Washington, Napoleon, the Pope and so forth. Delusions of grandeur mirror cultural values: in 1962, a hospitalized young patient was convinced that he was Elvis Presley (the other Elvis Presley being an impostor) and that his girl friend was Elizabeth Taylor in disguise.

Most delusions are marked by an intense personal conviction. There are several other misinterpretations of reality that may or may not occur at so high a level of intensity. These include *depersonalization,* the feeling that one's identity has been lost and that others as well as oneself are dreamlike and have no reality; *misidentification of other persons*—family, doctors, nurses or complete strangers; and *déjà vu* (already seen), the uncanny feeling that something seen for the first time has actually been seen before. The phenomenon of *déjà vu* is occasionally experienced by all normal individuals, but it seems to be more frequent among disturbed persons, both neurotic and psychotic. Similarly, the belief that one has previously heard, thought, told or done something—which is actually occurring for the first time—is experienced more often by disturbed than by other individuals.

Disordered Affect

Sensations, perceptions and thoughts are always accompanied by emotional reactions, sometimes experienced as clear, conscious feelings, sometimes felt only vaguely and sometimes completely inaccessible to consciousness. The disturbed individual's reactions of joy and grief, pride and shame, love and hate, delight and horror frequently differ in one or another way from those of relatively normal persons. For example, he may experience guilt reactions that are too frequent and intense or too infrequent and weak. He may be incapable of loving or he may be overwhelmed by the emotion of hate. Emotional difficulties—conscious and unconscious—are at the core of many psychological disorders.

Consciously experienced emotional reactions are often referred to as affective experiences or, simply, affects. An affect lasting over a period of time is a mood or average feeling-tone. Affects may deviate from normality in four ways: they may be unduly increased or decreased in intensity, in conflict with each other, increased or decreased in variability or inappropriate to the external situation.

Moderate feelings of well-being, sadness, fear or anger are experienced at different times by the normal individual. An excessive increase in affect is characteristic of many psychological abnormalities and may take the form of euphoria, depression, irrational anxiety or pathological anger. An extreme decrease of affect is apathy.

In *euphoria* or *elation,* frequent in mania and paranoid disorders, exaggerated feelings of well-being take possession of the individual along with a pleasant feeling of liberation from the restraints of conscience. The euphoric individual is confident and energetic, and believes he is capable of achieving great things. He describes himself as sitting on top of the world. Despite its intensity, a disturbed individual's euphoria is quite shallow, for if he is frustrated his mood rapidly shifts to irritability.

All intense affects other than euphoria are unpleasant. In *depression* there is morbid sadness and dejection, an increased perception of physical pain and a guilt-ridden, remorseful oversensitivity to conscience. The depressed person's facial cast and voice are mournful and he may repeat morbid phrases such as "What have I done?" and "I don't deserve to live."

The affect found in *anxiety* consists of apprehension, tension and uneasiness. The anxious individual anticipates a danger or disaster that he may or may not be able to describe clearly: he may apprehend it only as something vague and nonspecific.

If a specific danger is feared, the anxious affect is accompanied by the phobic symptoms discussed in the previous section. When an individual cannot specify the object of his fears, his anxiety is referred to as free-floating. It has already been pointed out that anxiety is a very complex phenomenon. It is an affect, a drive or motivating state and also an excessive reaction to a danger anticipated consciously or unconsciously. Both normal and disturbed persons defend themselves against anxiety by a variety of mechanisms—repression, projection, rationalization and many others—which are discussed in the next chapter.

Anger is closely related to aggression, one of the basic components of human motivation. Pathologically intense anger may be expressed as a generalized disposition to be aggressive toward everyone and everything, or it may be focused on specific persons.

In *apathy,* on the other hand, the individual is neither euphoric, depressed, anxious nor angry, but manifests a decrease in affect and an emotional "flatness." Apathy is most commonly observed in patients with organic brain syndromes or schizophrenia.

Ambivalence refers to the simultaneous existence of conflicting feelings or emotional attitudes toward the same object, person or goal. A neurotic female patient, for example, was simultaneously attracted to and repelled by her husband. She loved, admired, pitied and felt hostile to him, all at the same time and, in consequence, she did not know how to behave toward him. Ambivalence hampers efficiency of thought and action; in its most severe form it may lead to inability to make decisions. Some degree of ambivalence is found in every functional disorder.

Affects may be excessively *labile,* that is, unstable and inordinately variable, or they may vary to a less than normal degree. Every individual has a characteristic pattern of variation about his average affective level or mood. The normal pattern and three deviating patterns are schematically illustrated for the dimension of euphoria vs. depression in Figure 3–2. As can be seen at the left of the figure, the normal individual is likely to vary moderately about a level that is neither markedly euphoric nor markedly depressed. The second diagram illustrates the rapidity with which a prevailing mood

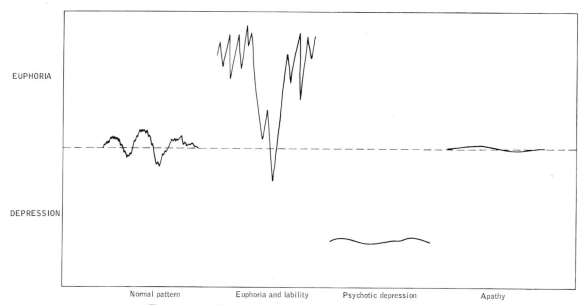

EUPHORIA

DEPRESSION

Normal pattern   Euphoria and lability   Psychotic depression   Apathy

Figure 3–2.   Four patterns of affective tone and variability.

of euphoria may suddenly change into depression, for euphoria is usually associated with excessive variability. The third diagram, in which there is an absence of variability around an intensely unpleasant average level, is characteristic of psychotic depression. Last, in apathy, as in normal affect, the average affective level is neither elevated nor depressed, but, as in psychotic depression, there is little lability. In addition to the absence of lability, apathy is qualitatively different from a normal balance between euphoria and depression. The figure illustrates only the quantitative relationships among affects along one dimension.

An *inappropriate* affect is qualitatively different in a gross sense from that experienced by the majority of people in a given situation—for example, joy where most people experience grief, or vice versa. Inappropriate affects are most characteristic of a schizophrenic and reflect a basic incongruity among his emotions, ideation and overt behavior. If a schizophrenic is told that a friend has died, he is aware that something sad has happened but his affective functioning and overt responses may be so poorly integrated with his cognitive awareness that he will laugh instead of expressing sorrow.

Disordered Motivation

A motive may be defined as a readiness or disposition to respond in some ways and not others to a variety of situations. The individual with a strong aggressive motive responds to threats by lashing out at them; the individual motivated by fear tries to escape. Motives, unlike stimuli and responses, are not observable but must be inferred from their effects on the individual's perceptions, thoughts, feelings and overt actions.

Motivation has a number of important properties that hold true for both normal and disturbed individuals. For example, they are either physiological or psychogenic (psychological) in origin. The physiological motives include hunger, thirst, excretory needs, need for oxygen, warmth, rest and sleep, avoidance of pain and sexual drives. Physiological needs serve to promote survival; the organism can live only a very limited period if its physiological needs are thwarted. The only exception to this generalization is the sexual drive, which guarantees the survival of the species rather than of the individual organism. The sexual drives also differ

from the other physiological drives in being almost infinitely plastic and modifiable by experience. Sexual gratification may be indefinitely delayed without harming the organism physically or it may be satisfied by a variety of activities and goal-objects. Human sexual motivation would not have such enormous psychological significance if it did not have so great a range of effects on human behavior.

Like sexuality, but unlike the other physiological motives, psychogenic motives are readily modifiable as a cumulative result of individual experiences, and may be strengthened, weakened, displaced, distorted or prevented from direct expression. How—and whether—the organism expresses curiosity, competitiveness, need for self-actualization, need for social status, independence, affiliation with others and many other psychogenic motives depends on his life experiences. To take one example, the direction and strength of the need for achievement depend on the rewards and punishments the individual has received for past achievements and failures.

One special subgroup of psychogenic motives seems to be as ingrained in the human organism as the basic physiological drives. All human beings need a modicum of affection, a feeling of personal adequacy and self-esteem, a sense of emotional security and a freedom from strong feelings of shame, guilt and anxiety. If these needs are frustrated, behavioral difficulties result.

A need is experienced by the organism as a state of tension. The need energizes the individual to strive toward some goal-object; reaching the goal gratifies the need and reduces the state of tension. The hungry animal hunts, eats and then sleeps. The lonely human being feels restless until he finds people with whom to talk.

Motivated behavior does not, however, consist solely in reducing unpleasant tensions, for behavior is also influenced by the positive attractiveness of goals. The organism seeks intrinsically satisfying experiences as well as tension reduction. Food reduces hunger pangs but it also produces pleasurable taste sensations. A distinction should thus be made between negative and positive motivation. Positive motives are expressed in such behaviors as the pursuit of pleasurable or novel sensations, the establishment of warm relationships with others and the attempt to understand the environment or respond to it esthetically. Negative motives include hunger and other physiological deficiency states, avoidance of physical suffering, fear of physical situations or others' disapproval, fear of one's own drives and avoidance of inferiority feelings. Positive motives are usually coupled with a favorable attitude toward oneself and others. Negative motives are marked by a need to escape or avoid punishment and by an unfavorable evaluation of oneself and others. A motive does not cease to exist when it is unconscious: on the contrary, when it is not under the organism's conscious control it can affect behavior compellingly. The unconsciously aggressive individual may feel compelled to behave in a hostile fashion while denying that he is aggressive.

The physiological needs, the universal psychogenic motives (e.g., need for affection and self-esteem) and the nonuniversal psychogenic motives (e.g., need to achieve, compete etc.) may be thought of as constituting three successive levels of a hierarchy. Physiological needs insist on being satisfied first; the energy used in efforts to satisfy them limits the energy available at the higher levels. At the second level, self-esteem, affection, avoidance of internal distress and emotional security must be at least minimally gratified before the organism can expend much energy at the third level to satisfy his unique, self-actualizing motives. Of course, human motives, like other organismic processes, are closely and complexly integrated so that higher level motives may lead to behavior that helps gratify lower level motives also. Achievement and altruistic behavior, for example, usually bolster self-esteem, and adequate self-esteem aids in successful striving for physiological gratification.

Motivational Disturbances. In theory, a distinction may be made between a disturbance of motives and a disturbance of the behaviors that spring from motives. This distinction cannot be pushed too hard, however, for it is sometimes impossible to specify whether the difficulty is in the motivational state, the consequent behaviors or, as is most likely, both. Furthermore, behavior may become *functionally autonomous* (Allport, 1961): it becomes independent of the drive from which it originated and then functions as a potent motivator in itself. An individual who acquires a skill may in time find that he is motivated to use it for its own sake instead of for the rewards that originally motivated its acquisition. The distinction between disturbances of motives and disturbances of motivated behaviors is therefore purely a matter of convenience.

Motives may be too negative, too strong or weak, too immature, too variable or in conflict with each other.

Excessively negative motives. A preponderance of negative motivation marks neurotics and many psychotics. Neurotic individuals suffering from anxiety reaction, phobic reaction or obsessive-compulsive reaction are primarily motivated by anxiety, fear and guilt; positive motivation plays a lesser role in them than in normals. Schizophrenics have a basic and deep mistrust of other people and depressives are often afraid of others' intentions, even when they believe that other persons would be justified in punishing them.

Excessively strong or weak motives. A motive may be strong to the point of insatiability or weak to the point of atrophy. Endocrine imbalances or emotional disturbances may lead to abnormal motivational states such as *bulimia,* a condition of insatiable hunger, or *anorexia,* a loss of appetite that in some cases is fatal. Drug addiction — an emotional and physiological dependence on alcohol, morphine, sedatives or other drugs — is a special case of an intense drive. Strong aggression is characteristic of antisocial sociopaths and of paranoids who develop delusions of persecution as a projection of their own hostility.

In hysterics and individuals with various personality disorders, the motive of emotional independence is relatively weak and dependency needs are strong. The hysteric with a functional paralysis or visual difficulty must be cared for; his symptom guarantees that his dependency needs will be gratified.

The moral standards of the superego constitute a motivational force. A person's moral standards can constitute a strong motivational force, particularly if these standards have been carried over from childhood with little modification (superego). The typical neurotic has primitive or childlike moral standards which prohibit almost all expression of impulses. A crucial characteristic of the sociopath, on the other hand, is the extreme weakness of his superego or moral restraints, evidenced in a lack of control of impulses and an inability to delay gratifying them.

Motivational immaturity. In the normal individual, motives develop and mature with increasing chronological age due to physiological factors and social pressures. In motivational immaturity the individual manifests a discrepancy between the norm for his age and the level of development of an important motive. The adult who resembles a pre-adolescent in displaying a lack of interest in the opposite sex, in seeking security through strong identification with heroes or in fearing to be "different" from others is motivationally immature. In Freudian theory, emotional disorder is basically an immaturity of sexual motives resulting from psychological trauma.

Narcissism, or excessive love of self, is an indicator of motivational immaturity. The normal individual moves from childhood love of self to adult concern and love for others, from narcissism to some degree of altruism. The disturbed and immature individual usually remains overconcerned with himself.

Excessively variable and changeable motives. Motives may be too variable and changeable. A sociopath is often characterized by impulsive variability in his sexual, aggressive and other motives. His sexual behavior may run the gamut of promiscuity, sexual assault and homosexuality. Manics and other individuals whose affect is labile are also motivationally variable.

Conflict. The most important of all motivational disturbances is conflict. Several types are common.

In the type termed approach-approach conflict, two positive motives clash. For example, the individual may be forced to choose between gratification of sexuality and personal achievement or between intellectual and social motives. Such choices are usually made consciously and rarely play a central role in serious disturbances. Approach-approach conflicts tend to be resolved by first satisfying one motive and then the other.

More important is an avoidance-avoidance conflict between two negative motives. The individual caught in a double-negative conflict has a choice, or believes he has a choice, between the frying pan and the fire. To go to the dentist may mean pain and to stay away means continued discomfort. To seek psychotherapy may threaten the psychic pain of disclosing unlovely aspects of oneself, but not to seek it means a continuation of emotional distress. Obsessive-compulsive neurotics are often caught in a conflict between the shame aroused in them by their obsessions and compulsions and the anxiety they feel when they try to inhibit the obsessive thoughts or compulsive acts. Not surprisingly, the individual caught in an avoidance-avoidance conflict tends to vacillate between the two paths open to him.

Even more important for abnormal psychology

are approach-avoidance conflicts between negative and positive motives. Approach-avoidance conflicts are found in every emotional disorder and are accompanied by the ambivalent affects discussed earlier. The child whose need for affection conflicts with an unconscious hostility toward his parents is in a psychological trap.

Behavior Disturbances. Viewed with reference to motivation, behavior may be disturbed in either of two fundamental ways: it may fail to gratify basic needs or, alternatively, it may gratify them in ways inappropriate to the individual's cultural group or to society in general.

Environmental or personal difficulties may prevent satisfaction of sexuality or psychogenic needs. An impoverished environment, physiological difficulties, physical defects, low I.Q., lack of skills or social techniques, or paralyzing internal problems often interfere with need-satisfying behaviors.

The most extreme form of lack of gratification is found in *abulia,* an absence of energy so profound that the individual cannot carry out voluntary actions or make decisions. It is rarely found in disorders other than schizophrenia.

Society permits some forms of gratification of every motive and interdicts other gratifications. Murray (1938) refers to the allowed expressions of needs as the *tpmo* (time-place-mode-object):

A child is allowed to play during the day but not the night (time). He may defecate in the toilet but not on the floor (place). He may push other children but not hit them with a mallet (mode). He may ask his father but not a stranger in the street for money (object). No need has to be inhibited permanently. If the individual is of the right age and chooses the permitted time, the permitted place, the permitted mode and the permitted object, he can objectify [gratify in action] any one of his needs.

Murray's statement does not contradict the fact that needs may be chronically inhibited and unsatisfied if external or internal factors prevent a serviceable choice of time, place, mode and object.

Disordered Verbal and Motor Behavior

Verbal behavior—a form of motor behavior—includes speech and writing. In disturbed individuals both the content and manner of verbal behavior may be disordered in many different ways. *Stuttering* and *stammering* are more common in neurotics than in relatively normal individuals. *Mutism,* the complete inability or refusal to speak, is found in depressive and schizophrenic psychoses. An opposite symptom is *logorrhea* or excessive speech, often incoherent, which accompanies the symptoms of euphoria, flight of ideas and motor overactivity.

Verbal peculiarities are especially common in schizophrenia. These include *neologisms,* the coining of new words (such as "radimony," a word coined by a patient as a fusion of "radio" and "money"); *verbigeration,* the monotonous repetition of words or sentences, often without apparent meaning; *echolalia,* the echo-like repetition by the patient of what has been said to him; and *word salad,* an unintelligible mixture of real words and meaningful phrases with neologisms.

One of the most common nonverbal motor disturbances is a *compulsion,* an overwhelming urge to perform an act or ritual, such as continually washing one's hands, while knowing that the act is irrational. Compulsions are to obsessions as acts are to thoughts, and both compulsions and obsessions are by definition found in the neurosis called obsessive-compulsive reaction.

In hysterical neurosis the motor disturbances known as tics and choreas are often found. A *tic* is a periodic muscular twitch, especially facial. *Chorea* is an irregular, involuntary, spasmodic movement; it may be hysteric or organic in origin. *Tremors,* continuous involuntary, spasmodic contractions, or trembling, in a small group of muscles, are found in neurotic anxiety and hysteric reactions and also in organic difficulties.

The majority of motor disturbances are found not in the neuroses but in the organic disorders and functional psychoses. *Retardation* of movement sometimes reaches the point of *stupor,* a state of lethargy and immobility in which it is very difficult to arouse the patient. Motor *restlessness,* agitation or excitement, invariably accompanied by severe insomnia, is the opposite of retardation. Either of these symptoms may occur in organic brain disorders, affective disorders or the type of schizophrenia known as catatonia. *Catalepsy* is an increase in muscle tone with fixity of posture and occurs in schizophrenic (or severe hysterical) states. In catatonic schizophrenia a type of catalepsy called *waxy flexibility* occurs in which the patient permits his limbs to be molded into any position and then holds the position for long periods despite discomfort. He does not dare to initiate behavior nor resist another person.

Automatism is mechanical, repetitious motor behavior, carried out unconsciously, that may occur in schizophrenia and sometimes in amnesic states. The patient may repeatedly clench his fist or move his hand stiffly to his mouth and touch his lips without being aware of what he is doing. Also frequently associated with schizophrenia, especially the catatonic type, are *stereotyped mannerisms* in which the patient consciously grimaces, gestures or moves his entire body stiffly and repetitively; *negativism* in which the patient refuses to cooperate with a request or behaves in a manner opposite to that requested (for example, he may stand up only if told to remain seated); *echopraxia,* a compulsion to imitate the movements of another person; and *posturing* in which the patient assumes an unusual posture and maintains it over a period of time.

In general, verbal and motor symptoms are more dramatic and striking than other types of symptoms. The popular conception of "crazy" consists of peculiar speech, violent movements, extraordinary facial expressions and bizarre gestures. For some patients this picture is accurate, but for most the deviations from normality are more subtle.

THE SYNDROMES OF ABNORMAL BEHAVIOR

The various symptoms of abnormal behavior just described often occur in clusters called syndromes. Various classifications of these syndromes have been attempted since the humoral theory of the ancient Greeks. The two most widely used modern systems of classification today are those adopted by the World Health Organization (1967) and the American Psychiatric Association (1968) which largely parallel each other.

As we shall see later, there are many difficulties with the current system of classification and diagnosis of abnormal behavior. For the present we can simply point out that both of the current systems are firmly based on a disease model of abnormality. In this definition abnormality is an illness like any other while normality is the absence of illness. As was discussed in Chapter 1, this is only one of many methods of conceptualizing abnormality. Up to now, however, no widely accepted comprehensive system of classification has been proposed by proponents of other conceptual schemes. In many respects diagnosis, which gives differing individuals the same labels, is anathema to conceptual schemes which emphasize the uniqueness of each person. However, this view has not yet achieved the widespread acceptance of the disease model.

The official diagnostic manual of the American Psychiatric Association lists ten major groups of disorders and numerous subgroups. A brief outline of the major groupings is presented below:

I. *Mental Retardation.* Subnormal general intellectual functioning, originating during the developmental period, and associated with impairment of either learning and social adjustment or maturation, or both.

II. *Organic Brain Syndrome.* Disorders caused by or associated with either permanent or temporary impairment of brain tissue function. Impairment of all intellectual functions, memory, orientation and judgment, together with lability and shallowness of affect.

III. *Psychoses Not Attributed to Physical Conditions Listed Previously (The Functional Psychoses).* Mental functioning is sufficiently impaired to interfere grossly with the individual's capacity to meet the ordinary demands of life. The impairment may involve marked distortion of socially accepted interpretations of reality. Frequently accompanied by severe distortions of perceptive, intellectual functioning, affect, motivation, and behavior.

IV. *Neuroses.* The chief characteristic is anxiety, which may be consciously experienced or unconsciously controlled by means of various psychological self-protective or defense mechanisms. There is no gross distortion of reality nor disorganization of personality.

V. *Personality Disorders and Certain Other Non-Psychotic Mental Disorders.* Characterized by deeply impaired maladaptive patterns of behavior that are perceptibly different in quality from psychotic and neurotic symptoms.

VI. *Psychophysiological Disorders.* Group of disorders characterized by physical symptoms that are caused by emotional factors and involve a single organ system. Physiological changes are those that normally accompany certain emotional states, but the changes are more intense and sustained.

VII. *Symptoms.* A category for the occasional patient whose psychopathology is manifested by a single specific symptom such as speech disturbance, learning disturbance, enuresis and the like.

VIII. *Transient Situational Disturbance.* More or less transient disorders of any severity, occurring in persons without any apparent underlying mental disorders, and representing an acute reaction to overwhelming environmental stress.

IX. *Behavior Disorders of Childhood and Adolescence.* Disorders occurring in childhood or adolescence that are more stable and resistant to treatment than transient situational disturbances, but less so than psychoses, neuroses and personality disorders.

X. *Conditions Without Manifest Psychiatric Disorder and Nonspecific Conditions.* Includes social maladjustment without manifest psychiatric disorder, such as marital or occupational maladjustment, as well as nonspecific conditions with no mental disorder or maladjustment.

Many of the syndromes are discussed in detail later in the book.

SOME PROBLEMS IN CLASSIFICATION

When the major psychiatric syndromes were first defined, each syndrome was regarded as a separate disease, mutually exclusive of other diseases and—in the case of chronic syndromes—unchanging during the patient's lifetime. It was believed that each syndrome had a unique cause that prevented the development of any other syndrome; for example, each of the disorders that we now consider to be caused by psychological factors was presumed to be due to a specific constitutional or hereditary vulnerability. Neurotic and psychotic symptoms could not be present simultaneously; neurosis could not change into psychosis (nor one neurotic reaction into another); borderline cases between two disorders and combinations of two disorders were believed to be impossible.

However, it was soon recognized that patients simultaneously or successively may manifest symptoms of more than one diagnostic category. An individual may be born mentally defective, in time develop sociopathic symptoms and simultaneously or later also display signs of schizophrenia. Diagnosis is a summary of the *predominant symptom pattern at a given time.* It is not a label excluding all other syndromes.

The main purposes of a classification or diagnostic schema are: to determine the etiology or causes of specific syndromes, to determine the

Not long ↑

course and probable outcome (prognosis) of differing abnormalities, and to select those treatments or interventions which have the highest probability of achieving favorable results. Perhaps the most practical and immediate reason for diagnosis is the selection of the appropriate treatment. In recent years the modes of treatment have expanded greatly in number, particularly with the advent of ataractic drugs and an increased variety of psychotherapeutic methods. It is becoming increasingly necessary to identify and select the most appropriate treatment for each syndrome.

In fact, the matching of treatment with diagnosis is often difficult partly because experts cannot always agree on the proper diagnosis. Two diagnosticians evaluating the same patient may assign him to differing diagnostic categories. The reasons for such disagreements are numerous but may be grouped under three broad general headings: (1) patient variables, such as occur when the patient manifests different behaviors at different times; (2) diagnostician variables, such as two diagnosticians attending to different aspects of the patient's behavior or weighting the same behavior differently, and (3) inadequacies in the present diagnostic schema.

It is important to know how much agreement or reliability there is in assignment to diagnostic groups. Several methods have been used to investigate the reliability of diagnosis. One method is to examine the percentage of agreements between two or more diagnosticians assessing the same patients. Table 3–1 presents summary data of six studies which have used variants of the agreement method.

As can be seen from the data presented, the percentage agreement between observers is rather high for the organic psychoses (85 to 92 per cent) but is low (52 per cent agreement) for the psychoneuroses. In general, the more severe the diagnosis (organic or psychotic), the greater the agreement. Patients suffering from severe disorders often display more obvious symptoms which are easily apparent to the observer, while the symptoms of the neurotic are often more subtle. In addition, for certain organic syndromes there are specific laboratory tests, which further reduce the possibility of human error in diagnosis.

The data in Table 3–1 point out another interesting fact. The overall average agreement for the broad general categories (i.e., organic disease, functional psychosis) is much higher than the average agreement for specific syndromes within the general category. Thus, diagnosticians find it easier to agree that someone is psychotic than it is to agree that a particular subtype of psychosis is present.

Table 3–2 presents data from studies using another method of investigating the reliability of diagnosis: the stability or concordance of diagnosis over time. As can be seen, the broad diagnostic categories display a low order of consistency over time. However, it is important

TABLE 3–1.   Summary of Studies on the Percentage Agreement on Diagnosis by Observers*

	Ash (1949)	Seeman (1953)	Schmidt (1956)	Krietman (1961)	Beck (1962)	Sandifer (1964)
Description:						
Number of patients	52	6	426	90	153	91
Sex	M	(Not recorded)	M/F	M/F	M/F	M/F
Method of selecting patients	Selected patients	Selected patients	Successive admissions	Successive admissions	Random selection	Selected patients
Interval between diagnostic interviews	Same day	Same day	2 weeks	1 week	Same day	Same day
General Diagnostic Categories:						
Organic psychoses			92	85		
Functional psychoses			80	71		71
Characterological disorders			71			74
Psychoneuroses				52		
Average Agreement on General Categories	64		84	78	70	
Average Agreement on Specific Categories	38	66	55	63	54	57

*Adapted from Zubin, J. (1967). In Annual Review of Psychology, Volume 18, page 382.

TABLE 3–2. Summary of Studies on Consistency of General Diagnosis over Time

	Hunt (1953)	Norris (1959)	Kaelbling (1963)
Description:			
Number of patients	794	6263	218
Sex	M	M/F	M/F
Sampling method	Successive admissions	Successive admissions	Successive admissions
Interval between contacts	—	2 to 4 weeks	1 day to 26 weeks
Time of diagnosis	At admission	At admission	At discharge
General Diagnostic Categories:			
Organic psychoses		53	65
Functional psychoses	59		43
Psychoneuroses	24	46	49
Personality and character disorders	74	46	58

*Adapted from Zubin, J. (1967). Annual review of Psychology, Volume 18, page 385.

to remember that changes in diagnosis over a period of time may reflect changes in the patient's symptoms rather than inconsistency in diagnostic evaluation. Patients often change dramatically after only a few days in the hospital or soon after the initiation of drug treatment. This argument finds support in the fact that the diagnoses which should be less subject to change show little variability over time. For example patients diagnosed as having a chronic brain syndrome (a disorder due to permanent brain tissue damage) usually receive a similar diagnosis on subsequent evaluations (92 per cent agreement in a study by Babigian, 1965). Over short time periods disagreements in diagnosis tend to be lessened. For example, Schmidt and Fonda (1956) found that when only two weeks elapsed between diagnoses, agreement reached the satisfactory figure of 80 per cent between two independent diagnoses of hospitalized patients as suffering from organic, psychotic or character disorders. Agreement for specific syndromes was also investigated; it was 91 per cent for schizophrenia but only 51 per cent for specific subtypes of schizophrenia. As in other studies, the more narrow the category, the less reliable the diagnosis.

Another method for studying diagnostic reliability is to examine the frequency in occurrence of various diagnostic categories in two samples of patients drawn from the same general population. If the distribution of diagnostic categories in the two samples is similar, it may be concluded that the diagnostic schema being used is reliable. In a study whose findings are typical for investigations using this approach, Pasamanick (1959) examined the diagnoses assigned to female patients admitted on three comparable psychiatric hospital wards. The patients assigned to each ward were comparable in age, place of residence, education, type of admission, and marital status. An examination of the distribution of individual diagnostic categories on each ward revealed marked differences in the occurrence of schizophrenia and psychoneuroses. Such differences should not have occurred by chance since all patients were assigned randomly to the wards. Further, it was found that on one ward where there had been three different administrators, a marked discrepancy existed between the distribution of diagnoses made by one administrator and those of the other two.

The somewhat limited reliability of diagnoses of functional disorders over short time periods and their almost complete instability over long time periods have led some psychiatrists and psychologists to believe that it is really pointless to try to distinguish among different functional syndromes. It has even been suggested that all functional disorders represent a single abnormality whose external manifestations vary quantitatively in severity but not qualitatively. As far back as 1859 the German psychiatrist Heinrich Neumann wrote:

. . . We consider any classification of mental illness to be artificial, and therefore unsatisfactory [and] we do not believe that one can make progress in psychiatry until one has resolved to throw overboard all classifications and to declare with us: there is only one kind of mental illness. . . .

The major objection to this point of view is that research on causation, effectiveness of treatment and many other aspects of abnormal psychology and psychiatry can be carried out scientifically only on the basis of diagnosis. One cannot investigate any aspect of mental disorder unless the nature of the sample to be studied is first specified. Research on a sample of miscellaneous patients of unspecified diagnosis is likely to be meaningless because different kinds of patients behave differently. Furthermore, with all its imperfections, diagnosis is necessary as an everyday guide to treatment and other practical matters. A depressed patient, for example, responds much better than a schizophrenic to electroconvulsive therapy; in order to prescribe the proper treatment for depressives, it is first necessary to diagnose them as such, even if some cases are misdiagnosed. Diagnosis is not completely unreliable, and a number of studies now in progress have as their aim the improvement of diagnostic reliability and accuracy.

In spite of the low reliability of classification, studies on the subsequent history of people receiving various diagnoses have shown that the diagnostic schema does have some predictive validity. In other words, for all its shortcomings the present diagnostic schema has proven useful in making general prognostic statements. In a classic study of patients in London mental hospitals, Norris (1959) found that diagnoses were highly related to outcome as measured by length of stay in the hospital. Manic-depressives and neurotics remained in the hospital for relatively short periods of time while schizophrenics tended to be hospitalized much longer. Approximately one-third of all schizophrenic patients remained in the hospital longer than five years. Psychoneurotics, on the other hand, were rarely kept in the hospital as long as two years. (only 5 per cent). These figures are comparable with data collected in the United States and other countries. The average duration of the psychoneuroses is two years, whereas schizophrenia tends to be a long-term disorder which requires continuous hospitalization for a significant proportion of its victims.

Table 3–3 presents the results of 364 studies summarized by Zubin et al. (1961) which related diagnosis to favorable or unfavorable outcomes for various subcategories of schizophrenia. As can be seen, the diagnoses of catatonia and undifferentiated schizophrenia are associated with favorable outcomes in the large majority of studies. Hebephrenia and catatonia in later life, on the other hand, have been typically found to have unfavorable outcomes.

Clearly, if diagnosis were completely unreliable or meaningless, such relationships between classification and prognosis could not occur. The present system has many shortcomings. Improvements will have to be made in order to reach acceptable standards of scientific exactitude. But for the present, we do have a system which is modestly reliable and which does have some predictive ability.

Apart from the issues of diagnostic agreement and stability, opponents of diagnosis often stress the importance of a psychodynamic rather than a diagnostic approach to the patient. They urge that instead of attaching a label to a patient, efforts should be made to understand him as a unique individual with a unique past and a unique pattern of conflicts, anxieties and goals. Considering the patient *as a person* is claimed to be irreconcilable with considering him as a member of a class, not so much because classification has limited reliability as because it is purportedly inimical to dynamic understanding. A dynamically oriented psychiatrist, J. C. Nemiah, has stated this position well

TABLE 3–3.   Summary of 364 Studies on Outcome in Schizophrenic Diagnoses*

	Number of Studies Reporting Favorable Outcome	Number of Studies Reporting Unfavorable Outcome
Types of Schizophrenia:		
Catatonia	119	2
Reactive	2	0
Schizo-Affective	3	0
Schizo-Depressive	1	0
Mixed	5	1
Undifferentiated	15	0
Simple	1	33
Paranoid	55	39
Catatonia in later life	0	15
Hebephrenia	13	57
Process	0	3

*Compiled from Zubin et al. (1961).

(*Foundations of Psychopathology,* 1961). Referring to a patient correctly classified as a paranoid schizophrenic, he asserts:

Unfortunately this sort of categorization tends to fog a more complete understanding of the mental disorder at hand. Once sorted and labeled, the patient is swallowed up in an ocean of schizophrenia. As one of thousands of roughly similar cases, her own peculiar manifestations of the illnesses are lost from sight.

There is no logical contradication between the dynamic and diagnostic points of view, however. A patient shares some characteristics with all human beings, some characteristics with members of his diagnostic class only and still others—his unique characteristics—with no other patient. Diagnosis is a useful way to summarize the characteristics he shares with the members of a class *at a given time.* In psychiatry and psychology both the diagnostic and dynamic approaches are needed.

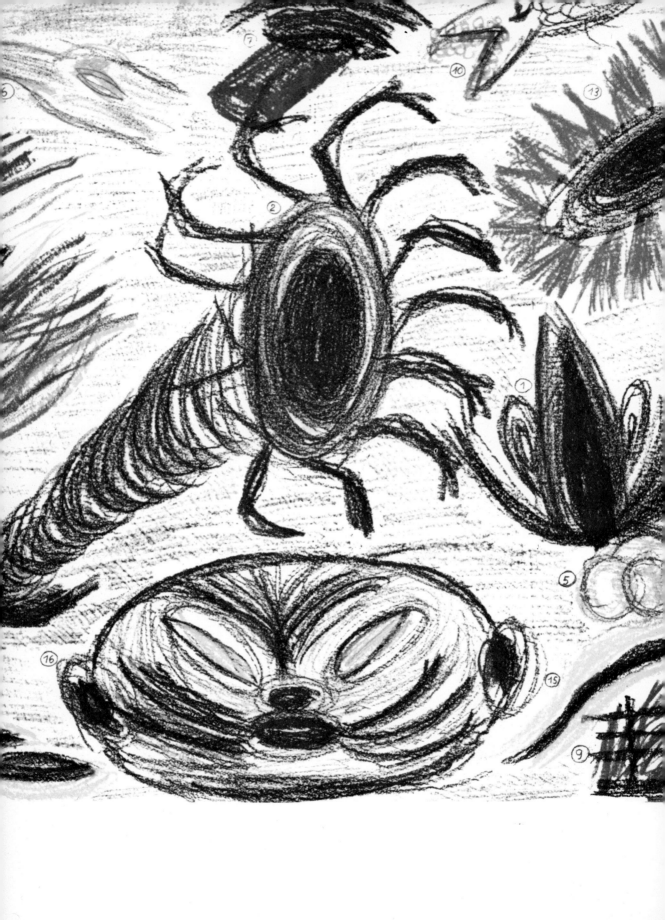

Man, one of those amphibious creatures who are plunged simultaneously
in the past and in the reality of the moment . . .
Marcel Proust, *Remembrance of Things Past*

DEVELOPMENT OF THE
NORMAL PERSONALITY

As we have seen, emotional problems in some form or another have always been with us, and so have explanations as to their causes. At the turn of the century the most popular theory was that emotional problems were the direct result of organic disturbances. But through his study of neurotic patients, Freud became convinced that the current problems being manifested were more or less the direct outgrowth of traumatic childhood disturbances which had caused a departure from normal, emotional maturation. He formulated a now famous dictum to the effect that there can be no adult neurosis without an infantile neurosis. In other words, mental disturbances were seen as the logical outcome of the individual's instinctual development and thus potentially understandable and preventable. No longer was mental illness viewed exclusively as some mysterious disease process, visited on the person without explanation. This conclusion led Freud to the development of a basic theory of personality development which has been continuously elaborated and modified over the past seventy years.

THE PSYCHOANALYTIC THEORY
OF DEVELOPMENT

This *dynamic* approach places special emphases on the continuity of personality de-

velopment, beginning with early infancy, and on emotional reactions to the multitude of forces and challenges which all growing persons must encounter. Freud's original formulations are still highly useful but have been modified considerably by subsequent theoreticians such as Sullivan, Adler, Jung, Horney, Erikson and others.

Freud (1949) himself was impressed by the instinctual aspect of man's development and particularly with his sexual drives. His theory of personality development consequently was organized around vicissitudes in the development of the sexual instinct. While this view has proved too restrictive to many scientists, Freud did call attention to the fact that psychological development begins at birth, passes through predictable stages, and is molded for good or ill by the emotional climate surrounding significant developmental milestones. The child's success in coping with the various developmental milestones largely dictates how adequate he will be in meeting life stresses as an adult.

The sexual instinct, as Freud (1938) saw it, was not something that suddenly appeared with physical maturity. Rather, vague, poorly differentiated sexual instincts were present in infancy and gradually developed into the mature sexuality of the adult. In fact, attitude and emotions acquired during childhood toward the child's own sexual instincts largely determined

51

not only his view toward adult sexuality but also his tendency either to trust or fear his inner instinctual life. Such attitudes were the cornerstone on which were erected neurotic conflicts, self-doubts and maladaptive compensatory behaviors.

The psychoanalytic theory of personality development which Freud postulated was based almost exclusively on the sexual instinct which was invested in various pleasurable zones as the individual grew. Initially, gratification and pleasure is focused in the mouth, later in the anus and finally in the genitals. Interpersonal and social influences were acknowledged but received little emphasis. Later writers (such as Erikson) have tended to retain Freud's psychosexual developmental stages as focal points in total development while adding the previously missing emphasis on psychosocial factors (see Maier, 1965). As one prominent psychologist, Freida Fromm-Reichmann (1949), put it:

. . . modern developmental psychoanalytic theory is characterized by the maintenance of the paramount significance of the total developmental history and by the negation of its classical psychosexual interpretation.

Let us look at the sequence of infantile development as Freud saw it, without ignoring the totality of the child's interpersonal and cultural milieu which later writers have emphasized.

The Oral Stage $O - 1\frac{1}{2}$

At birth, the infant is totally dependent upon his environment for nurturance and support. Without a mothering person, the infant's survival time would be only a matter of hours. Visual and auditory discrimination are almost absent, motor control is quite limited, and voluntary communication is undifferentiated. Primarily the infant relates to his environment with his mouth. Freud saw the obvious pleasurable reactions of the infant to the use of his mouth as the first source of bodily pleasure and thus the primitive forerunner of adult sexuality. To use his terminology, libido or sexual energy is invested in the oral zone. The mouth and its related activity, such as sucking, quickly come to be associated with pleasure, the diminution of hunger pangs, comfort and a sense of well-being.

Freud saw the oral period, or infancy, as an extremely important one in the subsequent

development of the individual. Fundamental attitudes toward the environment and the self are established which prove all but unshakable later in life. Probably this is due to the fact that these attitudes and ideas are acquired before the development of language and thus are preverbal apprehensions outside the pale of our typical modes of thinking.

As Erikson (1950) and others have pointed out, the attitudes acquired during infancy come about through the influence of the total emotional climate. The infant relates to his world through an incorporative mode. He is largely a passive recipient taking in what the world has to offer through his mouth, through sounds, and through tactile sensation. Feeding is associated not only with a nipple and hunger satisfaction but also with the soothing noises of the mother, with closeness, touch, body contact, warmth, the mother's smell and a general sense of well-being. Likewise, if the infant is cold or wet his cries often bring warmth, closeness, and comfort. While some discomfort and frustration is inevitable, the infant's view of the world is largely shaped by his experience in having his needs met at this early period. If discomfort usually leads to reassurance, comforting, and pleasurable sensations, he comes to see the world as a safe and supportive place. Contrariwise, if tension frequently leads to further frustration or displeasure, the environment acquires threatening rather than reassuring qualities. A sense of basic trust or basic mistrust is established. If the mother is chronically tense, insecure, or erratic in relation to the child, she fails to provide the warm and protective atmosphere which is essential to the acquisition of basic trust. Basic trust in others and self-esteem are closely associated. An infant who experiences his mother's attitudes and feelings as good, accepting, and gratifying is likely to come to see himself as worthwhile and worthy of love.

It is important to remember that it is the total mothering environment over time which is crucial to the acquisition of basic attitudes about the goodness of the world and the self. Frustration is inevitable. Often the baby's cries fail to bring the immediate desired effect and the mother grows progressively less available on demand. The infant is forced to tolerate more and more delays and frustrations. What is crucial is the total emotional atmosphere, the constancy of the mother's positive reaction and feedback to the child. What he is acquiring through her at this point can be stated quite

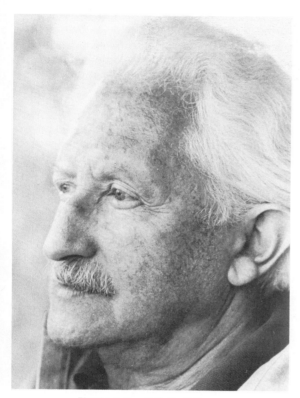

Figure 4–1. *Erik H. Erikson.*

seen as the all-powerful providers of whatever the child wishes. They emerge as separate entities who begin to make demands of their own in exchange for satisfying the child's needs. In Western cultures much of this socialization process revolves around the child's learning to voluntarily control his sphincter muscles. The primary site of body pleasure shifts from the mouth to the genital region but is centered in the eliminative organs rather than the genitalia. The child experiences pleasure in the alternative withholding and relaxing of the sphincters. Pleasurable sensation, relief, and praise follow relaxation; increasing tension, expectancy, and disapproval precede it.

EXPEL
RETENT

Depending upon the child's relationship with his parents as established during the oral period, he is either relatively eager to win approval by complying with their wishes or he obstinately begins to resist such outside controls. This is the child's first encounter with the demands of society. He can resist and frustrate his parents or submit to their demands in exchange for their approval and esteem. For the first time he is expected to give up some of his own self-centeredness and acknowledge the demands of reality. If he has had adequate mothering during his early days the child can learn to relinquish some of his own inclinations and accept the demands which can be placed on him. But if he's had very little experience with real need gratification he is quite likely to be resistive and stubborn. Some lifelong character traits such as negativism, stubbornness, rigidity, and frugality were believed by Freud to originate with attitudes established during the anal period.

NB

The retentive-eliminative mode or holding on and letting go characterize many of this period's psychosocial contacts. The child is engaging his environment in ever widening circles and ever increasing distance, both psychologically and physically, from his mother. He retains and releases perceptions, objects and interpersonal relationships. In so doing he is developing his own sense of autonomy and control. He demands increasing freedom to form his own opinions, to manipulate objects for himself, and to dress himself. But since he is still quite young and poorly developed, his increasing autonomy is also a threat to the comfortable dependency and love of the oral period. He tends to doubt his own abilities at the same time that he insists on trying them out. Each move toward independence also means looser ties to

simply as a fundamental sense of the world as either a friendly or a hostile place.

As the child grows he continues to relate to the world primarily through his mouth. New objects are explored by tasting them, putting them in the mouth, and later by biting as the infant becomes more active and less passive. After about the first year of life the infant begins to change from a passive recipient of care and affection into an active and increasingly autonomous being. Speech begins to acquire importance, other persons come to be seen as separate objects, and there is increasing control of the skeletal musculature including the anal and urinal sphincters. This is the second phase in Freud's theory of development.

The Anal Period $1\frac{1}{2} - 4$

During the period from roughly eighteen months to four years the child is being increasingly socialized and subjected to external demands and authority. Parents are no longer mother. There is some shame over revolting against the previously much enjoyed dependency. It is the struggle for autonomy in the face of doubt over his abilities and shame in rejecting the warm dependency toward the parents which Erikson sees as primary during this phase of life. The struggle is easily observed in young children as they stubbornly insist "let me do it" one minute only to become hopelessly frustrated and in need of support and comforting the next.

The Phallic Period 3-6

During the phallic period (covering roughly the preschool and kindergarten years) sexual feelings and excitement are finally localized in the genitalia, although the child's sexual feelings are still quite immature and unfocused. Children develop a keen interest in the genitals of both sexes and become especially aware of differences. Children imagine that something has happened to the female's penis and that something can happen to that of the male. During a playful, teasing "doctor game" a girl was overheard telling a boy that she would cut off his penis and make him a girl. When queried as to whether she believed that this was how

girls became girls, she replied that she did not but once believed it to be true.

Although both sexes evidence an active, aggressive engaging with the environment during this period of development, shifts in emphasis for the two sexes begin to emerge. Males begin developing an intrusive mode of engaging the world which involves thrusting themselves physically and emotionally into space, into people's lives, into problems, and into play. Female intrusiveness on the other hand emerges as the active passivity which is characteristic of the later mature woman. This includes making herself attractive, learning to be endearing, and, in short, discovering how to get others to include her into their lives.

This is a period of energetic learning, increased activity with peers and with the testing of new experiences and skills. Learning to take initiative and to sense oneself as an active, decision-making organism is the keynote. But learning to take initiative also involves some guilt. The child fears going beyond his rights and beyond the limits of acceptable behavior, and frequently he does. Questions arise as to whether this is acceptable behavior for a boy or for a girl. Giving in to passivity and guilt means denial of self while acting too readily on his own initiative can lead to pain, punishment,

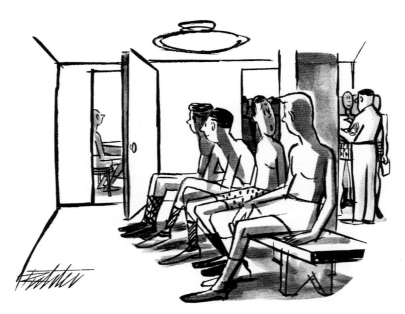

"If you tell him you hate your mother, you know what that means, and if you tell him you love her, it's even worse."

Figure 4–2.   *(Drawing by Richter; © 1962 The New Yorker Magazine, Inc.)*

or unintended hurt to others. The development of a proper balance between a sense of initiative and a sense of guilt is the major conflict which Erikson sees in this period.

Desires for the expression of genital affection appear for the first time and color the child's relation to both parents. The psychological interrelationships surrounding the parent-child relationship along with its sexual undertones were labeled by Freud the *Oedipal complex.* Specifically, Freud was referring to the child's growing attachment and sexual feelings for the parent of the opposite sex along with concomitant feelings of rivalry with the parent of the same sex. The feelings do not so much relate to incest as they do to the fact that the child tends to attach his sexual desires to the most trusted and available man or woman he knows. The woman a young boy knows best is his mother. However he gradually learns that mother is not an appropriate love object. Freud postulated that the learning was motivated out of fear that the father would retaliate against the son for his transgression by cutting off the boy's penis. ⟶FREUD Erikson emphasizes the child's learning that his chosen love object is simply unobtainable. He⟶ERIKSON discovers the persons closer to his own age and more accessible and not already taken. Further, he comes increasingly to appreciate the physical, social and sexual inequality between himself and his ''rival.'' With the renunciation of his mother as a primary sexual object and the acceptance that sexual gratification must be delayed, the child begins to channel much of his energy into other pursuits. Sexual drives are subordinated to intellectual and social pursuits. Freud labeled this the latency period.

Latency, Adolescence and Adulthood 6-12

Psychoanalysis has distinctly less to say about personality development following the Oedipal period. Beginning around age 5 or 6 the child's active interest turns increasingly outward. His energies are channeled into intellectual pursuits, curiosity, interactions with peers, and adaptation to more and more social demands. Interest in the opposite sex per se is at a low ebb. In short the only thing latent during the latency period is the child's striving toward ultimate involvement with a member of the opposite sex. The child attempts to excel, to prove himself, and to develop a sense of industry or competence. Competition with peers

is intensified in many pursuits, not so much to reduce the rival as to win the acceptance and esteem of friends.

During adolescence play begins to lose its importance. A sense of the person's unique identity begins to be forged. Sexual feelings reappear with new intensity and in more mature form. The individual must establish himself anew with his peers in a manner more closely approximating the adult role which will soon be his. In an effort to establish his own identity and separateness as a person it becomes crucial for the person finally to separate himself from his parents. In a sense it is vital to find some fault with parents and parent figures in order for the adolescent to reassure himself that he is capable of independent judgment, that he does not have to continue to rely on the parents, and that he is now ready to assume responsibility for himself. It is of necessity a strong period marked by a breaking of old patterns and experimentation with many alternatives. But it is also a time of great excitement, change and challenge.

Typically, further delay is also involved. The person is required to wait for sexual gratification even though he is capable of mature heterosexual behavior. Participation in certain privileges of society (such as voting, ownership of property) are denied him even though his understanding of the process is excellent.

It should be clear by now that a primary *cognitive framework with a no. of ideas* theme in Freud's developmental schema is renunciation and delay. The child's ability to give up the gratifications of one period in life in favor of promised but unguaranteed greater rewards lays the foundation for his whole later development. Difficulties at any one level affect all subsequent ones. A child who does not successfully master his dependency needs may remain a clinging, helpless person all his life. Without the basic trust in himself and others which is learned during the oral period he lacks the necessary maturity to cope successfully with the stress of the next period. The child must learn to give up the secure dependency of the oral period in order to become a more separate person, but then society imposes further rules and he must give up some of his stubborn independence in certain areas (such as eliminative functions) in order to be allowed even greater autonomy in others. Having learned to control both dependency needs and eliminative-retentive functions, the child finally must learn to give up his first love object. Naturally the process does not end there. Frustration, delay and the ability to accept realistic limitations without sustaining crippling blows to one's self-esteem are challenges that remain all through life. Freud's major contribution was to call attention to the importance of our early experiences on later development.

In adulthood a person begins to answer the responsibilities dictated by his social-cultural environment. He is faced with the need to develop the capacity for intimacy with other persons. This is not an easy task. It presupposes a more or less successful mastery of the previous developmental stages. Intimacy means there must be a basic trust in one's own worth and a lack of fear of others. Intimacy is not possible without a well-developed sense of autonomy and independence. An ability to take the initiative without fear, to see oneself as a competent person, and to see oneself as a unique and separate person are all implied in the ability to have psychological intimacy with another. The challenge is to be able to relate to others without mistrust, without self-doubt, without guilt, without inferiority and without losing one's own sense of uniqueness. Obviously it is impossible for anyone to be all of this, all of the time, with all people. Maturity is a relative matter which can change with added experiences in adult life.

The Defense Mechanisms

As we have seen development is not a smooth process. Numerous frustrations, deprivations and threats to one's self-esteem are inevitable. The individual is in a constant struggle to maintain his autonomy against society's demands for conformity and to respect his instinctual life without giving into to it completely. The struggles between conflicting needs are often intense. Many internal compromises in the face of conflict, of necessity, occur in childhood before mental and physical maturity have been achieved. The child is incapable of the balanced, reasoned approach to difficulties that marks the mature adult. He often perceives himself to be in greater danger than is actually the case and the anxiety generated is extremely frightening. Methods of protecting himself against anxiety are developed. These habitual modes of protecting oneself from anxiety are referred to as mechanisms of defense.

The infant is almost completely dominated by instinctual strivings. Tension discharge and need satisfaction are experienced as "good" while tension accumulation and frustration are experienced as "bad." The striving for need satisfaction is intense, with little regard for the rights of others, the reality of the situation, or the ability of the parents to guarantee a perpetual tensionless state. It is an approach which states "I want what I want when I want it because I want it." Everything which contributes to need satisfaction is experienced as good while the converse applies toward anything which leads to frustration. The child gradually sees adults in the same terms. Mother emerges more and more in the child's perception as a total person who is either associated primarily with satisfaction ("good mother") or frustration ("bad mother"). Impulses which the child expresses likewise come to be regarded by him as either good or bad, depending on how the mother and, later on, other adults respond to them. Those impulses which lead to praise from nurturing adults are felt to be good, while those which are disapproved of are experienced as bad and thus pose a threat to the child's continued need for nurturance. If he displeases mother she may not give the food (or later the acceptance and warmth) which he needs. It is important to note that all of the instinctual strivings are natural but some come to be labeled as "good" or as "bad" depending on the reaction of the environment. The atmosphere in which such learning or labeling takes place is of crucial importance for later development. If some of the child's instinctual needs are met with harsh punishment and disapproval rather than with gentle but firm limitations the child can come to view himself as a "bad" person. Self-acceptance and self-esteem are thus deeply embedded in the child's early experiences with need gratification.

The child's task is to establish a mode of living which steers a middle course between the pressures of instinctual strivings from within and the often conflicting socio-cultural pressures from without. Essentially there are only a limited number of courses open to the child in the face of conflicting demands:

1. He can leave the field in order to escape the dilemma. For obvious reasons this is in reality only a theoretical possibility.

2. He can attempt to modify the demands of the parents to make them more achievable. This is a course of action frequently chosen by children, as any parent can testify.

3. He can try to change himself so that the

external demands become less troublesome. This is the most common solution adopted. Indeed, Freud saw the child's willingness to relinquish pleasurable gratifications in order to secure the approval of adults as the foundation on which all socialization is built.

4. Finally, if the conflicting demands are too severe and other alternatives prove unworkable, the child can protect himself psychologically by excluding the entire situation from awareness and thus convince himself that the problem does not exist. Insofar as he is aware, there is no problem. The conflict excluded by this unconscious forgetting is referred to as having been *repressed.*

Repression is the earliest method of defense which the child utilizes to reduce the anxiety generated by conflict and make an otherwise intolerable situation tolerable. As a thoroughly dependent organism the child must have his parents' approval. If parental displeasure with instinctual strivings is extreme so that virtually no instinctual discharge is allowed, the child is forced to deny a part of his own real experience. The anxiety generated in such situations is intense and is experienced as overwhelming and life-threatening. The solution in repression is to forget the entire problem. Parenthetically, it may be said that all psychological defenses begin at the point where the individual perceives or in effect tells himself, "I have an emotional experience which is too much to bear. I cannot tolerate this much discomfort or I will die." The defense then is a way of remaining in a situation without being aware of the extreme discomfort which is generated. All defenses serve the function of protecting the individual from what appears to be overwhelming anxiety or fear and all lie outside of the individual's awareness.

Several factors about repression need to be emphasized. Repression is motivated forgetting followed by a motivated continuation of the inability to recall. Since a return of the repressed conflict would subject the child to further experiences of overwhelming anxiety, the material is continuously kept from awareness. Another feature of the repressed material is that its power to stimulate anxiety is not diminished over time. Adult patients who recover repressed childhood memories during psychoanalysis experience a great deal of discomfort and anxiety. In large measure this is true precisely because the issue is so long responded to as if it could not be conceived. The very act of avoiding an

emotionally charged subject tends to reinforce its anxiety-producing qualities. Thus the adult represses out of fear that he would respond in the same manner to the conflict as he did as a child. His very fear that this is so prevents him from testing alternatives. In addition, repression occurs outside of awareness, or unconsciously, so that the adult is in a poor position to undo a repression. The defense of repression is triggered automatically by an anxiety signal that is typically too brief to be apprehended consciously. Not only is the defensive individual unaware of his defenses but usually also of the forces in himself that produce his anxiety, and sometimes even of the very fact that he tends to be anxious. In other words, he lacks insight into both the existence and motivation of his defensive behavior. A final feature of repression is its pervasiveness. The entire conflict and events surrounding it are excluded from awareness so completely that it is as if they had never happened. As the individual matures he develops more sophisticated defense mechanisms which are less global or more specifically aimed at the core of the anxiety-producing situation. In this manner there is less need to exclude the totality of certain significant experiences from existence.

Repression is the basic defense on which many others may be built. In development, subsequent experiences may threaten to revive or remind the person of previously repressed material and other defenses are utilized to help maintain the original repressions. It also happens, of course, that new conflicts can emerge when the child is psychologically more mature and when it is more likely that defenses other than repression will be used. Repression is characteristically employed more often before verbal skills are well developed and is therefore more typical of early childhood than of the latency period.

A concept such as repression is difficult to prove or disprove. By definition a person cannot validate from his own experience that something is repressed. The fact of his failure to remember may be proof of its existence! However, in the clinical practice of psychotherapy patients often do recall previously forgotten material with a great deal of accompanying anxiety. In addition, a number of studies have attempted to demonstrate the existence of emotionally motivated forgetting. Literally hundreds of these experiments relevant to the concepts of repression have been performed and the majority—but not all—have produced results consistent with psychoanalytic theory. To cite only a few, Sharp (1938) found that neurotic subjects recalled emotionally disturbing words (—) more poorly than words connected with the gratification of their needs. Diven (1937) used a conditioning procedure to associate selected words in a list with electric shock. The next day the subjects recalled the words that had not been associated with shock better than the anxiety-producing shock words. Subjects were then told that there would be no more shock and their recall of the previously threatening words immediately increased. Zeller (1951) found a decrease in the recall of nonsense syllables that had been experimentally associated with failure on another task. These and similar experiments deal with secondary repression; the primary repression of pregenital sexuality postulated by Freud cannot be directly experimented upon, for ethical and practical reasons.

Displacement. The mechanism of displacement consists of directing an emotion toward a safe or acceptable object as a substitute for a dangerous or unacceptable object. To quote Samuel Johnson, "A man will sometimes rage at his wife when in reality his mistress has offended him, and a lady complain of the cruelty of her husband when she has no other enemy than bad cards." Frequently the emotion in displacement is a hostile one; the hostility is vented on a scapegoat in overt action, emotional attitude or fantasy. It is dangerous to clash with a business superior but not to reprimand an assistant. A dependent child may experience more anxiety than he can tolerate if he feels angry with his mother; instead he gets angry with his siblings or playmates.

In an ingenious experiment, Miller (1948) demonstrated the role of displacement in animal subjects. He trained rats to strike each other when an electric shock was administered. If the shock was then administered to a rat placed in the shock box with a celluloid doll, aggression was displaced to the doll; the rat struck at it and knocked it down. Miller views displacement as an instance of generalization and believes that several principles of stimulus-generalization also hold for the displacement mechanism: First, if the original object of the impulse is absent, the strongest displaced response occurs to the most similar object available, just as generalization occurs to the most similar stimulus. Second, if the original object is present but a

direct response to it is prevented by conflict or potential anxiety, then generalization—or displacement—will occur even to objects quite different from the original one. Third, the stronger an impulse, the more likely it is that generalization or displacement will occur to very dissimilar objects. Thus, with intense but inhibited feelings of hostility the most trivial incident may trigger an emotional explosion.

Sublimation. Sublimation consists of gratifying frustrated psychosexual or aggressive impulses by channeling them into socially approved activities. Psychoanalytic theorists have suggested that sadism may be sublimated into the skilled work of a surgeon, exhibitionism into acting or dancing, voyeurism into scientific or artistic curiosity and anal retentiveness into financial acquisitiveness. Sublimation is unique among the defenses in that it is defined with reference to social standards; sublimation characterizes the successful, socially approved, well-adjusted adult. In the framework of psychoanalytic concepts, sublimation is viewed as a mark of emotional stability, and one of the aims of psychoanalytic therapy is the replacement of other defenses by successful sublimations.

Freudian theory and empirical evidence both suggest that pregenital impulses may be sublimated, but not the genital impulses. Genital sexuality may be inhibited but it cannot be gratified through substitute activities in the same manner as infantile orality, anality and so forth (Kinsey et al., 1948).

Reaction Formation. This mechanism is a kind of "repression plus." The individual reinforces his repressions by developing conscious attitudes and patterns of behavior that are the antithesis of his unconscious and unacceptable tendencies. Through the mechanism of reaction formation the messy child becomes fussy and neat at the close of the anal stage, the sexually preoccupied individual becomes prudishly oversensitive and hostile to sex and the aggressive individual displays an excessive kindness such as taking great pains to avoid stepping on insects. Fenichel (1945) cites the example of a dedicated vegetarian leader who became a butcher; in cases of this sort it is likely that the first pattern of behavior represents a reaction formation, later abandoned, against the second pattern. Reaction formations can be distinguished from genuine neatness, modesty, kindness or any other nonreactive trait by three qualities. First, reactively motivated behavior is excessive. The individual who makes a fetish of cleanliness as a reaction against sinful and "dirty" impulses keeps things clean to a ridiculous extent. Second, the objectionable impulse occasionally breaks through the reactive facade, often in response to a minimal precipitating stimulus. Third, the individual manifests a strong stress reaction when his reactive behavior is blocked by circumstances; he responds with anger, anxiety and sometimes irrational excitement.

An interesting and sometimes amusing aspect of reaction-formation is in the nature of the internal compromise. Continual reassurance that one is clean, virtuous or morally upright is ensured by the behaviors. At the same time, there is no surer way to be in constant contact with dirt than to seek it out and clean it, nor to remain close to illicit sex than by such activities as censoring obscene films or writings!

Projection. The attribution of an unwanted trait or impulse to others and denying it in oneself clashes with external reality more sharply than the other mechanisms do. A male psychotic with unconscious homosexual tendencies may have the delusion that men are trying to seduce him or that radar is being used to implant homosexual ideas in him. In a far milder form, projection appears in a very young child who is given two toys, one more attractive and one less so, and told to give one toy to another child. If the child gives away the unattractive toy he is likely to justify his behavior by claiming that the recipient would have done the same. If he gives away the attractive toy he makes no such claim, i.e., he has no need to project blame.

Many social-psychological studies have provided evidence that prejudice against racial, religious and other minority outgroups involves a projective process (of course, economic, sociological and other variables also affect prejudice). In prejudice, unacceptable wishes and traits are not only attributed to other people but further removed from oneself by choosing people outside one's own group to focus upon and reject. In both projection and prejudice, as id or superego elements are cast out and attributed to external objects, the scope of rational ego processes shrinks.

Introjection and Identification. These terms are often used synonymously to mean a self-expanding process of internalizing others' attributes into oneself. Sometimes, however, only the term "introjection" is used to refer to the process and "identification" is used to refer to the end result of introjection. Introjection is the opposite of projection. In the Oedipal stage, the boy defends himself against his overpowering father by introjecting his father's qualities into his own ego and superego, so that he too may feel powerful; he is then said to have effected an identification with his father. "If you can't beat them, join them," is the formula for introjection and identification. In the Nazi concentration camps and the prisoner camps of World War II, a number of inmates responded to the extreme stress of incarceration by identifying with their captors. They eagerly wore bits of guards' uniforms and adopted some of their behavior and attitudes.

Minor identifications abound: both children and adults enhance their self-concepts by identifying with admired heroes (or heroines) of fiction, films and real life. In such cases, the fantasy identification is not confused with reality, but the psychotic who attempts to enhance his self-concept and allay anxiety by identifying with the President of the United States may believe he really is the President.

Fixation and Regression. In fixation the individual persists in a behavior pattern or stage of development—sexual or otherwise—after the time has come to move to a more advanced level. In regression he returns to an earlier level. Temper tantrums, baby talk, oral dependency, sibling rivalry or Oedipal attachments, for example, are not outgrown in fixation; in regression they are dropped but later resumed.

Fixation and regression are actually intertwined: under stress an individual regresses to behaviors on which he had previously become partially fixated. Fixation, whether partial or fairly complete, is a defensive safety maneuver, since the fixated organism does not have to face the possible dangers of new modes of behavior but is safe with behavior that has been strongly gratified. Strong frustration leads to the same result in some cases. People apparently need a minimum of gratification at a given stage before they are ready to try the next one.

A classic case of regressive behavior appears in the three photographs of Figure 4–3 reproduced from Masserman (1961). The following case description accompanies the photographs:

A 17-year-old girl (A) was brought to a psychiatric clinic by her mother with the complaint that for the preceding five months her behavior had become increasingly irrational and destructive. The history revealed that after the patient was about four years old her parents had begun to quarrel violently, making her early environment extremely contentious and unstable.

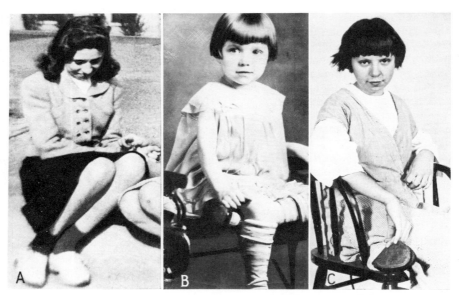

Figure 4–3. *Thanks are due to Drs. John Romano and Richard Renneker for providing the photographs and data. (From Masserman, J. H. 1961. Principles of Dynamic Psychiatry. 2nd Ed. Philadelphia, W. B. Saunders Co.)*

"bedwetting"

At about this age she first developed various neurotic traits: nail-biting, temper tantrums, enuresis and numerous phobias. When the patient was seven the mother refused further sexual relations with the father and left the marital bed, but the patient continued to sleep with the father until she was thirteen. At this time the mother suspected that the patient was being incestuously seduced, obtained legal custody of the girl and moved away with her to a separate home. The patient resented this, quarreled frequently with her mother, became a disciplinary problem at home and at school and acquired a police record for various delinquencies. Three years later, at the patient's insistence, she and her mother paid an unexpected visit to the father, and found him living with another girl in questionable circumstances. In a violent scene, the mother denounced the father for unfaithfulness and, again, contrary to the patient's wishes, took her home. There the patient refused to attend school and rapidly became sullen, withdrawn and non-communicative. During her mother's absence at work she would keep the house in disorder, destroy clothes her mother had made for her, and throw her mother's effects out of the window. During one of these forays she discovered a photograph of herself at the age of five (*B*), which, incidentally, was so poorly lighted and faded that, for one detail, it did not show her eyebrows. Using this as a pattern, she shaved off her own eyebrows, cut her hair to the same baby bob, and began to affect the facial expression and sitting posture of the pictured child (*C*). When brought to the hospital her general behavior was correspondingly childish; she was untidy and enuretic, giggled incessantly or spoke

in simple monosyllabic sentences, spent most of her time on the floor playing with blocks or paper dolls, and had to be fed, cleaned and supervised as though she were an infant. In effect, she appeared to have regressed to a relatively desirable period in life antedating disruptive jealousies and other conflicts; moreover, she acted out this regression in unconsciously determined but strikingly symbolic patterns of eliminating the mother as a rival and regaining the father she had lost in her childhood.

Denial and Emotional Withdrawal. Denial appears in myriad forms. The individual unable to tolerate his anger denies that he feels angry. The student who is afraid his grade will be poor protects himself by denying that he wants a good grade. People deny external reality as well as emotional responses: under stress, they may deny the existence of a carefully diagnosed illness and even deny for many years the death of a loved person. Denial is an attempt to minimize the impact of past, present or future hurtful events.

Withdrawal is closely related to denial. The individual may withdraw in advance by refusing to compete when he fears losing or by refusing to become emotionally involved with another person if past involvements have been painful. In an extreme case withdrawal may be total and reality may be shut out by taking to one's bed and being "sick," or by apathy, resignation and flat affect. An apathetic attitude is a defensive surrender before the battle starts; there can be no victory but there can also be no defeat. Denial and withdrawal are equivalent to asserting, "It hasn't happened"; or, "It isn't happening"; or, "It doesn't matter to me if it does happen"; or, "I will hide so it won't happen."

Defensive denial, repression and reaction formation are manifestly present in the following sentence completion test responses of a hospitalized 20-year-old married student. (A sentence completion test consists of a series of opening phrases which the subject completes with whatever comes to mind. The completions may be analyzed for such variables as mode of defense, affect, intense feelings and conflicts, attitudes to oneself and others, goals and peculiarities of thinking). The patient was anxious and depressed. For some months prior to testing she had been separated from her husband who attended a university in another city. She was failing in her classes despite an extremely high I.Q. She unsuccessfully attempted to cope with these stresses and with a variety of fears and conflicts by a rigid defensive pattern. Many of her problems are visible in the test completions just beneath the defense surface.

Marriage . . . has brought to me more happiness than I ever dreamed possible. *RF*

Most women . . . should strive to remember to be feminine, though capable and not overly feminine. *RF*

My body . . . satisfies me the way it is. I won't let it be defiled. I know I must not be ashamed of it. *RF*

Most bosses . . . aren't nearly as nice as mine. He is the best in the world, I'm sure. *?*

* A husband . . . must be prepared to stand by and understand through thick and thin—as mine *D* *D or RF?* is doing now. His love for his wife must take second place only to his love for God.

I like . . . to like people and to be liked by them. Perhaps love would be a better word. I like *REP.* to be in the wild free outdoors and to run uninhibitedly.

My mother . . . is one of the dearest, most precious persons in the whole world. I'd do almost anything to make her happy.

If I were in charge . . . of the world, I'd arrange things so that everyone loved everyone else all of the time.

My father . . . has always and still does refuse to let me grow up. At least he won't admit to himself that I have.

Most men . . . are wonderful, fascinating creatures who never forget that women are female. *RF.*

This place . . . is wonderful. It is more like a hotel than a hospital and does everything possible to prevent us from thinking we're really very, very sick. *RF₂*

My job . . . is perfect. Though the work gets boring, the people are wonderful beyond words. *RF₁*

It is easy for me to . . . love many people and animals and friends all at the same time. *RF-D*

My health . . . is good and bothers me only when I think something is psychosomatically wrong again. *D.*

Nothing cheers me up as much as . . . my husband or a good talk with God. *RF*

I am the sort of person who . . . is so full of love it just bursts out and sometimes in the wrong ways. *RF*

I am ashamed when I think of . . . my past relations with a man named X—also hurt and regretful. *R*

Things look hopeless when . . . I'm all depressed, excited, angry and don't know why. Really, I don't think things have ever looked really hopeless! *D*

I need . . . help to understand myself and loads of love.

Most of the time, I am . . . a very pleasant, likeable (I think and hope) person.

If I saw a fire truck . . . I'd like to follow it and always hope no one was hurt and that it wasn't too bad.

Everywhere . . . around me I find people who love me and want to help me now when it's so important.

If I were the boss, I . . . would arrange for everyone to love everyone else.

I really think my place in life . . . is and will be wonderful and satisfying. *D*

Some people don't like me because . . . I don't know of anyone who dislikes me. *D*

Rationalization. Rationalization is an attempt to bolster self-esteem by substituting "good" reasons for real ones. It is a very pervasive defense and quite often occurs when the individual tries to justify his own behavior and prove that others are wrong.

Rationalization may be dramatically demonstrated in hypnosis. Under hypnosis, a subject is told to remove his necktie when the hypnotic session is over but he is given no reason for the action. Everyone present is wearing a necktie. When the subject begins to remove his necktie he may try to avoid being judged eccentric by volunteering the rationalization that it is too tight, or that he had not tied it correctly and had better do it over, or that it has an interesting design which someone may wish to examine.

Two special kinds of rationalization are the

so-called sour-grape and sweet-lemon varieties. The individual who fails to get the grapes— whatever he had striven for—tells himself they are sour and inedible. Conversely, the lemon— an unsatisfactory outcome of one's hope—is really sweet and after all tastes fine.

Fantasy. Daydreams, reveries or fantasies gratify drives in imagination and replace the unsatisfactory world of reality. They defend the individual against frustration by an autistic process. For the normal and neurotic individual it is easy to shift from the fantasy world back to the real one, but for the psychotic the shift may be impossible.

A classic example of fantasy in literature is James Thurber's "The Secret Life of Walter Mitty." The sheeplike, henpecked and inept Mitty has an unsuspected inner life in which he takes on new roles: commander of an eight-engine plane in a hurricane, the world's greatest surgeon or crack pistol shot and great lover. These are "conquering-hero" fantasies. Mitty also has "suffering hero" fantasies; in these, a great affliction or injustice is borne with such stoical courage that the hero's basic nobility cannot be challenged:

> He put his shoulders back and his heels together. "To hell with the handkerchief," said Walter Mitty scornfully. He took one last drag on his cigarette and snapped it away. Then, with that faint, fleeting smile playing about his lips, he faced the firing squad; erect and motionless, proud and disdainful, Walter Mitty the Undefeated, inscrutable to the last.

Isolation. There is a similarity between isolation and repression. In repression the individual is not aware of the motives behind his be-(UNCONS.) havior; in isolation he has some insight into his motives but cannot see their connection with his behavior, although the connection is often obvious to others. A young man who readily admitted that he tended to be hostile reported a recurrent fantasy in which a machine gun was mounted on the hood of his car and sprayed bullets into passersby as he drove; yet he failed to see any connection between his hostile drives and his fantasy. His explanation of the fantasy was that it was interesting to speculate on the correct angle for mounting the gun and the arc through which it should sweep for maximum efficiency; besides it kept him from being bored while driving. By substituting these intellectual reasons for the motive of hostility, he made it easy to express his hostility in fantasy without feeling guilt. Isolation is often

aided, as in this case, by a process of intellectualization.

A related defense isolates contradictory attitudes or behaviors from each other. An assaultive individual may be extremely kind to animals and not realize that his behavior is internally inconsistent. Exhibitionists and persons with other sexual perversions frequently have moralistic attitudes, even on matters of sex. A paranoid schizophrenic may assert grandiosely that he is enormously wealthy and then ask to borrow a dollar; his mental organization has logic-tight compartments that isolate his delusion from the rest of his behavior. If challenged, he may rationalize that his enemies keep him from access to wealth.

Undoing. A magical attempt to wipe out a real or fancied guilt is termed undoing. The individual engages in ritualistic behavior such as repetition of a magic phrase or performance of a ceremonial act. Lady Macbeth tried to undo her guilt by removing imaginary spots of blood from her hands while sleep-walking. A patient decided that he had been unjustifiably stingy in not permitting his wife to buy an item of jewelry she wanted but felt it would be humiliating to admit his stinginess to her. Instead, for several successive days, he gave away small sums of money; he was not being genuinely charitable but was attempting to atone for his guilt and thus undo it. Another example is that of some compulsive individuals who have a strong need to count the people near them. This behavior may represent an attempt to cancel out and undo hostile death wishes against people by making sure that they are all present and therefore still alive.

SUPPRESSION - (cons.)   *Do one thing to make up for another.*

Defenses and Psychopathology

The defenses just discussed are found in both disturbed and relatively undisturbed persons. A completely defenseless person could not cope with emotional and social pressures. However, defenses play a role in normal behavior different from that in disturbed behavior. The normal person's defenses are relatively successful; the disturbed individual's defenses fail, despite the fact that in some forms of disorder, particularly the neuroses, defenses are very strong. When defenses are no longer adequate to keep unacceptable impulses and anxiety at bay, psychopathological symptoms flourish and intensify.

won't use them excessively or in wrong places, etc.

A second difference between normal and non-normal defensiveness is that certain defenses are strongly undesirable when employed excessively, because of their effect on other people. Regression to infantile hostility, reaction formations that limit others' freedom and projections may easily become damaging to society. The consequences of Hitler's infantile rages and paranoid projections were world-shaking.

The phrase "paranoid projections" indicates that although nonparanoids also project there is an intimate link between a paranoid disorder and the particular defense of projection. This type of link is present in several disorders: The hysteric represses and denies whereas the obsessive-compulsive defends himself by reaction formation, isolation and undoing. Of course each type of patient utilizes other defenses too, but in many disorders some one defense, or a small group of defenses, plays a central role and the others are secondary. A hysteric's repressions explain more of his behavior than his other defenses do.

A very basic problem is that of distinguishing defensive from nondefensive behavior. It is as foolish to call all behavior defensive—e.g., to explain all generosity as a reaction formation against stinginess, all reasoning as rationalization and all criticisms of others as projection—as it is naïve to take all behavior at its face value and overlook its defensive components.

The distinction between defense and nondefense is basically a distinction between two kinds of motivation. Defensive motivation is present if the individual is driven, impatient, overemphatic and easily frustrated. These characteristics affect the *manner* of behavior as much as its content. The individual who hammers the table with his fist and shouts, "I'm not angry!" is angry but cannot admit his anger and defensively denies it. A classic instance of defensive denial is that of the patient who reported dreaming about a shadowy female figure, "I don't know who it was, but it certainly wasn't my mother!" Projection is often revealed by the excessive intensity with which an individual states his opinion. Nondefensive behavior, on the other hand, is usually relatively relaxed, because it is not primarily motivated by anxiety or guilt. Differences in motivation and manner of behaving distinguish constructive imagination from defensive fantasy, intellectual analysis from intellectualizing isolation, patience from resigned withdrawal, or any other nondefensive behavior from its defensive counterpart.

Some Criticisms of Psychoanalytic Theory

The preceding discussion of psychoanalytic developmental theory and defense mechanisms is exceedingly abbreviated and simplified. Freud's collected works alone run to 23 volumes, not to mention the countless volumes of his many colleagues, ideological heirs, and modifiers. We have attempted merely to present in outline form some of the basic ideas which have achieved widespread acceptance in clinical settings.

Although psychoanalysis is one of the most comprehensive personality theories yet formulated, it is far from complete. Freud himself was continually revising his ideas up until the time of his death. Further modification and clarifications have been proposed by theorists such as Erikson (1950) and Rapaport (1960), to name but two. Nevertheless, some psychoanalysts have tended to regard Freud's formulations as final teachings rather than as tentative theoretical formulations and have thus laid themselves bare to charges of being unscientific.

Another criticism already mentioned was Freud's relative lack of emphasis on the sociocultural determinants of behavior and development. While Freud himself was well aware of the importance of the emotional climate in which the child was reared, he tended to focus mainly on the internal, psychological state of the developing organism.

A related criticism was Freud's emphasis on the sexual drives and sexual energy as the primary motivating force in development and in psychopathology. To many modern theorists the emphasis seems unnecessarily narrow.

Since Freud attributed great importance to the early vicissitudes of the sexual instincts, most of his development speculations focus on the first six years of life. For Freud, patterns laid down in these early years can be traced through all subsequent stages of life. Persons suffering severe deprivations during the oral-dependent stage are apt to be emotionally crippled and resistant to corrective emotional experiences for the remainder of their lives. For some theorists the view that unsuitable patterns we establish in infancy can be only slightly modified later seems unnecessarily pessimistic. In fact, many persons can be found who have made significant and striking changes for the better from previously crippling life styles.

Another criticism of the theory concerns the difficulty in testing many of its basic hypotheses.

The experimental evidence is not all in and more sophisticated research will be necessary before many aspects can be tested. To take but one example, many of the processes which Freud described cannot be observed directly but have to be inferred from the patient's behavior. Inference, however, is a tricky process and different consequences can be inferred from the same behavior, even using the same theory.

Other criticisms will be explained as we look briefly at two competing theories for the explanation of the development of psychopathology: existential theory and learning theory.

AN EXISTENTIAL APPROACH (MONistic)
Not to explain but to understand.

The existential approach to the explanation of psychopathology takes its departure from the philosophical writings of various authors, such as Kierkegaard (1954), Sartre (1956), Tillich (1952) and Camus (1946). The movement began as a European phenomenon in the later 1940's based on the experiences of clinical observers such as Frankl (1955), to name but one of several. One of the chief spokesmen for the existential approach in the United States is Rollo May (1969) and it is principally his writings which provide the basis for the following discussion.

For May, the primary focus of attention in understanding psychopathology should be on those aspects of existence which are uniquely and individually human. Focusing on the unique leads to a deemphasis of systematized, all-encompassing and highly structural theories of dynamics, forces, or energies which pay little or no attention to the individual's present phenomenological world. The existentialist takes exactly the opposite approach. He seeks a more unique, more subjectively humanistic approach to explanation in order to complete his understanding of an abnormal personality. May (1969) states it thus:

We do not deny dynamism and forces; that would be nonsense. But we hold that they have meaning only in the context of the existing living being—if I may use a technical word, only in the ontological context.

This approach is more than a play on words or a slight shift in emphasis to supplement psychoanalytic theory. Existentialism has implications for psychological theory building and

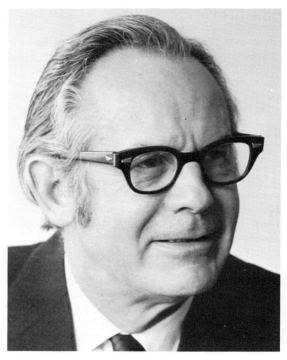

Figure 4–4. Rollo May.

scientific investigation of far-reaching significance. This is easily seen in terms of the approach to the understanding of a patient. Whereas Freud placed primary emphasis on the patient's problem as the proper unit of study and concluded that the present problem properly could be understood only in terms of the person's past developmental history, May points out that such an approach ignores the here-and-now experience of the patient in relation to others around him. The psychoanalytic view, with its emphasis in the past, thus ties itself to the conventional biological approach to the study of organisms. In this view, the more complex or more highly developed organism can be understood in terms of its evolutionary precursors. May asserts that this approach lends only to partial understanding of more complex organisms. With evolution or growth new skills and experiences appear which exert a reorganizing pressure on all the simpler elements previously in the organism. Understanding of the adult neurotic is thus a two-way street for May. We can only partially understand the adult by looking from the past to the present (à la Freud). We must also look from the present to the past in terms of how present experience tends to shape and distort and reorganize previously learned patterns of adjustment. It is precisely these larger meanings and reorganizations which constitute the uniquely human for May and which in his view are distorted in psychopathology. To quote him further:

I argue only against the uncritical acceptance of the assumption that the organism is to be understood only in terms of those elements below it on the evolutionary scale, an acceptance that has led us to overlook the self-evident truth that what makes a horse a horse are not the elements it shares with the dog but what constitute distinctively "horse!" *Now, what we are dealing with in neurosis are those characteristics and functions that are distinctively human.* It is these that have gone awry in disturbed patients. [May, 1969].

What are the unique characteristics of the human experience? May postulates six characteristics or processes arising from his clinical experiences as a psychotherapist:

1. Every existing person is centered in himself and experiences an attack on this center as a threat to his very existence. The natural tendency of organisms is toward growth or maintenance of their individual integrity. Neurotic symptoms are methods by which a person seeks to preserve at least part of his unique existence. A patient who has difficulty in expression of hostility may avoid situations which appear to risk anger-producing behavior. In so doing, he restricts himself in one area of life in order to live comfortably in others. Neurotic symptoms then are seen as methods by which the individual preserves at least part of his own center (being) rather than as deviations from some theoretical norm. Rather than defining neurosis as a failure of adjustment, the existentialist sees adjustment as exactly what neurosis is. It is precisely this point which makes neurotic behavior so difficult to change. It is an adjustment by which the individual manages to preserve some aspect of his being.

2. Every existing person has the character of self-affirmation or the need to preserve its centeredness. All persons have the potential of self-affirmation or courage. By courage May refers to the individual's willingness to accept responsibility for his own choices and decisions, and it is a lack of such self-affirmation which characterizes the neurotic patient.

3. All existing persons have the need and possibility of going out from their centeredness to participate in other beings. This involves two kinds of risk: (a), the person can shrink

back or withdraw from others in order to protect his own conflicted center and face a narrow, shrunken world; or (b), a person may lose his own identity through overdispersal of self in the lives of others. May believes the latter to be particularly relevant with the modern emphasis on conformity and other-directedness.

4. The subjective side of centeredness is awareness. Here May refers to vigilance toward the outside world and its perceived threats.

5. The uniquely human form of awareness is self-consciousness. This is an extremely important concept in May's theory. Consciousness of the self implies affirmation of one's uniqueness and separateness. It implies the ability to affirm all of one's desires and needs as well as the ability to see that each of us is completely unique and thus utterly alone.

6. The final characteristic of the existing person is anxiety. As May sees it, man is in a constant struggle in which he must either grow, reach out to the world, and risk failure or shrink into himself and give up aspects of his own being. Anxiety then is "the state of the human being in the struggle against that which would destroy his being." Full existence is possible only to the extent that a person can accept the anxiety which naturally results from having to make choices even though he can never have absolute certainty about the choices. ↗

EX. GUILT —
change neurotic to normal anxiety.

Some Criticisms of Existentialism

In a world beset by rapid change, difficult choices, and seemingly overwhelming problems, May's contentions that anxiety is a natural state of existence and that man has an innate capacity for self-destruction has a certain face validity. At the same time, his emphasis on the simultaneous potential for self-affirmation and grandeur seems to place man on a somewhat higher plane than has typically resulted from traditional scientific approaches. The existentialists stand almost alone against a science of persons which sometimes seems bent on seeing man exclusively as a series of traits, motives and part processes and thus losing sight of his unique humanness. Existential psychology has called attention to major shortcomings in our present theories through their insistence that man is more than the sum of his traits, motives and defenses.

While existentialism has intuitive appeal, many of its basic tenets are extremely difficult to test. In itself such a criticism need not be telling, since it may say more about present inadequacies in measurement than about short-comings of the theory. But it is a fact that up to now the theory has failed to generate the large body of experimental studies which have flowed from other explanatory systems. Until a better research base is established, existentialism is likely to be limited in its appeal to behavioral scientists. In fairness, it should be noted that existentialism, being only recently divorced from philosophy, is historically speaking roughly in the equivalent position of psychoanalysis in the early 1910's. Empirical laboratory investigation of psychoanalytic postulates did not occur with any great frequency until around the middle of this century, or some 40 years after the theory was first developed.

A LEARNING THEORY APPROACH

The application of learning theory to the study of emotional disorders is of fairly recent origin. As mentioned in an earlier chapter, it was Pavlov who first labeled the so-called "experimental neurosis" in laboratory animals and suggested some parallels to human behavior. In this country, Pavlov's experiments have been extended and replicated with both animals (Liddell, 1944) and human subjects (Wolpe, 1958). Many modern-day theorists lean heavily on Pavlov's conception of learning as modified by Hull (1951). Essentially, such theorists (i.e., Wolpe, Eysenck) define neurosis as "persistent unadaptive habits that have been conditioned (that is learned)" and the learned habits persist because they are anxiety-reducing. Adherents to this approach subscribe to an S-R (stimulus-response) model of learning which places emphasis on the conditioning of a particular response so that it will occur in the presence of a particular stimulus.

Another broad school of learning theorists take their departure from the work of B. F. Skinner (1938) who has postulated an S-S (sign-significate) model of learning. This model is antitheoretical and pragmatic in outlook. Those behaviors are repeated which are reinforced. Thus symptoms are seen as one class of behavior which have been learned through a history of reinforcement and which continue to exist because of their effects. Proponents of this approach (i.e., Krasner, 1958) emphasize the discovery of the reinforcement contingencies which maintain the "neurotic behavior." Once known, the reinforcers are withheld and positive reinforcement is applied to more socially desirable behaviors. In this manner, new behavior is "shaped," and old responses or symptoms are extinguished through lack of reinforcement.

In the present discussion we will use as an example the work of H. J. Eysenck, a British psychologist, and Joseph Wolpe, an American psychiatrist, who subscribe to a Pavlovian-Hullian approach to learning.

For Eysenck (1959) neurotic symptoms are simply learned patterns of behavior which are, for one reason or another, unadaptive. The prototype for the acquisition of a neurotic symptom can be found in the famous case of little Albert reported by Watson and Raynor (1920). Albert was a nine-month-old boy with no fear of white rats. A phobic response to white rats was established by a simple process of Pavlovian conditioning. Each time the boy reached out toward the rat the experimenter, who was standing behind the child, made a loud noise by banging an iron bar with a hammer. After a few pairings of the rat followed by the loud fear-

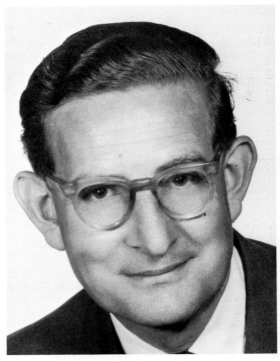

Figure 4–5. Hans J. Eysenck.

producing noise, the unconditioned response of fear became conditioned to the stimulus of the rat. Albert not only developed a phobic-like terror response when faced with a white rat, his response also *generalized* to other furry objects. Eysenck regards such a fear response to be unadaptive and hence neurotic, since white rats are not actually dangerous. However, if the conditioning had happened to take place with respect to a snake or scorpion the response would be adaptive. Thus chance happening may play a large part in the acquisition of neurotic symptoms and such symptoms need not imply a psychic trauma of the kind postulated by Freud.

Some conditioned responses are so unadaptive that they lead to social isolation or hospitalization, but Eysenck feels that much of the conditioning process is essential to effective socialization. Most children are conditioned to inhibit, or at least control, the direct expression of powerful emotions such as sex and aggression. If this were not the case, civilized society as we know it would not be possible. The overt expression of hostility toward another person is typically severely punished, thus producing a conditioned fear response (anxiety) to situations in which aggression is likely to occur. Thus, from a learning theory viewpoint, the child avoids aggressive response not out of fear of some anticipated, possible retaliation or loss of love, as Freud would say, but rather because it is only through avoiding such situations that he can relieve the painful conditioned response of anxiety.

To account for individual differences in the acquisition of conditioned responses, Eysenck points to the fact that people differ in the speed and firmness with which conditioned responses are built up. There are demonstrable individual differences in the speed with which conditioned responses are learned. In addition the strength of the conditioned stimulus has much to do with how firmly a conditioned response is established. Thus in the example of little Albert, the louder the noise, the greater the fear response and the stronger the phobia. Further differences can be accounted for by the number of pairings between the conditioned and unconditioned stimulus. Up to a point at least, the more times the loud noise has been paired with the rat, the stronger the learned or conditioned response. Finally, Eysenck points out that people differ widely in terms of autonomic reactivity. The same amount of noise may produce quite unequal amounts of autonomic upheaval in different children.

This approach to the explanation of emotional disorders contrasts sharply with the psychoanalytic developmental theory discussed earlier in this chapter. Eysenck has summarized the crucial differences as he sees them in a table which is reproduced here (Table 4–1). Among

TABLE 4–1. Differences Between Freudian Psychotherapy and Behavior Therapy*

Freudian Psychotherapy	Behavior Therapy
1. Based on inconsistent theory never properly formulated in postulate form.	Based on consistent, properly formulated theory leading to testable deductions.
2. Derived from clinical observations made without necessary control observation or experiments.	Derived from experimental studies specifically designed to test basic theory and deductions made therefrom.
3. Considers symptoms the visible upshot of unconscious causes ("complexes").	Considers symptoms as unadaptive conditioned responses.
4. Regards symptoms as evidence of *repression*.	Regards symptoms as evidence of faulty learning.
5. Believes that symptomatology is determined by defense mechanism.	Believes that symptomatology is determined by individual differences in conditionability and autonomic lability, as well as accidental environmental circumstances.
6. All treatment of neurotic disorders must be *historically* based.	All treatment of neurotic disorders is concerned with habits existing *at present*; their historical development is largely irrelevant.
7. Cures are achieved by handling the underlying (unconscious) dynamics, not by treating the symptom itself.	Cures are achieved by treating the symptom itself, i.e., by extinguishing unadaptive conditioned responses and establishing desirable conditioned responses.
8. Interpretation of symptoms, dreams, acts, etc. is an important element of treatment.	Interpretation, even if not completely subjective and erroneous, is irrelevant.
9. Symptomatic treatment leads to the elaboration of new symptoms.	Symptomatic treatment leads to permanent recovery, provided autonomic as well as skeletal surplus conditioned responses are extinguished.
10. Transference relations are essential for cures of neurotic disorders.	Personal relations are not essential for cures of neurotic disorders, although they may be useful in certain circumstances.

*Reprinted by permission from Eysenck, H. J. 1959. Learning theory and behavior therapy. J. Ment. Science. *105*:61–95.

the most important differences are the manner in which the neuroses are viewed, the treatment approaches dictated, and the different explanations of symptoms. For the learning theorist the symptom *is* the neurosis. There is no presumed underlying disorder or cause other than a past learning history which is of no current relevance. Since psychoanalysis sees neurosis as a process of which the symptom is a sign, the theory leads to the conclusion that removal of the symptom without attending to the basic disturbance has little value and, furthermore, other symptoms may soon appear to take the place of the one eliminated. The complex, though hidden, still exists and will seek outlets in other symptoms. Eysenck correctly points out that the data do not support such a view. Typically the alleviation of painful or disruptive symptoms leads to a reduction in anxiety, greater harmony with one's environment, and general improvement in behavior. A study of patients successfully treated for symptom removal fails to show that alternative symptoms are developed (Mowrer 1950). For Eysenck, the neurosis is "cured" when all the symptoms are removed, including all conditioned autonomic responses.

Some Criticisms of the Learning Theory Approach

The learning theory approach presents some exciting challenges to traditional concepts of abnormality. By relating symptoms and neurotic problems to processes that can be demonstrated with normal subjects in the controlled conditions of the laboratory, learning theorists open the door to rigorous, scientific study of formerly elusive problems. In addition, there can be little doubt that the treatment approaches which the theory dictates are effective for many types of patient. In fact, Wolpe (1958) claims a success rate of 90 per cent, which is far superior to the claims thus far advanced for any other treatment approach. While these claims may be exaggerated, as we shall see later, few would question the fact that in the right situation "deconditioning" can be a very effective treatment.

Probably the most thorough critical evaluation of learning theory applications to the study of abnormal behavior is that of Breger and McGaugh (1965). These authors make a number of interesting points:

1. In part, behavioristic theory may appear more scientifically respectable than it is because of the language used. Terms such as "laboratory-based," "experimental," "systematic" and "control" are often used somewhat loosely and may create an impression of greater scientific precision than the data actually warrant.

2. The so-called "laws of learning" on which Eysenck's approach is based are not always easily explainable or clear-cut. To take but one example, a conditioning model is hard pressed to explain the phenomenon of generality of behavior whereby what seems to be learned is a "set" to respond in a particular manner rather than in a highly specific response. Thus it is easier to explain a phobia, which implies a specific response to a specific stimulus, than to explain a depression, in which there is a general attitude which arises from many different types of stimuli. Even with rats, behaviorists have had to move away from a simplistic S-R learning model to explain the observed behavior. Behaviorists wishing to apply the "laws of learning" to humans often are more simplistic than the data warrant, even with white rats!

3. The claims of success for the treatment methods used are probably exaggerated. For example, in the often quoted instance of Wolpe's (1958) 90 per cent success rate, Breger and McGaugh point out, there are sampling biases, observer biases, and improper use of controls; any one of these factors would spuriously inflate the quoted success rate.

The evidence is clearly not all in. Charges, countercharges, and studies which contradict each other abound. It is natural for the student to feel somewhat bewildered and to want to know "which is right." Each has its appeal and each seems to explain certain aspects better than any other theory. To add to the problem, the list of theories discussed here is incomplete and by no means exhaustive. We have merely presented examples of divergent viewpoints to convey some of the flavor of the problems which are of current concern in abnormal psychology. There are theorists not discussed here who have earned the allegiance of many followers—Harry Stack Sullivan, Erich Fromm, Sandor Rado, Hobart Mawrer, Otto Rank, Carl Jung and Karen Horney, among others.

The solution to the bewilderment engendered by this multiplicity of viewpoints is the substitution of better questions for the premature query, "Who is right?" A single theory consists of a number of hypotheses; some of these may be correct, some half correct and some incorrect. The questions to ask are therefore: What are the hypotheses of each theory? What do the hypotheses mean? How are the hypotheses of different theories alike and how do they differ? What are the strengths and weaknesses of the hypotheses in each theory? What is the evidence for the hypotheses? Given this approach, there is no need to accept or reject a theory prematurely and *in toto.* In the last analysis, each hypothesis of each theory will stand or fall on slowly accumulated empirical evidence, and it will undoubtedly be found that in each theory there are both valid insights and some errors.

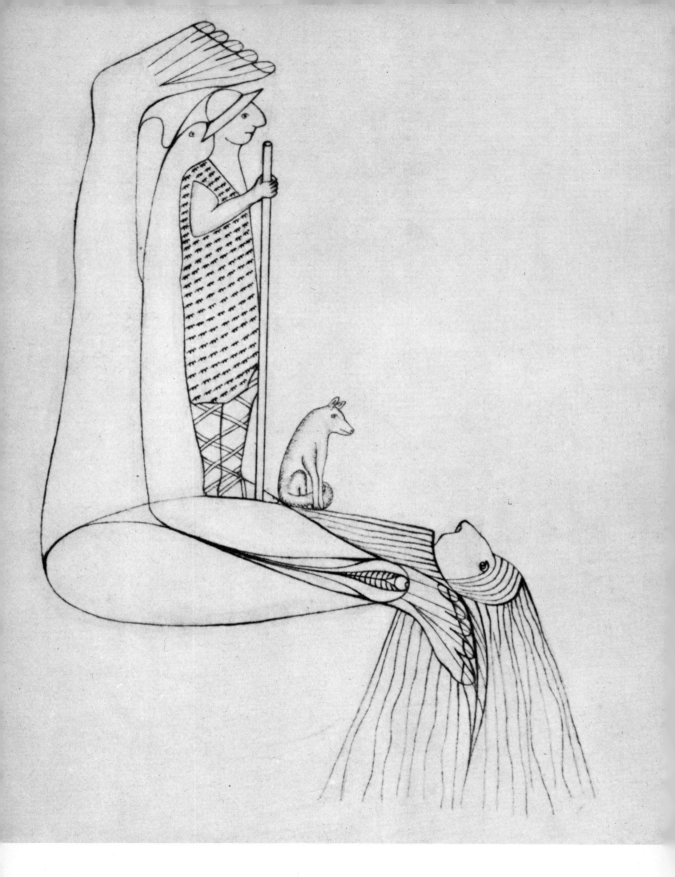

For want of a nail, the shoe was lost,
For want of a shoe, the horse was lost,
For want of a horse, the rider was lost,
For want of a rider, the battle was lost,
For want of a battle, the kingdom was lost,
And all for the want of a horseshoe nail.

Oxford Dictionary of Nursery Rhymes,
Edited by Opie, I., and Opie, P.

5

THE NATURE OF CAUSATION

It is usually necessary in science to answer such questions as "What" and "When" before the more difficult "Why." In Chapter 3 the "What" of deviant behaviors was described and classified; in Chapter 4 the developmental "When" was explored and an analysis of the "Why" of abnormality was begun in the discussion of sexuality, aggression and the defenses. In the ensuing several chapters, the crucial "Why" is further considered in a systematic survey of the various causes of abnormal behavior.

Etiological investigations may be pursued by various methods such as analysis of case histories, reconstruction of past experiences through interviews or controlled experimentation. Whatever method is used, the identification of causes is a complex endeavor in which it is easy to err and arrive at false conclusions. The errors one may make are of various types; perhaps the most common consists of errors in logic. In the rest of this chapter we shall discuss the *logic of causation* in relation to abnormal psychology.

CATEGORIES OF CAUSATION

The simplest category of causation consists of a single determinant leading to a single result. Frequently, however, a single cause leads to multiple consequences. Sometimes there is a chain of consequences following each other in sequence (as in the progression from the missing nail to the lost kingdom in the nursery rhyme quoted at the beginning of this chapter). In other instances the multiple end results of a single cause are concurrent. Chained and concurrent effects may occur together. Psychological cause and effect are often interlocked in a fashion so complex that it is generally unsound to expect a psychological cause to have only one effect.

In another pattern of causation frequent in biology and psychology, a single end result can be reached through different and mutually exclusive pathways. For example, choriodoretinal degeneration, an inherited disease of the eye, may be transmitted through any one of five different and alternative genetic mechanisms. In abnormal psychology there are countless examples of alternative causal paths to a particular end. Thus, let us consider three possible sources of pathological fear of social interaction. ① One causal pattern begins with economic or geographic factors that result in enforced social isolation in childhood; isolation then leads to a lack of opportunity to master social techniques; social ineptitude, in turn, leads to social fear. ② Alternatively, either parental influences or constitutional factors may be responsible for an acute sensitivity to social rebuffs from one's peers in childhood and this may result in a conviction of personal inferiority and fear of other people. ③ Third, parental rejection may lead to a generalized hostility which the individual cannot tolerate and accept in himself; he may then fear social interaction because it raises his hostility level.

Two or more concurrent causes may interact in more than one way. Their possible interrelations are schematically diagrammed in Figure 5–1. Interaction between causes is represented by an area falling within two or more intersecting circles. A completely shaded circle represents a single *sufficient* cause, that is, a cause adequate in itself to produce a given result, although other causes might also lead to this result. In Diagram I of Figure 5–1 either A or B is sufficient to produce a given result, and hence neither A nor B is *necessary*—that is, given A, B is not necessary to produce the result; given B, A is not necessary. For example, either brain degeneration (A) or emotional conflict (B) is sufficient to produce some cases of mental disorder; neither is a necessary cause of every case of mental disorder. In Diagram II, A is both necessary and sufficient, whereas B is neither. For example, a single dominant gene (A) is necessary in the causation of Huntington's chorea and is sufficient by itself to produce the psychosis. No other variable (B) is either a necessary or adequate cause of Huntington's chorea. In Diagram III, only the interaction of A and B is sufficient to produce the required results and hence both A and B are necessary. Thus, one theory of the etiology of the disorders termed reactive is that they are a

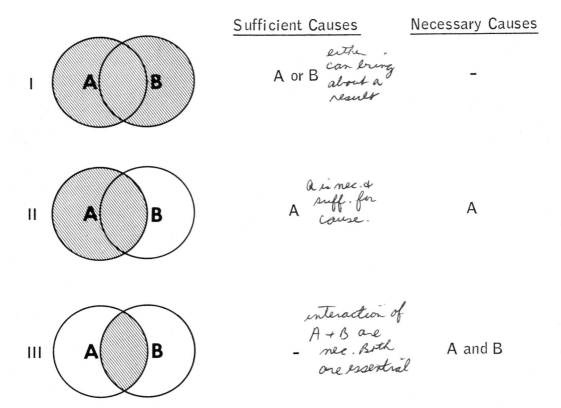

Figure 5–1. *Patterns of interaction of two independent variables (A and B). A completely shaded circle represents a sufficient cause. A single shaded circle, as in II, represents a cause that is both sufficient and necessary. A shaded area of overlap of two circles, as in III, means that the causes represented by both circles are necessary.*

reaction to environmental stresses (A), but the reaction occurs only in individuals who had experienced too much frustration (B) in childhood.

As the number of independent variables increases, the number of types of causal interaction increases even more rapidly. Two consequences for abnormal psychology flow from this complexity of interaction. First, one must not think of the causes of a symptom or syndrome as isolated from each other: biological, psychological and cultural factors all interact. Second, in order to make etiological research in the biological and social sciences feasible, causal factors must be organized in a model that usually oversimplifies reality; more complex models are too unwieldy. In psychiatry, the most frequently used model divides causes into the three categories of predisposing, precipitating and perpetuating. In psychology many causal models have been constructed. The one we shall follow borrows the concepts of predisposing and precipitating causes from psychiatry and combines them with four classes of determinants—hereditary, biological, psychological and sociocultural.

A *precipitating* cause occurs immediately or shortly before its effects. A *predisposing* cause is relatively remote in time from its effects. Predispositions set the stage for the triggering action of precipitants. However, since the time difference between the two types of causes is relative rather than absolute, predispositions shade into precipitants. Hereditary causes always consist of predispositions, whereas the other three classes—biological nonhereditary, psychological and sociocultural—include both predisposing and precipitating causes, the former resulting in increased vulnerability to the latter.

The ensuing chapters therefore discuss (1) hereditary predispositions; (2) other biological determinants, precipitating and predisposing; (3) psychological determinants, precipitating and predisposing; and (4) sociocultural determinants. (As we shall see, it is difficult to separate sociocultural precipitants and predispositions from each other.) As an introductory example of the operation of these determinants, let us consider the etiology of a common and apparently simple piece of behavior—the wearing of sunglasses. To begin with, one finds a hereditary factor interacting with the obvious external cause, the intensity of light. Albinism, a hereditary condition, results in a lack of pigment in the iris and an extreme sensitivity to light. Inheritance of blue eyes is associated with a relative lack of pigment in the iris, and blue-eyed persons are therefore more likely to wear sunglasses than brown-eyed persons.

Apart from heredity, other biological variables may play a causal role in several possible ways. First, infection may make the retina very sensitive. Second, toxic factors may be present; the visual sensitivity of the "morning after" is a case in point. Third, individuals with protruding eyes are more sensitive.

Psychological factors enter in many ways. Some paranoids wear sunglasses because they wish to hide their facial reactions; schizoid individuals because they tend to seek isolation; depressives because they wish to keep tears or a mournful expression invisible; neurotics because wearing sunglasses may be fashionable among their friends and they are too anxious and conforming to resist cultural pressures; and individuals with character disorders because for them the behavior symbolizes a rebellious nonconformity to the majority, who, after all, do not wear sunglasses.

Finally, sociocultural factors directly affect the phenomenon. In some cultures, the vast majority of inhabitants cannot afford to wear sunglasses despite the intensity of the sun, e.g., in Southern Italy. Within Italy, the peasantry does not wear them; the upper classes do, and this not alone for economic reasons: the peasantry considers the behavior alien and the upper classes consider it fashionable. (One of the authors once observed a very elegantly dressed individual who wore a sunglass monocle.)

It should be noted that biology, psychology and culture interact in this behavior. In Southern Italy the predominance of brown eyes lessens the need for protecting the retina and reinforces the cultural sanctions of the majority against wearing sunglasses. A blue-eyed, upper-class paranoid living in a region of strong sunlight might wear sunglasses because of the convergence of many causes.

SCIENTIFIC PROOF AND ITS DIFFICULTIES

A scientific hypothesis gathers support from its ability to predict and explain phenomena and from successful efforts to replicate the phenomena experimentally and control them in a manner consistent with the hypothesis. None of these is sufficient by itself to prove a hypothesis, but one—the ability to predict—

provides relatively strong support for it. Kline (1961) has elaborated these points in the following discussion, here somewhat abridged:*

. . . In point of fact, we are never able to "prove" anything; we can only accumulate more and more evidence that our hypothesis is not *incorrect*. There are a number of ways of doing this; although some of the methods are contributory they are not, of themselves, sufficient.

Explanation Is Not Sufficient

To explain, *post hoc,* what psychodynamics were involved or how a molecule broke down to produce a particular effect, can be done in dozens or hundreds of different ways. If mere explanation were sufficient, all of these ways would be "true." . . . Embellishment, "interpretation," or extension of a theory to meet the nonconforming cause is usually a reason for suspicion and closer examination.

Regularity Is Not Sufficient

Because a certain event in, let us say, the psychological area regularly follows or occurs simultaneously with a neurophysiological event is no proof that the two are directly—or even indirectly—related. Such a correlation certainly constitutes an invitation to investigate if there is a common causal nexus, but a theory relating the two is suitable only as a working hypothesis. All too often we have been told that this or that chemical (or sociological factor or electrophysiological event) is the *cause* of some mental state or feeling tone, simply because the two were associated. Even the existence of such pairing has usually been shown to be false when more extensively and intensively investigated.

Replication Is Not Sufficient

. . . To stimulate the globus pallidus [a nerve nucleus in the cerebrum] and produce symptoms of parkinsonism [a disorder involving tremors and rigidity, possibly due to lesions in the globus pallidus] does *not* prove that a disorder of the globus pallidus is the cause of the disease. This nucleus may be involved only as an intermediate step, or may not be involved in the causal chain at all, and the fact that stimulation reproduced certain symptoms may be artifactual. Similarly, the chemical structure of drugs that are known to produce psychoticlike behavior is no demonstration that a similar type of chemical structure occurs in the human patient and produces mental disorder. The fact that electrical activity of the reticular activating system [a system of neurons in the brain] is markedly different during sleep, wakefulness, and under a variety of specified conditions does *not*

of itself prove it is the alertness center of the brain. It, too, may only be part of the causal chain, or it may be coincidentally involved. All of these findings are, however, invitations to further investigation, since they constitute preliminary but insufficient "proof."

Control Is Not Sufficient

A patient is treated by a psychiatrist who believes in Pavlovian theory (or Freudian theory or Jungian theory) and who uses techniques compatible with his theory. The fact that the patient recovers does not constitute a "proof" of the psychiatrist's beliefs. The same holds true in the more "exact' disciplines. . . .

Even Prediction Is Not Sufficient

At the core of the scientific method is the ability to predict, and if this is done with two special qualifications observed it is the strongest evidence that we can educe for correctness. The first qualification is that the prediction must be in respect to an irregularly occurring, rare, or new event. [Kline makes this qualification because the more irregular, rare, or new the event, the more difficult it is to predict it and therefore the stronger is the evidence provided by a correct prediction. Predicting that a regular, frequent or customary event will occur—for example, that the sun will rise tomorrow or that a very neurotic child will develop into an emotionally immature adult—is too easy to prove anything.] The other qualification is that the prediction should be disjunctive, that is, that various incompatible alternative possibilities are enumerated, and the ones that will *not* occur, as well as the one that will occur, are specified.

Hence it is not sufficient to say that if a patient has a severe psychic trauma his condition will change. Specifically, what he *will* do and what he *will not* do must be described. . . .

. . . There are many occasions in which theory is not adequately developed nor techniques available for proceeding in this manner. Under these circumstances it is perfectly legitimate to base our working hypothesis and our practice on such evidence as is available. We should, however, strive to develop theory and technique to the point at which new and disjunctive events are predicted and their occurrence empirically verified.

There are difficulties in the investigation of causation in addition to those already discussed.

1. Retrospective information concerning antecedent factors—for example, childhood experiences—that may be significant in the development of a disorder is often extremely difficult to obtain and subject to error, particularly when a long time has elapsed since the antecedent event. Informants may also distort information because of their emotional involvement.

2. Prospective or anterospective information—

---

*Excerpted by permission from Kline, N. S. 1961. On the relationship between neurophysiology, psychophysiology, psychopharmacology, and other disciplines. Section on "Scientific 'Proof.'" Ann. N.Y. Acad. Sci. Vol. 92, Art. 3., pp. 1009–1011.

the accumulation of current information over a period of time—requires long-term and extensive observations of large numbers of individuals. Only a small proportion may be expected to develop the abnormality under study. For example, to investigate the antecedents of schizophrenia by this method, approximately 100 children must be studied for every one who will eventually develop the disorder.

3. Exact experimental replication of a psychiatric disorder or of various hypothetical causal situations is usually not possible. Attempts to reproduce psychiatric syndromes such as schizophrenia by means of various toxic agents or biological deprivation (e.g., deprivation of sleep, oxygen or vitamins) result in incomplete replication of syndromes. The experimental and the natural syndromes have some similarity, but they are not identical. Reasoning from the artificial to the real syndrome is argument by analogy.

CAN ABNORMAL BEHAVIOR BE EXPLAINED?

The difficulties of establishing causation in abnormal psychology are so great that it might be concluded that the task is impossible and ought to be abandoned. Fortunately, this cynical conclusion is unjustified.

Two general truths about causation are well established. First, it is clear that naturalistic theories explain abnormal behavior better than non-naturalistic theories and that several naturalistic types of causes—hereditary, psychological and so forth—affect behavior concurrently. Second, for a number of disorders, specific causation is also well established. We know the cause of Mongolian idiocy, Huntington's chorea, paresis and a great number of other conditions, most of them of organic origin. It is the functional disorders that are most troublesome to explain, but even here there is good evidence that a hereditary factor operates in some functional disorders; that identifiable, physiological factors precipitate, and probably also act as predisposing causes of, some functional disorders; that psychological stress results in disturbed behavior; and that cultural and class variables also result in disturbance. The task of etiological theory is to evaluate these causal factors and construct tentative explanations on the basis of our incomplete and partial evidence, avoiding both cynicism and dogmatism.

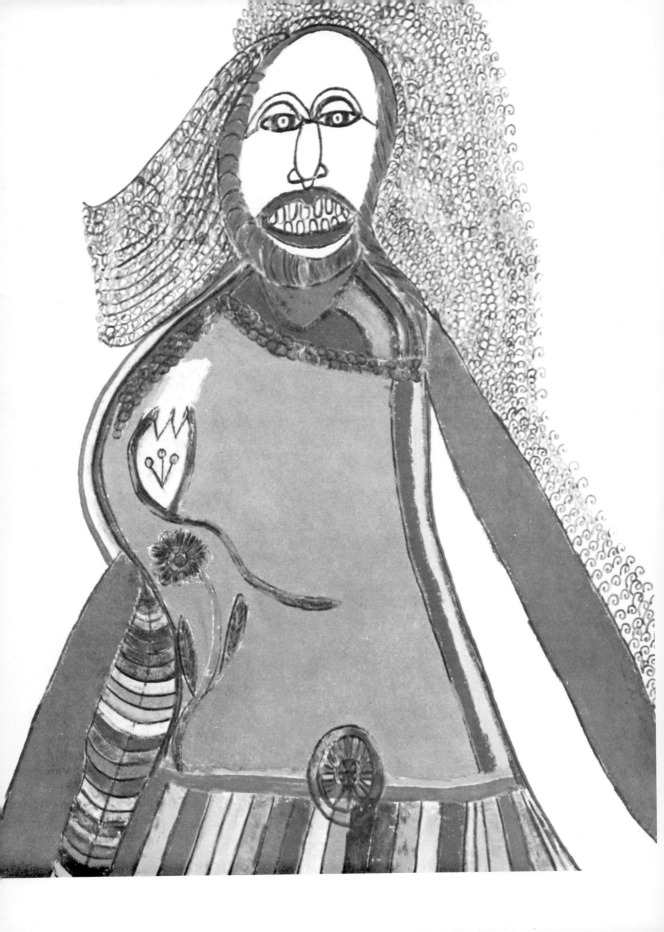

Cruelty and compassion come with the chromosomes.
Aldous Huxley, *Ape and Essence*

6

HEREDITARY AND BIOLOGICAL DETERMINANTS

It is widely believed by laymen that many kinds of emotional disturbances are inherited. References to a patient's "bad blood" or labeling him a "bad seed" reflect a belief that mental illness is passed on from parent to child by inheritance. Extreme proponents of this belief often hold that, since abnormalities are fixed by heredity, they are unchangeable and incurable. A widespread counterview is that psychological difficulties result from unfortunate environment and experience. At the most extreme, this view leads to a belief that abnormalities can be alleviated, or even completely eradicated, by adequate corrective life experiences.

Behavioral scientists have argued the relative merits of hereditary vs. environmental causal explanations for many decades. The nature-nurture issue is still unresolved and it is becoming increasingly clear that neither view can explain all the relevant data. Both causal factors are needed to understand the majority of abnormal behaviors. Mostly it is a matter of relative emphasis. Some scientists are more impressed with the evidence for a hereditary factor in mental disturbances while others tend to emphasize the weight of significant life experiences. Every characteristic of every individual depends upon an interaction between a hereditary predisposition and environmental influences. Our starting point is the observation that all behaviors are a result of both heredity and environment.

However, some behavioral *variations* among individuals are determined mainly by differences in hereditary predisposition, some by differences in the environment and some by an inextricable combination of both. A trait or behavior may be called hereditary if all or most of its interindividual variation results from differences in genetic endowment (for example, the determination of blood groups). A trait or behavior may be termed environmental or acquired if it has little or no genetically determined variation (for example, social customs and language). All other traits and behaviors are markedly influenced by both heredity and environment. For example, body height and weight, intelligence and temperamental variables like emotionality, irritability and energy level seem to be affected strongly by both genetic and nongenetic determinants.

While it is true that the word hereditary has some connotations of fixed immutability, there is no necessary connection between heredity and prognosis. A disorder may have a strong hereditary component and yet be amenable to treatment. Tuberculosis, known to have a hereditary predisposing element, is curable and

77

even preventable. Conversely, a disorder largely due to environmental factors may have a negative prognosis. For example, the effect of continuous, stressful, environmental pressures on some psychotic patients could be so strong that no known method of treatment would suffice to overcome the overwhelming weight of the past. The hereditary-environmental problem is quite different from the problem of curability.

In this chapter we shall be concerned not only with heredity but with the broad range of nonenvironmental contributions to behavior.

Nonenvironmental, biologically based contributors may be differentiated into hereditary, innate, congenital and constitutional factors. Qualities transmitted through the genes by the parents are referred to as hereditary. However, some genes in the germ cell at the moment of conception are not exactly like those of either parent but result from mutations. Strictly speaking, these genes are not inherited in the sense referred to above. The hereditary components plus the changes traced to mutations make up the group termed innate. The term congenital is a broad one used to refer to something present at birth. It thus includes hereditary and innate factors as well as any changes acquired between conception and birth. Finally, constitutional contributors are defined even more broadly, encompassing all the above plus all in life experiences that is physiological or somatic in the determination of changes in the body state.

HEREDITARY FACTORS

Although hereditary contributions to behavior have been studied for many years, the precise mode of inheritance for many disorders has never been determined. A few characteristics are known to be linked to the effect of a single dominant gene while others apparently result from the pairing of recessive genes. Some of these characteristics are sex-linked and others are not. A complication, even with single gene theories of inheritance, is that some genes show partial dominance and partial recessivity. Single gene theories are useful in explaining the occurrence of those characteristics which are identifiable and can be determined to be either present or absent. However, many behaviors occur on a continuum—relatively more or less of a given characteristic may be present. For example, intelligence cannot be said to be either

completely present or completely absent in a given individual. What we observe from a large, random sample of I.Q. scores is, in fact, a normal curve distribution of scores. Height and weight, to take but two other examples, are similarly distributed in the general population. A single gene model of inheritance simply does not fit the facts of such a distribution. To explain characteristics such as height, weight, intelligence and many of the behaviors important in abnormal psychology, it is necessary to utilize a polygenic model of inheritance. Polygenic mechanisms are believed to be involved in continuous, approximately normally distributed characteristics and are due to the combined effects of many minor genes which can join in a large number of combinations.

The Role of Heredity in Sensory and Perceptual Processes

Certain forms of gross defects such as blindness and deafness, which have important psychological consequences, are due to simple mendelian inheritance (i.e., a single dominant or recessive gene). A variety of other major or minor defects in the several senses are also related to genetic endowment.

A well known example of inherited sensory variation is red-green color blindness, frequently quoted as an example of simple sex-linked inheritance. This is an oversimplification of the true state of affairs, however, for no less than four types of color difficulty can be distinguished, suggesting that several genes may be responsible.

In night blindness the rods of the retina are slow to adapt to darkness. This defect exists in a number of forms, either as an isolated trait or in association with various genetically determined eye diseases.

There is reason to believe that differences in sensitivity to smell, taste, touch, pain and temperature stimuli may in part be genetically determined. Some years ago it was discovered that a substance known as phenylthiocarbamide (PTC) was tasteless to some people but very bitter to others. The distribution of taste sensitivity to PTC is bimodal rather than unimodal; it therefore appears that one major cause of individual differences in taste sensitivity to PTC is a single recessive gene.

Finally, some evidence exists for a genetic basis in some—but by no means all—cases of a complex perceptual defect known as *dyslexia*, a persistent inability to read and spell even when general intelligence is high.

Summing up the role of inheritance in sensory and perceptual processes, Fuller and Thompson (1960) state that, "Sensory and perceptual processes are generally more alike in related individuals. Heritability is not limited to anatomical defects (blindness, deafness) or to chemical defects (color blindness), but is found less clearly in more complex perceptual processes." Since sensation and perception are the basis of intellect and emotional behavior, it is at least possible that they also have a hereditary component.

Hereditary Influences on Intelligence, Motor Responses, Temperament and Interests

Some of the most pertinent studies of the relative importance of heredity and environment in the determination of intelligence (as measured by scores on intelligence tests) were performed a generation ago on foster children. Two studies which are quite sound methodologically are summarized in Table 6–1. In both, the correlation between the intelligence scores of children and true parents is consistently higher than the correlation between the intelligence scores of children and foster parents. The findings suggest that heredity is of considerable importance in determining parent-child similarities in intelligence.

Twin Studies. Twins have been used extensively in investigations of the effect of heredity on intelligence as well as on personality characteristics and behavior disorders. In humans, twins may originate as a result of either the separate fertilization of two different ova or the fertilization of one ovum which at a subsequent, but still early, stage of development divides into two separate individuals. Binovular (two-egg) twins are called dizygotic, DZ or fraternal. They may be alike or unlike in sex. Monovular twins, arising from a single fertilized egg, are called monozygotic, MZ or identical. They are always of the same sex.

The relative importance of heredity and environment in determining a given trait may be assessed by comparing the magnitude of trait differences between monozygotic twins with the magnitude of differences between dizygotic twins, preferably like-sex pairs. Since MZ twins have identical genetic structures, any difference in externally manifested characteristics in an MZ pair must be due to environmental influences. In contrast, differences between a pair of DZ twins may be due to either hereditary or environmental influences. It would therefore seem that the relative size of the MZ and DZ differences should reflect the contribution of heredity accurately, but the procedure frequently suffers from methodological difficulties which are described below.

First of all, the determination of zygosity may be incorrect if it is not based on modern serological (blood) tests, which alone permit accurate calculation of zygosity. Prior to the development of the serological tests, it was common to decide that twins were monozygotic (identical) on the basis of fingerprints, physical resemblance or heresay. Gottesman (1961) has shown that such methods often resulted in errors of up to 30 per cent in classification of zygosity. Secondly, in studies of heredity in schizophrenia it has been often the case that the same investigator made the diagnosis of both the index case and the co-twin. Unless co-twins are diagnosed without reference to the index cases there is a danger that the investigator may, out of bias, make the same diagnosis for a pair of MZ twins and a different diagnosis for DZ twins. Such studies may tell us a great deal about the effects of personal bias on judgment while contributing little to our understanding of the influence of heredity. Finally, there are several statistical problems in estimating concordance rates (concordance refers to incidents in which both twins develop the trait under study) and these problems can

TABLE 6–1. Correlations of Intelligence between Parent and Own Children and Parent with Foster Children

	Foster Group: Children and Foster Parents		Control Group: Children and True Parents	
	r	N	r	N
(a) Data of Burks (1928)				
Father's MA	.07	178	.45	100
Mother's MA	.19	204	.46	105
(b) Data of Leahy (1935)				
Father's Otis score	.15	178	.51	175
Mother's Otis score	.20	186	.51	191

Reprinted from Human Heredity by J. V. Neel and W. J. Schull by permission of The University of Chicago Press. Copyright 1954 by The University of Chicago, p. 113.

TABLE 6–2. Correlation Coefficients between Monozygotic and Dizygotic Twins for Intelligence and Other Psychological Tests

Test and Investigator	r_{MZ}	r_{DZ}	H*
Intelligence tests			
Wingfield (National Intelligence Test and McCall's Multimental Scale)	0.90 ✓	0.57	0.77
Herrman and Hogben (Otis)	0.84	0.48	0.69
Newman, Freeman and Holzinger (Binet)	0.88	0.63	0.68
Blewett (factor score)	0.76	0.44	0.57
Eysenck (data of Blewett and McLeod) (factor score)	0.82	0.38	0.71
Other psychological tests			
Mechanical aptitude (Brody)	0.69	0.28	0.57
Motor skills (McNemar)	0.79	0.43	0.63
Bernreuter's neurotic inventory (Carter)	0.63	0.32	0.46
Woodworth-Matthews' neurotic tendencies (Holzinger)	0.56	0.37	0.30
Strong's vocational interests (Carter)	0.50	0.28	0.31
Autonomic factor (Eysenck, data of Blewett and McLeod)	0.93 ✓	0.72	0.75
Neuroticism factor (Eysenck and Prell)	0.85	0.22	0.81 ✓
Extraversion factor (McLeod)	0.77	0.03	0.76 ✓
Extraversion factor (Eysenck, data of Blewett and McLeod)	0.50	−0.33	0.62

*H = estimated heritable component
Modified after Shields, J., and Slater, E. Heredity and psychological abnormality. *In* Eysenck, H. J. (Editor). 1960. Handbook of Abnormal Psychology. London, Pitman Medical Publishing Company, p. 333.

result in either overestimating or underestimating the influence of heredity.

While there are difficulties and many misleading studies, some of the twin study results are impressively consistent. The upper portion of Table 6–2 summarizes the findings of five studies investigating the contribution of heredity to intelligence. The heritable component for intelligence ranges from 57 per cent to 77 per cent.

In the study reported in 1937 by Newman, Freeman and Holzinger (Table 6–3) comparisons were made for height, weight and intelligence in 19 pairs of MZ twins reared apart since early childhood (MZA), a larger sample of MZ twins reared together (MZT) and also a larger sample of DZ twins. The resultant estimates of the environmental determinants of variation (E) were derived from comparing MZA and MZT twins, and the estimates of H (a statistic for estimating the proportion of variance which can be attributed to heredity) from comparing MZ with DZ twins. It should be noted that a negative value for an estimate of environmental or hereditary influence is meaningless. Furthermore, if it is assumed that the effects of environment and heredity are *additive* (other assumptions are possible), then E + H should add up to exactly 1.00 for any given characteristic; that is, 100 per cent of the total variance should be attributable to the sum of the hereditary and environmental contributions. It may be seen from the table that a negative value occurs, and E + H do not add to 1.00, thus emphasizing the fact that the figures are subject to various errors, including these due to small sample sizes. Since the number of twin pairs used to estimate H was considerably larger than the number involved in estimating E, the values for H can be regarded as somewhat more reliable than those for E. Heredity seems to have contributed more heavily to height and weight than to measured I.Q.

Foster child and twin studies cannot provide information from which to deduce the probable mechanism of inheritance. To infer the mechanism, a comparison may be made of the fre-

TABLE 6–3. Degree of Similarity between Monozygotic Twins, Reared Apart or Together, and Dizygotic Twins*

Charac-teristic	Correlation			E	H
	MZA	MZT	DZ		
Height	.969	.932	.645	−0.544	0.808
Weight	.886	.917	.631	+0.272	0.775
I.Q.	670	.881	.631	+0.639	0.678

*Data of Newman, Freeman and Holzinger (1937).
Reprinted from Human Heredity by J. V. Neel and W. J. Schull by permission of The University of Chicago Press. Copyright 1954 by The University of Chicago, p. 276.

quencies or correlations for the characteristic in various classes of relatives with the frequencies or correlations to be expected when some specified mechanism of inheritance is hypothesized. Intelligence test scores are distributed throughout the general population in very close approximation to the normal curve, and correlations between various classes of relatives roughly correspond with those expected on the assumption that the genetic component of intelligence is polygenic (Table 6–4). Siblings correlate highest (.51), then parents and children, then uncles or aunts and nephews or nieces, then grandparents and grandchildren, and lowest of all first cousins (.29). The only departure from the expected order for a polygenic trait is that grandparents and grandchildren do not show the expected higher correlation than uncle or aunt with nephew or niece; instead, the respective correlations are .34 and .35, for all practical purposes identical. Note that for stature there is no departure from the expected order of correlations. For both stature and intelligence the evidence for a polygenic mechanism of inheritance is thus quite impressive.

Comparisons between MZ and DZ twins have been made for a wide variety of psychological tests other than those designed to measure intelligence (see lower portion of Table 6–2). In the tests designed to measure mechanical aptitude, motor skills and temperamental traits, a strong heritable component is suggested by the size of H. The mechanism of inheritance involved is probably polygenic. For neuroticism and neurotic tendencies the findings are inconsistent and for vocational interests H is quite small. However, the tests used are not necessarily the best available to tap the traits under

TABLE 6–4. Correlations for Stature and Intelligence, According to Degree of Relationship

Degree of Relationship	Correlation for Stature	Correlation for Intelligence
Siblings	.54 ✓	.51
Parents and children	.51	.49
Grandparents and grandchildren	.32	.34
Uncles (or aunts) and nephews (or nieces)	.29	.35
First cousins	.24	.29

Data from Burt, C., and Howard, M. 1956. The multifactorial theory of inheritance and its application to intelligence. Brit. J. Statist. Psychol., 9:59.

TABLE 6–5. Heritability of CPI Extraversion-Introversion Scales

Factor	CPI Scale	H	F
Extraversion	Sociability	0.49	1.97+
	Self-acceptance	0.46	1.85+
	Social presence	0.35	1.55+
Introversion	Dominance	0.49	1.95+

+ = significant at the 0.01 level;
Reprinted by permission from Gottesman, I. 1966. Genetic variance in adaptive personality traits. J. Child. Psychol. Psychiat. 7:199–208. Copyright Pergamon Press.

consideration and the studies need replication with better measures.

Gottesman (1966) compared the responses of 79 MZ twins with 68 pairs of DZ twins on the California Personality Inventory (CPI). Those CPI scales which have been found to relate to an Extraversion-Introversion factor were highly related to genetic inheritance (see Table 6–5).

These results may be compared with the findings relevant to a different extraversion measure summarized in Table 6–3. It may be, as these and others suggest, that the tendency to seek out or avoid other people is linked to a genetic inheritance which determines the reaction range of the person to different types of environments.

It is uncertain to what extent the findings from animal experimentation are relevant to the genetics of human intelligence and temperament. A great many interesting animal studies have been carried out to test the inheritance of learning ability, problem-solving ability, emotionality and a variety of different animal behaviors (e.g., Tryon, 1942; Thompson, 1954). In the majority of instances, the heritable determinant of such behavioral characteristics seems to be polygenic in nature. In general the studies indicate that the genetic determination of behavior at the subhuman level is very real and is responsible for much of the variance of behavior.

The Role of Heredity in Behavior Deviations

A large number of degenerations of the central nervous system in man are hereditary, for example, certain types of *ataxia* (incoordination and inability to maintain balance in standing or walking). Various degenerations of the neuromuscular apparatus such as muscular dystrophies (disorders involving paralysis of muscles) and neural atrophy (degeneration of peripheral nerves) are also inherited. These disorders are determined by a variety of single genes—dominant and recessive, sex-linked and autosomal (non-sex-linked). The major manifestations of the disorders are abnormalities of sensation and motor functions rather than intellect or affect.

Epilepsy appears to be partially hereditary. Epileptic seizures sometimes occur as a consequence of structural brain pathology and sometimes in the absence of an identifiable basis in the brain. Twin studies appear to discriminate between these two categories. *Idiopathic epilepsy,* in which there is no identifiable brain damage, seems to have a major heritable component. *Symptomatic epilepsy,* associated with various forms of brain disease, apparently has a relatively small heritable component. Family studies of the idiopathic variety indicate that there are considerably higher frequencies of epilepsy among close relatives of epileptics than among the general population. The frequencies among relatives are smaller than those associated with transmission by a single dominant or recessive gene, and it is therefore probable that the heritable component is polygenic. The hypothesis that proneness to seizures is determined in part by the cumulative action

of multiple minor genes also receives support from animal experiments in selective breeding for vulnerability to seizures. In these experiments it has been found that seizures progressively increase over several generations, as would be expected in the case of polygenic determination of a quantitatively continuous characteristic.

Several of the adult organic brain syndromes which involve behavior symptoms are believed to have a strong heritable component. One of these, Huntington's chorea, is unique in that the mechanism of inheritance has been established beyond reasonable doubt to consist of a single, autosomal, dominant gene with a high rate of expression (Fig. 6–1). Huntington's chorea is marked by speech impairment, intellectual impairment and emotional disturbance. The same mechanism of inheritance has been postulated in the case of a presenile psychosis known as Pick's disease, in which atrophy of the cerebral cortex occurs. Polygenic transmission, on the other hand, is usually considered more probable for the genetic component of a form of presenile psychosis with atrophy of the cerebral cortex known as Alzheimer's disease and for psychoses due to deterioration in the senile period. The evidence in the case of these last three conditions is less clear, however, than for Huntington's chorea.

Among the large group of psychophysiologic disorders the significance of hereditary factors

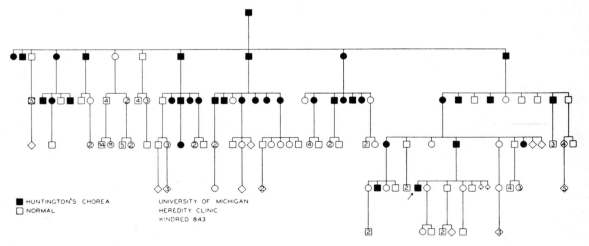

Figure 6–1. *"A pedigree of Huntington's chorea. A single dominant autosomal gene is responsible for the onset at about age thirty to forty of the degeneration of various areas in the brain. In many pedigrees there appears to be a deficiency of affected persons because of the death of carriers of the gene before the age of onset." (Reprinted from Human Heredity by J. V. Neel and W. J. Schull by permission of The University of Chicago Press. Copyright 1954 by The University of Chicago.)*

TABLE 6–6. Concordance for Mental Illness in Twins of Diagnosed Schizophrenia*

Status of Co-Twin	MZ		DZ	
	No. Pairs	%	No. Pairs	%
1. Hospitalized for schizophrenia	10	42	3	9
2. Other psychiatric hospitalization plus hospitalized for schizophrenia	13	54	6	18
3. Marked abnormality plus other psychiatric hospitalization, plus hospitalized for schizophrenia	19	79	15	45
4. Normal	5	21	18	55
Total	24	100	33	100

*Adapted from Gottesman, I., and Shields, J. 1966. Brit. J. Psychiat., *112*:809–818.

remains largely undetermined. Heredity is believed to contribute to the etiology of hyperthyroidism and peptic ulceration, at least in certain families. Persons of blood group O are about 40 per cent more susceptible to peptic ulceration than other blood groups, suggesting the importance of genetic factors. In the psychosomatic disorder known as essential hypertension, arterial blood pressure is high; arterial pressure itself is thought to have a hereditary predisposition.

The role of hereditary predispositions in determining vulnerability to the functional disorders is a matter of controversy and neither the exact importance of heredity and environment nor the specific mechanisms of inheritance have been conclusively established for them. However, there is strong evidence that heredity plays *some* part in functional disorders. The most extensive studies of psychological disorders using twins have been carried out for schizophrenia.

A study of Gottesman and Shields (1966) provides one example of the many which have been reported. They studied 77 pairs of twins in which one twin had been admitted to Mandsly Hospital with a diagnosis of schizophrenia. As can be seen from Table 6–6, 10 of the 24 MZ co-twins had also been hospitalized for schizophrenia, whereas only 3 of the 33 DZ co-twins had received a diagnosis identical to their index case. Seventy-nine per cent of the MZ co-twins and 45 per cent of the DZ co-twins either had developed schizophrenia or had been hospitalized for other emotional disorders or gave other evidence of marked abnormality.

Only 5 of 24 MZ co-twins appeared normal while 18 of 33 DZ co-twins had no detectable emotional disturbance.

Estimates of the heritable component in twin studies have consistently varied over the reasonably small range of 63 to 84 per cent. These figures are quite large, but owing to the methodological difficulties of twin studies emphasized earlier the precise importance of heredity in schizophrenia is unsettled; one can only say heredity makes *some* contribution to the disorder. The problem of the mechanism of transmission in schizophrenia is also unsolved.

It is important to keep in mind that heredity is a predisposition only. Stressful environmental events as well as a genetic predisposition seem to be essential for the development of most, and perhaps all, cases of schizophrenia. A hereditary predisposition may be a necessary cause of a disorder, yet not be sufficient. The lifetime expectancy for schizophrenia (i.e., the total percentage of persons who develop the disorder during their lifetime) has been estimated as approximately 1 per cent, but the genetic potentiality for schizophrenia is probably much more widely distributed.

A number of twin and family studies for other functional disorders such as manic-depressive psychosis and the neuroses have been based on small and often inadequate samples. In some studies, higher concordance rates for MZ twins have been reported for manic-depressive psychosis than for schizophrenia, but other studies of manic-depression have reported low rates. The estimates of H for manic-depression have varied from 0.39 to 1.00. On the other hand, familial frequencies for manic-depression—for example, parent-child and sibling-sibling combinations—have been consistently high. There seems to be a definite genetic factor in manic-depressive psychosis but it is of uncertain weight.

In Table 6–7, the expected percentages reported by Brown (1942) are given for parents of index cases categorized according to three types of neurosis. The results are quite different for the three types. Thus the lifetime expectancy—the probability of developing the

TABLE 6–7. Expectancy Rates for Various Kinds of Neurotic Disorders in Parents of Index Cases

Types of Index Cases	Per Cent of Affected Parents
Anxiety neurotics	21.4
Hysterics	19.0
Obsessionals	7.5

Modified after Brown, F. W. In Fuller, J. L., and Thompson, W. R. 1949. Behavior Genetics. New York, John Wiley & Sons, Inc., p. 295.

disorder at some time during the person's life—is 21.4 per cent that a parent of an anxiety neurotic also is or will be an anxiety neurotic, 19.0 per cent that a parent of a hysteric will be diagnosed hysteric and only 7.5 per cent for a parent of an obsessive. Hence, with respect to heredity, neurosis is not a unity and cannot be inherited as such. Insofar as neurosis may have a genetic component, each neurotic type is genetically different. Furthermore, the percentages are not too high to be accounted for by such processes as identification of a child with a neurotic parent, response to a common environment on the part of a parent and child, and direct parental reinforcement of those childhood modes of behavior that are similar to the parent's own neurotic behaviors. On the basis of this and other studies, it appears that although close relatives are more likely than members of the general population to manifest a disorder similar to that of a neurotic patient, hereditary determination in neurosis is unproved.

Geneticists consider it extremely unlikely that any of the functional disorders is determined by a single dominant gene or a single pair of recessive genes. Whatever genetic predisposition exists in any of these disorders is much more likely to be polygenic. One possibility, however, is that some of the functional disorders, as presently defined by clinical diagnosis, may eventually prove to consist of two or more subtypes, each with varying degrees of hereditary predisposition. If such were to be the case, then within one clinical disorder there could be a subtype transmitted by a single, rare gene, a subtype resulting from the cumulative effects of multiple minor genes and a subtype resulting primarily from environmental influences with no appreciable hereditary determination. Our present classification system is not final and it may be modified by future findings in genetics.

The promise of genetics in abnormal psychology is exciting. If the genetic components of a disorder can be isolated, then it becomes possible to identify the particular environment which may enhance or inhibit the development of the behavior in question. It may then be possible to develop treatments which are designed to maximize adaptive behaviors while minimizing the likelihood of maladaptive ones. At another level of prevention it would be possible to provide sound genetic counseling for couples identified as having a high likelihood of producing affected children.

In summary, the inferences we may make from the results of animal genetic studies and from studies of sensation, perception, intelligence, motor responses and temperament in humans suggest that it is reasonable to expect human behavior deviations to have a genetic component. This expectation has been confirmed for several organic syndromes and types of mental deficiency, some psychophysiologic disorders, schizophrenia and manic-depression. However, with a few exceptions the exact importance of heredity and the precise genetic mechanism in each disorder remain to be determined.

BIOLOGICAL DETERMINANTS OF BEHAVIOR

Nonhereditary biological determinants of behavior may be either predisposing or precipitating in character.

Biological precipitants consist of noxious agents, such as disease-producing bacteria, toxic chemicals and physical injury, and deprivation of necessary biological substances such as oxygen, vitamins, hormones and the like. Both noxious agents and deprivation may precipitate a functional disorder to which the individual is predisposed or may cause structural changes in the brain.

To explore the behavioral effects of predisposing or precipitating biological factors, several different lines of inquiry have been followed. The first approach attempts merely to correlate behavior with concurrent biological variables. A second research design attempts to correlate behavior with earlier biological events such as antecedent glandular changes or childhood diseases. Third, a number of investigators have studied the effects of the administration of toxic drugs and the deprivation of oxygen, vitamins and sleep on the behavior of normal individuals; some of these studies have been motivated by the desire to *reproduce experi-mentally* the symptoms of naturally occurring disorders, particularly schizophrenia. Fourth, *the behavior of animals* subjected to special biological conditions has been observed. Fifth, the effect of drugs and other biological agents in modifying *the behavior of patients* has been investigated. For the purpose of inferring causa-tion, none of these research designs is com-pletely free of the logical difficulties discussed in an earlier chapter. Nevertheless, the results of the different designs have been sufficiently con-sistent when taken all together to provide solid evidence of the importance of biological causa-tion in behavior disturbance.

The organism may be subjected to biological stress by more sudden or intense exposure to noxious agents or deprivation than it can tole-rate. Stress may be defined broadly as the *ex-ternal or internal stimulus conditions, noxious or depriving, which demand very difficult ad-justments.* Stress may consist of emotional trauma and emotional deprivation as well as biological conditions. A *stress reaction* is a severe disturbance of the balance and regulation of functioning that results from exposure to stress stimuli. The organism must always adjust to changing stimuli, but under stress the ad-justment is onerous or even impossible.

The precipitating biological causes of ab-normal behavior—both naturally occurring and experimentally induced—and the stress reac-tions of the organism to these precipitants are discussed in the following section, followed by a survey of the more remote, predisposing, biological causes.

Precipitating Causes

Noxious Agents

External noxious agents are necessary causes of various types of acute and chronic brain syndromes and mental deficiency. Functional disorders also are sometimes pre-cipitated by noxious agents. An individual may be genetically or psychologically predisposed to schizophrenia, depression or neurosis, but the actual symptoms of one of these disturbances may appear only after exposure to a noxious agent.

The three classes of noxious agents—dis-ease-producing microorganisms, toxic chemicals and physical injury—include a tre-mendous number of specific individual agents.

The brain may be severely affected by the microorganisms of general bodily infections, by infections mainly localized in the skull, or by a brain abscess. A variety of chemical poisons such as lead, carbon tetrachloride, carbon monoxide, methyl alcohol and many others may result in brain disorder. Structural or func-tional brain pathology may be caused by concussions, brain lacerations and other types of physical trauma. The brain may be damaged by these injuries either directly or through inter-ference with its blood supply.

The brain disturbances or syndromes pre-cipitated by these noxious agents may consist of a temporary and reversible disruption of mental functioning or a permanent and irrevers-ible impairment. In both cases disorientation, memory loss and other signs of intellectual difficulty occur. The brain syndromes called toxic psychoses, produced by toxic drugs, are marked by particularly vivid visual illusions and hallucinations as well as by the disorientation and memory loss common to all brain syndromes.

Drugs called hallucinogens or psychotomi-metics have been used experimentally to pro-duce disturbed behavior in normal persons. There are early accounts of certain Mexican Indian and Arabian cultures in which certain compounds were eaten or smoked for their hallucinogenic properties.

Within this century, several species of mush-rooms indigenous to Mexico have been found to possess hallucinogenic properties. Portions of a particular variety of cactus (mescal buttons or peyote) have been used by the Aztecs and subsequently by other residents of northern Mexico and the southwestern regions of the United States to produce intoxication. *Mesca-line,* a hallucinogen now widely used, was isolated from this plant in 1888. Mescaline pro-duces distorted and hallucinatory sense per-ceptions together with some degree of clouded consciousness, intellectual impairment and con-fusion, paranoid thinking and lack of emotional control. It has been claimed that the behavioral picture closely resembles an acute type of schizophrenia.

The particularly schizophrenic-like symptom induced by hallucinogens is the subject's feel-ing that he is simultaneously aware of occur-rences in both his inner and outer worlds; he experiences a kind of double consciousness. However, psychotomimetics do not produce the auditory hallucinations common in schizo-phrenia but, instead, result in vivid visual illusions and hallucinations, resembling the effects of toxic psychoses in this one respect. The other symptoms of naturally occurring schizophrenia—difficulty in communication with others and a tendency to inappropriate affect—can be induced by hallucinogens, but the induced verbal and affective difficulties differ considerably from the comparable schizophrenic symptoms. No known drug can reproduce *exactly* the manifestations of schizophrenia or any of the other naturally occurring emotional disorders.

Osmond and Smythies (1952) drew attention to some similarities between the chemical structures of mescaline and epinephrine (also known as Adrenalin; it is produced by the adrenal glands and increases heart rate and blood pressure). On separate grounds, the adrenal functioning of schizophrenics had previously been suspected by various investigators to be disturbed. The observations of Osmond and Smythies stimulated a search for components of epinephrine, or substances related to it, that would be capable of reproducing the clinical manifestations of schizophrenia. Several such substances have been reported; they induce temporary psychotic states but none has proved beyond doubt to be present at higher than normal concentrations in *natural,* acute schizophrenics. The experimental studies of the effects of mescaline have thus not provided convincing evidence of the role of toxic substances in the causation of schizophrenia, but current and future research may lead to a different conclusion.

One of the most commonly known hallucinogens is LSD-25 (lysergic acid diethylamide), which has been the subject of widespread, and often controversial press coverage in recent years. The hallucinogenic properties of LSD were discovered accidentally in 1938 by the Swiss research chemist A. Hofmann. Hofmann had hoped to combine in a new compound a uterus-contracting agent and a central nervous system stimulant. Indeed, LSD has these properties but, in addition, was found to have other, unexpected effects as well. Hofmann's account of his experience as the first man on an ''acid trip'' is informative:*

Being a cautious man, I started my experiment by taking 0.25 mg. of d-lysergic acid-diethylamide tar-

---

*Hofmann, A. The discovery of LSD and subsequent investigations on naturally occurring hallucinogens. *In* Ayd, F., Jr., and Blackwell, B. (Eds.) Discoveries in Biological Psychiatry. Philadelphia, J. B. Lippincott, 1970.

trate, thinking that such an extremely small dose would surely be harmless.

After 40 minutes I noted in my laboratory journal: slight giddiness, restlessness, difficulty in concentration, visual disturbances, laughing.

At this point the laboratory protocol ends. The last words are hardly legible and were written down only with greatest difficulty. It was now obvious that LSD was responsible for the earlier intoxication. I requested my laboratory technician to accompany me home. Since it was war time and no car was available, we went by bicycle. This trip is about four miles and I had the feeling of not getting ahead, whereas my escort stated that we were rolling along at a good speed. I lost all control of time. I noticed with dismay that my environment was undergoing progressive changes. My visual field wavered and everything appeared deformed as in a faulty mirror. Space and time became more and more disorganized and I was overcome by a fear that I was going crazy. The worst part of it being that I was clearly aware of my condition. The mind and power of observation were unimpaired. I was not, however, capable, by any act of will, of preventing the breakdown of the world around me. At home the physician was called.

At the height of the experience, the following symptoms were most marked:

Visual disturbances, everything appearing in impossible colours, objects out of proportion. At times the floor seemed to bend and the walls to undulate. The faces of the persons present changed into colorful grimaces.

Marked motor restlessness alternating with paralysis. Limbs and head felt heavy as if filled with lead and were without sensation!

Occasionally I felt as if I were out of my body. I thought I had died. My Ego seemed suspended somewhere in space, whereas I saw my dead body lying on the sofa.

When the physician arrived, approximately 2½ hours after I took the drug, he reported that my cardiac function was normal, pulse good, blood pressure normal, respiration deep and regular.

In the course of the evening, the symptoms subsided gradually and then disappeared completely. Only the visual disturbances persisted somewhat longer. It was particularly striking how acoustic perceptions, such as the noise of water gushing from a tap or the spoken word, were transformed into optical illusions. Then I fell asleep and awakened next morning somewhat tired but otherwise feeling perfectly well.

Hofmann's experiences have been replicated numerous times by subsequent investigators. Some people have such extremely unpleasant experiences that psychological or medical intervention is necessary in order to restore the individual to his pre-drug state. Others report intense dreamlike states which are filled with pleasant images and tender feelings of love and closeness. Whether the experience will be pleasant or unpleasant is heavily dependent on the individual's emotional adjustment and on the context in which the drug is taken. Thus, hallucinogens do not act by inducing unambiguous pharmacological effects. Rather, their effect is the result of an interaction between the chemistry of the drug, the personality of the subject and the setting in which the drug is administered (Blacker, 1969).

LSD, and indeed all hallucinogens, are potent chemicals about which current information as to their possible long-term effects is still incomplete. Some persons have argued that hallucinogens are harmless drugs which merely expand a person's consciousness and thereby free him for creative living. Others predict dire consequences and warn against any use of such drugs under any circumstances. Doubtless, the truth will be found to lie somewhere between these extremes. Nevertheless, the use and misuse of what are frequently impure preparations by the uninformed and the immature, the sensational press coverage devoted to some reported hallucinogenic drug effects, and the fact that much vital knowledge is still missing led to restrictions on the legal distribution of many depressant and stimulant drugs. Since 1966, LSD has been supplied only to qualified investigators registered with the Food and Drug Administration.

Biological Deprivation

Pellagra, a disease often accompanied by confused mental states, was attributed to poor diet as long ago as the eighteenth century and is now known to be due to vitamin deficiency. Vitamin deficiencies during early embryonic development have been shown to affect brain structure in experimental animals. It has been established that in human adults dietary deficiency of certain vitamins (particularly members of the so-called B-complex such as thiamine, niacin and B_{12}) may result in organic brain syndromes with gross impairment of intellectual functions or in the release of latent symptoms of functional psychosis or neurosis.

Among the substances necessary for adequate biological and mental functioning is *glucose,* a sugar derived by the body from carbohydrates. About 90 per cent of the energy used by brain cells is derived from glucose. A severe deficiency of glucose can be brought about by injections of the hormone insulin, resulting in a temporary, organic brain syndrome characterized by clouding of conscious-

ness, impairment of intellectual functions, release of latent behavior abnormalities and accentuation of abnormalities already present. The insulin coma treatment for schizophrenia, a very popular type of therapy prior to the discovery of tranquilizing drugs, deliberately induces a temporary deficiency of glucose.

Deficiencies of adrenal, thyroid, pituitary and other hormones, manufactured and secreted internally by the endocrine or ductless glands, may occur for a variety of reasons and may result in a diversity of abnormal behaviors. For example, *hypothyroidism* (insufficient thyroid activity) may stem from structural or functional pathology of the thyroid gland and may be responsible for the type of mental deficiency in young children known as *cretinism,* or for the equivalent disorder in older persons, *myxedema.* The latter is characterized by apathy and lethargy as well as mental dullness.

Neurosis has been experimentally induced by starvation. Keys (1952) observed 36 World War II conscientious objectors during a voluntary regimen of three months on an adequate diet, followed by six months of semi-starvation on an extremely low calorie diet and finally by several months of nutritional rehabilitation. In the semi-starvation period the men lost about one-fourth their previous body weight. Self ratings during the pre-starvation and semi-starvation periods are shown in Table 6–8. The ratings for depression, moodiness, irritability, apprehension, apathy and sensitivity to noise increased while ratings for desirable traits and affects decreased. Additional evaluation of emo-

TABLE 6–8. Average Self Ratings of the Subjects in the Minnesota Experiment During Pre-starvation Control Period (C) and After 12 and 24 Weeks of Semi-starvation.

Symptom	C	S12	S24
Depression	0	.69	1.38
Moodiness	0	.84	1.50
Irritability	0	1.31	1.81
Apprehension	−.03	.34	.41
Apathy	0	1.09	1.81
Sensitivity to noise	0	1.31	1.81
Ambition	0	−1.19	−1.75
Self-discipline	0	−.56	−1.72
Mental alertness	0	−.84	−1.53
Concentration	0	−.91	−1.66
Comprehension	0	−.44	−1.03

Reprinted by permission from Keys, A. 1952. Experimental induction of psychoneuroses by starvation. *In* The Biology of Mental Health and Disease. New York, Hoeber-Harper, p. 520.

tional states was obtained by administration of the Minnesota Multiphasic Personality Inventory. Figure 6–2 shows the mean profiles during the pre-starvation control period (C), after 24 weeks of semi-starvation (S24) and after 32 weeks of rehabilitation (R32). The most noticeable elevations during semi-starvation occurred on the scales for hypochondriacal bodily complaints (Hs), depression of mood (D) and hysteria (Hy). These three scales are ordinarily elevated in naturally occurring neurosis.

Anoxia—a deficiency of the oxygen supply to the tissues—has very dramatic and important effects on behavior. It is well established that structural changes in the adult animal brain result from anoxia which may be induced by an inadequate proportion of oxygen in the atmosphere, or by halting the circulation of blood to the brain or by deep and prolonged intake of nitrous oxide, an anesthetic popularly known as laughing gas. Nerve cells are very sensitive to lack of oxygen, and complete anoxia need be of only brief duration to cause profound and permanent damage. Milder degrees of oxygen deficiency over a longer period of time may also result in permanent brain damage in adult animals. Severe anoxia near the time of birth may result in either death, structural damage to the brain with consequent neurological symptoms (as in congenital cerebral palsy) or life-long mental deficiency. The maze-learning ability of experimental animals subjected to anoxia at birth is consistently lower than that of litter mates not so subjected.

Anoxia has a drastic effect on complex mental functions such as immediate memory. In addition, subjects note increased mental turpitude, greater criticalness of others, heightened sensory irritability, touchiness, frequently recurring ideas, and difficulty in concentrating.

Figure 6–3 shows the deterioration of handwriting during the course of an hour as the oxygen content of the atmosphere was artificially lowered from normal sea-level concentration to the concentration found at an altitude of 28,000 feet. The subject had no insight into his intellectual impairment. He remained cheerful for the whole hour and felt that he was performing adequately except for occasional temporary blanks. At 23,000 feet he stated that his feet felt a long way off and he was unable to orient other parts of his body. At 26,000 feet he was greatly incapacitated but appeared well satisfied with his performance. He was quite annoyed when removed from the apparatus at 28,000 feet and insisted that he could have gone much higher. Had the oxygen content been further reduced the consequences would have been unconsciousness and lasting brain damage or death.

Sleep deprivation has interested a number of investigators in recent years. As far back as the Spanish Inquisition sleep deprivation was used to impair personality function and extract confessions of heresy and evildoing. In the Korean War captured American fliers, deprived of sleep and subjected to other stress, sometimes confessed to having engaged in germ warfare. In 1896, Patrick and Gilbert kept three students awake for 90 hours and found decreases in sensory acuity, reaction time, motor speed and ability to memorize; hallucinations were reported in one subject. In more recent times, several studies were reported in which some subjects developed psychotic symptoms following prolonged, total sleep deprivation. Some investigators theorized that the ultimate result of prolonged deprivation (100 hours or more of wakefulness) was a temporary psychosis. Later studies have failed to confirm this hypothesis. The subject's response to sleep loss depends upon his age, physical condition, the stability of his mental health, expectations of those around him, and the support he receives from his environment (Johnson, 1969). Sleep loss may act like any other precipitating stressor by reactivating previous acute symptoms.

While psychosis does not inevitably follow prolonged total sleep deprivation, there often are pronounced and incapacitating behavioral changes. These changes include irritability,

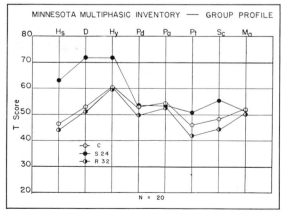

Figure 6–2. *(Reprinted by permission from Keys, A. 1952. Experimental induction of psychoneuroses by starvation. In The Biology of Mental Health and Disease. New York, Hoeber-Harper.)*

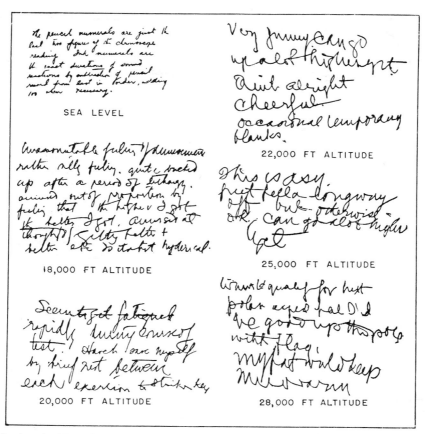

SEA LEVEL

18,000 FT ALTITUDE

20,000 FT ALTITUDE

22,000 FT ALTITUDE

25,000 FT ALTITUDE

28,000 FT ALTITUDE

Figure 6–3. *The handwriting of a subject gradually deteriorated at progressively higher altitudes (simulated). In comparison with the normal handwriting, that at higher altitudes shows an increase in size, muscular incoordination and omission of letters. (From McFarland, R. A. 1932. The psychological effects of oxygen deprivation (anoxemia) on human behavior. Arch. Psychol., 145.)*

feelings of persecution, inability to concentrate, and periods of disorientation or misperception. Illusions and hallucinations may be present and typically are visual or tactual rather than auditory. Behavioral changes become more pronounced as sleep loss continues and are usually more pronounced in the early morning hours.

Besides the behavioral changes, researchers have noticed mild neurological changes in healthy young adults. However, for persons susceptible to seizures sleep deprivation may be a highly activating stress. In addition to the aforementioned effects, there may be autonomic nervous system effects (i.e., constriction of peripheral blood vessels and reduced ability to respond to external stimuli), particularly as wakefulness exceeds the 200 hour mark.

Advances in sleep research technology have made it possible to distinguish between various stages of sleep which tend to repeat themselves throughout the night. One stage is called REM sleep, after the rapid eye movements which occur. Subjects awakened during REM sleep report having been dreaming about 75 per cent of the time. Persons awakened during non-REM sleep report dreaming only about 7 per cent of the time. These findings led investigators to study the effects of depriving subjects of different stages of sleep rather than of total sleep.

Initially, it was observed that subjects deprived of REM sleep spent more time in REM sleep in subsequent nights before returning to their typical base level. As subjects were continually awakened as they entered REM sleep they tended to slip into REM stage sleep more and more quickly so that awakenings were required more frequently. It was believed for a while that persons deprived of REM sleep were being dream-deprived and thus tried to make up dream time. Investigators began to look at the effects of "dream deprivation." Fisher (1965) summarized the early findings:*

As judged by frequent clinical interviews, the subjects tolerated the dream suppression procedure well and continued to engage in their usual school and work activities. However, a number of mild-to-moderate disturbances of certain ego functions developed in the subjects exposed to more prolonged periods of dream deprivation (four to seven days) . . . (*i*) moderate degrees of tension and anxiety with a major anxiety attack in one subject; (*ii*) brief period of depersonalization in one subject; (*iii*) disturbances in motor coordination, e.g., dropping of small objects; (*iv*) memory disturbances, e.g., forgetting appointment; (*v*) difficulty in concentration; (*vi*) increased startle reaction in one subject; (*vii*) development of irritability and hostility; (*viii*) disturbances in time sense in several subjects. . . .

Later investigators failed to support these findings and raised other hypotheses to account for the finding that subjects appear to try to make up lost REM sleep. It now appears that certain types of physiological activity, particularly in the brain, occur predominantly during REM sleep, and it is the "need" which subjects try to make up if deprived, though not on an hour for hour basis. More data will have to be gathered before definitive statements can be made about the effects of partial sleep deprivation. It does seem clear that REM sleep deprivation results in a hyper-response state (such as increased heart rate, increased activity, and increased sexuality), while stage 4 ("deep" sleep stage) deprivation results in a hypo-response stage manifested by decreased aggressiveness, increased physical complaints and withdrawal (Webb, 1969).

Luby and his associates (1959) have pointed out that sleep deprivation provides a unique opportunity for correlative studies of biochemical functions and behavior. In a carefully executed study they found that sleep deprivation produced a progressive depletion of the body chemical substances that are necessary for the production of energy. Similar, although not identical, chemical depletion has been reported in schizophrenic patients and in adult monkeys reared in isolation. The implication seems to be that the biological stress of sleep deprivation in normal humans and the psychological stress of isolation in monkeys lead to chemical reactions

*By permission, Fisher, C. 1965. Psychoanalytic implications of recent research on sleep and dreaming: Part I, Empirical findings. J. Amer. Psychoanal. Assn., *13*:197–205.

that conceivably are related to basic processes in schizophrenia. One of the difficulties of chronic schizophrenics may be their inability to mobilize the energy needed for adaptation due to a genetic defect or a history of overwhelming stress, or both.

The Stress Reaction

The great nineteenth century French physiologist Claude Bernard pointed out that the living parts of complex organisms are surrounded by an internal, fluid environment, such as blood and lymph, which must be constant for life to exist. The object of all physiological mechanisms, he hypothesized, is solely the preservation of this constancy. These concepts were elaborated by Cannon (1932), who gave the name *homeostasis* to the maintenance of internal constancy when the organism is disturbed by external and internal stress conditions. For example, homeostatic mechanisms come into play in an effort to maintain an optimal proportion of salt in the body fluids when one or another kind of stress results in a reduction of the total amount of fluid. More recently, Selye and his associates (1952) have provided a detailed and useful theory of the organism's reaction to stress. Selye's theory includes an account of how homeostasis breaks down—*the stress reaction*—under sufficiently severe conditions.

The basis of Selye's theory was his observation of the responses of various species of animals to such different conditions as infections, intoxications, physical trauma, heat, cold, muscular fatigue, x-rays and severe emotional pressure; in Selye's terminology these are referred to as *stressors.* No two of these agents have the same specific effect on the body, yet over and above diverse specific effects, they all result in a stereotyped reaction to stress per se. This reaction, termed the *general adaptation syndrome* by Selye, consists of three stages.

The first stage of the general adaptation syndrome consists of three organic changes. (1) The cortex or outer portion of the adrenal gland increases in size, becomes hyperactive and overproduces several hormones that help the body in its attempt to cope with the stressor. (2) The thymus and lymph glands decrease in size and function; concomitantly there is a reduction of certain white cells in the blood with a consequent loss of resistance to infection. (3) Signs of organic shock appear, such as a drop in blood pressure and ulceration of the stomach and intestines. It is striking that while reduction in size and degenerative changes occur in many organs of the body in this stage of the adaptation syndrome, the cortex of the adrenal gland alone increases in size and activity. Hence Selye suspected that the adrenal response plays the crucial role in the first stage of the general adaptation syndrome and that this stage is essentially a biologic defense mechanism which he termed the *alarm reaction.* It can be subdivided into two successive phases—an initial phase of disorganized shock and a second phase in which the organism counters the shock by attempting to restore its homeostatic balance.

The second stage of the general adaptation syndrome is that of *resistance.* In this stage, the organism's continued attempts to restore a physiological balance are fairly successful and an adequate adaptation to the specific stressor occurs. The third and final stage, following prolonged exposure to the stressor, is *exhaustion*; in this stage resistance and homeostasis can no longer be maintained. The three stages of the general adaptation syndrome are diagramed in the solid line of Figure 6–4; the dotted line shows that resistance to other or extraneous stressors simultaneously imposed on the organism decreases even in the second stage of resistance to the major source of stress. Thus, the organism may succumb to additional secondary burdens or stressors even while successfully resisting a primary stressor. It is as if energy is entirely used up in fighting the first difficulty.

Changes in bodily function and structure may occur in any of the three stages. Tissue degeneration, such as ulceration of the stomach and intestines, is most prominent in the initial phase of the alarm reaction and again in the final stage of exhaustion. Since it has been clearly established that these bodily changes may be caused by prolonged emotional as well as biological stressors, it appears that Selye's general adaptation syndrome is of great relevance to the development of human psychophysiologic disorders. The adaptation syndrome may also be applicable to the development of neuroses and functional psychoses under emotional stress.

PREDISPOSING CAUSES

Differences in Constitutional Predisposition

Responses to psychological stress differ considerably from person to person. In experiments in which subjects are required to carry out intellectual tasks while being criticized before an unsympathetic audience, threatened with electric shock for errors and distracted by intense visual and auditory stimuli, there are wide variations in performance from subject to subject. Most subjects display a decrement in performance as compared to the level achieved in non-stress conditions, but some maintain their prestress levels and some actually improve.

Responses to biological stress also vary widely from person to person. For example,

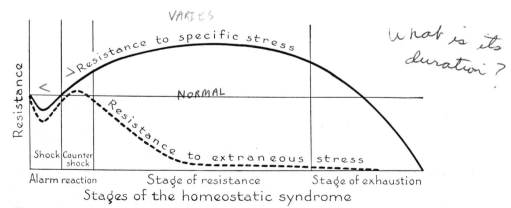

Figure 6–4. *Changes in resistance to specific and extraneous stresses during the general adaptation syndrome. During shock, the organism is less resistant to the specific and extraneous stresses. During countershock, the organism builds up a resistance to all stresses. During the period of resistance, there is an increase in the resistance to the specific stress. At the same time the resistance to other (extraneous) stresses decreases, so that the organism may easily succumb to them. (After Selye, H. 1946. General adaptation syndrome and diseases of adaptation. J. Clin. Endocrinol., 6:117–230.)*

deficient O₂ (handwritten note)

McFarland (1952) investigated differences in the responses of psychoneurotic patients and normal control subjects to anoxia. The neurotics' reactions were much poorer. Koranyi and Lehmann (1960) deprived six chronic schizophrenic patients of sleep for 100 hours and reported the reappearance of symptoms which had not been present since the early phase of the patients' breakdowns.

NB (handwritten note) These and many other observations indicate that reactions to psychological and biological precipitants are a function of both psychological and biological predispositions, often referred to as *constitution*.

Constitution consists of those *relatively enduring biological characteristics,* in part due to heredity and in part to experience, that influence responses to immediate stimuli. Defined this way, some aspects of constitution are more strongly affected by heredity than others. Research has focused on two classes of constitutional factors, *(1)* the morphological, or structural, and *(2)* the physiological. Morphological characteristics include body size; body structure or physique (also termed bodily habitus or somatotype); the distribution and relative development of muscle, fat, bone and connective tissues; disharmonious growth of body parts (dysplasia); and the balance of masculine and feminine physical characteristics. Of these, physique has been most studied, usually by correlating it with nonphysical variables. Investigations, for the most part, also correlational, into the physiological factors in constitution have explored the relation of behavior to autonomic, central and peripheral nervous-system processes; cardiac, circulatory and other visceral functions; and various biochemical and endocrine factors.

Physique or Body Structure

Belief in a correspondence between behavior and bodily configuration goes back to antiquity. The physicians of Greece and Rome postulated relations between body build and susceptibility to certain physical diseases. Modern studies have investigated the relations among three variables: (1) physique, (2) temperamental and personality traits and (3) psychiatric disorders. These studies were stimulated by the work of Kretschmer, who distinguished four main types of physique: (1) *The asthenic or leptosomatic type.* This individual is slender and has long bones and poor muscular development. Kret-

schmer considered this type to be almost invariably associated with schizoid personality (schizophrenic-like or "shut-in" personality) and to be vulnerable to overt schizophrenia. (2) *The athletic type.* This type is marked by sturdiness and strength, wide shoulders and well-developed muscles. (3) *The pyknic or pyknosomatic type.* This individual is stocky, plump and rounded. Kretschmer believed that pyknics almost invariably had cyclothymic personalities (extraverted, with alternating and changeable moods) and were prone to manic-depressive psychosis. (4) *The dysplastic type.* In this type endocrine disturbances occur and body development is disproportionate; an example is the body distortion due to disorders of the pituitary gland. (See Figure 6–5 for illustrations of the first three of these types.)

In a large-scale study of psychotics, Kretschmer reported that among asthenic patients there were 81 schizophrenics and only 4 manic-depressives, and among pyknics there were 58 manic-depressives and only 4 schizophrenics. Dysplastic and athletic types also tended to schizophrenia; only the pyknics had, in Kretschmer's phrase, a "clear biological affinity" for manic-depression. The results are consistent with Kretschmer's belief that mental disorder, the varieties of normal personality, and body type are systemically associated.

In recent years, it has been increasingly recognized that more than one scale or dimension is needed to describe physique. It has also become clear that the physical characteristics on which classifications of body type are based are continuously rather than dichotomously distributed, with most individuals falling near the middle of each distribution. Recent studies have therefore used classification systems that comprise several scales, each with several—rather than just two—steps.

Sheldon (1954) devised a system in which the individual is rated on a seven-point scale for each of three dimensions of physique and for each of three groups of temperamental characteristics. Ratings of physique are based on standardized photographs (see Fig. 6–6). Ratings of temperament are based on interview. The dimensions or components of physique are *endomorphy* (visceral development), *mesomorphy* (muscular development) and *ectomorphy* (linearity of physique). A three-digit code is used to describe each individual; the three digits run from 1 to 7 and refer, in order, to endomorphy, mesomorphy and ectomorphy. Thus, 6-4-1 describes an individual very high on

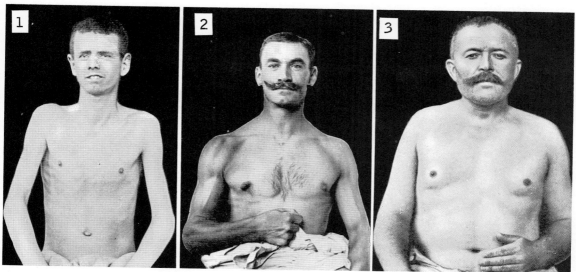

Figure 6–5. *1, Asthenic type; 2, athletic type; 3, pyknic type. (Reproduced by permission from Kretschmer, E. 1925. Körperbau und Charakter. Berlin, Göttingen, Heidelberg, Springer-Verlag.)*

endomorphy, medium on mesomorphy and very low on ectomorphy. Sheldon reports extraordinarily high correlations, of the order of +0.8, between ratings for these dimensions of physique and ratings of temperamental characteristics. Predominantly endomorphic body build is purportedly associated with *viscerotonic* temperamental characteristics (for example, relaxation, love of physical comfort and sociability), mesomorphic body build with a *somatotonic* temperament (for example, assertiveness, high energy level and competitiveness), and ectomorphic body build with a *cerebrotonic* temperament (for example, restraint in posture and movement, love of privacy and sensitivity). The major temperamental characteristics associated with the three somatotypes are listed in Table 6–9. The following anonymous verses which appeared some years ago illustrate the three physique-temperament correlations:

Oh, I'm a little endomorph asittin' in the sun.
I dote on beer and skittles; and I like my bit of fun.
I'm just a trifle lardy, just a trifle fat,
I may be somewhat tardy, but I like to be like that.

Oh, I'm a busy mesomorph encased in gorgeous muscle,
My thinking is a trifle short, I'm long on vim and hustle.
I'm a certified go-getter; I'm the boy who will succeed,
(Minus reason even better) perspiration is my creed.

Oh, I'm a spectral ectomorph, full of ratiocination.
The mind's my happy hunting ground and I loathe participation.
Lonelier than any cloud, I'm always quite superior
To the mouthings of the motley crowd and grunts of the inferior.

A study by Wittman, Sheldon and Katz (1948) investigated the relation between the three components of physique and three dimensions of mental disorders: disturbed affective behavior (typical of manic-depressive psychosis), paranoid behavior (typical of paranoid psychosis) and heboid behavior (manifested in the hebephrenic form of schizophrenia). On each of these psychiatric dimensions, 155 male patients were rated on the basis of case-history files alone. The correlations reported are very impressive: +0.54 between endomorphy and the affective component, +0.57 between mesomorphy and the paranoid component and +0.64 between ectomorphy and the heboid component. Two of these results are compatible with Kretschmer's conclusions: the endomorphy-affective correlation parallels Kretschmer's association of pyknic physique and manic-depression; and the ectomorphy-heboid correlation is parallel to the asthenic-schizophrenic association.

The results of studies of body build and behavior seem very impressive but they are open to several criticisms. (1) The methods of assessing physique are not beyond reproach.

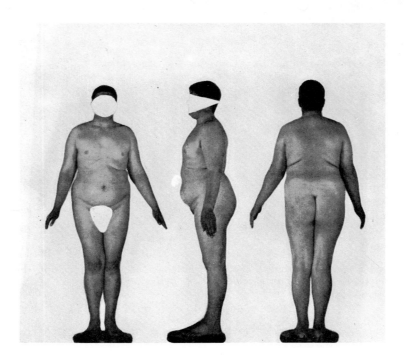

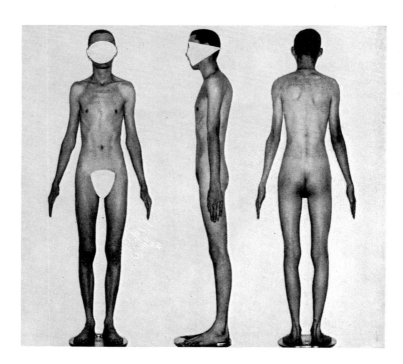

Figure 6–6.   *(From "Atlas of Men" by W. H. Sheldon, Copyright 1954 by Harper & Row, Publishers, Inc. Reprinted by permission of the publishers.)*

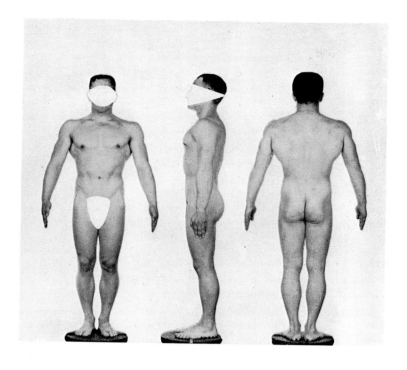

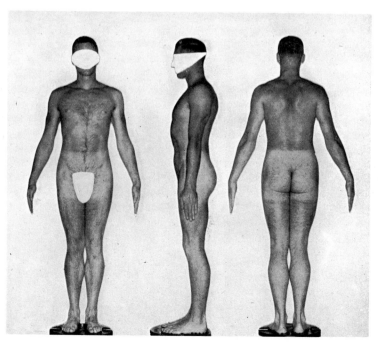

Figure 6–6. Continued.

TABLE 6-9. Sheldon's Scale for Temperament

I Viscerotonia	II Somatotonia	III Cerebrotonia
1. Relaxation in posture and movement	1. Assertiveness of posture and movement	1. Restraint in posture and movement tightness
2. Love of physical comfort	2. Love of physical adventure	2. Physiological over-response
3. Slow reaction	3. The energetic characteristic	3. Overly fast reactions
4. Love of eating	4. Need and enjoyment of exercise	4. Love of privacy
5. Socialization of eating	5. Love of dominating, lust for power	5. Mental overintensity, hyperattentionality, apprehensiveness
6. Pleasure in digestion	6. Love of risk and chance	6. Secretiveness of feeling, emotional restraint
7. Love of polite ceremony	7. Bold directness of manner	7. Self-conscious motility of the eyes and face
8. Sociophilia	8. Physical courage for combat	8. Sociophobia
9. Indiscriminate amiability	9. Competitive aggressiveness	9. Inhibited social address
10. Greed for affection and approval	10. Psychological callousness	10. Resistance to habit and poor routinizing
11. Orientation to people	11. Claustrophobia	11. Agoraphobia
12. Evenness of emotional flow	12. Ruthlessness, freedom from squeamishness	12. Unpredictability of attitude
13. Tolerance	13. The unrestrained voice	13. Vocal restraint and general restraint of noise
14. Complacency	14. Spartan indifference to pain	14. Hypersensitivity to pain
15. Deep sleep	15. General noisiness	15. Poor sleep habits, chronic fatigue
16. The untempered characteristic	16. Overmaturity of appearance	16. Youthful intentness of manner and appearance
17. Smooth, easy communication of feeling, extraversion of viscerotonia	17. Horizontal mental cleavage, extraversion of somatotonia	17. Vertical mental cleavage, introversion
18. Relaxation and sociophilia under alcohol	18. Assertiveness and aggression under alcohol	18. Resistance to alcohol and to other depressant drugs
19. Need of people when troubled	19. Need of action when troubled	19. Need of solitude when troubled
20. Orientation toward childhood and family relationships	20. Orientation toward goals and activities of youth	20. Orientation toward later periods of life

From William H. Sheldon, ''Constitutional Factors in Personality,'' in Personality and the Behavior Disorders, edited by J. McV. Hunt. Copyright 1944 The Ronald Press Company.

(1) Kretschmer's ratings of physique apparently were less careful and objective than is desirable, and other investigators have failed to replicate his ratings. Sheldon's photographic technique is an improvement over Kretschmer's procedure, but it may be less reliable than the most careful and objective direct measurement would be. (2) Kretschmer and many other investigators did not use statistical controls to correct for the tendency of people to get heavier and therefore less ectomorphic with age. Sheldon claims that his system is little affected by age but this assertion has been disputed. Since the onset of schizophrenia typically occurs at an earlier age than manic-depressive breakdown, the correlation of physique and diagnosis—especially in Kretschmer's work—may reflect the spurious contribution of age. Nutrition and a variety of environmental changes may also affect body type measurements. (3) Kretschmer included men and women in the same study. This procedure complicates body-type rating and makes it difficult to know just what the data mean.

However, Sheldon has avoided this difficulty by studying one sex at a time. (4) Perhaps most serious of all, the studies are almost never free of contamination by the fact that the investigator who rates personality variables can see the subject's physique and is familiar with the relation between physique and personality postulated by the theory. Hence it is difficult for a rater to be free of bias. A mesomorph may be called energetic, courageous, aggressive, indifferent to pain and callous precisely because he is mesomorphic, not because there are independent grounds for these trait descriptions. Similarly, in the case of a psychotic with both schizophrenic and manic-depressive features—a not unusual combination—the diagnosis may be affected by perception of the physique; or, if the diagnosis is made independently, the rating of body build may be affected by the diagnosis. Many psychologists have felt that the correlations between physique and temperament reported by Sheldon are unbelievably large and could be obtained only by contaminated procedures. It has also been claimed that some of the temperament variables are not independent *but* of physique but are really aspects of it, for example, overmaturity of appearance in the *are dependent* somatotonic temperament and youthful appearance in the cerebrotonic temperament.

It is not easy to devise experimental designs that would be free of contamination for the study of physique and personality. Some possible designs might employ objective personality tests, ratings on the basis of autobiographies and other documents (without seeing the subjects, and with care taken to eliminate clues that would indicate the type of physique) and interviews by persons who are unfamiliar with the physique-personality hypotheses or skeptical of their validity. A study by Hood (1963) which avoided contamination compared the scores of ectomorphic and endomorphic male college freshmen on the Minnesota Multiphasic Personality Inventory and found that ectomorphs had lower scores on impulsive excitability but higher scores on scales measuring depression, anxious compulsiveness and hysteroid defensiveness. Although the results were statistically significant and consistent in the main with Sheldon's hypotheses, the differences found between the ectomorphs and endomorphs were very small in a practical sense.

The consistency of the physique-behavior correlations found in a number of investigations has led many observers to conclude that after discounting the spurious effect of poor design a hard core of relations of unknown magnitude still remains. Several causal factors might account for the correlations. (1) Hereditary endowment may determine both physique and behavior via gene linkage. Just as there are sex-linked traits there may also be body-linked traits. (2) Environment may affect both physique and behavior. For example, extreme economic deprivation in childhood may lead to social seclusiveness, and the poor diet prevalent in economically deprived groups may lead to asthenic physique. (3) The culture has different expectations for different kinds of physique. People tend to conform to the social roles expected of them, so that the congruence of physique and behavior may be a function of social influence. A mesomorph is expected to be dominant; it is therefore easier for him to *be* dominant than to resist the culture and be submissive. (4) It is rewarding for the individual who has a particular type of physique to make certain responses and it is punishing for him to make certain others. By virtue of his body build

the mesomorph is likely to be successful if he is aggressive and dominant. The ectomorph often fails if he attempts to gain his ends through aggression and he must therefore learn other techniques. Persons with different physiques practice different responses and consequently develop different behavior and personality patterns.

The four possible explanations illustrate the gulf between causation and mere association. Physique and behavior may be correlated because heredity affects both, or because physique affects behavior via the intermediate variable of either social expectations or differential success and failure. A combination of all of these is also possible.

In addition to the components of physique studied in the Kretschmer-Sheldon tradition, structural variables such as body size, masculinity-femininity and physical immaturity have also been investigated. The relation of body size to mental defect was reviewed by Penrose (1954), who pointed out that all body measurements diminish slightly with decreasing I.Q. until the imbecile level is passed; below this level the decrease is rapid. Mental defectives are also much more susceptible to various forms of physical disability, both congenital and acquired after birth, than members of the general population. The reasons are not clear; we do know, however, that education and socioeconomic status seem to be involved in the chain of causation.

The dimension of masculinity versus femininity of bodily structure was correlated with homosexuality by Coppen (1959). A group of 41 male homosexuals was compared with 22 male heterosexual neurotics and 53 male heterosexual normals. Homosexuals were found to have a significantly more feminine structure than the normal controls, but the body structure of the heterosexual neurotics deviated from the controls as much as the homosexuals. It is possible that both neurosis and homosexuality are affected by causal factors similar to those discussed in connection with Sheldon's basic body components. A tendency to bodily femininity and a tendency to one or another kind of behavior deviation from the norm may be carried by the same genes; or body build and behavior deviation may be affected by the same environmental influences; or the effect of feminine body build on behavior may be mediated by social expectations or social reward and punishment. A male whose build is perceived as somewhat feminine may behave in either a nonmasculine or a neurotic manner if the masculine, nonneurotic behaviors he essays are not adequately rewarded.

Doust (1952) studied a variety of structural characteristics in a large sample of healthy adults and mixed psychiatric patients. He reported an excess of characteristics indicative of structural immaturity among the patients; for each patient group there seemed to be a distinct bodily pattern. Doust's conclusion was that delayed or deviant biological maturation contributes to the causation of presumably functional disorders. This conclusion has received some support from studies of peripheral blood capillaries in psychiatric patients, particularly schizophrenics. Many deviations from the normal number and structure of the small blood vessels have been reported and the findings have been cited as evidence of defects in development and maturation. However, structural peculiarities of this nature may result from environmental causes or from a physical disease occurring during the course of a mental disorder. Structural immaturity, masculinity-femininity and body size—like variation in the basic body types of Sheldon or Kretschmer—have not yet been *conclusively* proved to be related causally to psychological disorder, although there is some evidence—weakest for structural immaturity and strongest for physique—for each of these variables.

Bodily Functions

It will be recalled that a disturbance of both homeostasis and intellectual functioning can be precipitated by relatively small changes in the internal environment, for example, a change in the oxygen supplied to the tissues. It is reasonable to suppose that minor deviations in the chemical functioning of the body can also affect predisposition to various forms of disturbed behavior. Indeed, as pointed out earlier, when a hereditary influence on behavior can be demonstrated and no structural pathology exists, then it must be assumed that the hereditary determinants act through their effects on biochemical equilibrium, whether or not these effects have been identified and their nature specified.

Studies interrelating body function and behavior have multiplied rapidly in recent years but there have been few clear-cut results. Most of the studies are correlational, so that the task of explaining the findings causally has hardly

begun. Studies of physiological factors in disturbed behavior have failed again and again to be replicated successfully.

A great many investigations of metabolic processes in functional disorders have been carried out and abnormal metabolism has been reported frequently. For a number of reasons, however, it is no simple matter to summarize and evaluate the results of these studies. First, different investigators have reported noncomparable results. Not only have the findings been inconsistent for similar groups of patients studied by different investigators but in some cases there has been no consistency for the same investigator at different times. The phenomena appear to be very subtle, affected by many variables and hard to replicate.

A second difficulty is that, even if consistent metabolic findings were discovered, the nature of the operating causes would be uncertain since these might be genetic, or the result of biological experiences (diet, disease and so forth) or the result of emotional factors. It has been remarked by critics øf the biochemical investigations that trying to differentiate by biochemical tests between psychiatric patients and normal persons is comparable to trying to distinguish between different makes or models of automobiles by measuring gasoline consumption, engine revolutions per minute or speed. The biochemical differences between normals and schizophrenics or manic-depressives might be real but secondary and unreliable. Many of the metabolic peculiarities reported for patients with functional disorders have proved to result from nutritional intake; nutrition is affected by the mental hospital menu and by the behavior disturbance itself. Depressives and schizophrenics are quite likely to eat inadequately in the stage of breakdown prior to hospitalization. Metabolic peculiarities may ultimately constitute an effect, rather than a cause, of functional disorders. The evidence to date has fallen far short of proving that there is a biochemical predisposition to schizophrenia (the disorder that has been most studied) or any other functional disturbance, although it does seem that there are biochemical factors *associated* with disturbed psychological functioning.

Metabolic processes are regulated by the cooperative effort of the endocrine or ductless glands. It has therefore been suggested that from a research point of view it would be more economical to investigate the behavioral effect of endocrine disturbances than to try to relate behavior to those biochemical disturbances that are a secondary consequence of endocrine malfunctioning. A number of behaviors in different animal species are known to be strongly influenced by hormones; for example, tendencies toward dominance or submission, and the nature and frequency of sexual behavior can be regulated by hormone injections. However, in the course of evolution the extent to which gonadal hormones control sexual behavior has progressively weakened, so that human sexual behavior is largely independent of hormonal control. Although it is known that thyroid, parathyroid, adrenal and pituitary malfunction may lead to behavior disturbances, no one-to-one relationship has yet been found between a specific type of endocrine dysfunction and any of the common psychiatric disorders. To date, investigations of hormone-behavior relationships in humans have yielded few results relevant to abnormal psychology.

Studies of autonomic nervous system functioning have indicated that there is an overall increase of nervous activity in neurosis. The physiological signs of heightened anxiety common in neurosis, such as increased heart rate, cold sweats and inhibition of salivation (dry mouth) are accompanied by intense autonomic activity. Again, however, autonomic hyperreactivity may be a concomitant or consequence of neurosis, rather than a determinant of it.

Several types of evidence point to a statistical association between vulnerability to emotional difficulties and vulnerability to infectious and other diseases and to death. Unusually high rates of physical illness and death have been reported among psychiatric patients; conversely, there is a high frequency of psychopathology among patients who seek medical treatment for bodily illness. Both bodily illness and psychopathology are more frequent in individuals of limited intelligence and lower socioeconomic status. Furthermore, certain patients with psychiatric difficulty have a diminished capacity to develop the antibodies necessary for immunity against infections. It is possible that the association between vulnerability to psychopathology and inadequate resistance or immunity to bodily disease indicates a common constitutional predisposition, but of course many other causal links are possible. To mention one such possibility, emotionally disturbed individuals tend, as part of their disturbance, to take very poor care of their health over long periods of time.

Finally, it should be mentioned that a rela-

tively high frequency of electroencephalographic (EEG) abnormalities, indicating peculiarities in the electrical activity of the brain, has been reported for obsessive-compulsive neurosis and antisocial behavior disorders. The peculiarities of brain functioning may be due to a genetic or constitutional predisposition to the disorders or to predisposing past experience. EEG abnormalities may also result from psychological disorder, rather than reflect its causation.

SOME INFERENCES

A survey of the nonhereditary biological determinants of abnormal behavior leads to certain inferences and general conclusions.

Much more is known about precipitating than predisposing biological causes. The belief is widespread that predisposing causes are the more important and basic of the two; however, definitive and causal, rather than correlational, research on predispositions is difficult to design and carry out.

The belief that predisposing biological causes are real, that "something must be there," is not unwarranted despite the relatively weak results to date. First, since the organism is an interrelated system of biological and behavioral processes, it is plausible to assume that there *must* be biological predispositions to disturbed behavior. Second, since the existence of hereditary predispositions to certain behaviors is fairly well established, it follows that structural or functional dispositions should also exist, as connecting links between heredity and behavior. Third, although the results are weak, they have some degree of consistency: the studies have repeatedly demonstrated that, at the very least there are biological correlates of disturbed behavior. Some of the correlations that have been found undoubtedly reflect causation and some do not. The problems to be solved consist of determining which biological factors are predisposing causes as well as correlates, precisely which disorders are influenced by such biological causes and just how the biological causes interact with other etiological agents.

It is certain that research on biological factors in behavior abnormalities will continue, probably at an accelerated rate. As research techniques and designs improve, important etiological advances will be made.

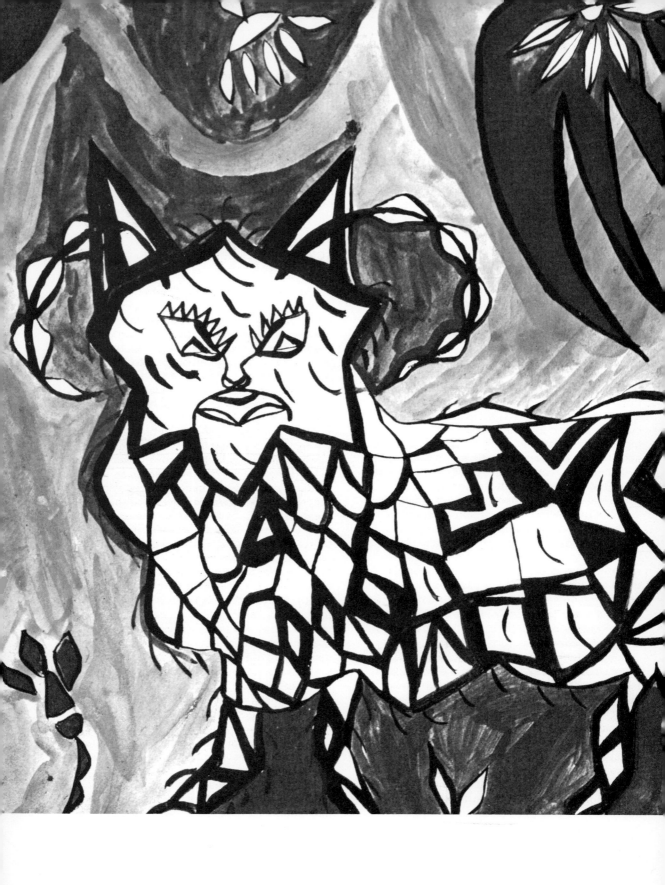

Our deeds still travel with us from afar,
And what we have been makes us what we are.

George Eliot, *Middlemarch*

7

PSYCHOLOGICAL DETERMINANTS

The behavior of the human organism is profoundly influenced by psychological as well as biological variables. Behavior disturbance results from severe frustration, emotional deprivation and conflict. The reactions to these determinants occur in accordance with the principles of learning.

LEARNING

We may define learning as a process by which changes in behavior result from experience. If a change does not occur there is no learning. If a change occurs because of maturation or such biological states as fatigue or physical damage rather than experience, there is no learning. The definition advanced by Hilgard (1956) covers these points:

Learning is the process by which an activity originates or is changed through reacting to an encountered situation, provided that the characteristics of the change in activity cannot be explained on the basis of native response tendencies, maturation, or temporary states of the organism (e.g. fatigue, drugs, etc.).

Several implications of the definition should be noted. First, the change in behavior need not be a desirable one. The acquisition of incorrect word usage, poor habits of social interaction or propensities for regression under stress indicate, as much as desirable changes do, that learning has occurred. Second, although teaching sometimes results in learning, most learning occurs without any form of planned guidance. Finally, it is important to realize that one may learn without being aware of it: learning is defined by objective behavior changes, not by consciousness of these changes.

Types of Learning

Two general models of learning have been distinguished: classical conditioning and instrumental learning.

Classical conditioning was described in Chapter 2. In this type of learning paradigm the organism simply learns (or is conditioned) to make an old response to a new stimulus, which prior to learning would not have evoked the response. For example, a hungry dog naturally salivates at the sight of food but not at the sound of a buzzer. By repeatedly sounding the buzzer just prior to the presentation of food it is possible to condition the dog to salivate at the sound of the buzzer (Fig. 7–1). For a time the animal will continue to salivate to the buzzer even when it is not followed by food. However,

101

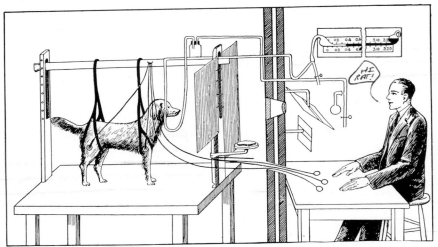

Figure 7–1. *Studying the conditioned reflexes of salivation. The dog and experimenter are in separate rooms. In front of the experimenter's hands are the controls for the conditioned stimulus (CS) which is tactile (note the attachments on the dog's shoulder and thigh) and the unconditioned stimulus (UCS), the food (the food dish swings around within the dog's reach). A tube attached to the dog's cheek by cement leads to the manometer (upper right), by which the amount of salivary secretion is measured. (From Pavlov, I. P. 1928. Lectures on Conditioned Reflexes, trans. by W. H. Gantt. New York, International Publishers, Inc.)*

after a period of such non-reinforcement, the conditioned response of salivation to the buzzer alone will extinguish.

In the early stages of classical conditioning there is a tendency to *stimulus-generalization,* and a dog conditioned to salivate at the sound of a buzzer may also salivate at the sound of a bell or almost any other noise made in the room. As conditioning continues, the dog learns to discriminate between the correct buzzer and other buzzers of higher or lower pitch. However, should the discrimination become too difficult, major and persistent changes in behavior, particularly emotional behavior, may occur. These changes constitute an experimental neurosis, discussed later in this chapter.

The classical conditioning paradigm is often evoked to explain or attempt changes in the so-called "involuntary" responses, which are innervated by the autonomic nervous system and effected by the smooth muscles and the glands. Thus, if a neutral stimulus is presented in temporal contiguity with an electric shock, the neutral stimulus will be conditioned to the involuntary increase in pulse rate and sweating normally evoked by the shock. At the same time, the neutral stimulus will become conditioned to more than these changes: it will generate fear because of its association with the shock and therefore will become a danger signal and will trigger attempts to avoid the feared,

noxious unconditional stimulus (UCS), shock. The same processes may occur when UCS is a social or emotional punishment or frustration rather than an electric shock. A child typically responds with physiological components of anxiety (pulse increase and other changes) to the UCS of sufficiently severe punishment, drive frustration or withdrawal of affection. Through temporal contiguity many previously neutral stimuli become associated with these painful stimulus situations so that the child learns to respond with anxiety to the CS of the sight or sound of a punishing parent and thence to the sight or sound of other people (because of stimulus generalization from the parent). He may also respond with conditioned anxiety to the thoughts and the drive stimuli—sex, aggression and others—that occurred at the time he was punished, frustrated or threatened. His conditioned anxiety leads to a conditioned avoidance of internal thoughts and impulses which is manifested as denial, repression, isolation, reaction-formation and the other defenses. Thus, classical conditioning may provide a theoretical basis for the explanation of many neurotic and defensive behaviors. The phenomenon of classical conditioning also suggests that an important part of psychotherapy consists of helping the patient to substitute nonanxious reactions for his neurotic anxieties. To achieve this substitution, the therapist may employ many procedures: for example, he may establish a warm and accepting therapeutic atmosphere, reinforce the nonanxious components of the patient's behavior, or interpret the meaning of his behavior so that the patient may gain insight into the source and nature of his anxieties.

A classical conditioning psychologist observes a particular behavior and asks himself what stimulus evokes this response. Once this information is obtained it is possible to condition another response to the stimulus or extinguish the present response. An instrumental conditioning expert looks at the same behavior and looks for the reinforcer which maintains the response in question. Knowing the reinforcing contingencies which maintain a behavior, it is then possible either to extinguish the response by withholding the reinforcer or to reinforce alternative behaviors and thus increase their likelihood of occurring.

A hungry rat placed in a small box with a lever may, in the process of exploring his environment, accidentally depress the lever. If he is immediately reinforced (fed) he is likely to continue exploring the cage and depress the lever again. Soon he learns that only pressing the lever brings food and consequently his other behaviors decrease in frequency of occurrence. The response is instrumental in securing the reward. It is possible to "shape" the animal's response more quickly by rewarding him for remaining in the end of the cage near the lever. Once this behavior is established, reward is suspended for merely being in the desired end of the cage but is given for being close to the bar, and so on until the desired behavior of bar-pressing occurs.

The difference between operant and classical conditioning may appear academic, but both models are useful in explaining different abnormal behaviors. A great deal of social learning seems to be basically instrumental in nature.

Keeping clean, waiting for mealtime, making decisions and inhibiting physical aggression are learned, instrumental behaviors that result in being rewarded. Failure to make approved responses is instrumental in bringing about punishment. The child who is rewarded for expressions of aggression or punished for all expressions of sexuality is likely to develop long-range social and emotional inhibitions and distortions. Family constellations and parental attitudes, obviously of prime im-

portance in maladaptive instrumental learning in childhood, will be discussed at a later point in this chapter.

Some Principles of Learning

Learning Varies with the Amount of Reward. A larger reward on each learning trial, or a larger accumulation of reward over a series of trials, increases the strength of learned habits and slows down the rate of extinction. The reward may be primary or secondary. Primary rewards are innately satisfying; food, for example, is a primary reward for the hunger drive. Secondary rewards acquire their value from association with primary rewards. Money, attention and approval have powerful secondary reward value by virtue of their repeated associations with many, different primary rewards.

There is a third kind of reward. It has been demonstrated that the brains of rats, monkeys, and other organisms contain centers which, when stimulated electrically, give the organism pleasurable or unpleasurable sensations (Olds, 1955). A rat will depress a lever over and over to obtain no reward other than electrical stimulation of a reward center in which the experimenter has implanted an electrode, and it will repeatedly make escape responses to stop the electrical stimulation of a punishment center. The punishment centers are not pain centers; there are no receptors for the pain sense in the brain. In one experiment Olds found that if rats were given the choice of a maze path leading to food and a maze path at the end of which pleasure centers were stimulated, they preferred the latter. A monkey stimulated in a punishment center shakes violently, wildly attempts to escape and bites and tears whatever object is available; for days thereafter he is irritable and eats poorly. These after-effects can be reversed by stimulation of a reward center. On the basis of observations of conscious humans electrically stimulated during brain surgery, it has been concluded that humans too have reward centers associated with intense feelings of well-being as well as punishment centers which, when stimulated, elicit intense anger or fear.

It has been speculated (Meehl, 1962) that proneness to schizophrenia may be characterized by excessive activation of punishment centers. For hereditary or constitutional reasons, or because of past experience, a schizoid individual's nervous system may function in such a manner that his own thought and memory responses lead to stimulation of his punishment centers; in a non-schizoid person the same thoughts and memories might lead to stimulation of neutral or reward centers. Although there is no direct experimental evidence to substantiate this theory of schizophrenia, it is compatible with such phenomena as the schizophrenic's fear, withdrawal and ambivalence and his tendency to anhedonia (failure to experience pleasurable affect under conditions that evoke pleasure in normal persons).

Learning Varies with the Length of the Temporal Interval between the Response and Its Reinforcement. The shorter the interval, the more rapidly learning occurs. This temporal factor is one reason why defenses become ingrained so easily in behavior: a repressive, projective or other defensive mechanism is immediately followed by a rewarding reduction of anxiety, and it therefore becomes a strong habit in a few trials.

Learning Varies with the Amount of Repetition. The more the organism practices a learned response, the stronger the learning. In intermittent or partial reinforcement only one trial in each block of several successive trials is reinforced. Learning with this kind of reinforcement is slower than with continuous reinforcement, but it is also slower to be extinguished since some nonreinforcement was a part of the original learning situation. The phenomenon of fixation on a stage of development may be due to such intermittent reinforcement: if the behaviors of a given stage are sometimes gratified but more often frustrated—i.e., if they are gratified intermittently instead of continuously—then they are difficult to extinguish and they persist as fixations.

Learning Varies with the Strength of Motivation. The stronger the drive, the stronger the learned response and the slower its extinction. Like rewards, drives may be primary or secondary. Innate drives like hunger, thirst or pain are primary. Learned drives like the need for status, peer acceptance or avoidance of guilt feelings are secondary.

Since anxiety is a drive, highly anxious individuals have a high drive level. It has been demonstrated experimentally that a number of responses condition more rapidly and extinguish more slowly in anxious individuals than in less anxious control subjects (Franks, 1960).

A stimulus constellation that is neutral for a nonanxious individual—such as talking to a stranger, being in a crowd, being alone, noise, quiet, darkness or a host of other stimulus conditions—may come to evoke a conditioned fear response or a conditioned, defensive avoidance of fear in an individual prone to anxiety; the conditioned fear or avoidance response then resists extinction. The neurotic's defenses and symptoms partly stem from the fact that a high anxiety drive has led to strong and maladaptive conditioning. Neurosis, from this point of view, is an overlearning of undesirable emotional habits motivated by a high drive state. An extremely high drive does not facilitate all types of learning, for it interferes with the learning of fine discriminations. Consequently, although the highly anxious individual overlearns maladaptive habits, it is difficult for him to learn to discriminate between the stimuli that truly warrant fear and the stimuli that should not be threatening.

The sociopath, in contrast with the anxious neurotic, conditions more slowly than normals (Lykken, 1957). His level of anxiety seems to be too low for successful acquisition of the conditioned responses and instrumental habits that constitute socialization. The anxious neurotic and the sociopath are opposites in certain respects and the normal falls midway between them.

Learning by Reward Is in Many Ways More Efficient Than Learning by Punishment. The inhibition of a response by punishment is temporary unless the punishment is very intense; a response inhibited by punishment at ordinary levels of intensity will return later if the organism is in a state of high drive and if no alternative response is available. Thus, although neurotic behaviors are often self-punishing, they may tend to persist because the neurotic has no other responses in his repertory. The overaggressive individual is punished by retaliation for his aggression, the phobic individual is repeatedly punished by experiencing an extremely unpleasant feeling of panic and the conversion-reaction patient is punished by the restriction on his freedom imposed by his symptoms; yet these symptomatic responses persist because the psychologically disturbed individual has not learned how to be anything but disturbed.

Mild punishment can serve as a reinforcer in learning new responses and maintaining them once they have been learned. If a hungry dog is fed after a mild electric shock, it soon learns to welcome the shock as a preliminary to feeding and it makes no avoidance response. In human infants resentment of a needle-prick vanishes if it is repeatedly followed by feeding. It may be that an individual who initially obtains sexual gratification under uncomfortable circumstances learns to associate sexual gratification with physical pain, as is found in masochism. It has been speculated that proneness to accidents may involve an unconscious, pleasurable response to punishment, perhaps as a prelude to the attention received when one is hurt.

On the other hand, the result of *very intense punishment* may be a generalized avoidance of many responses other than the one for which the individual is punished. Toilet training is a pertinent illustration of this principle: training by severe punishment may result in emotional avoidance of anything remotely connected with excretion, and the consequence may be the development of an extreme tendency to be orderly, neat and clean.

Dollard and Miller (1950) have offered a comprehensive explanation of neurotic behavior in terms of learning principles that summarizes several of the points so far discussed. According to Dollard and Miller, if an individual is severely punished, especially in childhood, for the responses that normally are effective in reducing drives such as sex and aggression, then the stimuli associated with these drives become associated with fear. This fear then motivates other responses that are incompatible with the punished, drive-reducing responses; consequently, the tensions of sex and aggression are not reduced. A child who is severely punished for exploratory sexual behavior, for example, learns to associate the sexual stimuli with fear; his fear motivates repressions of sexual thoughts, feelings or overt actions; and his repressions, continuing into later life, are incompatible with satisfactory interactions with persons of the opposite sex. The neurotic's inhibitions result in an accumulation of unsatisfied drive tensions which make him feel miserable. Furthermore, his fear-motivated repressions result in poor social and other discriminations because repression interferes with the higher mental processes that aid in discrimination. He therefore finds it increasingly hard to discriminate nonpunishing from punishing situations and to extinguish unrealistic fears. He is caught in a vicious circle in which learning results in maladaptive responses and these, in turn, prevent learning more adaptive ones.

PRECIPITATING PSYCHOLOGICAL STRESS

The individual subjected to severe conflict or frustration, long-continued vigilance, uncertainty, deprivation or threat may not be able to perceive a ready escape route; the result is a state of stress. Combat in war, serious illness, the prospect of dangerous but necessary surgery, a threatened shortage of food, deprivation of affection in childhood, unchangeable social isolation or a threatened, drastic loss of self-esteem are all psychologically stressful.

Stress varies in severity depending on a number of factors. It is more severe if an important need is frustrated rather than a relatively unimportant one; if the frustration, deprivation or other stressful determinant lasts over a considerable period; if it steadily mounts in intensity; and if a series of stress-producing events succeed each other with little time for recovery between them. Stress may involve objective and real threats or the organism may perceive a threat when none exists. The more severe the perceived danger or deprivation, whether the perception is objectively justified or not, the more stressful the situation. A moderate but sudden change for the worse may be perceived as disastrous, as in the case of a wealthy individual who suddenly undergoes mild financial losses and commits suicide although he is still far from poor.

The timing of successive stressful experiences is important in personality development. A 10-year-old boy suddenly became deeply depressed, failed in his school work and slept poorly. Investigation revealed that he had been very fond of his grandmother but had become angry with her after a trivial quarrel and had wished her dead. She died that day. He was an intelligent youngster and knew quite well that he was not responsible for her death, yet he could not shake off an irrational conviction of guilt. Neither the quarrel with his grandmother, nor the death wish nor her actual death was individually too stressful for him to cope with, but the juxtaposition of the three occurring in rapid succession was overwhelming.

A number of animal experiments have dramatically demonstrated how psychological stresses precipitate abnormal behavior. In 1914, one of Pavlov's students tested the ability of a dog to discriminate between a circle and an oval. The dog was trained to salivate in expectation of a food reward each time it was shown a card marked with a circle but not to salivate in response to a card with an ellipse. There was no punishment for errors. The ellipse was gradually made more circular; when it reached a shape so close to a circle that the dog could no longer discriminate between the two, its whole behavior suddenly changed. Instead of standing quietly in the experimental apparatus waiting for the next signal, it struggled and howled, salivated irregularly and ceased feeding. Instead of coming readily to the experimental room, it struggled to avoid the ordeal and its previously capable performance on simpler discrimination tests now became grossly impaired and disorganized. Even after a period of prolonged rest away from the experimental situation, the dog continued to be restless and agitated when reintroduced to the experimental harness. Apparently conflict and frustration had so profoundly disorganized its learned behavior and its capacity for new learning that the result has been termed an "experimental neurosis."

Liddell (1952, 1954, 1960), working with conditioned responses in sheep and goats, found that if the duration and number of daily laboratory tests were suddenly doubled, the animal developed a state of chronic agitation which made it useless for further testing. There were continuous movements of head, limbs and body, breathing became rapid and irregular, the heart rate was high and variable and frequent urination and defecation occurred. The agitated behavior persisted in the barn at night and the animal vigorously resisted being led back to the laboratory. When approached in the pasture it would dash away from the rest of the flock. This disturbed behavior remained unchanged even after three years away from the laboratory. The sheer pressure on the animal to remain vigilant a good part of the day was thus stressful enough to produce disturbance.

If a sheep or goat is repeatedly given a warning signal followed immediately by a mild electric shock to the forelimb, it soon begins to flex this leg each time it receives the warning signal, in anticipation of the shock to come. In the absence of warning signals, however, the animal remains in a state of alert vigilance and apprehension in which its respiration increases from about 40 per minute to as high as 135 per minute. Prolonged anticipation of danger or of unpleasant experiences may thus be much more stressful than the experiences themselves. Similarly, the fear of punishment in humans may be much more stressful than actual punishment.

The emotional stress resulting from standing and waiting may be additionally increased by giving the animal a series of signals without the reinforcement of the painful stimulus, after it has learned to expect a shock with each signal. Uncertainty regarding the future may be more stressful than an unpleasant experience that is certain. In children as well as in experimental animals, inconsistent punishment precipitates fear and anxiety more than consistent punishment.

The stressful effects of prolonged vigilance were illustrated by Brady's experiments (1958). Two monkeys, designated as an experimental and a control subject, were placed side by side in specially designed chairs. For 6 hours out of every 12 both monkeys received a mild electric shock on the foot every 20 seconds unless the experimental subject pressed a nearby switch at least once within the 20-second interval. The experimental subject was an "executive": he had to be vigilant, make decisions and act to avoid undesirable consequences to himself and his companion. The first experimental subject with whom this procedure was carried out developed signs of a stomach ulcer and died suddenly after 23 days. It will be recalled that the stress reaction, described by Selye and discussed in the previous chapter, is marked by degenerative tissue changes, including ulceration. In subsequent experiments several of the "executive" monkeys died, or if they survived were later found on autopsy to have developed ulcers, whereas none of the control subjects suffered ill effects. Since the shock was mild and administered to both experimental and control animals, the results are explainable only by the stress of prolonged vigilance.

In experiments with cats, Masserman (1961) produced a variety of symptoms including fear, vacillation and disorganized behavior. The role of motivational conflict in the production of an experimental neurosis is illustrated in Figure 7-3. A cat was trained to depress a switch when a light flashed or a bell sounded; the switch opened a box containing a pellet of food. The cat was then trained to press the switch and open the box as often as it wished, without waiting for the signal. It then was subjected to an air blast or electric shock at the moment of food taking and an approach-avoidance conflict arose between its hunger motivation and fear. It crouched, trembled, breathed rapidly, had an increased pulse and an elevated blood pressure and displayed all the manifestations ordinarily following generalized stimulation of the sympathetic nervous system. These manifestations increased when the light or sound signals

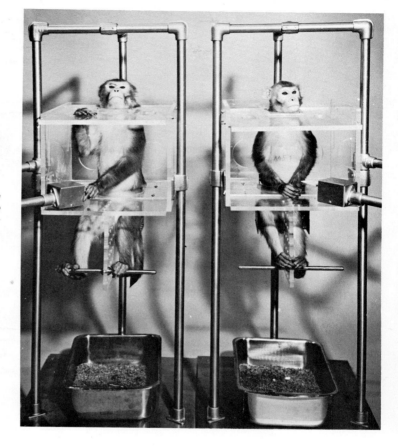

Figure 7–2. *(Reprinted by permission from Brady, J. V., et al. 1958. Avoidance behavior and the development of gastro-duodenal ulcers. J. Exp. Anal. Behav., 1:70.)*

were presented or when the cat was forced toward the food box by a moveable barrier or offered food pellets similar to those previously obtained from the food box. The animal's aversions readily became even more generalized and it tried to escape from the experimental cage and subsequently resisted returning to it. Its emotional and behavior disturbance persisted afterward even in comfortable and familiar surroundings.

Masserman has drawn an analogy between the motivational conflict in such experimental animal neuroses and in acute war neuroses (termed "shell shock" in World War I and "combat fatigue" in World War II). Acute war neuroses have often been precipitated by an approach-avoidance motivational conflict between the desire for the approval or satisfaction to be earned by doing one's duty and the fear of injury or death. However, other etiological factors are also often present in war breakdowns: prolonged sleep deprivation, excessive sensory stimulation in combat or excessive isolation in lonely posts, and separation from family and friends. Experimental neuroses in animals partially, but not wholly, parallel human neurotic reactions.

In general, the animal studies demonstrate that animal behavior patterns become disorganized and deviant if the learning required of the organism is too difficult and frustrating; if the learning tasks require too prolonged and intense a state of anticipation and vigilance; if the organism is subjected to too much uncertainty or inconsistency; or if conflicting motives are aroused, particularly between approach and avoidance motives. Each of these determinants is obviously important in the everyday lives of humans.

However, we should not be too quick to generalize from animals to humans or to accept without question animal studies of "experimental neurosis." Hebb (1947) has laid down several criteria which experiments should meet before one could confidently accept the fact that experimental neurosis does occur in animals. In

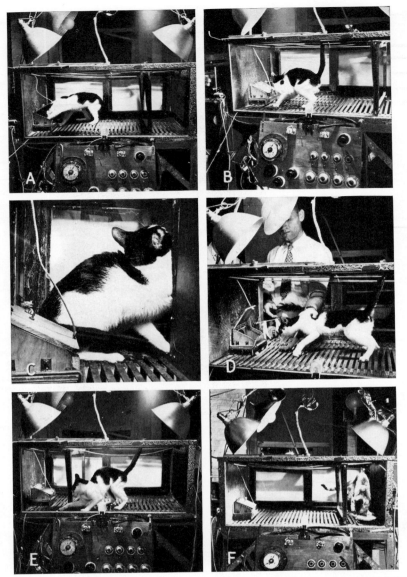

Figure 7–3. *"A. Control Observations. A cat has been trained to pass a barrier at a signal light (upper right flash) and open the food-box for a pellet of food. The animal's behavior is goal-directed and efficiently adaptive.*

"B. Conflictful Experience. At a later feeding signal the cat is subjected to a mild air-blast (12 lb.) at the moment of food-taking. The animal is shown recoiling from the traumatic situation.

"C. Neurotic Behavior. After five such experiences at irregular intervals the animal refuses to feed or approach the box and develops other neurotic aberrations of behavior. . . . The animal, though starved for 48 hours, is here shown in a typical phobic response to a feeding signal: crouched away from the food in cataleptic immobility (during 12 minutes) against an impassable barrier.

"D. Transference Retraining. After four months of neurosis, the animal is retrained by manual feeding and gentle guidance once again to feed from the box. At first, the animal does so only when being petted by the author; later, feeding responses may be reconstituted in response not only to the light but even to the air-blast (nozzle shown in deep left corner).

"E. Therapeutic Result. After 18 days of such retraining the animal's neurotic reactions largely disappear and it once again passes barriers for food at the light or air-blast signal.

"F. 'Masochistic' Patterns. Another animal, trained to depress an electric switch for its feeding signals, made experimentally neurotic by a mild electric shock at food-taking and then retrained as above to take the food despite the trauma, is here shown once again manipulating the switch with spontaneous avidity to experience the shock with or without the food reward." (From Masserman, J. H. 1961. Principles of Dynamic Psychiatry. 2nd Ed. Philadelphia, W. B. Saunders Co.)

control did the same as the exp. gr. so

fact, very few studies have met these criteria and many have contained major deficiencies in their experimental design. For example, in the Masserman study referred to above, the author failed to include a control group of animals who were given the noxious stimulus (air blast or shock) alone without the conflicting motivation of hunger. Wolpe (1952) repeated Masserman's experiment with this control and obtained similar results. Thus, it appears that a fear response to a threatening stimulus is sufficient to explain Masserman's results without postulating a conflict between the competing drives of fear and hunger. A fear response to a realistically obnoxious stimulus is hardly abnormal and cannot qualify as an experimentally produced neurosis. Animal studies which appear to produce behaviors similar to abnormal behaviors in humans raise intriguing possibilities but, thus far at least, the analogy must be accepted cautiously.

Frustration, Overgratification and Defense

Any response that effectively diminishes frustration will be reinforced because the lessening of the tensions and anxiety of frustration is rewarding. The response may then generalize and become a habitual pattern of behavior even in situations quite different from that in which it was first reinforced. The defense mechanisms outlined in Chapter 4 follow this sequence: a mechanism is tried under conditions of frustration, reinforced by the reduction of tension and anxiety and then rigidly used in many situations. It has been demonstrated experimentally that a severely frustrated organism is likely to become fixated and unable to learn further patterns of adaptation, i.e., it becomes inappropriately rigid. Maier (1949) trained rats to discriminate between light and dark cards placed side by side and to jump through a window in front of one of them in order to obtain a food reward. The window without a food reward was locked so that an animal jumping against it fell into a net below. If the animal jumped against the right window, it fell backward allowing him a foothold and a food reward. The experimenter then began to frustrate the subjects by randomly rewarding jumps to either card 50 per cent of the time. Faced with this insoluble problem, the animals developed a stereotyped habit of jumping to the same side every time; in

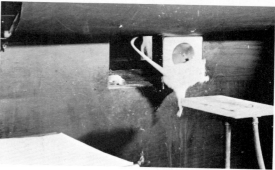

Figure 7-4. *"Fixation caused by conflict. The rat above was given an insoluble, conflict-producing problem. In this conflict, the rat developed the habit of jumping to the window on the right. Below, it jumps compulsively to that window, which is locked, while food in the left window is readily visible." (Reprinted from Frustration by N. R. F. Maier, by permission of The University of Michigan Press. New York, McGraw-Hill, 1949.)*

maybe the rat liked falling into the net..

a number of cases, this fixation continued even when food was placed on the other side in full sight of the animal. Like a defensive human, the rat had blindly adopted a fixed pattern of response under stressful conditions and had then stuck to it irrationally.

Traumatic experience

Solomon and Wynne (1954) performed an experiment with dogs that suggests that a sufficiently traumatic precipitant may result in virtually irreversible stereotyped behavior. A strong electric shock was the UCS in the first phase of the experiment. In the second phase the shock was discontinued, but even after hundreds of trials without it the dog still expected the shock on presentation of the neutral warning stimulus *CS* with which the shock had originally been paired, and it persisted in making an avoidance response to the warning signal. Since avoidance is a component of the defenses and since there is some similarity between emotional trauma and the trauma of severe electric shock, the experiment suggests one reason why defenses are often so difficult to extinguish. Another reason, mentioned earlier, is the short time interval between defensive behavior and its reinforcement.

In humans, there is much reason to believe that a reasonable degree of gratification of needs over the long run furthers maturity and emotional stability and prevents rigid defensiveness, whereas both excessively indulgent overgratification and severe frustration and rejection do the reverse. Overgratification, like frustration, leads to fixation. The individual who is rewarded over and over in a given stage of development may have no impetus to move on to the behaviors of the next stage. The familiar "spoiled-child" syndrome is an example; the child has no urge toward independence when dependency behavior is overgratified.

Parental overgratification often masks a subtle rejection. A parent may indulge dependency because of a wish that the child remain babyish, thus frustrating him by rejecting his potential maturity as a human being. On the other hand, insecure parents may overindulge a child merely to keep him quiet in the hopes that he will not make even more extreme demands, which the parents may feel are reasonable but which they are not capable of satisfying. Sometimes there is a pattern of public indulgence and private rejection which places the child in the difficult position of adjusting to conflicting parental messages. A four-year-old boy was brought to a clinic by his mother because of frequent nightmares, phobic fears of animals and people and undesirable feeding habits. During the clinic interview the mother smiled at the boy, spoke to him in an apparently loving tone, patted him, kept reassuring him that they would be out of the office soon (he was restless and very bored) and gave him candy from her purse. But as they were leaving the building she was overheard reproaching him. "What am I going to do with you? I'm so ashamed of you!" Her voice and expression were angry and she dragged him down the stairs faster than he could comfortably go. The emotional learning problems presented to this child by his mother were more than he could solve by normal behaviors.

Still another pattern consists of a sequence of frustrating rejection followed by indulgence. Sears, Maccoby and Levin (1957) found that mothers who scolded their children for dependency behavior and pulled away from them, but yielded after this initial resistance, had the most dependent children. The children clung to their parents, cried, demanded to be picked up and sought help for all their problems.

Rejection and overgratification both consist of special patterns of reinforcement. Since rejection is rarely total, a rejected child is sometimes rewarded although he is more often ignored or punished; in other words, he is reinforced intermittently. Since intermittent or partial reinforcement results in habits that are very resistant to extinction, it is not surprising that rejection and frustration should lead to developmental fixation. A child whose demands for help are usually rejected by his mother may keep asking for help long after such behavior is appropriate. This outcome is particularly likely to occur if he is not rewarded at all on the few occasions when he makes tentative efforts to be independent. Partial reinforcement of dependency, coupled with complete nonreinforcement of independence, are almost certain to lead to fixation on dependent behavior.

In overgratification, on the other hand, the individual overlearns habits. Reinforcement is so strong and repeated on so many trials that no competing responses can acquire much strength, especially if the competing responses that the child tentatively tries out are not reinforced at all.

Psychological Deprivation

There are many types of psychological deprivation; oral deprivation, deprivation of mothering, dependency deprivation, sensory deprivation and social deprivation (isolation) are among the most important. Levy (1928, 1934) demonstrated the stressful nature of oral deprivation and the substitutive behavior to which it may lead. He found that 25 per cent of a group of children deprived of pacifiers began to suck their thumbs, while children who were not deprived did not do so. In another study, Levy found that puppies who had been limited in sucking activities chewed at each other's bodies and at a proffered finger more than control animals who had been permitted to suck adequately. Like many other drives and needs, the oral drive seems to be displaceable from one activity to another when the first activity is inhibited.

Stresses instigated by deprivation of mothering in infancy have been much investigated. After studying 600 infants, Ribble (1944) concluded that emotionally disturbed mothers do not give their offspring enough tactual, kines-thetic or auditory stimulation. In consequence, infants either become negativistic, refusing to suck and displaying muscular rigidity, shallow breathing and constipation, or else they regress, becoming apathetic and depressive, showing no interest in food and evidencing a diminution of muscle tonus and reflex responses. An extreme form of regression is *marasmus,* in which the infant becomes flabby and lethargic and literally wastes away.

Ribble's observations have been supported by those of other investigators but such studies can be taken as suggestive only, since they present no statistical data. Others have arrived at similar conclusions through more careful study, although most of their methods are subject to criticism. Spitz (1949), for example, studied two groups: infants reared in a foundling home since birth who were impersonally handled by a nurse with many charges, and a control group institutionalized since birth in a nursery where each infant was visited and handled by his own mother. Physical care was good in both groups. Observation and testing over a two-year period revealed that the foundlings' development fell further and further behind the nursery children in bodily, manipulative, perceptual, memory, in-tellectual, imitative and social functioning. By age two, the foundlings had not learned to walk, talk or feed themselves and their be-havior resembled that of apathetic or agitated mental defectives.

A study by Spitz and Wolf (1946) reported that if emotional deprivation does not begin until late in the first year, the resultant infantile de-pression and arrested development may be re-versed, provided mothering is resumed within three months. However, if the infant is deprived for a longer period before the therapeutic re-sumption of mothering, his deterioration con-tinues. The study confirms the principle that stress increases with duration of deprivation and it points to the desirability of early therapy for emotional disturbances.

Spitz's findings have been questioned by Pinneau (1955) on the basis of several methodo-logical and statistical shortcomings. For ex-ample, the test used to measure intellectual functioning has never been adequately standard-ized even though it is widely used. Thus it is difficult to determine whether the observed losses in intellectual functioning were due to the effects of maternal deprivation or to short-comings in the measuring instruments.

In an ingenious animal study, Liddell (1952,

1954) found that withdrawal of maternal care during daily periods of stressful training greatly affected the behavior of lambs and kids and apparently increased their mortality. Twin lambs and kids were subjected every two min-utes to darkness signals of 10 seconds each, followed by a shock to the foreleg. One lamb or kid was tested in a room with its mother present, and its twin was simultaneously tested alone in an adjoining room. At the end of the test period the lone lamb or kid rejoined its mother and twin. In each instance the twin tested in the presence of its mother developed the usual anticipatory flexion of the forelimb prior to shock but showed no adverse effects of the training procedure and freely explored the room in the intervals between signals. The lone twin, on the other hand, showed progressive inhibition of movement and soon remained motionless, standing or lying on the floor when the lights were dimmed and hardly moving even when shocked. After a total of 1000 sig-nals, 20 each day, the animals were returned to the pasture. Both the lamb and kid trained in isolation died within a few months, whereas their twins were still healthy two years later.

Severe stress instigated by deprivation of the opportunity to gratify the dependency drive was found to occur in children who were separated from their mothers by evacuation from English cities during World War II. Anna Freud and Burlingham (1943) reported that the children who suffered most were aged one to two, the height of psychological dependency. They protested violently at the separation, went into a state of despair when their screaming was of no avail, then became either apathetic or thoroughly dependent on anyone who hap-pened to attend to their physical needs. The only exceptions were children who had a low level of maternal attachment to start with: they had had little experience of dependency and therefore suffered less.

The following case illustrates some of the effects precipitated by continued, stressful de-privation.

A five-year-old boy who resided in a children's village as a permanent ward of a children's agency was brought to a clinic after a long-standing history of emotional deprivation. Since his first year he had been considered a problem child. At the time of ad-mission to the children's village—six months before being brought to the clinic—he frequently screamed for long periods of time and was very destructive of property. Although these behaviors soon diminished he fought and quarreled a great deal with the other

CRIT. OF SPITZ

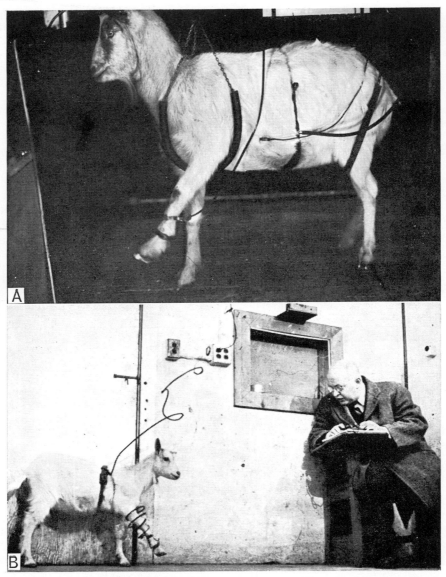

Figure 7–5. *"A, an 'experimentally neurotic' goat exhibiting behavior of the type characterized as tonic immobility. Note the awkward lifting of the rigidly extended left foreleg in response to the signal for shock. B, a goat 3 months of age exhibiting the characteristic neurotic reactions of tonic immobility. The lights have gone out for ten seconds as a signal for shock and this flash-bulb photograph shows the same awkward lifting of the rigidly extended foreleg as seen in the adult goat pictured in A. Here the goat has complete freedom of locomotion but has relinquished this freedom and become neurotic in consequence of a rigid time schedule of twenty darkness signals per day separated by two-minute intervals. This picture shows the reaction to the last signal of the twenty-third day of training." (From Liddell, H. S. 1952. Experimental induction of psychoneuroses by conditioned reflex with stress. In Milbank Memorial Fund. The Biology of Mental Health and Disease. New York, Hoeber-Harper.)*

children, ate poorly, slept little, sometimes wet the bed and on one occasion defecated at night and smeared the floor with his feces.

He was in good physical health. His I.Q. was 92, within the normal range. In the first clinic interview it was noted that he had a short attention span, was markedly restless and verbally uncommunicative. Although he was hostile, he hungered for physical contact: he shot a water pistol at the therapist but also held the therapist's hand.

He was an illegitimate child who had been cared for by his mother during his first two months and then placed in a private foster home. Eighteen months later his foster mother refused to keep him because of problem behavior. Between this point and his admission to the children's village he lived in three other foster homes and two institutions. One of the foster mothers was psychotic, with hallucinations and delusions. None of them could cope with his aggressive behavior.

He slowly began to establish a good relationship with the therapist. His expressions of hostility diminished, he began to communicate verbally and he reached the point of discussing the possibility that bed-wetting might be his way of getting back at authorities. Concurrently he became less aggressive to other children and more communicative with supervisory adults. It seemed clear that long-continued deprivation had resulted in a chronic state of stress and that aggression was his mode of response to deprivation; his relationship with the therapist filled some of the gaps left by the deprivations of his first five years.

Both the Liddell study and the Freud and Burlingham report raise intriguing possibilities, although neither can be taken as conclusive proof that maternal deprivation invariably results in psychological problems. Liddell's study fails to meet Hebb's (1947) criteria for proving an animal neurosis, and the Freud and Burlingham study did not employ objective measures of the changes noted. After a careful review of the literature, McCurdy (1961) concluded:

The existing data do not permit us to say confidently that early maternal deprivation has long-term deleterious effects. The hypothesis is clear-cut and subject to testing, it is based on reasonable theory, but the studies adduced in its favor are methodologically or factually weak. . . . We may only hope that adequate studies will be forthcoming [p. 146].

Inadequate sensory stimulation and social deprivation or isolation are still other types of deprivation. In recent years these have been much investigated. They are interrelated: social isolation is often accompanied by reduction of, or monotony in, the external stimulation impinging on the organism. Under conditions of isolation and reduced sensory input, normal individuals will develop psychopathological reactions.

The effects of a carefully controlled decrease in variation of the sensory environment were

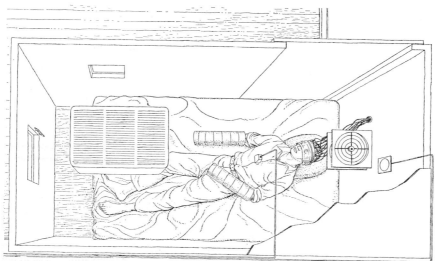

Figure 7–6. *The subject in the isolation experiment (seen from above, with the ceiling cut away). Cuffs prevented somesthetic perception by the hands; the plastic shield over the eyes admitted light but prevented pattern vision. A foam-rubber U-shaped cushion covered the subject's ears; here it has been removed so that EEG tracings can be taken. The air conditioner is on the ceiling (upper left), and just above the subject's chest is the microphone by which he could report his experiences. (From Heron, W. 1957. The pathology of boredom. Sci. Amer., 196, No. 1, p. 52. Reprinted with permission. Copyright 1957 by Scientific American, Inc. All rights reserved.)*

reported by Heron, Bexton and Hebb (1953). College students were paid $20 a day to do nothing but remain lying down on a comfortable bed with eyes, ears and hands shielded to minimize perception of their environment. The conditions were relaxed only to permit a subject to eat or go to the toilet. Most subjects could endure the experiment for only two or three days; the upper limit was six days. Among the effects noted were a significant decrease in the ability to solve problems and persistent, vivid visual imagery or hallucinations.

Hallucinations or hallucinatory-like experiences may be obtained through reduced sensory input alone without social isolation. The sensory input which comes from one's own motor movements is also involved since reduction of movement alone is sometimes sufficient to produce hallucinatory experiences (Zubek, 1963). Thus, sensory input, motor movement and social interactions all seem essential to the maintenance of rational, goal-directed thinking.

In prolonged solitary confinement, the individual attempts to compensate for the loss of human relationships by imagining that he has companions with whom he converses, plays or fights. As time goes on he becomes increasingly withdrawn into his inner world of fantasy and may have great difficulty in reestablishing his contact with reality when removed from isolation. A prisoner (Burney, 1952) spent 18 months in solitary confinement. When he was allowed to join his fellow prisoners he was afraid to speak to them for fear of showing himself to be insane. For several days he confined himself to listening, recaptured the usual criteria of sanity and then permitted himself to speak.

Living alone in the polar night, isolated in a small hut for weeks or months on end, is another experience that involves both absence of human contact and monotony in sensory stimulation. There are several detailed accounts of such experience; those of Byrd (1938) and Ritter (1954) are outstanding. In his book, *Alone*, Admiral Byrd included excerpts from his diary and analyzed his thoughts and behavior during four and one-half months of isolation in the Antarctic during the southern winter of 1934. After three weeks of isolation, he wrote:*

The morning is the hardest time. It is hard enough anywhere for a man to begin the day's work in dark-

---

*Reprinted by permission of G. P. Putnam's Sons from ALONE by Richard E. Byrd. Copyright 1938 by Richard E. Byrd.

ness; where I am it is doubly difficult. One may be a long time realizing it, but cold and darkness deplete the body gradually; the mind turns sluggish; and the nervous system slows up in its responses. This morning I had to admit to myself that I was *lonely.* Try as I may, I find I can't take my loneliness casually; it is too big. But I must not dwell on it. Otherwise I am undone.

The following day he wrote a passage that graphically illustrates the effect of sensory deprivation:

. . . I find that I crave light as a thirsting man craves water; and just the fact of having this lantern alive in the night hours makes an immense difference. I feel like a rich man.

His fantasy life became very active:

Yet, I could, with a little imagination, make every walk *seem* different. One day I would imagine that my path was the Esplanade, on the water side of Beacon Hill in Boston, where, in my mind's eye, I often walked with my wife. I would meet people I knew along the bank, and drink in the perfection of a Boston spring. There was no need for the path's ever becoming a rut. Like a rubber band, it could be stretched to suit my mood; and I could move it forward and backward in time and space, as when in the midst of reading Yule's *Travels of Marco Polo.* I divided the path into stages of that miraculous journey, and in six days and eighteen miles wandered from Venice to China, seeing everything that Marco Polo saw. And on occasion the path led back down the eons, while I watched the slow pulsations of the Ice Age, which today grips the once semi-tropical Antarctic Continent even as it once gripped North America.

The following month he wrote:

The senses were isolated in soundless dark; so, for that matter, was the mind; but one was stayed, while the other possessed the flight of a falcon; and the free choice and opportunity of the one everlastingly emphasized the poverty of the other. . . . I find, too, that absence of conversation makes it harder for me to think in words. Sometimes, while walking, I talk to myself and listen to the words, but they sound hollow and unfamiliar. . . . I've been trying to analyze the effect of isolation on a man. As I said, it is difficult for me to put this into words. I can only feel the absence of certain things, the exaggeration of others. . . . The silence of this place is as real and solid as sound. . . . It seems to merge in and become part of the indescribable *evenness,* as do the cold and the dark and the relentless ticking of the clocks. . . . I'm getting absent-minded. Last night I put sugar in the soup, and tonight I plunked a spoonful of cornmeal mush on the table where the plate should have been. . . . Well, this is the one continent where no woman has ever set foot; I can't say that it is any better on that account. In fact, the stampede to the altar that took place after the return of my previous expedition would seem to offer strong corroboration of that. Of the forty-one men with me at Little America, thirty were bachelors. Several married the first girls they met in New Zealand; most of the rest got married immediately upon their return to the United States.

There are numerous accounts of abnormal perception, cognition, affect and motor behavior among persons who have endured long periods of relative isolation at sea. From examining these accounts, it appears that individuals who survive in groups, even as small as two or three, are less apt to manifest signs of severe psychopathology than those who survive singly; the latter almost invariably show evidence of psychosis.

The underlying mechanism of such disturbances seems to be a tendency to project mental activity outward. Mental processes that are usually governed and bound by reality turn to fantasies and then to hallucinations and delusions. Subjective thought processes are superimposed on, and confused with, inanimate matter. Imagination absorbs more and more of the energy that normally is expended in interactions with the environment.

Interest in the consequences of social isolation was strongly aroused during the Korean War in an attempt to understand the

effectiveness of Communist techniques of so-called "brainwashing," extortion of false confessions and indoctrination (Lifton, 1961). The techniques employed in brain washing largely consist of the production of "debility, dependency and dread" (Farber et al., 1957). These are produced by the combined effects of physical pain and injury, malnutrition, disease, sleep deprivation, isolation, inability to satisfy the demands of interrogators and actual or implied threats of death, pain, nonrepatriation, deformity, permanent disability and harm to loved ones at home. Isolation is one component among these stress-inducing biological and psychological factors.

The mutual relationships among the three variables of (1) the degree of stress (brought about by frustration, deprivation, uncertainty, conflict or any other sufficient condition), (2) the degree of personality stability and (3) the resulting type of psychopathology have been diagramed by Marmor and Pumpian-Mindlin (1950); an adapted version is shown in Figure 7–7. The diagram does not consider quaitative variations in types of instability and stress, but indicates that from a quantitative viewpoint mental health requires considerable individual stability and not too much stress. Minor stress is sufficient to precipitate severe emotional dis-

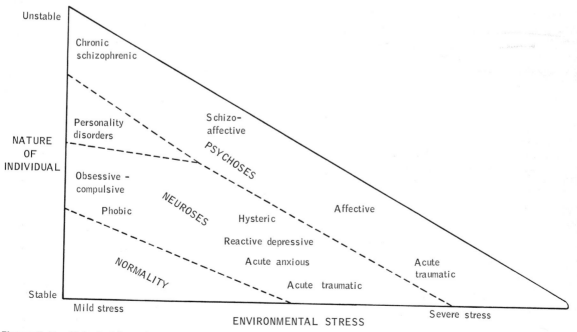

Figure 7–7. *(Adapted from Marmor, J., and Pumpian-Mindlin, E. 1950. Toward an integrative conception of mental disorder. J. Nerv. & Ment. Dis., 3:19–29.)*

order in an unstable individual, and sufficiently extreme stress will produce disorder in any individual, no matter how stable. As instability increases, the psychological disorders precipitated by relatively little stress shift from phobias and obsessive-compulsive reactions to personality disorders to chronic schizophrenia. With a stable personality, on the other hand, mental health is maintained for quite a period as stress increases, but eventually it too breaks down.

PREDISPOSING PSYCHOLOGICAL DETERMINANTS

Individual vulnerability to precipitating psychological stresses depends on the degree of personality instability. In turn, personality instability is affected by the psychological predispositions established early in the life of the individual.

A single psychological determinant may have both short-range precipitating and long-range predisposing effects. Childhood oral deprivation, for example, may precipitate immediate substitutive behaviors such as thumb sucking and also predispose the individual to pessimism in later years. Consequently, some of the stressful determinants whose predisposing effects we shall now explore have already been discussed as precipitants; some have also been touched on in the discussion of development in Chapter 4. (The student may wish to review Chapter 4 before reading further.)

The major psychological predispositions arise in the process of socialization. Child (1954) has defined socialization as "the whole process by which an individual, born with behavior potentialities of enormously wide range is led to develop actual behavior which is confined within a much narrower range—the range of what is customary and acceptable for him according to the standards of his group." Through socialization the child learns to make acceptable responses to other people as social stimuli and to conform to social rules. Socialization is learned in interactions with parents, sibs, peers, school teachers and various authority figures. In theory, the child can be socialized either because (1) he automatically responds to social rewards and punishments or (2) one of his motivations is a creative force which, by itself, leads to socialized behavior, provided his basic needs are not blocked. There is theoretical disagreement on which of these two explana-

tions is correct, but in either case the end result for most children is social conformity.

One of the means by which social norms are learned is nonverbal communication. Fear may be transmitted by example—flinching, changes in facial expression and so forth—as well as by verbal threat. Sexual attitudes are learned from parental embarrassment or evasion as much as from what parents say. There are many subtle ways in which the parents of delinquent children may communicate actual expectation and approval of antisocial behavior. Johnson and Szurek (1952) and Johnson (1959) have postulated that unconscious, permissive sanctioning by parents is a major and specific cause for children to live out antisocial impulses. The parents vicariously achieve gratification of forbidden impulses through the child's acting out.

performed in place of another.

Oral Deprivation and Later Personality

The methods used to socialize and train oral habits have several predisposing effects on later personality. Holway (1959) correlated ratings of the emotional stability reflected in the play of 17 children between three and five years old with ratings of the degree to which they had been indulgently permitted to suck in infancy. The rating of oral indulgence was based on interviews with mothers. The two variables correlated +0.78; the more indulged infant became the more stable, less destructive, more constructive and more affectionate child.

Sears et al. (1953) studied early oral deprivation, later dependency and later aggressiveness in 40 nursery-school children. Oral deprivation (sudden rather than gradual weaning, and scheduled rather than self-demand feeding in infancy) correlated with later dependency +0.40 for boys and +0.55 for girls. The orally deprived children sought attention, physical contact, help and praise from teachers and other children. Contrary to expectation, however, Sears did not find a relation between early oral deprivation and later aggressiveness.

Goldman-Eisler (1953) investigated the relation between weaning and optimism-pessimism many years later in a small sample of adults. A small positive correlation was found between late weaning and optimism in adult life (+0.31) and between early weaning and pessimism (+0.27).

However, several other studies have failed to substantiate the hypothesis of a specific relation between infantile oral deprivation and later personality. The area is a difficult one for research: there are problems of experimental control of variables, of accuracy of report of infantile experiences and of adequacy of the measuring instruments. There is also the ever-present question of whether causality may justifiably be imputed to developmental correlations. *A priori* it makes sense to hypothesize that the infant's first repetitive social relationship—his interaction with his mother while being fed—should be associated either with gratification or with ungratified and continued tension. It seems equally reasonable that this social relationship should generalize to a confident and optimistic or a fearful and pessimistic set of interpersonal attitudes and expectations. One of two cycles may then begin: confidence may breed skill and success in interpersonal relationships, or fear may breed failure, leading to still more fear and anxiety that culminate in emotional disturbance.

One theoretical qualification is in order, however. Although oral needs, because they occur so early, may have primacy in the development of affectional attachments and interpersonal relationships, they are not the only relevant variable. Recent observations of human and subhuman infants indicate that from a very early age the organism strives to explore, to manipulate and to touch with his whole body. The infant at times seeks arousal as well as a state of quiescence. It is possible that successful early explorations and satisfactory body contacts generate optimism, confidence, affection and stability as much as oral gratification does. Evidence on this point will be presented later in a discussion of the work of Harlow on monkeys and Levine on rats.

Parental Deprivation and Later Personality

The long-lasting effects of generalized deprivation of mothering in infancy are consistent with the short-term effects reported by Ribble and Spitz, discussed earlier. Goldfarb (1943, 1945) found that as late as adolescence children who had been institutionalized for their first three years were inferior in abstract reasoning and use of language to a control group of foster-home children. The intellectual deficiencies were not overcome by adoption into superior families after the age of three. As com-

pared to the foster controls, the institutionalized children manifested more behavior problems, anxiety, restlessness, difficulty in concentration, insatiable demands for attention and emotional coldness. Infants not placed in an institution until they were 11 months old did better than those placed at 6 months. The younger the organism, the harder hit it is by stress situations.

The effect of institutionalization on later personality and behavior is explainable in terms of generalization. The infant who is held carelessly, not attended to when uncomfortable and not fed when hungry (institutions must run on schedules and cannot use self-demand feeding) learns to associate pain with the adult who feeds him. The expectation of pain is generalized so that withdrawal from other people is really a withdrawal from anticipated pain and an avoidance of anxiety.

A corollary mechanism results from a habit of insatiably seeking attention. The habit develops easily in an overcrowded institution or any childhood setting in which ceaseless effort is necessary to make one's wants known. The attention-seeking generalizes to the responses of persistent restlessness, destructiveness and temper tantrums, since the child may not have learned to discriminate acceptable from unacceptable attention-getting techniques. Learning to discriminate between two similar responses depends on reinforcing one response but not the other. The conditions of institutional life often make it impossible for the institutional authorities to reward desirable techniques of attention-getting consistently and to withhold reward for undesirable techniques.

One method of investigating the effects of early deprivation on later personality is the retrospective investigation of the early histories of emotionally disturbed individuals. Barry and Lindemann (1960) retrospectively studied almost 1000 psychoneurotic and psychophysiologic outpatients and found a significantly high frequency of loss of the mother during the first five years of life. In another study of 216 depressed psychiatric outpatients, Brown (1961) reported that 41 per cent had lost a parent before the age of 15, as compared with less than 20 per cent for patients suffering from nonpsychiatric medical disorders and less than 17 per cent for the general population. In a review of various retrospective studies of adolescent and adult patients, Gregory (1958) concluded that the evidence shows abnormally high frequencies of parental death and parental separation during the childhood of individuals who subsequently manifest antisocial behavior, psychoneuroses and schizophrenia. Loss of both parents appears to be most common in the case of antisocial behavior, loss of the mother in schizophrenia, and loss of the father in psychoneuroses. One may speculate that loss of both parents particularly predisposes the individual to antisocial behavior because the absence of both parents makes socialization extremely difficult; that loss of the mother predisposes to schizophrenia because lack of mothering leads to mistrust, suspicion and social withdrawal; and that loss of the father, since it is psychologically less serious than loss of the mother, predisposes to neurosis rather than psychosis.

In a review of the effects of all types of maternal deprivation, Bowlby (1951) concluded that the evidence is ''. . . plain that when deprived of maternal care, the child's development is almost always retarded—physically, intellectually, and socially—and that symptoms of physical and mental illness may appear. . . . The retrospective and follow-up studies make it clear that . . . some children are gravely damaged for life. This is a sombre conclusion which must now be regarded as established.''

The effects of absence of the father due to separation or divorce are best understood in terms of the consequences for the child's self concept and his concept of others. The child may feel that he and his mother were abandoned because they were worthless, or alternatively that the mother abandoned the father and perhaps later might also abandon him. Too, he may feel that human beings as a whole are not trustworthy and that love relationships are hazardous and lead to hatred. The relationship with the mother is certain to change after the father has left the home. The mother may regard the child as an economic burden, as a reminder of her failure to retain her husband and home or as an embodiment of the father's undesirable characteristics. On the other hand, the mother may seek from the child the emotional satisfaction she could not obtain from her husband; she may overprotect the child and smother him with possessive demonstrations of affection which he is unable to reciprocate. Of course, parental deprivation does not inevitably lead to emotional disorder since adequate relationships may be developed with other persons important to the child, but it is one important source of psychopathology.

Anal Frustration and Later Personality

The predisposition to emotional difficulties arising from anal frustration has been studied by Huschka (1942, 1943). The case histories of 213 maladjusted children between 1 and 13 years old were examined. They had been referred to a guidance clinic because of restlessness, tics, pathological fear of school, speech disturbances and antisocial behavior. In over half the cases, bowel training had been coercive and had been begun at an age judged too early by the investigator. Most of the children reacted immediately with symptoms of distress, for example, fear of the toilet, anger, reactive and phobic overcleanliness and fear of wetness. Sixty-eight per cent had been started on bladder training too early; at age three, 58 per cent were still enuretic (bed-wetters), apparently as a protest against training. The author states that the responses of these coercively trained children constitute ''. . . a seed bed of psychopathology. Most if not all of them [the responses of the children] fall in the category of anxiety . . . the starting point in the genesis of much of the psychopathology observed in later life'' (1943, p. 261). Huschka's results are impressive, but it should be noted that the study has no control group. We do not know what per cent of well-adjusted children, equated with the experimental group on socio-economic status, intelligence and other major variables, has been subjected to coercive pressures in the anal stage. Hence, this and similar empirical studies are suggestive rather than conclusive and need further verification.

Sex Training, Infantile Stimulation and Later Adjustment

The attitudes toward sex learned in the process of socialization have profound effects on later adjustment. The child may acquire the belief that sex is shameful or fearful and then reflect this belief in diverse ways. One factor in some cases of homosexuality is fear of the opposite sex that has been engendered by threats associated with childhood sexuality. Complete sexual withdrawal may result from a fusion of sex impulses with inhibiting feelings of inferiority, guilt, disgust and fear. In the ''Don Juan complex,'' the individual attempts to ward off an unconscious feeling of sexual inferiority by demonstrating his sexual prowess in repeated and compulsive seductions.

Adult sexual behavior is also affected by other determinants. In a series of fascinating experiments on monkeys, <u>Harlow</u> and his associates made some important discoveries concerning <u>the relation between infantile interactions and subsequent sexual, maternal and social behavior.</u> The monkeys were divided into groups raised under different conditions. In one group, infant monkeys were raised and nursed by their mothers; in another, the infants were separated from their mothers 6 to 12 hours after birth and suckled on tiny nursing bottles. Among the latter group, some were raised in <u>isolation</u> in a wire cage and others were permitted to establish physical contact with, and emotional dependence upon, a cloth-covered substitute, or "<u>mother surrogate.</u>" Harlow and Zimmermann (1958) reported that the inanimate, cloth mother surrogate readily became an object loved with intensity and for a long period of time; in all instances it was preferred to a similar plain wire frame without the cloth covering. <u>The body contact possible with the cloth surrogate, but not with the wire surrogate, is an extremely strong affectional variable.</u>

place of a parent

The monkeys who lived with their own mothers and some of the monkeys reared with cloth surrogates were permitted to interact with other young monkeys of both the same and opposite sexes. In this situation male and female infants showed differences in sex behavior from the second month of life onward. Young males had a much higher frequency of threatening behavior toward animals of both sexes and young females had a much higher frequency of withdrawal and immobility. Young males initiated play contact with other animals much more frequently than did young females, while rough-and-tumble play was largely restricted to pairs of young males. In sex play, males rarely adopted a female sexual position. Females adopted female positions, and groomed and caressed other young monkeys more than young males did. In other words, <u>subjects permitted to interact with others normally or almost normally showed appropriate sexual behavior at a very early age.</u>

On reaching adult life, the male and female monkeys who had been <u>reared in isolation</u> and those reared with cloth surrogates *without* opportunity to interact with other infant monkeys showed an extraordinary pattern. They

① with
② with

what about control for faces here?

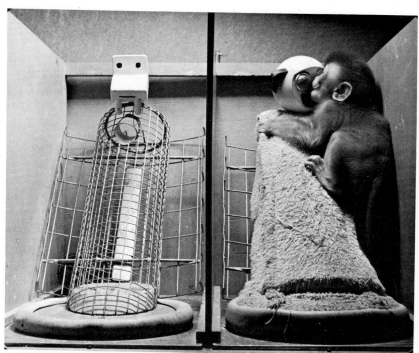

Figure 7–8. *Cloth and wire mother surrogates were used to test the preferences of infant monkeys. The infants spent most of their time clinging to the soft cloth "mother." (Courtesy of Professor Harry. F. Harlow.)*

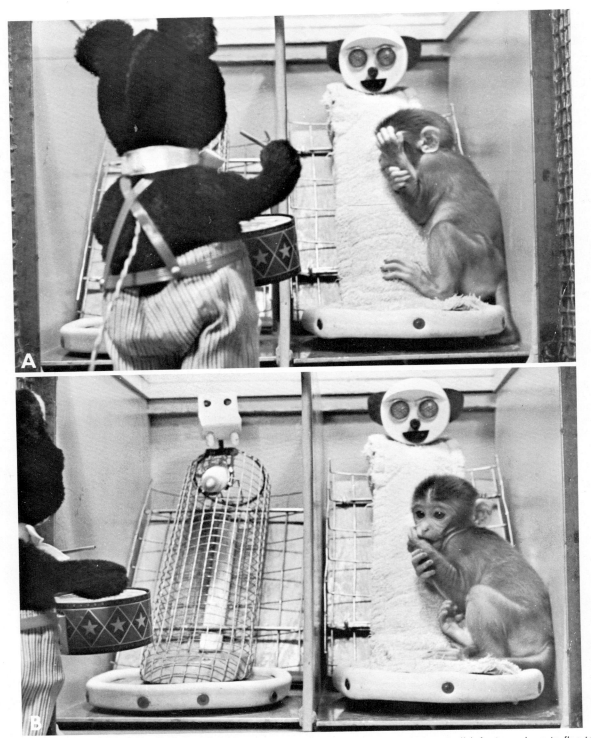

Figure 7–9.　*A, Frightening objects such as a mechanical teddy bear caused almost all infant monkeys to flee to the cloth mother. B, After reassurance by pressing and rubbing against the cloth mother they dared to look at the strange object. (Courtesy of Professor Harry F. Harlow.)*

now sat mutely, were indifferent and apathetic, and with heads in hands rocked back and forth repetitively. Sometimes they went into violent rages when approached or even when left alone; in their rage states they tore at and hurt themselves. They manifested no normal sex behavior whatsoever and had no offspring. Biologically mature adult males were passive in the presence of females or else engaged in violent fighting behavior. A few females were successfully retrained by a special program of social and sexual interaction with psychologically healthy animals of the opposite sex (retraining failed with most) and thereafter became mothers, but they were very bad mothers indeed and quite cruel to their infants (see Figure 7–10). Harlow (1962) calls them "helpless, hopeless, heartless mothers, devoid or almost devoid, of any maternal feeling."

The absence of opportunity for close interaction with other young monkeys thus appeared to have profound effects on the isolated subjects' subsequent sexual, maternal and social behavior. It may be possible to generalize

from these findings to the etiology of similar behavior disorders in humans, particularly schizophrenia. An interesting biochemical study by Beckett et al. (1962) suggests some similarities between Harlow's monkeys and human schizophrenic patients. Biochemical tests on the monkeys reared in isolation showed evidence of blood serum changes identical with some blood chemistry findings reported in human schizophrenic patients. The implication, tentative though it must be before corroboration by further experimentation, is that severe infantile deprivation in humans may lead to defects in physiological functioning which are responsible for some mental disorders.

The importance of stimulation in infancy has also been shown by Levine (1960) in experimental work with rats. Infant rats subjected to various stress stimuli but also handled by humans in order to give the animals body contact experiences did not show disturbances in adulthood. Infant rats who were not handled developed at a slower rate anatomically and physiologically, and were less tame and much more fearful. When placed in unfamiliar surroundings as adults they cowered in corners or crept about cautiously, frequently urinating or defecating. The implication is that rats, and presumably other organisms, may learn to develop a *normal* stress reaction—for example, the ability to cope with the stress of a new situation —provided there has been no deprivation of body stimulation in infancy. (Levine [1962] also demonstrated that the response to stress in rats is influenced by a hereditary component.) The effect of infantile exposure to stress on later ability to adjust to new stress situations may thus be a function of the context of other variables within which the original stress occurs. An emotional trauma in childhood may have little adverse effect if the child is basically secure.

The effect of human parental stimulation on the behavior of children has been studied extensively and the weight of the evidence seems to be that certain forms of parental stimulation have profound effects on the child's later development. For example, Baldwin et al. (1945) found the parents who were warm, democratic and indulgent had brighter children who were increasing in I.Q. during three years of observation, while children of parents who were cold, autocratic and nonindulgent were less bright and either remained stationary or decreased in I.Q. during the period of study. Other investigators have noted that the combination of close

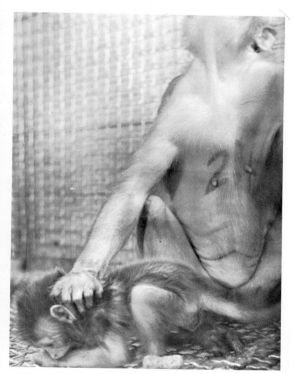

Figure 7–10. One of Harlow's "helpless, hopeless, heartless mothers," and child. (From Harlow, H. F. 1962. The heterosexual affectional system in monkeys. Amer. Psychol., 17:1–9.)

association with a devoted adult and a consequent reduction in peer contacts is associated with high intellectual performance and superior language skills in the child. McCurdy (1961) studied biographical data of 20 famous geniuses. He concluded that most of the 20 had received a great deal of loving, stimulating attention in early childhood from adults, that most grew up either primarily or exclusively in the daily company of these adults, and that their peer interactions had been either curtailed or nonexistent. Peer interaction seems helpful in developing social skills but too much emphasis on the peer group interaction may be at the expense of intellectual or creative activity. Conversely, an environment of rich parental stimulation seems associated with intellectual achievement, but without opportunity for peer group interaction the child may be a poor social animal. McCurdy (1961) summarizes the extreme alternatives as follows:

> A society which favors intelligence and individuality will approve of the hothouse effects of the loving family; one which favors horde life and group conformity will distrust the family influence and . . . [attempt] . . . to replace the influence of the small family devoted to its . . . few children with the influence of larger masses of age-equals such as are found in our public schools [p. 151].

Family Constellations and Parental Attitudes

Except for institutionalized children, human conflict and stress occur within a family context. Specific family constellations and parental attitudes have been shown by various investigators to have specific effects—both precipitating and predisposing—on behavior.

Three family constellations are particularly frequent in the background of disturbed individuals (Becker et al., 1959; Peterson et al., 1959; Liverant, 1959).

1. The parents are impulsive, inconsistent and arbitrary. They act out their unstable emotions on their children.

2. The father is preoccupied, weak and withdrawn; the mother is strong and dominant and the relationship between the two, not surprisingly, is poor. The father resents his strong wife and does not support her methods of disciplining the children.

3. The mother is average while the father is authoritarian, demanding and punitive. The children fear the father and tend to withdraw

from him; they are sensitive to threats and feel inferior.

A definitive investigation of the relation of familial constellation to aggression in children was made by McCord, McCord and Howard (1961). They intensively studied 174 lower-class boys over a period of more than five years by observation, home visits and reports of neighbors, police, YMCA officials, teachers and other sources. Twenty-five boys were consistently hostile and aggressive in response to all frustrations, 97 were sporadically or selectively aggressive and 52 were rarely or never aggressive.

The consistently aggressive boys, as contrasted to the others, were more often disciplined punitively. One or both parents of 95 per cent of the aggressive boys had rejecting attitudes. A particularly frequent constellation was a rejecting mother and an affectionate father. Aggressiveness was also positively correlated with lack of parental demands on the children to conform: for example, to be polite, attend Sunday school or keep their rooms clean. Inconsistency was noted in 78 per cent of the mothers of aggressive boys versus 48 per cent of the mothers of nonaggressive boys. Any paternal deviation—high aggression, passivity, escapist behavior, alcoholism, sexual promiscuity or psychosis—was associated with filial aggression. Parental conflict and mutual lack of respect as well as dissatisfaction of a parent with his or her role in life also correlated with filial aggression. The investigators interpreted their results on the premise that parental frustration increases the child's aggressive responses to his parents. The child's concept of the parents then generalizes to other human beings and his aggression is displaced to them. At the same time, the lack of effective parental discipline prevents the child from inhibiting his displaced, aggressive urges; on the contrary, should one of the parents be aggressive, he will set a model for the boy's aggressiveness. In such a case the boy's superego cannot easily adopt the moral values of the other, nonaggressive parent because the aggressive parent overshadows the nonaggressive one.

Family constellations are obviously quite complex. Parents interact with each other and children interact differently with each parent and, of course, with their siblings. The aspect of family interactions that has been most studied is that of parental attitudes to children. Four attitudinal dimensions have been suggested by various psychologists: care-neglect, dominance-submission, democracy-autocracy and accept-ance-rejection; the last is possibly the most fundamental of the four. Experimental studies and clinical experience indicate that parental acceptance is associated with friendliness, self-confidence and stability in children, and lack of acceptance with confusion, instability and either rebelliousness or apathy. Kanner (1957) has categorized parental attitudes into four basic types, each with a specifiable effect on the child. (Kanner's four types cut across the four widely recognized dimensions of parental attitude.) Three of these types are nonaccepting (see Table 7–1). Failure to accept a child emotionally may take the form of overt rejection, perfectionistic demands or overprotective spoiling or domination.

The form of discipline employed by parents may serve as a sensitive indicator of the parent's attitude toward the child. Greenfield (1959) studied the childhood discipline as recalled by 58 outpatients at a university student psychiatric clinic and 58 matched control subjects. Disciplinary techniques were categorized as direct (physical or otherwise unambiguous) on the one hand, and indirect on the other. The direct techniques consisted of scolding or reasoning, spanking, isolation from the group or denial of some pleasure. The indirect techniques consisted of guilt-inducing expressions of disappointment or denial of love by the parents. The patients reported significantly higher frequencies of exposure to indirect rather than direct forms of childhood discipline. Since the induction of guilt feelings in children is a more subtle form of nonacceptance than direct punishment, it may be that the more subtle the lack of acceptance the greater is the probability of later disturbance.

One other aspect of family interactions is often important in abnormal psychology: due to man's slow maturation, the human family is unique in that it frequently includes two or more dependent offspring of different ages at the same time. This situation breeds *sibling rivalry,* a competition primarily directed toward securing the affection, attention and approval of parents. The relationships among siblings frequently mirror the relationship of each sibling to the parents. After the birth of a new baby, sibling rivalry is particularly evidenced in the form of aggressive or regressive behavior in the child who was previously the youngest member of the family. Manifestations of sibling rivalry are more marked in the eldest child than in later children, for prior to the birth of a second child the eldest had no competition for his parents' attention and he is hit hard by removal from this unique position. Emotionally disturbed individuals who have siblings almost always have a history of some degree of sibling rivalry.

PSYCHOLOGICAL PREDISPOSITIONS TO ABNORMALITY: SOME CONCLUSIONS

The experimental and clinical data, both animal and human, are consistent enough to permit a series of general conclusions.

(1) Psychopathological behavior results from learning under conditions of frustration, conflict and deprivation. If all other variables such as heredity were to be held constant, then the

TABLE 7–1. Principal Types of Parental Attitudes*

Attitude	Characteristic Verbalization	Handling of the Child	Reaction of the Child
Acceptance and affection	"It's the child that makes the home interesting."	Fondling; play; patience	Security; normal personality development
Overt rejection	"I hate him." "I won't bother with him."	Neglect; harshness; avoidance of contact; severe punishment	Aggressiveness; delinquency; shallowness of affect
Perfectionism	"I do not want him as he is; I must make him over."	Disapproval; fault-finding; coercion	Frustration; lack of self-confidence; obsessiveness
Overprotection	"Of course, I like him; see how I sacrifice myself for him."	Spoiling; nagging; over-indulgence or hovering domination	Delay in maturation and emancipation; protracted dependence on mother; "spoiled child" behavior

*Reprinted by permission from Kanner, L. 1957. Child Psychiatry. 3rd Ed. Courtesy of Charles C Thomas, Publisher, Springfield, Illinois.

more stressful these conditions were the more severe the subsequent psychopathology would be.

2. Early experience is crucial. Severe and possibly irreversible damage may result from early childhood experiences; at a later period the same experiences have less serious effects.

3. Within childhood there are several critical developmental periods and several critical types of stimulation and experience. In the critical oral phase the infant is particularly sensitive to oral stimulation or deprivation (as well as to body contact); in the critical anal phase he is sensitive to the discipline of toilet training; and so forth. Specific types of stimulation in specific phases mold subsequent behavior.

4. Lasting psychopathology is less likely to result from a single traumatic event than from prolonged stress.

5. For normal development, children require close and enduring relationships with a parent or parent-substitute of each sex and with peers of both sexes. Deprivation of these relationships is an unquestionable cause of emotional disorder.

6. Parents and siblings may condition inappropriate affects or reinforce maladaptive behaviors by a variety of obvious and subtle means including nonverbal communication. Any parental attitude that deviates from acceptance of a child—overt rejection, perfectionism, inconsistency and overdominance—increases the probability that the child will develop an emotional disorder.

where?

check it

1) Liddell – remained after 3 years
2) Bradys – monkeys died
3) Harlows – heartless mothers
4) spitz & wolf – maternal dep.
5) Levine – handled rats

SINGLE TRAUMATIC EVENT

1) Massermans cat –
2)

8
SOCIOCULTURAL DETERMINANTS

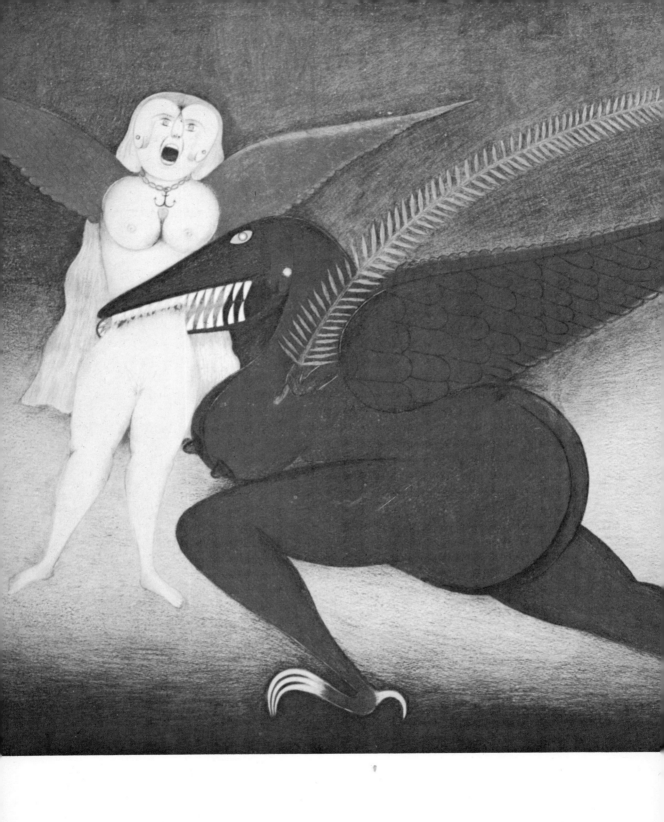

Society . . . requires that, forgetful of our own interests, we make ourselves
its servitors, and it submits us to every sort of inconvenience, privation,
and sacrifice, without which social life would be impossible . . . At every
instant we are obliged to submit ourselves to rules of conduct and of
thought which we have neither made nor desired, and which are
sometimes even contrary to our most fundamental inclinations and
instincts.

Emile Durkheim, The Elementary Forms
of the Religious Life

SOCIOCULTURAL
DETERMINANTS

The biological and psychological determinants of behavior act upon the human organism within a cultural environment—family, neighborhood, community, occupation, ethnic group, socioeconomic class and national culture. Often the sociocultural environment is stressful, for example, in times of unemployment, rapid technological change or war. Depending on the severity of sociocultural stress, biological and psychological determinants will have different effects on the individual.

Largely because they are not readily amenable to laboratory study, sociocultural determinants are difficult to divide into the two categories of predisposing and precipitating. An individual may behave in middle-class fashion because of an inextricable combination of predisposing childhood training and day by day social precipitants. Thus, after a war, emotional difficulties may occur as a residue of the war itself and also because of the later, postward stress of economic and vocational problems. In such a case, it is difficult to state whether war is a predisposing or precipitating

cause of disturbed behavior. To take one more example, a member of a minority group may be predisposed to anxiety by childhood deprivations associated with minority status; later, new stresses may precipitate additional anxiety.

CULTURE, SOCIAL
DISORGANIZATION AND CONFLICT

Society consists of interlocking formal and informal organizations—religious bodies, families, occupational groups, age groups, friendship groups and many others; each group is a cultural unit. A culture is composed of the patterns of perception, beliefs and goals shared by a group of people and of the social relations among these people. Each cultural group to which an individual belongs imposes obligations on him, assigns a status and a role to him, disciplines him by means of rewards and punishments, and—as the cultural pattern develops and changes over a time—alters his obligations and status. More than anything else, a culture demands from the individual some degree of conformity to its *social norms,* as these are expressed informally in folkways and mores or formally in laws.

The individual's status or position in the social structure may be ascribed to him on the basis of sex, age or kinship, or achieved through personal effort and success. In some societies and cultures, referred to as closed, the individual has very few opportunities for personal achievement of status. The Indian caste system and the medieval European feudal system are examples of closed societies. In open societies, the opportunities for personal achievement of status—through education or occupational striving—are considerable. The United States is generally considered to be a relatively open society. Both types have their advantages and disadvantages for mental health. A closed society has a great deal of stability since each individual knows precisely what his position is, but to a gifted individual this stability is frustrating. An open society, on the other hand, stimulates competition and permits gifted individuals to make maximum contributions and achieve changes in status, but the cost is insecurity, instability and often severe feelings of inadequacy.

A fundamental hypothesis linking the structure and functions of society to emotional disorders is that *social disorganization leads to personal disorganization.* The eminent sociologist Ernest W. Burgess (1955) stated this hypothesis as follows:

Mental ill health is a symptom and index of the malfunctioning of society. . . . Society . . . is a great organized structure of the social relations of its members. When society is well organized it provides through its institutions and groups the necessary roles to utilize the energies and to realize the wishes of its members. The thesis . . . is that an important factor, perhaps the most important single factor in mental disorders and disturbances, is the failure of society to provide adequately for the social roles essential for the mental health of its members. By its failure to devise and to maintain satisfying roles and relationships society creates and is therefore responsible for the misfits, the unadjusted and maladjusted persons who are or become either criminals or mentally ill or both.

L. K. Frank put the matter even more strongly in a statement (1936) that has since been widely quoted:

There is a growing realization among throughtful persons that our culture is sick, mentally disordered and in need of treatment. . . . The disintegration of our traditional culture, with the decay of those ideas, concepts, and beliefs upon which our social and individual lives were organized, brings us face to face with the problem of treating society, since individual therapy or punishment no longer has any value beyond mere alleviation of our symptoms.

Social disorganization is a matter of degree: a society or culture is more or less disorganized. The degree of disorganization may be indicated by phenomena such as widespread poverty, prostitution, alcoholism or drug addiction, sharp and disruptive ideological conflict, broken homes or other fractures of social relationships, poor community resources for education and recreation, lack of cooperation of individuals in voluntary associations, and widespread juvenile delinquency and crime. These phenomena tend to correlate with each other and with the frequency of mental disorder. As we shall see later in more detail, the neighborhoods with the highest rates of admission to mental hospitals have the most poverty, the poorest community resources, the highest crime rates and so forth. In a comparative study of disorganized and organized communities in the maritime regions of Canada, Leighton (1959) found a much higher prevalence of neurotic, psychophysiologic and sociopathic disorders, particularly the last, in the disorganized communities. Similar results were obtained in a study of organized and disorganized communities in Mexico (Murphy, 1962).

A corollary to the hypothesis that social disorganization leads to emotional disorder is that certain specific social conditions are required for mental health. It is widely assumed that in order to maximize the mental health of its members a society must satisfy their basic needs, make it possible for them to be and feel useful and provide them with opportunities for self-expression. A disorganized society fails in precisely these obligations and the result is conflict and emotional breakdown.

Even in the absence of marked disorganization, however, there are sociocultural forces conducive to personal conflict and emotional difficulty. The conflicts between subcultures may be internalized within the individual; for example, a first-generation offspring of immigrant parents may find himself exposed to simultaneous and incompatible pressures from his parents' immigrant culture and the native culture of his peers and teachers. In consequence, he may suffer from an inability to identify with either cultural model. A member of a socioeconomic class who is moving upward socially is likely to be caught in the conflict of trying to behave like a member of a higher class when he still belongs to the lower one economically. (Changes in the emotional and cognitive responses of upwardly mobile persons often precede changes in their economic conditions.) A conflict between drive expression and inhibition as well as a conflict of loyalties may result from socioeconomic mobility. The individual may wish to drink beer and play poker, for example, but feels that he should be reading "worthwhile" literature instead. More severe conflicts may arise among members of racial or religious minorities and among social nonconformists. The homosexual is often a social outcast and the political nonconformist is regarded with suspicion.

The conflicting demands of society as a whole may also breed personal conflict. Karen Horney (1937), a neo-Freudian analyst, believed that at the root of typical neurotic conflicts were three social contradictions: an emphasis on competition and success contradicts an emphasis on brotherly love and humility, cultural stimulation of needs is inconsistent with the frustration consequent on the actual difficulty encountered in attempting to satisfy them, and the alleged freedom of the individual is contradicted by the factual limitations to his freedom imposed by social reality and his own shortcomings. Horney wrote as follows:

These contradictions embedded in our culture are precisely the conflicts which the neurotic struggles to reconcile: his tendencies toward aggressiveness and his tendencies toward yielding; his excessive demands and his fears of never getting anything; his striving toward self-aggrandizement and his feeling of personal helplessness.

CULTURE AND PERSONALITY

The quotation from Horney's writings leads us into the problem of the relation of culture to relatively normal personality. Most investigators agree that cultural patterns profoundly and widely affect personality development; anthropologists have described many illustrative examples. The Zuni culture is so organized that lack of ambition is favored from an early age. In Bali, mothers stimulate their children emotionally and then callously ignore them; as a result, the children develop and maintain into adulthood the traits of self-defensive sullenness, seclusiveness and withdrawal from intense emotional conflicts. Among the Sioux Indians, children are incited to outbursts of rage; a seem-

ing consequence of this child-rearing pattern is an adult personality marked by quarrelsomeness, cruelty and hostility to outsiders.

Kardiner (1945) has formulated a theory that seeks to explain the culture-personality relation found in any society, whether primitive or advanced. In every culture, according to Kardiner's viewpoint, there is a *basic personality structure*—a modal norm of traits and behaviors shared by most members. The basic personality structure of a culture is formed by the action of its primary institutions—the particular type of family, the customary child-rearing patterns, the fundamental economic techniques and the like. The basic personality structure, in turn, is hypothesized to be responsible for such secondary cultural institutions as the prevailing religious beliefs, values and social attitudes. Thus, among the Alorese (inhabitants of the island of Alor in the East Indies) child rearing consists of sporadic and inconsistent care of the child. The mother is often absent, the child is weaned by being pushed away and he is frequently teased and deceived by adults. As a direct consequence, argues Kardiner, the modal Alorese personality is marked by feelings of self-inadequacy, isolation and worthlessness. The Alorese are easily discouraged, touchy, apprehensive, and both hostile and dependent. They are suspicious of each other in adult life; every member of the tribe is concerned with his own safety more than anything else.

The primary cultural institutions of Western society are undoubtedly just as important for personality development, but the variables are more difficult to disentangle and interpret than in more primitive societies. (Some effects of child-rearing practices on behavior in our culture were cited earlier, but the focus was on individual differences rather than on the prevailing practices and modal personality of an entire cultural group.) In any case, on the basis of studies of other cultures the hypothesis that culture guides the formation of personality traits—whether via its primary institutions or otherwise—seems sound. Hence there is a theoretical basis for investigating the sociocultural causes of the special variant of behavior and personality that we term "abnormality."

THE METHODOLOGY OF SOCIOCULTURAL STUDIES

The ideal method of studying sociocultural causation would involve controlled, experimental manipulation of families, neighbor-hoods, economic conditions or other cultural institutions and phenomena, and careful obser-vation of the resultant behavior. Some neighbor-hoods, for example, would systematically be dis-organized, while comparable neighborhoods would systematically be protected from disor-ganization. Obviously, this type of research design is unethical and impractical. The studies that have been carried out consist of nonexperi-mental observation of naturally occurring social phenomena and concomitant behavior. The studies are thus correlational and result in the standard problems of inferring causation from correlation. Nevertheless, almost all observers have concluded that sociocultural determinants have enormous effects on behavior disturbance.

Fundamental to the study of sociocultural causation are two basic questions: First, what are the *facts* about the frequency of abnormal behavior in any society or culture? Second, bearing in mind that the studies are correla-tional, how is it possible to *interpret* the facts to reach causal conclusions?

The Determination of Frequency

The factual determination of frequency is not easy. To begin with, it is affected by the behav-ior and attitude of a cultural group toward ab-normality. Reported frequencies of mental disorder differ radically depending on whether disturbed individuals are believed to be possessed by demons, as is still true in many primitive cultures, or perceived as criminals who should be jailed or as sick persons in need of treatment. If the members of a culture are ashamed of the existence of mental illness in the group, they will evade questions dealing with it. In the United States over the past few decades the stigma attached to emotional dis-turbance has markedly decreased and, con-comitantly, a larger and larger number of individuals have sought voluntary admission to hospitals while relatively fewer persons have been committed by court order or medical certification. Since persons admitted to hos-pitals voluntarily are usually less ill than per-sons admitted involuntarily, an increasing per-centage of hospitalized patients has been diagnosed neurotic rather than psychotic, thus causing a change in frequency data.

The determination of frequency is also af-fected by the very definition of abnormality. In cross-cultural research, for example, the prob-lem arises of whether to employ our own criteria of abnormality or those of the other culture. Behaviors that we perceive as abnormal may be adaptive in other cultures. For ex-ample, some of the behaviors we diagnose as hysterical, manic or even schizophrenic may help an individual to qualify as a medicine man in a primitive society. An Australian aborigine would undoubtedly consider working in an office, wearing a coat and tie and buying meat in a store instead of killing game very strange. Arieti and Meth (1959) point out that:

In the West, suicide is considered a sign of emo-tional disorder; in Japan, it is normal for a samurai in certain circumstances. Among the islanders of Dobu (Melanesia) no sane women leaves her cooking pot unguarded for fear of being poisoned. To us, this behavior would indicate paranoia. Among some Eskimo tribes, the mother accepts the killer of her son in her son's stead. Among the Papuans it is tradi-tional for an uncle and nephew (mother's brother and son) to practice homosexuality. In Tibet a group of brothers inherit their father's second wife when he gets old. A Navajo male may marry a widow with a daughter; later he discards the mother and marries the daughter. It is not unusual for an Arapesh to marry simultaneously a mother and her daughter. These are a few behavior patterns which we consider ab-normal, but which are entirely normal in other civilizations.

However, despite these variations there ap-pears to be a certain degree of cross-cultural agreement. For example, studies of mental dis-order among the Eskimos and the Yoruba tribe of Nigeria (Murphy, 1962) have suggested that the majority of individuals perceived as deviant in these cultures would be categorized as deviant by our own criteria. When the native Yoruba healers were asked to identify the mentally ill members of their community, they reported no cases that we would classify as psychophysiologic, neurotic, sociopathic or senile, but there were many that we would diag-nose as schizophrenic, mentally deficient or brain damaged. Based on a review of available knowledge of disorders among a wide variety of peoples, Arieti and Meth arrived at the con-clusions that, "Actually, there is a great uniformity in the psychiatric nosology of people whose cultural norms vary widely . . . the majority of psychiatric cases of all times and all places are similar to ours." It would therefore appear that cross-cultural comparisons can be meaningfully made.

Within a single culture, frequency determina-tion is affected by time changes in prevailing *are they all estimates?*

classification practices. A large number of cases of alcoholism or sexual deviation that formerly were considered to constitute delinquency or criminality are now included in the category, "personality disorders." Patients not long ago classified as manic are now often labeled schizo-affective. Hence, a study that employs frequency data for different points in time must take changes in classification procedures into account and try to correct for them. An extreme instance of the effect of historical events on classification occurred in Germany in 1850. Following the widespread European revolutions of 1848, in which democratic ideology played a large part, a medical student named Groddeck wrote a doctoral dissertation entitled "On the Democratic Disease, A New Form of Insanity." After some dispute among the faculty, the dissertation was accepted and the candidate was awarded a doctorate (G. Rosen, 1959).

The minimal degree of abnormality necessary for inclusion in frequency measurements must be decided arbitrarily. If we ask the seemingly simple question, "What per cent of the population of the United States is disturbed?" we get completely different answers depending on our criteria of disturbance. (See the discussion in Chapter 1 of the statistical criterion of abnormality.) If the criterion is admission to a mental hospital at least once during a lifetime, the answer is between 15 and 20 per cent; but if the criterion is a research worker's identification of any degree of symptoms of psychopathology in persons living at home, the answer yielded by a recent survey in New York City was 80 per cent (Srole et al., 1962).

Four different statistical measures of frequency, each of which is appropriate for a different purpose, must be carefully distinguished.

Three of these measures—incidence, prevalence and expectancy—are used to indicate what proportion of the general population manifests a disorder (or all disorders combined). Incidence rates describe how many persons *become* disturbed or ill within a given time (say, one year); prevalence rates describe how many *are* ill at a given point in time; and expectancy rates estimate how many *will* become ill during an entire lifetime. The fourth measure—percentage frequency—indicates what per cent of a group of patients belongs to a given diagnostic category.

Let us consider each of these measures more fully. An *incidence* rate is computed by dividing the number of new cases coming from a specified segment of the general population by the total number of persons in that segment. The traditional basis for estimating the number of new cases is the number of first admissions to hospitals in a year, that is, the number admitted during the year who had never before been hospitalized. Thus, for the year 1968 the rate of first admissions for all mental disorders in the United States was 84 per 100,000. By dividing the number of new cases in a given age group (e.g., aged 55 through 64) by the total number of individuals in that age group in the propulation, age-specific rates may be obtained. Thus, in 1968 the first admission rate, for persons aged 65 and over, for all mental disorders in the United States was 156 per 100,000; i.e., of every 100,000 persons aged 65 or more, 156 were admitted to hospitals as psychiatric patients for the first time in their lives. Table 8–1 presents first-admission rates, separately for various age groups and for all age groups combined, for the year 1968. The higher rates for older people are noteworthy; this is mainly a result of the greater incidence

BW

IE

Table 8–1. Estimated First-Admission Rates per 100,000 for State and County Mental Hospitals by Age and Diagnosis, U.S., 1968

Diagnoses	Under 18	18–64	65 and Over	All Ages
Acute and chronic brain syndromes	1.3	16.9	132.7	22.3
Psychotic disorders	3.7	34.0	7.2	20.4
Psychophysiologic, autonomic and visceral disorders	0.0	.2	0.0	.1
Psychoneurotic disorders	1.1	15.5	3.2	9.1
Personality disorders	3.1	36.4	4.2	21.3
Transient situational personality disorders	5.5	2.6	1.1	3.5
Mental deficiency	1.6	2.9	.3	2.2
Without mental disorder	.6	2.7	1.6	1.8
Undiagnosed	1.0	4.9	6.2	3.6
Total	17.9	116.1	156.5	84.3

Adapted from National Institute of Mental Health Statistics: Patients in State and County Mental Hospitals, 1968. Series A, No. 2, 1969.

of the brain syndromes, some of which are secondary to the effects of advancing age. The importance of chronic brain syndromes and the psychoses is also clear in the table; these two categories together comprise roughly one-half of all admissions in the United States. First admission rates are, of course, an underestimate of true incidence. Admission rates are influenced by availability of hospital accommodations, availability of other facilities for psychiatric treatment, social attitude toward mental disorder and hospitalization, and variations in diagnostic criteria. In addition, while some disorders are quite common, they usually do not require hospitalization. First admission rates to hospitals would give an underestimate of the true incidence of such disorders.

In Table 8–2 the percentage of all first admissions for various diagnoses are given for both sex and age. From this table it is clear that the incidence of some diagnoses is related to age or sex, or both. Acute and chronic brain syndromes comprise 26 per cent of all first admissions, but over 14 per cent of such admissions occur in persons over 65. Personality disorders account for 25 per cent of all first admissions if we combine figures for both males and females. From the table it can be seen that 20 per cent of the admissions diagnosed as personality disorders are males—mostly adult males in the 18 to 65 age range. Men are more likely than women to come into conflict with society and be diagnosed as sociopaths (one of the personality disorders), and this may help explain the higher incidence of this disorder in males.

Prevalence rates are computed by dividing the number of existing cases (in a single diagnostic category or in all categories combined) in a particular segment of the population by the total number of persons in that segment. For example, of every 100,000 persons belonging to the lowest socioeconomic class in the city of New Haven, Connecticut, on a specified day in 1959, the number in treatment for psychosis was 1505, i.e., the prevalence rate was 1505 per 100,000. This rate was approximately 10 times as large as the incidence of new cases of psychosis in the same class in New Haven during 1959. Reported prevalence underestimates true prevalence. In an investigation carried out in Sweden, for example, it was concluded that the number of patients with manic-depressive psychosis was only about one-seventh the total number of manic-depressives in the general population (Larson and Sjögren, 1954).

Expectancy rates define the probability that a member of a population will develop a disorder during his entire lifetime or a sizeable part of it. Expectancy is cumulative incidence over the years. In Table 8–3, the expectancy rates for ages 10 through 54 are shown for the inhabitants of the Danish island of Bornholm. The rates were computed by Fremming (1951) on the basis of an investigation of mental disorders in a very large sample of the inhabitants of the island. (No figures are given after age 55 when many cases first occur.) The figures concur with a number of studies carried out in other European communities. According to the table, no single disorder had an expectation as high as 3 per cent, but more than one-tenth the population could expect to be affected by one or another kind of emotional disorder prior to reaching the age of 55. In the United States, one out of every twelve persons can expect to spend some time in a mental hospital and a larger percentage can expect some form of severe psychological difficulty.

Percentage frequency is illustrated by Table 8–4. Percentages are given for first admissions in each category and for resident patients in each category. There is a large disparity between the first admission percentage (18.0) and resident percentage (48.7) for schizophrenia because this disorder is usually chronic: schizophrenic patients stay in the hospital a long time and therefore come to constitute almost half the total hospital population. On the other hand, patients with personality disorders—mostly sociopathy—and psychoneuroses come and go quickly, and their resident percentages are therefore much lower than their admission percentages.

The percentage frequencies for various diagnostic categories are different for different types of hospitals. Psychiatric hospitals affiliated with universities tend to accept fewer patients with organic brain syndromes or addiction to alcohol or drugs than state hospitals. Private sanitoria admit relatively fewer schizophrenics but relatively more depressives and neurotics than state hospitals. Unlocked psychiatric wards in general hospitals also admit a high proportion of patients with affective disorders or neuroses.

The Interpretation of Frequency Data. As a rule, it is unjustifiable to infer sociocultural causation from any single study. To illustrate, let us consider the fact that in 1957 the prevalence rate for mental disorder in New York was 648 per 100,000, whereas in Arizona it was 144

Table 8–2. Percentage of First Admissions to Public Mental Hospitals by Diagnosis, Age and Sex, U.S.

Diagnosis	Under 18		18–24		25–44		45–64		Over 65		All Ages	
	Male	Female	Male	Female	Male	Female	Male	Female	Male	Female	Male	Female
Acute and chronic brain syndromes	.4	.2	.5	.2	2.6	1.0	4.4	2.0	7.4	7.4	15.0	11.0
Psychotic disorders	1.0	.7	2.5	1.9	4.9	6.0	2.5	4.2	.3	.5	11.0	13.0
Schizophrenia	(.8)	(.5)	(2.4)	(1.6)	(4.4)	(4.6)	(1.3)	(1.9)	(.1)	(.1)	(9.0)	(9.0)
Psychophysiologic, autonomic and visceral disorders	–	–	–	–	–	–	–	–	–	–	.1	.1
Psychoneurotic disorders	.2	.2	.7	1.2	1.9	3.5	1.1	1.5	.1	.2	4.0	7.0
Personality disorders	1.0	.4	3.2	1.2	9.0	2.5	6.2	1.1	.4	.1	20.0	5.0
Transient situational personality disorders	1.4	.9	.4	.4	.3	.3	.1	.1	.1	–	2.0	2.0
Mental deficiency	.5	.2	.5	.2	.4	.3	.2	.2	–	–	2.0	1.0
Without mental disorder	.2	.1	.4	.1	.6	.2	.2	.1	.1	.1	1.0	.3
Undiagnosed	.3	.2	.4	.3	1.0	.6	.6	.4	.4	.3	4.0	2.4
	5.0	2.9	8.6	5.5	20.7	14.4	15.3	9.6	8.8	8.6	59.1	41.8

Adapted from Reference Tables on Patients in Mental Health Facilities—Age, Sex and Diagnosis, United States, 1968. National Institute of Mental Health, 1969.

per 100,000. It would be naive to interpret these data as meaning that social conditions in New York are more than four times as unhealthy as in Arizona; the difference in rates is due largely to the much greater availability of hospital facilities in New York. The data cannot tell us whether the rates in New York would be higher, lower or the same as in Arizona if all variables such as hospital availability were controlled.

However, *the weight of all the correlational studies combined* make it quite certain that sociocultural variables affect functional disturbances to a very great degree. Cultural causation also has powerful effects on organic disorders. For example, sociocultural conditions influence the frequency of syphilis and hence of paresis. In underdeveloped countries high rates of psychiatric disorder result from malaria, sleeping sickness (trypanosomiasis) and nutritional disorders such as pellagra. Protein deficiency, common in underdeveloped areas, brings on a psychiatric disorder known as kwashiorkor which has a high rate of incidence among African children. Organic psychoses due to alcohol and toxic industrial chemicals occur in western countries, in contrast to psychoses due to various exotic drugs in primitive tribes. Finally, the fact that people live longer in more industrialized and urbanized countries leads to

Table 8–3. Expectation of Mental Disorders during Ages 10 to 54 Years among Fremming's Sample of Danish Population*

Type of Mental Disorder	Expectation Expressed as a Per Cent of the Sample
Schizophrenia	0.88%
Manic-depressive psychosis	1.64
Epilepsy	0.35
General paresis	0.27
Reactive psychosis	0.93
Other psychoses	0.50
Mental defect	1.33
Dull (underestimate)	1.67
Psychopathy (minimal figures)	2.95
Alcoholism	1.74
Psychoneurosis	2.22
Minor affective disorders	0.26
Total	14.74%†

*5500 persons born in the island of Bornholm 1883–1887; 4130 remained available by start of eleventh year and 2710 were still domiciled in Bornholm at time of death or Fremming's inquiry.

†Over-all expectation allowing for multiple disorders in the same person was 11.9 per cent of the sample.

Adapted from Fremming, K. H. 1951. The Expectation of Mental Infirmity in a Sample of the Danish Population. Occasional Papers on Eugenics, No. 7. London, Eugenics Society and Cassell & Co.

Table 8–4. Percentage Frequency of First Admissions and Resident Patients in Mental Hospitals, U.S., 1968.

Diagnosis	First Admissions	Resident Patients
Acute and chronic brain syndromes	26.0	25.8
Psychotic disorders	24.0	56.1
Schizophrenia	(18.0)	(48.7)
Psychophysiologic, autonomic, and visceral disorders	.2	.1
Psychoneurotic disorders	11.0	1.9
Personality disorders	25.0	4.4
Transient situational personality disorders	4.0	1.1
Mental deficiency	3.0	8.6
Without mental disorders	1.3	.1
Undiagnosed	6.4	1.9
Total	100.0*	100.0
Total Number of Patients	154,098	340,235

*Column does not total 100 per cent because of rounding errors.

Adapted from Reference Tables on Patients in Mental Health Facilities—Age, Sex and Diagnosis, United States, 1968. National Institute of Mental Health, 1969.

a far greater frequency of disorders associated with the older ages, such as psychosis with cerebral arteriosclerosis and senile disorders.

From the point of view of research design, three types of sociocultural studies should be distinguished: cross-cultural studies, comparisons of abnormal behavior across time periods that are characterized by different social conditions (e.g., the 1840's and 1940's), and comparisons within a single society for a single variable (e.g., socioeconomic class, war vs. peace, marital status). The single variable type of investigation is pursued in one of two ways: either samples of two groups in the population at large, for example, rural and urban, are compared for behavior disturbances; or the rural-urban composition (or status on any other sociocultural variable) of a patient sample is studied.

CROSS-CULTURAL STUDIES

During the romantic movement of the eighteenth and nineteenth centuries it was widely believed that primitive life led to mental stability and civilized life to mental disorder. In 1828, Sir Andrew Halliday wrote:

The finer the organs of the mind have become by their greater development, or their better cultivation, if health is not made a part of the process, the more easily are they disordered. We seldom meet with insanity among the savage tribes of men; not one of our African travelers remark their having seen a single madman. Among the slaves of the West Indies it very rarely occurs; and, as we have elsewhere shown from actual returns, the contented peasantry of the Welsh Mountains, the Western Hebrides, and the wilds of Ireland are almost free from this complaint.

In the same year, George Burrows wrote:

. . . many of the causes inducing intellectual derangement, and which are called moral, have their origin not in individual passions or feelings, but in the state of society at large; and the more artificial, i.e., civilized, society is, the more do these causes multiply and extensively operate. The vices of civilization, of course, most conduce to their increase; but even the moral virtues, religion, politics, nay philosophy itself, and all the best feelings of our nature, if too enthusiastically incited, class among the causes producing intellectual disorders. The circumstances influencing their occurrence are to be sought in all the various relations of life, in constitutional propensities, and, above all, perhaps in education.

In 1873, W. A. F. Browne, a superintendent of a Scottish asylum, cited figures that appeared to indicate a much higher frequency of insanity in the United States than in Europe and offered the following interpretation:

This disparity probably depends on the rapid acquisition of wealth, and the luxurious social habits to which the good fortune of our trans-atlantic brethren has exposed them. With luxury, indeed, insanity appears to keep equal pace. . . . With civilization . . . come sudden and agitating changes and vicissitudes of fortune; vicious effeminacy of manners; complicated transactions; misdirected views of the objects of life; ambition, and hopes, and fears, which man in his primitive state does not and cannot know.

Writing in 1855, Samuel Woodward, an American psychiatrist, nominated competition as the villainous element in our civilization.

Here [in Massachusetts] the mind, and body, too, are often worked to an extreme point of endurance. Here wealth and station are the results of well-directed efforts; as the general diffusion of intelligence among the whole people stimulates a vast many of them to compete successfully for these prizes. But in the contest, where so many strive, not a few break down. The results on their minds may not, perhaps, be any less disastrous, whether wealth and station are obtained or not. The true balance of the mind is disturbed by prosperity as well as adversity.

More recent observations and studies have not attempted grandiose comparisons of civilized vs. primitive society, but have concentrated on one culture at a time or a comparison of a small number of them. Malinowski (1927) studied the Trobriand islanders and claimed that not a single individual manifested hysteria, nervouc tics, obsessions or compulsions. Faris (1937) found few or no psychoses among natives of the Congo and attributed this finding to the simple and integrated social organization of the Congolese. Carothers (1953) reported that mental hospital admission rates in Kenya were only a fraction of the comparable rates for England, the United States and Canada. Such findings must, of course, be treated with skepticism because in primitive cultures facilities are lacking for the care of disturbed individuals, families may view mental disorder as a disgrace and conceal it, and troublesome psychotics may be allowed to die if they cannot take care of themselves or they may be killed if they become violent. It has been definitely established, however, that certain disorders found in various primitive societies do not occur in Western society at all. Among these are *latah*, found in Malaya and characterized by echolalia, echopraxia and extreme obscenity of language; *amok*, a sudden homicidal mania occurring in Malaya, the Philippines and parts of Africa; *koro*, a phobia observed in the East Indies which consists of the fear that the penis will disappear into the abdomen and result in death; *witigo*, an Eskimo psychosis involving melancholia, fear of becoming cannibalistic due to supernatural possession, and sometimes actual cannibalistic behavior; and *voodoo death*, a widespread phenomenon among many primitive peoples in which the affected individual actually dies after transgressing a taboo or becoming convinced that he has been bewitched. The phenomenon of voodoo death appears fantastic to Westerners but it has been thoroughly and repeatedly authenticated. The mere fact that these disorders occur in some cultures and not others demonstrates the causal importance of culture.

It has also been established that hospitalized schizophrenics are less aggressive and assaultive in India and Japan than in Western mental hospitals and that the content of schizophrenic delusions is related to the cultural milieu. In primitive tribes, schizophrenics tend to complain of being bewitched or poisoned, whereas in highly developed cultures they are apt to believe they are being persecuted by radio, television or various other impersonal devices.

Cross-cultural comparisons have often been made within Western society. In a study of northern vs. southern Italians, Rosen and Rizzo (1961) found that material and cultural differences between the geographical regions were associated with large differences in Minnesota Multiphasic Personality Inventory scores. The southern regions' lower level of education, lower standard of living and poorer communication facilities were reflected in marked tendencies to psychopathy—anxiety, depression, bizarre thinking, suspiciousness and other indices of disturbance. On all psychopathological scales in the inventory, the northern Italians had significantly healthier scores.

An important sociocultural study by Eaton and Weil (1955) measured the prevalence and estimated the lifetime expectancy of various disorders among members of the Hutterite sect, a relatively isolated rural group resident in Canada and South Dakota. The outstanding finding was the high frequency of depression, coupled with low frequencies of schizophrenia and antisocial behavior. These results were attributed by the authors to the Hutterites' extreme emphasis on communal cohesiveness, strict morality and self-blame:

There is much stress on religion, duty to God and society, and there is a tendency in their entire thinking to orient members to internalize their aggressive drives. Children and adults alike are taught to look for guilt within themselves rather than in others.

It was striking that no cases of suicide occurred, despite the frequency of depression. The Hutterite culture is far more closed than the open culture of the United States and Canada, and there is reason to believe that the less sophisticated, urban and open a culture, the lower its suicide rate. For example, suicide is lower in southern than in northern Italy, despite the southerners' greater tendency to emotional difficulties. It is also lower among Negroes than whites in the United States, apparently as a reflection of differences in economic and cultural advancement.

The cross-cultural studies, in summary, amply demonstrate that a number of syndromes reported in various primitive cultures do not occur in Western society; that cultural differences affect the particular manifestations of universal disorders such as schizophrenia; and that prevalence rates vary for different Western cultural groups. It has not been demonstrated, however, that civilization *per se* is either good or bad for mental health. The stresses of civilization may be outweighed by the beneficial effects of a higher standard of living, adequate nutrition, control of physical disease and similar factors.

STUDIES OF TEMPORAL CHANGE

The outstanding study of long-term trends is that of Goldhamer and Marshall (1953). A careful analysis of all available data for Massachusetts from 1840 to 1940 revealed that admission rates approximately doubled during this period, but the increase was entirely accounted for by a rise in rates for persons aged 50 or more. A century ago, senile individuals were very likely to be cared for at home; as urban life replaced rural life, families and living quarters became smaller and the rate of hospitalization for senile individuals increased. Concurrently, the proportion of older individuals in the general population has increased due to longevity. For psychoses occurring before the age of 50, the rates of admission have been remarkably constant over the 100 years of the study, despite the increasingly favorable attitude in the later decades toward hospitalization and the concomitant increase in availability of hospital facilities. Studies of hospital records in other states have corroborated Goldhamer and Marshall's major finding: there is *no* evidence that the rates of admission for psychoses have been increasing in younger and middle life.

These results are open to two interpretations. It may be that the stresses of modern life breed mental disorder but that these stresses had already reached a plateau, for practical purposes, by 1840. (Reliable hospital records are not available to check earlier trends.) Massachusetts was somewhat industrialized by 1840, was rapidly changing and had a large influx of immigrants. These three social characteristics have all been linked with emotional disorder, as we shall see later. An alternative interpretation is that there are pluses for mental health in our modern society which cancel out the minuses of increased cultural stress. It was mentioned earlier that an adequate standard of living, good diet and control of physical disease—all of which have greatly advanced since 1840—seem to be beneficial to mental health, although they also lengthen life and therefore lead to the psychoses of old age. In addition, with increased longevity fewer children are orphaned and it is known that loss of parents is inimical to mental health. Still another factor that may conduce to mental health in modern society is that the lower class is relatively smaller and the middle class relatively larger than some decades ago; as we shall demonstrate later, the incidence and prevalence of psychosis are highest in the lowest socioeconomic class. It is not certain which interpretation of the facts is correct, but it is certain that there is no empirical basis for the widespread belief that modern civilization has been taking an ever increasing toll of severe mental disorders.

Comparisons over time for specific diagnoses have revealed some striking findings. In World War I, a great many soldiers developed conversion symptoms, but in World War II conversions were fewer and anxiety and psychophysiologic reactions were more frequent. The change may be related to the differences in the nature of the two wars. In the first war soldiers sat and waited in trenches, whereas the second war was one of movement and sudden, rather than continuous, danger. It is possible that interminable boredom and danger, combined with acutely uncomfortable living conditions, are most readily defended against by the denial and repression of conversion hysteria, whereas periodic and violent dangers cannot be defended against by primitive, hysterical defenses but instead precipitate anxiety that is felt directly or is manifested viscerally. Even in civilian life, however, there is reason to believe that conversion reactions have decreased over the past several decades but that anxiety, obsessive-compulsive reactions and psychophysiologic reactions have increased. One suggested explanation is that conversion is so primitive and simple a reaction that it does not "fit" into the increased sophistication of the contemporary world. Sophisticated cultures breed sophisticated and complex disorders.

An interesting time change has been noted in the relative frequency of ulcers in men and women. Prior to 1900, about as many women as men suffered from severe stomach and duodenal ulceration, but since then a far higher frequency for men than for women has been reported in various Western countries. A highly speculative but plausible sociocultural explanation is that the double standard of morality and suppression of feminine freedom in the Victorian Age bred ulcers in women. As women became more free in the twentieth century the frequency with which they developed ulcers decreased. Meanwhile, men

became less free to make unchallenged, authoritarian decisions in the family and home; frustrated, they became more vulnerable to ulcers.

A number of studies have revealed that in the past 50 years large scale changes have occurred in the first admission rates for various diagnostic categories. The data reported by Malzberg (1959) for New York State are typical. Admission rates between 1914 and 1950 increased tenfold for psychoses with cerebral arteriosclerosis, almost tripled for schizophrenia and decreased to about one-third for paresis and manic-depression.

It appears that some disorders have been increasing faster than can be accounted for by longevity, greater hospital availability and so forth, and other disorders have been rapidly declining. The decrease in paresis has been due to better control of syphilis, and the increase in psychoses with cerebral arteriosclerosis has been at least partly related to an increase in circulatory disorders noted in the general population. It is more difficult to explain why manic-depressive reaction should decline and schizophrenia multiply rapidly. In part, changes in diagnostic criteria have been responsible: individuals formerly classified as manic-depressive are now often labeled schizo-affective. But over and above this factor, there seems to be a genuine movement away from mood-swing disorders toward schizophrenic isolation, suspiciousness and bizarre thinking. A possible explanation—admittedly speculative—is that the increasingly extraverted nature of our society, oriented as it is toward social adjustment, puts too much pressure on individuals who are not predisposed by biological makeup or childhood learning experiences to easy interpersonal interactions. They respond by emotional withdrawal. On the other hand, individuals with a predisposition to extraversion can function well in an other-directed society; extraversion and cyclothymic mood swings tend to be correlated.

Apart from diagnostic changes, observers have noted alterations in the characteristic behavior of individuals within various diagnostic categories. Violent behavior—whether manic, paranoid or other—was common in hospitals 25 years ago. Today such behaviors are seen less often. The difference is due to earlier recognition of disorders, earlier treatment, tranquilizing drugs and, perhaps also, broad sociocultural factors. The increased tractability and docility of patients may be a reflection of the emphasis on social adjustment mentioned earlier. Even when they are hallucinatory and delusional, most patients do not wish to be troublesome.

SINGLE VARIABLE STUDIES

The majority of single variable studies have been carried out within Western society. Some of the variables that have been studied are racial origin, native vs. immigrant status, urban vs. rural dwelling, war, unemployment, marital status and family instability, residential mobility, technological complexity and change, socioeconomic class and type of neighborhood (degree of neighborhood disorganization).

Race. In the United States, mental-hospital admission rates are higher for Negroes than whites in all diagnostic categories. The difference may be due to several factors: the stresses associated with minority status, the economic handicaps of Negroes and the tendency of our society to hospitalize Negroes more readily than equally disturbed whites. An interaction between biological and cultural factors may also play a role.

Native vs. Immigrant. Admission rates in the United States for schizophrenia, manic-depression, senile disorders, alcoholic psychoses and paresis are higher for immigrants than for the native-born population. It has been suggested that selective factors may operate in the case of schizophrenia: a large proportion of the individuals who choose to emigrate from their native lands may be motivated by the social isolation and alienation characteristic of the schizoid personality. On the other hand, the responsible variables may be the minority status and economic handicaps of immigrants in the United States. There is some evidence that immigrants in former generations, as compared to more recent times, had higher prevalence rates. This change correlates with the fact that the average socioeconomic level of earlier generations of immigrants was lower than the level of more recent immigrants.

Urban vs. Rural. For all mental disorders, urban admission rates are approximately twice as high as rural rates, and the larger the city the higher the rates. There is no reason to believe that mental disorder is really twice as prevalent in urban areas; the urban-rural differences merely reflect availability of facilities. For senile psychoses it has been shown that the closer a patient lives to a mental hospital, the more likely he is to be hospitalized rather than cared for at home.

War. The effects of war on mental disorder have been subject to observation for a long time. In 1794, Benjamin Rush, the so-called father of American psychiatry, wrote, in a discussion of the effects of the American Revolution: "An uncommon cheerfulness prevailed everywhere among the friends of the Revolution. Defeats, and even the loss of relations and property, were soon forgotten in the great objects of the war." Many sick persons, according to Rush, were restored to perfect health, including a number of women with hysterical symptoms. In sharp contrast was the high frequency of mental and physical breakdown among the colonists who remained loyal to England. The latter frequently suffered from a form of hypochondriasis which Rush termed *Revolutiana*. It was popularly known as "protection fever" because it appeared to arise from the loyalists' concern for the protection of their persons and possessions. The loyalists were also disturbed by their loss of power and influence, the suspension of the established church, changes in manners and diet, and the legal and extra-legal oppression to which they were subjected.

These observations indicate the complexities of assessing the effects of war on emotional disturbance. In addition to the direct stress of physical danger, war may entail economic, family and geographic dislocation, biological deprivation and political oppression. But it may also boost the morale of participants so long as the war is going well; temporary decreases of mental disorder and suicide have often been noted among civilian populations during wars. (Among combatants, the rates of psychiatric breakdown are high.) At the conclusion of wars, on the other hand, mental disorder shows a tendency to increase. French psychiatrists reported an increase in the number of psychoses requiring hospital admission after the French Revolution, the Revolution of 1848, the Franco-Prussian War and the ensuing civil war of 1871.

Unemployment and Economic Distress. The effects of long-term unemployment on the individual are almost always unhealthy. Apathy and despair, rage reactions and escapism, often taking the form of alcoholism, have been frequently observed. The unemployed individual's children are affected by these reactions so that unemployment may predispose the next generation to psychological difficulties.

Variations in suicide rates appear to reflect

economic distress, including unemployment, more than any other factor. As shown in Figure 8–1, suicide in the United States has increased in times of great economic difficulty, for example in 1907 and the immediately following years, and again in 1929 to 1933. The sharp decrease in suicide during wartime may be due in part to full employment. The relative stability in the total suicide rate over the past 20 years results from the offsetting of substantial decreases in the death rate for persons 45 years of age and over by steady increases in the rate for persons under 45 years. The decline in the suicide rate for older persons started in the mid-1930's, concomitant with the establishment of broad Social Security programs for the nation.

Marital Status and Family Instability. Mental disorder is closely related to marital status. A study of the first-admission rates in Canada among married, widowed, single and divorced persons in 1950 noted the following rates per 100,000: for married persons, 56 per 100,000; widowed, 89; single, 115; divorced, 286. The findings of investigations in the United States have been similar. The variation in rates is not due to age differences among the four groups since the figures have been adjusted to correct for different rates of mental disorder at different ages. The data do not simply mean that marriage prevents mental disorder and disruption of marriage precipitates it. Marriage may, indeed, act as a protection against stress for many individuals, and divorce, which terminates approximately one in four marriages, may be a precipitant to breakdown. More important, however, is

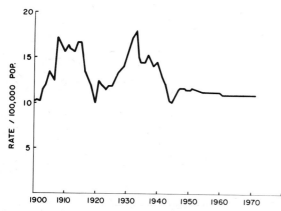

Figure 8–1. *Suicide rates per 100,000 population, United States, 1900–1970. (From Vital Statistics of the United States, 1970. National Office of Vital Statistics, Federal Security Agency, United States Public Health Service.)*

the factor of selection: preschizophrenic and mentally defective individuals, particularly males, rarely marry. The somewhat higher rate for widowhood may also reflect selection, since widowed individuals vulnerable to mental disorder are less likely than more stable persons to remarry. Similarly, divorce may result from instability. In sum, marital status is undoubtedly a causal factor in disturbance, but it is even more a reflection and effect of it.

Sociocultural factors also affect abnormal behavior in families not disrupted by death or divorce. So-called problem families, characterized by the simultaneous presence of subnormal intelligence in one or both parents, instability of character, economic poverty and neglected children occupy much of the attention of welfare agencies and contribute heavily to psychopathology. In a study of a large Midwestern city, Buell (1955) reported that 6 per cent of all the families constituted a "multiproblem" group. They accounted for 77 per cent of the relief load, 51 per cent of the community health service recipients and 56 per cent of the clientele of mental health, casework and correctional services.

Better functioning families, however, also have their problems. In contrast to the strong, colonial family of bygone generations—in which the father was the unchallenged decision maker, the family was the unit of both production and consumption, the marriages of children were arranged, and the concepts of respect and duty regulated the family closely—many families today tend to be organized on a basis of companionship. The contemporary family is an interpersonal net rather than an authoritarian structure. One of its principal functions is to give and receive affection. Decisions are made by consensus in which the children begin to participate when still fairly young. This shift in function results in many gains for mental health, since there is evidence that democratic structures are emotionally healthier than authoritarian ones, but it also precipitates new problems. In many democratically organized families, conflicts arise between husbands and wives over decision making, male and female roles are not clearly defined and children have severe problems of sex identification.

Residential Mobility. Communities in which the rate of movement from one residence to another is high have relatively high rates of disorder. The rates are also higher for individuals who move from city to city than for those moving within a city. As with several other variables, effect as well as cause may be involved: the disturbed individual may move about a great deal because of his very instability.

Technological Complexity and Change. In a study of five Virginia communities varying in technological complexity and rapidity of social change, Sherman and Henry (1933) reported more neurosis in the more complex, faster changing communities and more sociopathic behavior in the less advanced, more static communities. In the latter, lying, stealing, absence of guilt reactions and shallowness of interpersonal relations were common. The authors interpreted the findings causally by hypothesizing that complex, changing cultures breed inhibitions that lead to neurosis whereas simpler cultures breed emotional immaturity.

Many sociologists have analyzed the impact of technological change in broader terms than Sherman and Henry and have concluded that change may create adjustment problems in two different ways. First, it is well known that the institutions of society usually fail to keep up with technological change so that the phenomenon of *cultural lag* occurs. The traditional cultural values, ideas and beliefs lag behind social reality and therefore cease to serve the function of organizing and giving meaning to the individual's life. He lacks the guidance of a clear and consistent pattern of loyalties and ideals and becomes conflicted, confused and sometimes antisocial. Some sociologists, ignoring the noncultural determinants of mental disorder, have gone so far as to hypothesize that in times of considerable cultural lag, mental disorder is solely a reaction to the disintegration of the traditional culture. Short of so extreme a hypothesis, however, there is no doubt that cultural lag may be one root of emotional disturbance.

Second, apart from cultural lag, rapid sociocultural change itself demands difficult adjustments not required in a static society. In a rapidly changing society the individual must be vigilant and ready to meet crises. Since a changing society tends also to be an open one, the individual must make many occupational, educational, marital, residential and friendship choices. Furthermore, technological mechanization and automation may make him feel unimportant and even useless. In summary, although technological advancement is in many respects beneficial to physical and mental health, it may also be reflected in conflict, lack of emotional security, the stress associated with

continuous decision making and a feeling of uselessness.

Socioeconomic Class. A number of careful studies have conclusively demonstrated that mental disorder is closely associated with socioeconomic class. Frumkin (1955) found that first-admission rates in Ohio were inversely related to income and occupational prestige. Many causal factors may operate to produce such results; one possibility is that low-prestige occupations may not provide enough ego-satisfaction to maintain mental health.

Hollingshead and Redlich (1958) carried out an extensive and important study of the social class membership of all residents of New Haven, Connecticut, who were in treatment at a designated time (prevalence) and of all new patients added during a period of six months (six-month incidence). Included in the study were patients receiving treatment outside as well as in New Haven. All patients were categorized into five socioeconomic classes, based on the standard sociological criteria of income, residential area, education, occupation and so forth. The rates of six-month incidence and total prevalence in each class were computed separately for neuroses and psychoses. As shown in Table 8–5, adapted from Hollingshead and Redlich's data, the incidence of new cases of neuroses was fairly evenly distributed across the five classes, but prevalence for neurotics receiving treatment was far higher in Classes I and II (the upper groups) than in Class V (the lowest group). The incidence of neurosis is apparently independent of class, but

TABLE 8–5. Incidence and Prevalence Rates per 100,000 for Neuroses and Psychoses (New Haven, Conn., Receiving Treatment, 1950)

Class	Six-Month Incidence	Prevalence
Neuroses		
I-II	69	349
III	78	250
IV	52	114
V	66	97
Psychoses		
I-II	28	188
III	36	291
IV	37	518
V	73	1505

Adapted from Hollingshead, A. B., and Redlich, F. C., Social Class and Mental Illness. Copyright 1958 by John Wiley & Sons, Inc., p. 235.

Define upwardly mobile

upper-class neurotics are far more likely to be in treatment. Neurosis remains hidden in the lower strata and is more open in the upper class. (The findings are reminiscent of George Bernard Shaw's remark in *Heartbreak House,* "There are only two classes in good society in England: the equestrian classes and the neurotic classes.") For psychosis the results were quite different: the incidence of new cases in the lowest class was two and one-half times as large as in the two upper classes and the prevalence of psychosis in treatment or receiving custodial care was eight times larger in the lowest than in the upper groups. The disparity between incidence and prevalence indicates that hospitalization for psychosis in the lowest class is particularly long lasting, perhaps as a reflection of inadequate treatment. Social class not only affects who gets treated, but also how and by whom he is treated, and the probable outcome of treatment. The higher the class to which a patient belongs, the more likely he is to be treated by intensive psychotherapy aimed at modification of personality rather than by exclusively medical measures or by brief psychotherapy aimed solely at removal or suppression of symptoms. Furthermore, the higher the class, the more likely treatment is to be conducted privately rather than in a hospital or clinic, and the more likely the patient is to improve or recover.

Myers and Roberts (1959) selected 50 New Haven patients and undertook an intensive analysis of each. Half belonged to Class III (middle) and half to Class V (lowest); half of each group were neurotic and half schizophrenic. Among the Class III patients, it was found that respectability and success had been the values most emphasized during the patients' socialization. Three stressful consequences seemed to have resulted from this emphasis: a conflict between drives and moral values, frustration when the patient was unable to

achieve respectability and success, and tension arising from upward mobility striving. In contrast, the Class V patients had been exposed to adverse economic conditions and isolated from community institutions. Five stressful consequences were noted for these patients: a childhood environment containing little love, protection and stability; a childhood relationship with parents marked by constant defensiveness; a feeling of neglect or rejection lasting through an entire lifetime, first by parents and siblings and later by the institutional representatives of society and higher status persons in general; a lifelong economic insecurity; and the experience of retribution by others when the patients directly expressed their instinctual impulses, particularly hostility. It was also noted that Class III patients were more upwardly mobile than their siblings or comparable nonpatients, whereas Class V patients had achieved no more success than nonpatients in the same class. This interesting finding suggests that psychopathology is sometimes associated with an upward mobility that expresses middle-class aspirations but not with the kind of mobility that is driven by a desire to escape from lower-class economic insecurity.

Of equal significance with the New Haven studies is an investigation undertaken by Srole and his associates (1962) of mental health in an area within New York City. A sample of more than 1600 residents, living at home, was interviewed at considerable length. Dividing the sample into six socioeconomic groups and four mental health categories (well, mild symptoms, moderate symptoms and impaired), the investigators found (Table 8–6) that at any socioeconomic level only a minority of the subjects could be considered well. A lack of symptoms was observed in only 24 per cent of the highest and 10 per cent of the lowest socioeconomic groups. Definite impairment—the poorest of the four mental health categories—

TABLE 8–6. Distribution of Mental Health Classification (Home Survey Sample)

Mental Health Classification	A (Highest)	B	C	D	E	F (Lowest)
Well	24%	23%	20%	19%	14%	10%
Mild symptoms	36	38	37	37	37	33
Moderate symptoms	22	22	23	20	20	25
Impaired	18	16	21	24	29	33

Because of rounding of decimals, some columns do not add to 100%.
Adapted from Srole, L., et al., 1962. Mental Health in the Metropolis: The Midtown Manhattan Study, Vol. 1. New York, McGraw-Hill Book Co., Inc., p. 213.

varied from 18 per cent in the highest to fully 33 per cent in the lowest socioeconomic stratum. (Precautions had been taken to minimize the investigators' class biases in the interviews.)

The investigators also divided the men and unmarried women in the sample into the occupational mobility categories of mobile upward, stable or mobile downward (Table 8–7). Mental health was poorest and impairment greatest for the downward group. Another finding was that the older members and immigrants in the sample had relatively high rates of impairment. Apart from the biological effects of aging, some of the variables accounting for the total pattern of the results are a lack of gratification of needs due to poverty; the disruption of life at the lowest socioeconomic levels when the family is hit by unemployment, parental disability or other critical factors; the minority status of lower-class and immigrant groups and their rejection by the community; and the difficulties of older individuals in shifting to new roles when they are no longer needed to raise children.

Neighborhood Disorganization. This variable is closely related to socioeconomic class and economic deprivation. In a classic sociological study, Faris and Dunham (1939) analyzed the distribution of mental-hospital admission rates for different areas within the city of Chicago. Overall rates were highest for residents of the center of the city and declined progressively with distance from the center. The pattern of decreasing admission rates correlated with the residential structure of Chicago: dividing the city into five concentric zones, it was found that the central zone was populated by many hoboes, drug addicts, prostitutes and other fringe members of society, the second zone was a slum

TABLE 8–7. Distribution of Mental Health Classification of Men and Single Women, by Occupational Mobility Types (Home Survey Sample)

Mental Health Classification	Mobility Types		
	Up	Stable	Down
Well	21%	23%	13%
Mild symptoms	42	37	34
Moderate symptoms	24	17	23
Impaired	14	24	30

Because of rounding of decimals, two columns do not add to 100%.

Adapted from Srole, L., et al., 1962. Mental Health in the Metropolis: The Midtown Manhattan Study, Vol. 1. New York, McGraw-Hill Book Co., Inc., p. 226.

area; the third consisted of low cost private homes; the fourth of higher cost homes; and the outermost zone contained wealthy residents. Social disorganization was at a maximum in the center and a minimum at the periphery, with a few exceptions. The pattern was fairly consistent: for example, new immigrants in zone two had a high crime rate (a good index of disorganization), but when they moved to zone three their crime rate dropped and they were replaced in zone two by a newer immigrant group with a high crime rate.

In addition to admissions for all mental disorders combined, the distributions of admissions for the specific diagnoses of schizophrenia, alcoholic disorders and paresis all corresponded to the zonal pattern, but manic-depression was randomly distributed throughout the city. A repetition of this study in half a dozen other cities has confirmed the main findings. Schizophrenia and organic disorders are closely related to social disorganization and manic-depression is not.

Two different hypotheses have been suggested to account for the relationship between schizophrenia and residence in disorganized neighborhoods. The hypothesis of *downward drift* postulates that disturbed individuals, particularly schizophrenics, drift to disorganized neighborhoods because their emotional instability makes them mobile downward. The finding in the New York City home survey that impairment is more frequent in persons who are mobile downward is consistent with this hypothesis. However, downward drift is not consistent with the fact that many schizophrenic patients are born and remain in deteriorated areas. Furthermore, foreign-born individuals have high rates for schizophrenia, but tend, on the average, to be mobile upward. Another fact contradicting the hypothesis is that in the New Haven studies the middle-class patients, whether schizophrenic or neurotic, were mobile upward.

An alternative hypothesis is that a disorganized neighborhood imposes a state of *social isolation* on its most vulnerable residents. A sensitive, timid individual is likely to feel alienated from a harsh, brutal environment and withdraw from the people around him. His withdrawal is both a cause and an effect of his inability to compete, loss of confidence and feeling of failure. Withdrawal protects him from the negative evaluation he fears others make of him. The culmination of this process is the schizophrenic's construction of a unique world not shared by others.

THE INTERACTION OF SOCIOCULTURAL AND OTHER CAUSES

Even in the most disorganized of neighborhoods only a minority of residents become disturbed to the point of requiring hospitalization. Obviously, other factors interact with culture to determine who will and who will not become mentally disordered.

The interaction of sociocultural with other causes may be illustrated by a number of examples. It was mentioned earlier that culture affects diet and disease, thus precipitating mental disorder via biological processes. Another example is the mutual interaction of socioeconomic class, psychiatric disorder and intelligence. In the discussion of development in Chapter 4, data were cited to demonstrate that intelligence is correlated with superior development and adjustment, and also with higher socioeconomic status. There is a considerable genetic component in intelligence; hence it is conceivable, although unproved, that the relationship between socioeconomic class and psychiatric impairment is partly due to genetic factors.

As a final illustration, a study bearing on the outcome rather than the occurrence of psychiatric disorders may be cited (Zigler and Phillips, 1961). The likelihood that a schizophrenic patient will improve sufficiently to be released from the hospital was found to increase with his degree of social competence, the latter being judged by the criteria of education, occupational status, stability of employment history and married rather than single status. But improvement also was more likely for younger patients and for patients with higher I.Q.'s, that is, improvement was affected by a combination of social competence, the biological factor of age and the partly genetic factor of intelligence.

SUMMARY: CAUSATION IN ABNORMAL PSYCHOLOGY

The discussion of causation in the last four chapters may be summarized as follows:

The Nature of Causation

1. Behavior is typically the result of several causes. A single cause may lead to multiple consequences and may be sufficient or necessary, predisposing or precipitating. Hereditary causes always predispose. Nonhereditary causes either predispose to psychological disorder or precipitate it. Nonhereditary causes of psychological disorder include various biological, psychological and sociocultural determinants.

2. Correlation is not causation. However, a network of correlations that are consistent with each other and with theoretical considerations permits us to make tentative causal inferences.

3. In the literal sense of "proof," a causal hypothesis cannot be proved. However, the probability that it is correct increases the better it can explain and predict phenomena and the more successfully the phenomena can be controlled or replicated experimentally in a manner consistent with a specific hypothesis. The more irregular the phenomena that are accurately predicted by the hypothesis, the stronger the evidence for it.

4. Causal investigations in abnormal psychology are rendered difficult by the problems of obtaining reliable retrospective information, by the enormous effort required to accumulate prospective (anterospective) information and by the failure of experimental replication of a disorder or a cause to be exact.

5. Nevertheless, the specific causes responsible for many disorders, mostly organic, are well established. For most functional disorders causal explanations are at present incomplete and tentative.

Hereditary Determinants

1. All behavior is a result of both heredity and environment. Some behavior and symptomatic *differences* among individuals are due mostly to heredity, some mostly to environmental factors and some depend heavily on both.

2. There are many genetic patterns of inheritance: for a given trait the genes may be sex-linked or autosomal, single or multiple, dominant or recessive and rare or frequent. For each pattern, different criteria are used to assess the contribution of heredity to the trait.

3. The two major methods of investigating animal inheritance are selective breeding and the method of pure strains.

4. Several methods of investigating genetic factors in humans—in particular, statistical comparisons among relatives, foster child methods and twin studies—are very useful. Each method has well-defined limitations, however,

and the findings obtained by each must be evaluated critically. Twins have been used either to compare monozygotic (MZ) and dizygotic (DZ) twins or to compare MZ twins reared apart and MZ twins reared together. For the first of these two comparisons, a rough estimate of heritability (H) may be obtained by a formula that takes into account the percentage of concordant MZ and DZ twins or the correlation between MZ and DZ twins. For the second comparison, a rough estimate of environmental contribution (E) is obtained by a simple formula.

5. The evidence of heritability in animal behavior, certain human sensory and perceptual processes, intelligence, motor responses and temperament is very strong and provides a basis for the hypothesis that behavior disorders also have a genetic component.

6. There is evidence for a hereditary component in several organic syndromes, some types of mental deficiency, schizophrenia and manic-depression. However, the precise magnitude of the hereditary components and the specific mechanisms of inheritance remain undetermined for all but a few disorders.

7. The evidence for a genetic component in the causation of neurosis is far weaker than for mental deficiency or psychosis.

stronger in ↑

Other Biological Determinants

1. Biological precipitants of psychological disorders are better understood than non-hereditary biological predispositions.

2. Noxious agents and biological deprivations can precipitate an organic disorder by causing brain pathology, or can precipitate a functional disorder to which the individual is predisposed. A noxious agent injures the organism; a deprivation is the absence of a needed substance such as oxygen or a vitamin.

3. The younger the organism at the time of injury or deprivation, the more severe the effects.

4. Hallucinogens precipitate symptoms similar to, but not identical with, some of the naturally occurring symptoms of schizophrenia. No disorder has as yet been completely replicated experimentally.

5. Any type of noxious agent (disease-producing microorganisms, toxic chemicals and physical injuries to the brain) as well as any type of biological deprivation—of vitamins, glucose, hormones, food, oxygen or sleep—

may lead to a variety of consequences such as intellectual decrement, psychotic reactions or neurotic reactions.

6. A severe noxious agent impinging on the organism or deprivation leads to a disturbance of homeostasis, a stereotyped stress reaction and a failure to adapt described in detail by Selye as "a general adaptation syndrome." A number of disorders, especially psychophysiologic disorders, resemble this syndrome.

7. There is some evidence that the body build component of constitution is correlated with temperamental characteristics and types of mental disorder in certain specifiable ways. However, there are several methodological difficulties in establishing these correlations and the explanation of the correlations is uncertain. The evidence accumulated to date for the causal role of bodily functioning—blood circulation, blood chemistry, basal metabolic rate and so forth—in functional disorders is even weaker.

Psychological Determinants

1. Abnormal behavior is learned in accordance with the principles of classical conditioning and instrumental learning. The amount, type and schedule of reinforcement, the temporal interval between response and reinforcement and the strength of drive are variables relevant to abnormal behavior.

2. The stimulus situations that precipitate abnormal behavior are characterized by conflict, frustration, long continued vigilance, uncertainty, deprivation or threat. A number of animal experiments have demonstrated that under these stressful conditions behavior modifications occur.

3. Both excessive frustration and overgratification in childhood may lead to fixation, defensiveness and neurotic behavior. The effects of frustration and overgratification are explainable in terms of reinforcement and generalization.

4. Deprivations of maternal care, dependency behavior, sensory stimulation or social interaction are particularly likely to precipitate psychological disturbance, varying from mild difficulties to severe psychosis.

5. A stable individual breaks down only under severe stress; an unstable one often breaks down with mild stress. For a given amount of stress, the severity of disorder will vary with the degree of personality instability.

For a given amount of instability, the severity of disorder will vary with the severity of stress.

6. Early psychological experiences are crucial and may lead to severe damage. The same experiences at a later period of life have lesser effects.

7. In childhood, certain phases and types of experience—oral, anal and phallic—are particularly crucial determinants of later behavior.

8. Severe, long continued psychopathology rarely results from a single traumatic experience.

9. Close relationships with parents and peers in childhood minimize the probability that emotional disorder will occur. Lack of acceptance by parents that takes the form of rejection, perfectionism, inconsistency or over-dominance increases this probability. Indirect discipline is more damaging than direct discipline.

Sociocultural Determinants

1. Culture shapes relatively normal personality; it is reasonable to infer that it also has great effects on emotional disorder. There is evidence that it affects both organic and functional disorders.

2. The attitudes of different cultural groups toward deviant behavior vary enormously. A type of behavior accepted in one culture may be completely rejected in another.

3. In a number of cultures there are unique disorders found nowhere else. The manifestations of widespread disorders such as schizophrenia are to some extent different in different cultures. But a great deal of cross-cultural consistency may also be found: schizophrenia, mental deficiency and a number of other disorders seem to occur universally.

4. There is no proof that civilization *per se* is bad for mental health and there is some reason to believe that its beneficial effects outweigh the negative ones.

5. There has been no overall increase in psychosis in the last century, except that due to longevity. The tendency to hospitalize older individuals who are disturbed has also increased greatly.

6. Certain syndromes—e.g., conversion hysteria and manic-depression—seem to have decreased in recent decades while others such as obsession-compulsion, psychophysiologic disorders and schizophrenia seem to have increased.

7. Urban hospital admission rates are about twice as high as rural rates, but the difference is apparently a reflection of hospital availability.

8. The effect of war on emotional disturbance is complex. Depending on whether an individual is a combatant or a civilian, on the character of the war and on the particular time period—whether during or immediately after hostilities—war has quite different effects.

9. Social disorganization, cultural conflict and economic deprivation and other undesirable aspects of membership in the lowest socio-economic class are the major sociocultural variables affecting various mental disorders, including schizophrenia. For manic-depression, however, a correlation with neighborhood disorganization has not been demonstrated. A mechanism by which social disorganization seems to conduce to schizophrenia is that of social isolation and withdrawal.

10. Minority status and family instability—both of which are known to be associated with disorganization, low socioeconomic status and cultural conflict—are inimical to mental health.

11. Stressful and critical situations—unemployment, family disintegration due to divorce or death, rapid technological change and residential mobility—have negative effects on emotional functioning.

12. Finally, since sociocultural determinants act on an individual with a given heredity, constitution and learning experiences, it follows that genetic, biological nongenetic, psychological and cultural factors always interact in the etiology of abnormality.

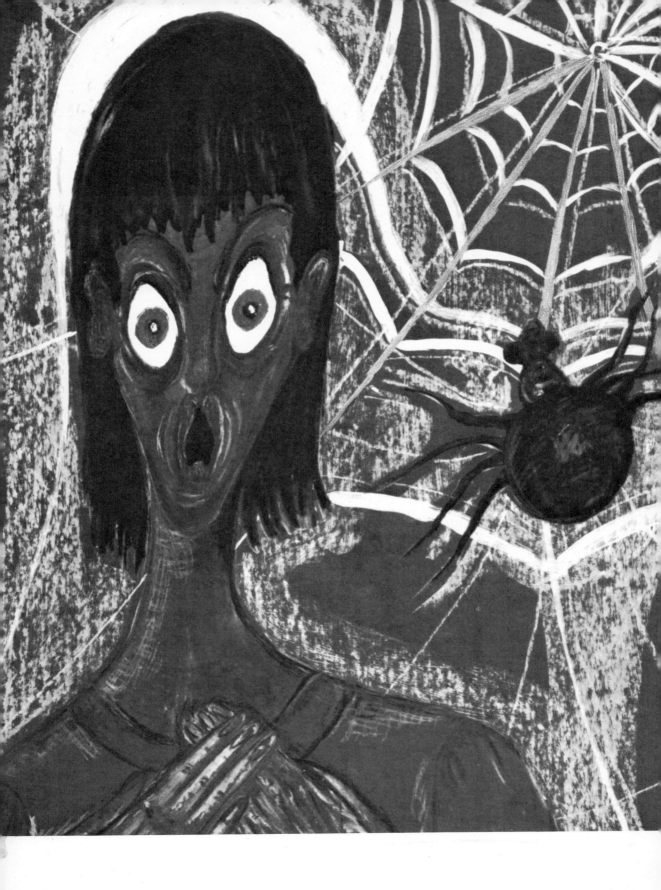

> Guilt is the source of sorrow, 'tis the fiend,
> Th'avenging fiend, that follows us behind
> With whips and stings.
>
> Nicholas Row, *The Fair Penitent*

> Fear and guilt
> Are the same things, and when our actions are not,
> Our fears are, crimes.
>
> Sir John Denham, *The Sophy*

PSYCHONEUROTIC DISORDERS

Obsessive Comp
Phobic } *psychasthenic rns.*

Ours has been labeled the age of anxiety and anxiety is the cardinal feature of the neuroses. Anxiety may take any of several forms. It may be experienced as a feeling state characterized by extreme dread or fear without apparent cause or as excessive fear of some object or situation. It may be experienced purely as a physical reaction without the accompanying feeling state; or as both physical sensation (such as increased respiration and heart palpitations) and an overwhelming feeling of apprehension. There are many other possibilities. But as Fromm-Reichmann (1954) concluded:

In going over the literature on anxiety in children and adults . . . it seems that the feelings of powerlessness, of helplessness in the presence of inner dangers, which the individual cannot control, contributes in the last analysis the common background of all further elaborations on the theory of anxiety.

In a follow-up study of former psychiatric outpatients, Strupp, Fox and Lessler (1969) asked the subjects to list the complaints which had led them to seek help. Over 50 per cent reported having felt overwhelmed and powerless to cope with the daily responsibilities of life. A sense of helplessness and hopelessness seems ubiquitous in the neuroses.

All human beings need affection, emotional security and self-esteem as well as a reasonable degree of freedom from anxiety and guilt. A neurosis may be viewed as a disorder in which these needs are insufficiently gratified. The neurotic usually feels unloved, anxious, guilty and unhappy even though he makes defensive efforts to subdue or control these feelings. Typically, he is basically lacking in a belief that he can win love or esteem by his own efforts or on his own merits. In other words, he feels basically helpless to effect those interpersonal relationships and support systems which he considers essential.

In spite of his extreme anxiety, the neurotic's personality is not disorganized and his relation to reality is not defective. He talks rationally and without excessive retardation or blocking. It is not difficult to follow his train of thought, for he is free of bizarre ideas, halluci-

147

nations and delusions. Except for those suffering from dissociative reactions, neurotics are also free of memory and orientation difficulties.

SYMPTOM NEUROSES AND THE NEUROTIC PERSONALITY

A distinction should be made between a symptom neurosis and a neurotic personality. Symptom neuroses are characterized by overt, identifiable symptoms of the anxiety, conversion, phobic, obsessive-compulsive or other reaction types. The term "neurotic personality," on the other hand, refers to a constellation of personality traits and interpersonal difficulties. A symptom neurosis may or may not evolve from a neurotic personality. Thus, the individual who tends to be compulsive—cautious, orderly, fussy and so forth—may at some time develop clinically identifiable obsessions and compulsions or may simply continue to have compulsive traits. A neurotic personality, in other words, is the basis of a potential or actual symptom neurosis. Of course, there are many borderline cases that consist of neurotic traits combined with a minimal degree of symptomatology. In symptom-oriented therapy, only the symptom neurosis is treated; in uncovering procedures, the symptom neurosis is largely by-passed and the underlying neurotic personality becomes the focus of therapy.

There are really a number of neurotic *personalities* rather than a single one; two neurotic individuals may manifest quite different and even opposite traits and behaviors. Thus, some neurotic patients appear tense, fearful, tremulous and easily startled by unexpected stimuli. They pour out their misery to an interviewer in a quavering voice and are preoccupied with their troubles to the exclusion of other interests. They may be depressed as well as anxious, show evidences of chronic fatigue, state that they don't care what happens to them and weep during interviews. But, on the other hand, many neurotic patients ward off enough of their anxieties and fears to appear outwardly calm and even indifferent to their difficulties. The conversion hysteric may appear almost unconcerned as he describes, with little affect, a paralysis or anesthesia. The obsessive-compulsive often strives for complete self-control and denies the anxiety that constantly threatens to erupt in him. A mixture of overt anxiety and defense is most common of all: the patient manifests denial, repression, reaction-formation,

isolation or other defenses but they are only partially successful and some anxiety appears at an overt, as well as at a deeper, level.

However, in addition to the traits that distinguish one kind of neurotic individual from another, there are a number of traits that characterize most neurotics, regardless of subtype. The "typical" neurotic tends to have a rigid superego; that is to say, his attitudes and behaviors are dominated by questions of what one should or ought to do. Despite his inner turmoil he is usually perceived by others as moral, reliable, responsible, truthful and conforming. Most neurotics are overly inhibited and have difficulty in recognizing or tolerating sexual and hostile impulses in themselves and others. The neurotic is likely to feel as guilty over mere impulses to unacceptable sexual or aggressive acts as a normal person would over the acts themselves. Male neurotics frequently suffer from some degree of impotence and female neurotics tend to be frigid. The neurotic's sexual inadequacy may be expressed in a variety of outward forms: avoidance of the opposite sex, rationalization of sexual inadequacy by blaming it on a marital partner or on the opposite sex in general, an unhappy, desperate type of promiscuity, or any of a number of other deviations —sadism, masochism, voyeurism and so forth.

Neurotics try not to express anger or hostility directly, yet they frequently frustrate and hurt others by passive stubbornness, clinging overdependence or indirect and displaced aggression. They are ambivalent to other people, for their interpersonal attitudes are compounded of hostility, fear and a need for affection; they simultaneously wish to be assertive and compliantly yielding. They want to feel loved but cannot easily love in return; they withdraw from people or try to unload their psychological burdens onto a stronger person. Quite often a neurotic expects the support and strength of a marital partner to overcome his own unhappiness. This rarely works, as his expectations prove to be constricting to both partners. It is constricting to the neurotic, for he is never forced to face and overcome his own perceived shortcomings. It also is constricting to the spouse, for if he attempts to change or grow psychologically such changes may be perceived as a threat by the neurotic partner. The fundamental error is in assuming that a continuing sense of adequacy or confidence or freedom from anxiety can be obtained from another person.

Another common feature of the neurotic is

hypersensitivity to the opinions and criticisms of others. He perceives himself as falling far short of his ideals and ambitions, and fears that everyone else will perceive his failure. He has an unstable self concept and is unsure whether he is an unusually good and sensitive person made of finer clay than others or whether he is really evil, inconsiderate and weak. Many neurotics devote a great deal of energy to the future, either making plans that are mingled with doubts and fears or daydreaming of great accomplishments and thus momentarily freeing themselves of the sense of failure.

The neurotic individual knows something is wrong although he may be reluctant to accept the existence of an emotional basis for his symptoms. Conversion patients are especially prone to believe that their troubles are purely physical, since a major function of the conversion mechanism is precisely to provide a rationale for this belief. The neurotic frequently gives a history of medical treatment, including surgery, for a variety of bodily complaints due to real or imagined illnesses. In one study (Gregory, 1959), it was found that female neurotic patients had had almost twice as much surgery as the average of other female psychiatric groups. Surgery for male neurotics was similarly higher than for other male psychiatric patients, but the difference was not as large as for females.

The transition from a neurotic personality to overt symptomatology may be precipitated by factors that differ somewhat from one neurotic reaction to another. In general, three types of precipitants may be distinguished. First, a breakdown may occur when the individual's life situation changes, usually in the direction of added responsibilities. Until he is promoted to a new position, or marries or becomes a parent he functions well enough and may even use his neurotic traits for adaptive purposes—e.g., a certain degree of neurotic aggressiveness may stand the individual in good stead occupationally. But he may perceive a change in his situation as threatening and dangerous. He may be reminded of childhood dangers; for example, parenthood may revive long dormant conflicts with his own father or marriage may revive unacceptable childhood sexual impulses or a fear of inadequacy. To quote Fenichel (1945): "Most precipitating factors are experiences that are (objectively or subjectively) somehow similar to the childhood events that gave rise to the decisive conflicts." In the case of precipi-

tation due to occupational success, a frequent additional factor is that the individual's achievements may be far less satisfying than those he had pictured in fantasy. Paradoxically, his success leads him to feel that he has failed.

A second type of precipitant consists of a progressive undermining of previously adequate defenses by physical illness, biological deprivation, actual failure, the death of a loved person or some other severely stressful condition; the precipitating traumas of combat neurosis are special cases of this type. Defenses are normally intensified under stress, but if it is sufficiently prolonged and intense the energy needed to maintain the defenses may be depleted.

A third and quite different pattern is that of the individual who from year to year expends more and more energy on the maintenance of defenses. As the burden of maintaining them increases, he becomes more tense, fatigued and unable to behave spontaneously or enjoy himself. Eventually, he breaks down and develops overt symptoms. A long series of difficulties rather than a single event is responsible for his neurosis.

THE MAJOR SYMPTOM NEUROSES

Each of the categories of neurosis to be discussed in this section refers to a *dominant pattern of symptoms at a given time*; it is rare for all of a patient's symptoms to fall into one category and it is not uncommon for the dominant symptom pattern to change from one category to another over time, e.g., from an anxiety reaction to an obsessive-compulsive reaction.

A neurotic symptom may have any of three related functions. It may mirror and express the patient's underlying anxiety (or guilt), or his defenses or the impulses that arouse his anxiety. A physiological anxiety reaction—sweating, shaking and so forth—directly and obviously expresses anxiety; compulsive hand washing represents a defense against anxiety; and certain obsessions—such as one patient's urge to repeat obscene words whenever he attended church—are impulse expressions. Usually, however, a symptom reflects some combination of impulse, anxiety and defense, all at the same time. For example, a patient who, for religious reasons, lived a life of celibacy began to manifest the conversion symptom of uncontrollably and repeatedly thrusting his pelvic area forward. Although to an observer the symptom was an obvious expression of sexuality, the patient was unaware of its significance; it represented his anxiety-motivated repression as well as the repressed drive.

Anxiety Neurosis

The neurotically anxious individual is tense and apprehensive. He experiences a vague, free-floating anxiety whose source he cannot specify. The childhood of an anxiety reaction patient is often marked by parental demands for perfectionism yet at the same time the child is kept in a state of uncertainty so that he does not know which behaviors will lead to approval and affection and which will lead to punishment. A common consequence of this background is the development of chronic fear, low tolerance of frustration and a predisposition to evaluate the world as basically threatening and cruel. The individual is uncertain of his ability to handle even the mildest of stress situations. He finds it hard to concentrate. Sometimes he feels as if his thoughts and actions are not really his own, as if he has somehow changed and is not really himself. These feelings of unreality should not be confused with a psychotic's defective relation to reality, for the anxiety neurotic is well oriented and basically in good contact with reality. Experimental evidence has demonstrated that subjects who are high in anxiety condition more rapidly than low-anxiety subjects, extinguish more slowly and perform more poorly on difficult tasks, particularly under conditions of stress (Jenness, 1962). High-anxiety subjects overestimate the physical size of pictures depicting failure situations, whereas low-anxiety subjects underestimate it (Zahn, 1960). High-anxiety subjects are more apt to experience symbolic sexual imagery when listening to music (Wallach and Greenberg, 1960). They recall more night dreams (Schonbar, 1959) and they daydream more (Singer and Schonbar, 1961). In sum, anxiety is not narrowly circumscribed but pervades many different aspects of the anxious individual's personality and functioning.

Neurotic anxiety is an exaggeration of so-called normal anxiety or fear, just as depression exaggerates normal grief. As contrasted with normal fear, neurotic anxiety is irrational in the sense that it is either completely unjustified by an actual, objective danger or else it is a disproportionately strong reaction to an objective but quite minor danger. Normal fear reactions end when the danger ends, but a neurotic anxiety reaction is not altered much by an improvement in the objective situation. The neurotically anxious individual tries to avoid situations that trigger his anxiety; he retrenches and inhibits his activities and thus loses many potential satisfactions. What he really fears is unconscious and within him, but his fear is displaced onto a variety of external situations or onto a vague "everything and nothing."

The onset of a neurotic anxiety reaction may be either sudden or gradual. In either case, the chronic state of anxious apprehension is periodically punctuated by intense *anxiety attacks*. These appear suddenly, mount to extraordinary heights and subside after a few minutes or at most a few hours. In an anxiety attack the individual is flooded by terror and panic. His sympathetic nervous system becomes extremely overactive and he sweats profusely, his heart pounds frighteningly and he cannot get enough air. In some cases, patients describe a voice "silently screaming" in the brain, or a feeling that the ground under them is slipping and cracking or a sense of being crushed and overwhelmed. The individual's mouth becomes dry, he shudders and shakes and he becomes dizzy. Diarrhea, an urgent need to urinate, blurred vision and loss of appetite—or paradoxically an intense hunger—are common. The individual feels that he is losing his mind and that his heart or head will burst. He may feel convinced he is dying and at the same time wish that he would. He is helpless and out of control and he can do nothing but wait out the attack. Afterward he is exhausted and limp, drained of both emotion and physical strength.

An anxiety attack may be precipitated by some behavior that is unacceptable to the ego—for example, masturbation and consequent guilt feelings, a sexual adventure, an episode of stealing or cheating, or hostility expressed toward someone whose support the neurotic individual needs. The attack may, however, precede the unacceptable behavior, e.g., it may anticipate and forestall a contemplated antisocial episode and thus save the ego from further pain. Sometimes, fantasies of unacceptable behavior break through the individual's defenses and precipitate severe anxiety even if he has no intention of translating the fantasies into action. The heightened anxiety then leads to new repressions so that the individual is never aware of the significance of fantasy in precipitating his symptoms. An expectation of punishment, taking such forms as an expected rejection by others or a feeling that one is being judged harshly may also precede an anxiety attack. In many individuals, anxiety mounts to great intensity with the approach of an examination or a social gathering in which it is important to make a good impression.

The following case illustrates a fairly common type of anxiety reaction. It will be noted that in addition to her basic pattern of anxiety the patient also manifested a transient conversion symptom (inability to move her legs) and a temporary neurotic depression.

A 28-year-old married woman was admitted to a state hospital because of severe anxiety. She was animated, talkative, neatly dressed and except for being apprehensive and jittery appeared quite capable. She described her anxiety as follows: "All of a sudden everything went wrong. It started with small things bothering me that I had done before—religion and bad dreams, and not feeling sure of myself and being afraid of this and that. . . . Everything got on my nerves and I didn't want to be alone and I didn't seem to want to take on responsibility at all. One thing that frightened me very much was those panic seizures I've had—attacks of shaking. . . ." When asked if she had ever thought of suicide she replied, "I have thought of it but I haven't the courage. The first time I ever felt like that was two or three weeks ago and I felt that way for two or three days running, but then I found out that I would be coming to the hospital soon and I felt better. I am unhappy about the way I am, I guess. I'm frightened about so many things."

It was learned that the patient was the eldest of three girls reared by emotionally immature parents. The mother was described as a "nervous" and "high-strung" person who had suffered from stomach ulcers. The father was a harsh disciplinarian who gambled, drank heavily and was sexually promiscuous. The patient feared her father but did not express the anger which she felt toward him. The parents divorced when the patient was in her twenties.

As a child and young adult the patient was nervous and frightened. She quit school in the tenth grade because of anxiety over school work and examinations. Afterward she held a series of jobs only briefly, leaving each one because of dizziness and panic when there were many people around her.

Socially and sexually she led a restricted life. She dated little and feared sexual contact. She had so little sexual information that she once believed she was pregnant as the result of an episode of mild petting. At the age of 19 she became engaged but "went to pieces" a week before her marriage. She was unable to move her legs and had to be taken home from work. This conversion symptom soon vanished and she was able to get married but cut her honeymoon short so as not to remain away from her mother too long. She was frigid and had sexual relations only three or four times a year.

She mentioned a close, dependent relationship with her mother after marriage. She had a daughter of her own but found it impossible to discipline her. Over a period of years she developed many physical complaints which appeared to be emotionally based. Because of these complaints and increasing anxiety she was referred to a psychiatrist at the age of 26. For 18 months she received psychotherapy and minor tranquilizers but became mildly depressed and dependent on the drugs. The depression and drug dependency were then treated by three electroconvulsive treatments. When her anxiety recurred three months later she was admitted to the hospital.

Hysterical Neurosis

Hysterical neurosis has as its chief characteristic an involuntary loss or disordering of functioning of the voluntary nervous system or state of consciousness. Often the symptoms appear suddenly in emotionally charged situations, such as happened in the case just described when the patient temporarily lost the use of her legs. Sometimes the symptoms disappear just as suddenly as they appeared and often they can be modified by suggestion alone. There are two types of hysterical neurosis: conversion type and dissociative type.

Conversion Hysteria. This neurosis has been studied more intensively than any other type. It is more frequent in females than males, but in recent decades it has been declining in frequency, possibly due to a decrease of prudery and an increase in the psychological sophistication of our culture. New cases of conversion usually are diagnosed only after the patient and his physician(s) have failed to find a physical basis for his difficulties. It is not unusual for such patients to have seen several physicians of various specialties who put the patient through numerous physical tests and sometimes even unnecessary operations.

Conversion patients tend to come from lower socioeconomic levels. An investigation by Miller and Swanson (1960) found that the defense mechanism of denial, which is characteristic of conversion reactions, is typically found in the lower socioeconomic levels. Members of the middle class, on the other hand, tend toward defenses such as displacement, projection, isolation, reaction-formation and hostility turned against the self. The middle class mechanisms are found in disorders other than conversion reaction, whereas denial is always present in conversion.

Conversion symptoms are enormously varied. Their common denominator is an involuntary disturbance of physical functions that are normally under voluntary control. The onset of the symptoms is usually rapid and occurs in response to recognizable emotional stress. Three main symptom subtypes may be distinguished: sensory symptoms, motor paralyses and disordered movements.

(1) In any of the *senses*—vision, touch, taste, smell, hearing and so forth—there may be anesthesia (total loss of sensation), hypoesthesia (reduced sensitivity), hyperesthesia (excessive sensitivity) or paresthesia (unusual sensations such as tingling or distorted vision). For example, in the visual modality the patient may be blind in one or both eyes or in half of each eye; he may have double vision (diplopia); he may have tunnel vision in which he can see straight ahead, as if he were wearing blinkers, but not in the periphery of the visual field; he may complain that things are too bright or dim; or things may seem either too small (micropsia) or too large (macropsia). The symptom of tunnel vision, although rare, is particularly interesting, for it is a symbolic expression of the patient's narrowed field of consciousness, his tendency to exclude or deny large segments of reality, especially internal and psychological reality.

In the auditory modality, deafness is the most common symptom. In the touch modality, "glove" and "stocking" anesthesias are sometimes seen: the patient does not respond to touch or pain stimuli in the areas normally covered by these articles of clothing. Anesthesia of other skin areas, such as the trunk or head and neck may also occur.

Perhaps the most common of all sensory symptoms is *vague pain* in which the patient has painful sensations that are difficult for him to describe in some area of the body; especially when the area is stimulated. If the patient is distracted during stimulation, the pain response is much reduced; this fact is consistent with an emotional basis for the pain. Conversely, a stimulus applied to an anesthetic skin area may produce a response if the patient is simultaneously distracted. If the anesthesia were due to nerve destruction there could be no response to stimulation under any conditions.

(2) *Motor paralyses*. The patient's ability to perform voluntary movements is diminished. If his fingers, knees or elbows are paralyzed for very long periods of time they may become permanently, or almost permanently, contracted. A paralysis of both legs or of one side of the body sometimes occurs. A loss of motor functions may affect the voice so that the patient is unable to speak or can whisper but cannot speak at normal volume.

(3) *Disordered movements*. Among the great variety of disordered movements seen in conversion patients are tics, tremors, seizures resembling those observed in epilepsy, choreas, stammering and stuttering. An interesting symptom is that of *astasia-abasia:* the patient cannot stand (astasia) or walk (abasia) but he can perform complex movements of the legs such as "pedaling a bicycle" while lying on his back.

In addition to these three main types of conversion symptoms, certain visceral symptoms are sometimes included in the category of conversion reaction. Respiratory difficulties, a sensation of a lump in the throat, vomiting, anorexia nervosa, excessive appetite, constipation and countless other such symptoms quite often occur in conjunction with sensory and motor symptoms. Janet (1920) felt that the hysterical conversion process could simulate any disease or physical condition involving the viscera—tumors, intestinal obstructions, tuberculosis and so forth. A number of cases of "hysterical pregnancy," in which menstruation ceases and the patient's abdomen swells, have been well authenticated. Because visceral symptoms involve the autonomic nervous system and the involuntary muscles of the body, they are somewhat arbitrarily classified as psychophysiologic disorders in present classification schema.

It is sometimes difficult to distinguish between a conversion reaction and an organic disease process. For example, a female patient with some anxiety and a tendency to use denial as a defense may develop a temporary weakness of an arm or leg with no neurological signs, symptoms which appear to be conversion symptoms. However, her symptoms may herald the beginning of multiple sclerosis. There are some signs which help in making such distinctions. First, the conversion patient with a symptom such as paralysis or deafness often manifests an attitude of blandness and indifference to his difficulties—"la belle indifférence"—whereas the organic patient is usually anxious and upset. The blandness of the hysteric stems partly from the secondary gains that accrue from his symptom and partly from the fact that his symptom, like the defense mechanisms, wards off anxiety: the patient has a conversion symptom *instead* of being anxious.

Second, anesthesias, paralyses and many other conversion symptoms may be induced, diminished or even removed, at least temporarily, by hypnosis or waking suggestions.

Third, the specific nature of many conversion symptoms does not conform to the anatomy of the nervous system. There are no nerves whose degeneration would result in a pattern of stocking or glove anesthesia (see Fig. 9–1).

Fourth, conversion symptoms are usually more inconsistent than organic symptoms. For example, in astasia-abasia the patient can make some complex movements but not simple ones. In conversion blindness the patient rarely bumps into objects.

Finally, there are various examination pro-

cedures that distinguish between functional and organic cases. Dorcus and Shaffer (1950) describe a procedure for diagnosing the functional nature of monocular blindness. Alternating red and green letters are shown on a dark background; together, the letters spell a meaningful word, but the red or green letters alone are meaningless, e.g.:

red: P Y H L G
green: S C O O Y

The patient wears special glasses with one red and one green lens, so that with one eye he sees only the red letters and with the other only the green ones. If his monocular blindness is organic he sees the letters of one color only. If it is functional he sees the whole word, for his visual system is anatomically intact.

The conversion patient also shows certain personality characteristics with a fair degree of frequency, whereas organic patients have no particular personality pattern. Both male and female hysterics tend to be dependent, immature and suggestible. In some respects they resemble the traditional "spoiled child" with his overstrong need for affection and fear of rejection. There is often a history of overprotection accompanied by the reward of extra attention when ill. Many female hysterics are extraverted, talkative and flirtatious; some are histrionically dramatic. They are often optimistic to the point of being Pollyannas who ignore all unpleasant aspects of reality. Male hysterics, on the other hand, tend to be relatively colorless individuals.

Conversion symptoms are usually precipitated by emotional stress and a need to escape from it. Symptoms may also begin as a functional continuation of a temporary organic condition, or a continuation of a violent motor reaction to a frightening situation, or a consequence of a physician's remarks or questions. e.g., "Do you have any pains in your legs?" Such a question may be sufficient to precipitate a symptom in a highly suggestible individual, especially when he is in the worried frame of mind characteristic of many people visiting a physician. The physician's high prestige in our culture reinforces the suggestive effect of his questions and comments.

The dynamic function and symbolic meaning of a conversion symptom depends on the individual's history. It should be understood that conversion is not a mysterious chemical process by which an instinct or anxiety is literally converted into a symptom. Rather, a symptom is *an automatic response to the stimuli of unconscious impulses or the anxiety associated*

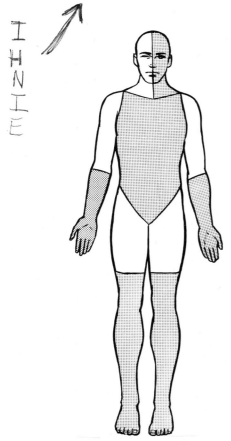

Figure 9–1. *Unusual pattern of sensory loss (anesthesia) in one patient with conversion hysteria. He was unable to feel pain in any of the shaded areas, which show a typical "glove and stocking" distribution, as well as involvement of half the head and neck and all the trunk.*

with them; the response is symbolically expressed by what has been called the "language of the body." A chronic, uncontrollable contraction of the hand into a clenched fist, for example, may symbolize hostility as much as angry words do.

The past history of the individual determines precisely which symptoms he will manifest as well as their significance. Thus, the organs that have played an important part in the patient's fantasies seem to be particularly vulnerable to the conversion process. Sometimes a symptom occurs in an organ that was active in the particular situation in which the patient experienced an unacceptable impulse. For example, a severe internal conflict felt while running may precipitate a functional weakness of the legs. In addition, there may be a constitutional factor: symptoms may attack those organs that are physically weakest and therefore most prone to difficulties.

In the following case of conversion reaction the patient had a history of unusually severe emotional stress dating back to her early childhood. Perhaps because the stress was so strong and began so early, a number of her personality traits were quite different from those of more typical conversion patients.

The patient was a 27-year-old married woman who had suffered from headaches for eight years. She was referred to a neurologist by her family physician. Three months before the referral she had begun to experience nausea, vomiting, blurred vision and generalized uncontrollable seizures. The latter consisted of a period of rigidity followed by rhythmical, violent jerking movements. Unlike epileptic convulsions, however, she did not lose consciousness nor the ability to talk; she had never fallen, become blue, frothed at the mouth, bitten her tongue, otherwise injured herself, or lost control of her bowels or bladder, nor was there post-seizure amnesia. The neurological findings were negative and she was referred for psychiatric evaluation.

She had been the eldest of four girls whose parents continually quarreled. Her father drank excessively. He molested her sexually when she was four years old and she contracted gonorrhea. This led to her being removed from her home by a welfare board for treatment; she was then placed in a foster home with two elderly women and no other children. She was frequently kept alone in a fenced yard and was not permitted to play with other children in the neighborhood. Her social isolation lasted until she returned to live with her mother at the age of six and began to attend school. Meanwhile the father deserted the family. The mother repeatedly told the patient that she was just like her worthless father. The mother remarried when the patient was nine, but this marriage

was also unsuccessful and soon ended in divorce. The patient did not get along with the stepfather.

She was no happier in school than at home; she found the work difficult, was shy and introverted, and had never learned how to make friends. In the 10th grade, at the age of 16, she complained of abdominal pain (possibly of emotional origin) and her appendix was removed. She did not return to school but took a series of brief jobs as a salesgirl. She began to date a young man living next door who was five years older than she. Her need for affection had been frustrated all her life and she did everything to please him; she soon became pregnant. On being told, her mother responded, "You made your bed, now lie in it." The pregnancy led to a forced marriage and during the next eleven years the patient had eight children. (Prior to evaluation she was asked if she had any problems and she replied, "Eight of them"; clearly, escaping from the drudgery of caring for her family constituted an important secondary gain.) Her headaches had begun when her second child had been only five months old and she had found to her distress that she was pregnant again.

Despite this history of stress she stated during the psychiatric evaluation that she had no problems other than the desire to avoid further pregnancies. She described her husband as a good provider who was considerate of her. It was difficult for her to accept the idea that her physical complaints had an emotional basis but she came regularly for weekly interviews and some of her emotional problems soon came into the open. She and her husband were Catholic but occasionally they used contraceptives and then felt guilty. She quarreled with him without realizing that the quarrels indicated their hostility to each other. Her unconscious hostility to him had led her to have an extramarital affair several years previously which she believed had led to one of her pregnancies. This, in turn, led to considerable guilt.

In the hope of modifying the couple's attitudes and behavior toward each other, it was suggested that the husband also be treated in psychotherapy and he accepted the suggestion. In therapy the wife gained considerable insight into her hostility and began to understand that it represented both a displacement from childhood attitudes toward her father and stepfather and a reaction to the reality problems of her marriage. For a brief period her anxiety mounted as insight grew and there was an increase in the severity of her seizures and headaches. This change necessitated temporary hospitalization, but she was soon discharged and for the next several years was able to maintain a more mature adjustment with fewer bodily symptoms.

Dissociative Hysteria. The major symptoms of dissociative reactions are amnesia, fugues, somnambulism and multiple personality. These symptoms often involve considerable personality disorganization that superficially may appear to be schizophrenic. However, unlike typical schizophrenic reactions, dissociative reactions usually have an abrupt onset as a response to obvious stress and they usually clear up fairly quickly, although they may later recur. As compared to the other neurotic reactions, dissociative reactions are relatively rare, but because of their dramatic nature have attracted considerable public and scientific attention. Reports of amnesic episodes, fugues and multiple personality frequently appear in the newspapers. A classic scientific account of multiple personality was given in Thigpen and Cleckley's *The Three Faces of Eve* (1957), later used as the basis for a feature film.

The *amnesia* of the dissociative-reaction patient usually occurs suddenly and covers a circumscribed, definite period of time, sometimes several years in length. The amnesia of organic brain syndromes, in contrast, may or may not have a sudden onset, tends to be diffuse rather than circumscribed, and is maximal for events of the very recent past. A prototype of amnesia and multiple personality may be observed in a normal individual who is given a post-hypnotic suggestion that on awaking from hypnosis he will not recall the hypnotic session. In a subsequent hypnotic session he may recall the previous session, almost as if in hypnosis he had a special set of reactions and memories separate from those of his waking state. Another dissociative prototype may be observed in the individual who responds to a severe emotional shock by a brief period of automatic behavior in which he does not know what he is doing. A neurotic dissociative state is more prolonged and uncontrollable than this, however, for the individual cannot snap back into a stable awareness as the normal individual does.

Dissociative amnesia may be partial or complete. The patient may forget only his address or name or he may forget all the events of a particular period. He does not, however, lose his learned basic habits: he can walk, talk, read, write and so forth.

A *fugue* is a combination of amnesia and physical flight. The individual flees from his customary surroundings; what he is really trying to escape is his own fear. Some individuals show recurring fugue episodes, indicating a predisposition to the habitual occurrence of the symptom. In some instances a wish-fulfilling component is clearly present, for the individual flees to a place where he has fewer responsibilities. In criminal trials, defense attorneys sometimes attribute the crime to amnesia or a fugue, but in actual fact few crimes are committed in these states.

The case cited below illustrates the motivational factors and sequence of events in a fugue. The patient also manifested some signs of depression which are not uncommon in fugue cases.

A woman was found by the police one night in an empty parking lot. She was untidy in appearance and carried no purse or other possessions. She had no idea who, where or how old she was. Taken to the emergency department of a hospital, it was found that her feet were blistered and swollen and that she was dehydrated, but no other physical or neurological difficulties were evident. She was admitted to a psychiatric ward where she dressed neatly, ate and slept well and socialized with other patients. In interview she appeared somewhat anxious, unhappy, depressed and dependent. She complained of a lump in her throat and stated that she felt as though she were "looking through a wet windshield." However, she answered questions as best she could, was soon correctly oriented for time and place and was able to remember most of the events that had happened after she had been found by the police. Prior to this event she vaguely recalled having walked through the woods, but could remember no other details of her past life. She could form a mental picture of her mother but not of her father and she angrily stated, "I don't want to know about him." She had a pervading feeling of personal loss but no idea as to what she might have lost.

Three days after admission to the psychiatric ward she was hypnotized and she vividly recalled the details of her previous life. She was 43 years old and had been an only child who had never known her father. Her mother had been a domestic servant in private homes and hotels and the patient had been able to live with her for only a few months at a time. The remainder of her childhood had been spent with an aunt and uncle, a middle-aged couple without children of their own. Until the age of 10 she had assumed that her father was dead, but then she learned from her mother that her father had deserted them before she was born. The information came as a shock to her. When she was 14 her mother committed suicide and the patient recalled having been so unhappy that she wished her mother had taken her too. She had made a number of friends in the few years previous to her mother's death, but then she withdrew socially.

At 18 she married a factory worker but their marriage was unsuccessful from the start. Sexual relations were unsatisfactory, the husband was unfaithful and drank excessively, and finances were uncertain. After three children and several separations the husband left her. The patient left her children with her in-laws and went to work. She never got around to actually obtaining a divorce although she led people to believe she had.

In her late thirties she met a married man to whom she became very much attached. His wife was a chronic patient in a mental hospital and he was unable to obtain a divorce. The patient lived with him as his wife, but she experienced a great deal of guilt and wished they were both free to marry each other. Twice she left him and returned to live with her in-laws but she felt unwanted in their home. On the second such occasion she had an episode of amnesia and was found by the police walking down a highway. The episode lasted for only three days, after which she returned to live with her male friend. Once again the conflict proved too much for her and she left him to work in another city. While there she received word that he had finally obtained a divorce and wished to marry her. She felt unable to tell him that she was not free to marry and was ambivalent about returning to live with him on the previous basis. She was trapped in her conflicts and her lie: she packed all her belongings in a suitcase, checked it in a railroad station locker, put the key in a purse which also contained all her money—needed to buy a railroad ticket—and then lost her purse and also her memory. It was summertime and for the next several weeks she slept outdoors and in abandoned houses. She was afraid of people and came out mainly after dark when she would walk aimlessly for hours. She was unable to recall eating or drinking. She was picked up by the police on her 43rd birthday close to a house where she had lived with her husband.

Somnambulism consists of behavior—walking, talking, eating and so forth—in a sleeplike state for which the individual is afterward amnesic. The most common type of somnambulistic activity is walking. The individual's eyes are open and he responds more or less well to commands, yet he is not awake. In some cases he goes outdoors in this state and may injure himself. Somnambulistic episodes may occur in childhood or puberty and then be outgrown, or they may recur in a pattern that continues into adult life. It has been estimated that at least 5 per cent of the general population is subject to occasional somnambulistic episodes. The symptom has been variously attributed to emotional trauma, guilt and sexual conflicts and to a clash between dependence on the family and a drive to be independent and flee the family environment.

An individual with a *multiple personality* manifests different, relatively complete systems of emotional and cognitive reactions at different times. The reaction systems are usually very unlike each other because each contains elements repressed by the other. Multiple personality is the rarest type of neurosis and should not be confused with the much more common "split personality," as it is often called, of the schizophrenic. The schizophrenic's cleavage is not between one personality and another but among various psychological processes; for example, his affect may be incon-

gruous with his thinking and motor responses. It has been estimated that fewer than 100 cases of multiple personality have been fully authenticated in the last century.

One of the most celebrated cases of multiple personality on record is that of Miss Beauchamp, a young woman who was treated for several years by Morton Prince (1906). Three major personalities were uncovered in the course of the therapy. The following account is a résumé of the outstanding features of the case.

As a child she was dreamy, lonely and "shut-in." She spent vacations from school reading and daydreaming. She reported having had visions of the Madonna and Jesus. During her mystical experiences she felt "saintly" and began to aspire to live like a saint. She cultivated meekness, humility, prayer and fasting and she strove never to have wicked thoughts. She was terrified of her father and adored her mother but felt that her mother did not love her in return. In her thinking, the Madonna and her mother became fused into one figure and she had an obsessive idea that if her behavior were perfect she could safeguard her mother against all dangers.

Her mother fell ill and the child blamed herself. She had no insight into the aggression implied by her feelings of guilt and instigated by her belief that her mother did not love her. Her mother's death when the child was 13 was a traumatic event. For the next several years she lived with her father in a constant state of unhappiness and then ran away and became a nurse. At 18 she fell in love with an older man whom she thought of as a "messenger from heaven" and worthy of all her trust and confidence. A second trauma now occurred: during a thunderstorm he attempted to kiss her at the entrance to the hospital where she worked. She was horrified by his facial expression and began to brood and to live in a solitary fashion as she had in childhood. An important factor in her reaction was guilt, for against her will she had felt sexually aroused by him.

It was at this point, aged 18, that the dissociation of her personality began. One personality, referred to by Prince as "The Saint," remained dominant until age 24. The Saint was somewhat sickly—undoubtedly due to a conversion process—and also hesitant, shy, altruistic, quiet, reserved and kind to children and old people. When her therapy began at 23 there was no indication that any other personality existed, but one year later she received a letter which revived the memory of the episode at the hospital entrance. She thereupon became excited, agitated and depressed; she hallucinated the earlier episode and suddenly manifested a second personality, "The Realist." This personality was sociable, self-assertive, easily angered, impulsive and resolute. It was quite unsaintly and represented the traits repressed by the Saint. The Realist disliked church and old people but liked reading newspapers, which the Saint disliked.

Both personalities could recall the 18 years ending just prior to the sexual trauma, but the Realist had complete amnesia for the ensuing six-year period. For about a year after the discovery of the Realist, the two personalities alternated, with reciprocal amnesia for events that occurred while the other was dominant. At the end of this period Prince discovered a third personality who called herself Sally and referred to the Saint as "she." Sally appeared only when the Saint's eyes were closed, knew what the Saint did and thought—although the Saint was unaware of Sally—disliked the Saint and sometimes discomfited her by making her lie. Sally was *coconscious* with the Saint, to use Prince's term. If the Saint read material that was boring to Sally, the latter thought of other things. The Saint could read French but Sally could not.

Eventually Sally forced the Saint to open her eyes; Prince felt that this was motivated by Sally's desire to see and control more of the external world. Sally began to dominate the Saint more and more, writing messages to her and mischievously destroying her knitting. Even when dominated, however, the Saint was not aware of Sally. Sally also tried to trick the Realist but the latter knew of Sally's existence through the consequences of her maneuvers and managed to resist and thwart them.

Prince's treatment, largely hypnotic, attempted to merge the Saint and the Realist and to repress the mischievous and impish Sally. The integration succeeded and Sally was "killed"; Miss Beauchamp was thereafter unable to recall Sally. A follow-up several years later revealed that Miss Beauchamp had married and was well.

Many persons who have reviewed this famous case have been troubled by the question of why Miss Beauchamp developed a multiple personality instead of schizophrenia. Childhood visions and a shut-in personality are commonly supposed to be signs of the individual's predisposition to break with reality and be subject to delusions and hallucinations. Although she experienced one hallucination, she showed no other psychotic symptoms as an adult. The question must remain unanswered, but one possibility is that the dissociation *prevented* schizophrenia: a psychotic response to the stresses she encountered may have been forestalled by stabilization at a severely neurotic level.

Phobic Neurosis

Phobias are characterized by intense fear of an object or situation, fear which the patient may recognize as unrealistic. In spite of his rational knowledge that the feared object presents no real danger the patient experiences great apprehension and symptoms associated with severe anxiety attacks in its presence.

A phobia includes several components: an expectation of panic if a feared situation should be encountered, an avoidance of the situation, and the actual panic reaction when the situation is encountered. Phobic individuals often go to great lengths in regulating and restricting their activities to avoid a panic.

A phobia is often accompanied by dependence and helplessness. Thus, an individual with acrophobia—a fear of heights—may be willing to descend a long staircase only if accompanied by someone he trusts. Another characteristic of a phobia is a tendency to generalization: a phobia may start as an irrational fear of cats, for example, and then begin to include the word "cat" and the sound of a cat as well as the sight of it, other animals of the cat family and even "catlike" persons.

Phobias arise in more than one way. A traumatically frightening experience may become the basis for a strong conditioned fear reaction. For example, an individual who in childhood was bitten on the hand by a dog may, decades later, automatically become tense and put his hands in his pockets at the approach of a dog.

A more important source of phobias consists of fear of an instinctual impulse, repression of the impulse, and displacement of the fear to an external object or situation. For example, a child's fear of his own hostility to his parents, and his fear of their anger should his true feelings be discovered, may be displaced and result in a phobic reaction to guns or other weapons. Fear of either anal or genital impulses may result in a phobic reaction to dirt, germs or disease. Phobias of this type serve a protective function, for they prevent awareness of threatening impulses. The individual can perceive no motivation for his fear and he feels that it has descended on him by some strange quirk of fate.

The symbolic meaning of a phobia, just like the meaning of a conversion symptom, depends on the individual's past history. Fear of heights, for example, may in one case unconsciously represent fear of abandonment, in another an overwhelming ambition, in a third a fear of sexuality and in a fourth a hostile or suicidal urge. Since repression is usually involved in a phobia, it may be very difficult to trace it to its source and tease out its symbolic meaning.

In the following case of agoraphobia, fear of open spaces, the patient had no insight into the roots of his symptom.

A 41-year-old married man of average intelligence was referred for evaluation because of a fear of being outdoors. Since he was a salesman, this symptom greatly interfered with his work. He had to force himself to leave home and frequently convinced himself that calls on customers were unnecessary. On weekends he would not leave the house except for rare instances and then only when accompanied by his wife.

He had obtained his present job six years earlier with the help of his older brother who was a successful salesman for the same company. He admired and looked up to the brother but was constantly less successful. His work as a salesman was marginal from the beginning and was getting worse at the time he developed his phobia.

In interview, his outstanding traits appeared to be insecurity, a complete lack of confidence, and an apologetic, fear-ridden manner. He was a passive and submissive person married to a rather dominant and capable woman. The standards he set for himself were very high for his abilities. He was supersensitive to criticism, unable to take any kidding or practical joking from colleagues on the job and very worried about his future. Some signs of depression were present and at times he wept. Another symptom consisted of headaches originating in tension. He was a very good mechanic who enjoyed tinkering with automobiles, but he considered mechanical work too dirty and too lacking in prestige to be pursued as an occupation. It was acceptable to him only as a nonserious hobby.

His phobia seemed to be motivated by a need to escape from a job situation in which he was inferior to his brother, without admitting defeat and quitting.

⑤ Obsessive-Compulsive Neurosis

A number of so-called "normal" obsessions and compulsions are very common. A tune that runs through one's mind repeatedly, a habit of counting the number of letters in words or the number of telegraph poles along a highway, and a child's care to avoid stepping on sidewalk cracks, are all instances of obsessive and compulsive, yet "normal," behavior. In comparison with these examples, neurotic obsessions and compulsions are more intense and persistent, for they are motivated by unconscious conflicts.

Obsessions and compulsions usually are found together, although one or the other may be more prominent in a given case. They are often also accompanied by phobias and by physiological signs of anxiety. The range of possible obsessions and compulsions is infinite: any idea or act can become the basis of a persistent and repetitive symptom.

An obsession or compulsion may be a direct expression of an antisocial impulse not accepted by the ego. Examples are obsessive fantasies of aggression, pyromania (compulsive

setting of fires) and kleptomania (compulsive stealing). Alternatively, an obsession or compulsion may result from a reaction-formation against an unacceptable impulse and express an attempt to expiate guilt or undo evil. Obsessive thoughts are frequently antisocial, but fortunately for society most compulsive acts embody reaction formations.

A special type of obsession or compulsion is excessive doubting: when a decision is necessary, the individual cannot make up his mind in thought or action. For example, he may spend hours ruminating whether to read a book or make a telephone call. An extreme instance is evident in a patient who parked his car and left it because he was unable to decide whether to turn right or left in order to circle the block and reach his home.

The personality of the majority of obsessive-compulsives is very striking. They tend to be obstinate, stingy, neat, methodical, rigid and perfectionistic. These are all traits which are associated with the anal-retentive level of development. Rigidity in handling details is evidenced by isolating and compartmentalizing them. Obsessives tend to be relatively cool intellectualizers; their speech is typically marked by many qualifications. Their detail-mindedness and insistence on qualifying everything tend to irritate other people intensely. They avoid affect by isolating it from ideas. Overcontrolled and unable to react spontaneously to other people, they try to live by rules and regulations; they are unconsciously afraid of flexible interactions in which decisions must be made from moment to moment.

In most obsessions and compulsions there is a disproportion between the overwhelming strength of the individual's urge to think his obsessive thoughts or perform his ritual acts and the triviality of the thoughts or acts themselves. For example, he feels a terrific need to repeat a foolish, nonsensical or infantile phrase over and over or to walk from home to office by one certain route although a number of other routes are just as good. (Because they are infantile, the obsessive's conscious thoughts have been likened to the unconscious of hysterics and the dreams of normals.) Since on rational grounds we would expect strong urges to be associated only with important ideas and actions, we must conclude that obsessions or compulsions are a distorted expression of important ideas or impulses that do not appear on the surface.

The distortion may occur in several ways: one

possibility is distortion through repression and displacement. Freud recounts the case of a patient who repressed a fear of insanity and instead continually brooded over such questions as "Why must I breathe?" She had substituted a trivial idea for a dangerous and feared one. Kleptomania may be a displacement of a repressed need for affection; the trivial objects that many kleptomaniacs steal may unconsciously stand for love, much as gifts are consciously used to express love and affection. It has been speculated that pyromania is related to regressed sexual impulses since the tension build-up, excitement and release which such persons describe seems quite similar to the mounting excitement and release of the sex act.

In a second type of distortion, the symptom arises from isolation of affect rather than repression. An obsessive fantasy of aggression or a ritual act of hostility, for example, may be felt by the individual to force itself upon him against his will, so that he himself does not "really" have strong hostilities. His impulses are strong, but through no fault of his.

In a third type, the superego gives rise to obsessive or compulsive reaction-formations. Examples are hand washing or an obsessive struggle to think only pure thoughts, arising out of guilt.

It is the impression of many experts that obsessive-compulsive patients tend to have had parents who were themselves perfectionistic, meticulous in their attention to detail and intolerant of noise and disorder. Often they turn out to have been overambitious for their children, as indicated by premature attempts to elicit behavior appropriate to a later stage of development. Premature toilet training, stressed by the Freudians, is only one area in which parents hurry children and push them into an obsessive-compulsive pattern.

An example of a severe obsessive-compulsive reaction in a basically obsessional personality is the following case of a 37-year-old unmarried woman. It should be noted that the patient's childhood was not "typical" for obsessive-compulsiveness; she was subjected to overt rejection rather than perfectionistic demands. The etiological determinants of her difficulties included biological and psychological deprivations, severe childhood frustrations, sociocultural stress and possibly heredity.

A 37-year-old woman was admitted to the clinic with complaints of many compulsive symptoms which had developed since her emigration to this country the previous year. She reported a compulsive urge to steal, although the items taken were of little value (pencils, pens and small amounts of money). She expressed no guilt in connection with her stealing but was disturbed over the intensity of her urges. A phobia of electricity, especially electric light sockets, had also developed and with it a compulsive need to check and recheck whether various lights and electric appliances had been turned off. She also had to check that all doors were shut and reported washing her hands and genitals many times each day in order to be sure that they were clean. Whenever one obsessive thought or impulsive action ceased another took its place; she had a generalized compulsion to do anything that was explicitly forbidden. On one occasion she felt that her compulsive behavior was under the control of some external force, but this transient delusion of influence persisted only briefly and there was no other evidence of psychotic distortion. Sometimes she felt depressed, but her depression was not severe enough to be considered psychotic and there were no thoughts of suicide.

She had sought help for similar symptoms in her native country of Austria four years previously. After two years of psychoanalysis, there was a diminution of her symptoms but a remaining dependency on the drugs which had been prescribed for her anxiety and insomnia. Following her move to a new country, the symptoms returned.

Her history revealed a lifelong pattern of severe emotional deprivation and stress. She was the product of wealthy but unstable parents. The father was syphilitic and had many attendant physical and emotional problems. The mother was afflicted with severe tuberculosis which resulted in frequent and prolonged hospitalizations. During these times, the patient usually stayed in a boarding home. In addition, the mother suffered from migraine headaches and was described as nervous, high-strung, quarrelsome, friendless, overly strict, and not close to her children. Some of her actions were quite bizarre; for example, she did not wash for long periods of time and invariably used a wash basin as a toilet.

The patient was weak and sickly as a child. Because of severe vitamin D deficiency, she was unable to walk until the age of four.

Her mother was so cruel and harsh in her discipline that the patient came to hate her and to pray for her mother's death. She was often told by her mother that she was weak, stupid and ugly.

The patient's sexual experiences included being left in boarding homes, in one of which she shared a single bedroom with the landlady and three other boarders, with the landlady entertaining men at night. Once she shared a room with an older girl who introduced her to mutual masturbation and stealing. After returning home she would stay awake at night until her parents went to bed. If either parent went to the room of the other she would scream and cry, and this resulted in severe reprimands or punishments by the mother. At 13 she began to masturbate and to have migraine headaches for the first time. When she later confessed her masturbating practice to her mother she was told the practice would result in insanity, that she would never be clean again and that she was just like her diseased father. The patient became afraid to go to sleep at night for fear of having erotic dreams and she felt so dirty that she began to wash her hands and genitals "hundreds of times a day."

As an adult, the patient gradually overcame some of her intense shyness and compulsive behaviors but remained lonely and meticulously tidy. Between the ages of 26 and her early 30's she developed a repetitive pattern of dating a man just to have "someone to talk to" but ending up having sexual relationships. Typically she would choose a married man and consent to sex when he promised to divorce his wife. Each time she was flattered by the man's attention and apparent concern for her. She was "engaged" five times, four of them to married men. During these years she had three pregnancies but had an induced or spontaneous abortion in each case. The compulsive sexual behavior appeared to have a number of antecedents including insecurity and a need for affection, rebellion against her mother's strictures against sexuality, a repetition of the disordered sexual behavior to which she was exposed in childhood, and fear of permanent entanglement with a man in marriage.

Depressive Neurosis

Normal grief or sadness is a response to an external, consciously recognized loss or frustration. A neurotic depressive reaction, frequently termed "reactive depression," is also precipitated by an external loss or frustration such as the death of a loved person, an occupational failure or a financial setback, but it differs from a normal reaction in two respects: It is disproportionate in intensity and duration and it occurs in an individual predisposed to it by certain personality traits.

In a neurotic depressive reaction the individual is listless and dejected. He feels lonely and helpless, weeps on slight provocation, and may eat either too little or too much. The individual is not as incapacitated as in a psychotic depression and does not manifest the retardation, agitation, delusions or other malignant symptoms often found in psychotic states. He may think of committing suicide but he is, in most instances, less likely to do so than a psychotic depressive.

The major predisposing personality traits are conscientiousness, dependency, inability to express anger directly and outwardly, and intropunitiveness, that is, a tendency to blame oneself rather than external factors for failures.

Depression may be viewed as a turning of hostility or anger against the self instead of outward. The formula for reactive depression is thus self-hate plus an external loss. A tendency to orality may be present: in psychoanalytic theory, pessimism, helpless dependency and appetite disturbances are associated with the oral-incorporative phase of development. In addition, many depressives are introverted and shy.

Depression is the most common of all the psychoneurotic disorders. Over 50 per cent of the neurotics seen, both in outpatient clinics and hospitals, are diagnosed as depressed. Women depressives are twice as common as males. Why this is so is unclear, but it is interesting to speculate that our culture does not provide its women with the outlets for aggression which are readily available for males. Competitive sports, career strivings and the like are generally regarded as more appropriate for males than for females. Such sociocultural factors may be important in the etiology of a disorder which has as its cardinal feature the tendency to blame the self rather than to be openly hostile and aggressive.

The personality characteristics and symptoms of the patient in the following case are fairly typical.

A 35-year-old unmarried private secretary requested therapeutic help. She appeared for an interview carelessly dressed and without makeup; her manner was listless and she wept quietly as she talked. She had long been dissatisfied with herself and her lot in life. She had always felt inferior and insecure with other people and was distressed over her inability to attract an acceptable husband. She was conscientious and very attentive to the details of her job but unable to enjoy it. Several months before coming for help she had begun to lose weight and feel increasingly tired. It had become very difficult for her to sleep at night and also to get up in the morning and go to work. Daily contacts with fellow employees had become increasingly threatening. She responded with irritation to a male friend and to her parents with whom she lived, yet these were the people she said she loved the most. Often she wondered if life was worth living but she reported never having seriously considered suicide.

The patient and her older sister had grown up in a middle-class family with anxious, conforming and overprotective parents. The father was a conscientious, hard-working manager of a small business who worried excessively about small details. He was able to assert himself only in the security of his own home where he was frequently irritable and would shout at the children with little provocation. The mother, who had suffered several brief "nervous breakdowns" during her life, continually worried and nagged both him and the children.

Asked about her early life at home, the patient hastily replied that it was "nice" but then said, "I was quite happy, I think. Mother was very, very fussy about the house—the housework was the most important thing in the world—she couldn't give the love a child needed. Nothing satisfied her. She was always nagging my father." Further, "Mother would say, 'You'll have to do this or your father will take care of you.' He's kind but had a very bad temper. He'd scream and yell and I was afraid of him. I was the good one. Everyone would say how sweet and quiet and good I was. My sister was the problem—she'd have temper tantrums."

She was asked if she ever got angry and replied, "It's hard for me to get angry at anybody. Sometimes at my mother but not outwardly. It's usually better not to say anything. If I get angry with her, I feel real bad afterwards—she always makes me feel wrong. I still feel she is my mother and I owe her respect. Everything I do, I'm trying to please her but then I can't. I can't feel like an adult in that household."

Both parents were overly concerned about the patient's physical health and repeatedly cautioned her to be careful of accidents. Neither provided her with any useful sexual information. "I always had a lot of dates —I always wanted to get married badly, but when I get close to it I can't. I was always naive and over-protected about sex—I'm sure this must have a lot to do with it—sex was never discussed at home. I never knew how a baby was born until I went to college. I never thought much about it. I was so innocent I'd flirt and not know what it was all about. I like to be loved or feel there's someone around. I like to be kissed at the time, but afterwards I get upset, like it was wrong or bad. My present boy friend has emotional problems and doesn't earn enough to support us if we got married, unless I also worked. We're both Catholic and we couldn't afford to have any children. When I see him I want to be close to him but I think it's wrong. I think we should stop seeing each other but then I miss him terribly."

The denial and repression of both sexual and aggressive impulses, apparent in these excerpts, failed to provide her with a workable way of life with her parents or in marriage. Some months previously her mother had become more difficult to live with, her father had begun to worry more and more as he approached retirement and it had become increasingly clear that her friend was unstable. The loss of the little security she possessed precipitated her depressive reaction. An added difficulty was that her supervisor, a rather demanding woman, stirred up her lifelong conflicts with her mother. One year previously she had tried living away from home but her dependence was so strong that she soon became more anxious and unhappy away from her parents than with them. She returned home, her ambivalent feelings of love and hostility, accompanied by guilt and self-blame, unresolved.

Other Neuroses

Other neuroses which will not be discussed in detail here include hypochondriasis, neurasthenia and depersonalization. In the latter, the individual does not feel real or feels that the situation in which he finds himself is not real or seems like a play rather than a real life event. The predominant feeling state is one of unreality and estrangement from the self or from the environment.

The neurasthenic individual is tired both mentally and physically and unable to concentrate. He complains that he "can't get started" and he feels very inadequate. He is irritable, sensitive to noise and prone to headaches. His fatigue stems from the general bodily tension that accompanies his worries and fantasies. Excitement is likely to snap him out of his fatigue, but it recurs when routine activities are resumed. Neurasthenia is observed with such frequency in housewives who are bored and feel neglected by their husbands that it has often been called "housewives'" neurosis. Since he is often unaware of being under any mental strain, the individual is able to blame his troubles on bodily fatigue instead of emotional factors.

Hypochondriacal concern with one's health tends to increase with age. The hypochondriac is not much interested in other people but is always ready to describe in detail his own bodily sensations. When medical examinations are negative, he is convinced that the doctors have erred. A severe hypochondriac has a conviction that he will not recover. Such persons merely substitute one worry for another. In a sense they very much resemble obsessive patients in that they ruminate excessively over a substitute for the emotional problems which they wish to avoid. Many depressives also report both hypochondriacal and neurasthenic symptoms.

THE CAUSAL DETERMINANTS OF NEUROSES

Despite the differences among the various neurotic reactions, there seem to be some etiological factors common to neurosis as such. In the case summaries that we have used to illustrate different neurotic reactions, several themes recur; the patient's parents and siblings were often also emotionally disturbed; the patient usually had a childhood history of rejection, sexual repression and trauma; and strong pressure was exerted on the patient to be "good." These background factors appear again and again in any large sample of neurotics.

Heredity

In Chapter 6 it was stated that there is little empirical proof that heredity is an important contributing cause of neurosis. Let us look at the evidence on which this statement is based.

Gregory (1959) studied the mental health of the families of 142 hospitalized neurotic patients (median age 35). Among the fathers, 9.1 per cent were reported to have consumed alcohol excessively; other significant behavior deviations were reported from 7.8 per cent. Among the mothers, significant deviations were reported for 18.3 per cent. These percentages are considerably higher than would be expected in the general population.

In considering these findings it should be noted that if a hereditary factor is present it could not be neuroticism as such but rather a general tendency to psychopathology, expressed in various deviant behaviors in parents and in neurosis in children. More important, as was pointed out in Chapter 6, a higher incidence of some variable among relatives of affected persons than among the general population may be taken as evidence of a hereditary component only if it is shown that environmental factors cannot account for the increased incidence. Parental alcoholism and emotional instability provide a poor environment for a child and may result in neurosis simply as a reaction to external stress.

However, a study by Brown (1942) provides evidence that the hereditary factor in neurosis— if it exists at all—may consist of specific predispositions for different types of neurotic reac-

tion rather than of the general psychopathological tendency indicated in Gregory's study. In Table 9–1, the expectancy rates reported by Brown for the relatives of patients with three types of neurosis are shown. Two inferences may be made from the data. First, if there is a genetic component in neurosis, it is of differential strength for different neurotic categories, since the per cent of parents who manifest the same type of neurosis as their children varies from 21.4 for anxiety neurosis to 7.5 for obsessives; the per cent of affected sibs also varies considerably, again being highest for anxiety neurosis (12.3). Second, anxiety reaction is the most common form of neurosis among the relatives of anxiety-reaction patients, hysteria is most common among relatives of hysterics and obsession among relatives of obsessives. These results are consistent with the hypothesis of a specific genetic predisposition in the various types of neurosis. But, as in Gregory's study, the results can also be accounted for without recourse to hereditary mechanisms. The child can learn the specific kind of maladaptive behavior he observes in his parents. The obsessive parent may consciously or unconsciously "train" the child to be obsessive, the hysteric parent may reward hysteroid behavior, and similarly for the other neurotic reactions.

Using psychological tests to measure the degree of neuroticism in a sample of 25 monozygous (MZ) and 25 same-sexed dizygous (DZ) pairs of school children from the general population, Eysenck and Prell (1951) reported that the correlation coefficient for degree of neuroticism in pairs of MZ twins was +0.85, whereas in pairs of DZ twins it was only +0.22. Applying the formula for H (the contribution of heredity toward the variance of a trait),

$$H = \frac{r_{MZ} - r_{DZ}}{1 - r_{DZ}} = \frac{0.85 - 0.22}{1 - 0.22} = 0.81$$

TABLE 9–1. Expectancy Rates for Various Kinds of Neurotic Disorders in Parents and Sibs of Index Cases

Types of Index Cases	Per Cent of Affected Relatives					
	Anxiety Neurotics		Hysterics		Obsessives	
	Parents	Sibs	Parents	Sibs	Parents	Sibs
Anxiety neurotics	21.4	12.3	1.6	2.2	0	0.9
Hysterics	9.5	4.6	19.0	6.2	0	0
Obsessives	0	5.4	0	0	7.5	7.1

Modified after Brown. 1942. *In* Fuller, J. L., and Thompson, W. R. 1960. Behavior Genetics. New York, John Wiley & Sons, Inc.

81 % = to heredity

This result suggests that no less than 81 per cent of the variance in susceptibility to neuroticism is attributable to heredity. However, the sample consisted of relatively normal children from the general population. It is not legitimate to generalize from normal children to neurotic adults and thus conclude that heredity makes a large contribution to neuroticism in the latter. Furthermore, other studies based on tests of neuroticism administered to twins selected from the general population have yielded estimates of H as low as 0.30 (Holzinger, 1929), a figure not too high to be accounted for by the greater similarity of experience in identical than in non-identical twins.

Other Biological Determinants

The precipitation of neurotic reactions by starvation, vitamin deficiency, sleep deprivation or oxygen deprivation was discussed previously. Sometimes, noxious agents also act as precipitants, for example, when psychological defenses break down during physical illness.

It has been suggested by some investigators that neurosis has somatic predispositions as well as precipitants. Rees and Eysenck (1945) compared 200 soldiers diagnosed as neurotic with a control group of 100 normals and reported that the body build of the neurotics was more variable. Hysterics tended to be endomorphic while anxiety neurotics, depressives and obsessives tended to be ectomorphic. It will be recalled that Sheldon reported a high correlation between endomorphy and the viscerotonic characteristics of sociable extroversion and need for affection, and also between ectomorphy and the cerebrotonic characteristics of restraint, inhibition, physiological overresponse, apprehensiveness, self-consciousness and introversion. Since hysterics tend to be extroverted, whereas patients who are anxious, depressed or obsessive tend, on the average, toward cerebrotonia, the data of Rees and Eysenck are consistent with Sheldon's basic scheme. However, no final judgment can be made with respect to the relation of body build to neurosis, since body build studies are subject to the various difficulties discussed previously.

Although no consistent structural differences have ever been found between the brain tissue of neurotics and normals, the activity of the neurotic's nervous system apparently differs in certain respects from that of the normal individual.

First, a number of obsessive-compulsives have EEG abnormalities. Second, increased sympathetic and parasympathetic activities of the autonomic nervous system of neurotics have been reported (Gellhorn, 1943). Sympathetic overactivity is manifested in increased heart rate, blood pressure and respiration; in dilation of blood vessels in the striped muscles and constriction of blood vessels in the skin and intestines; and in pallor, cold sweats, erection of hair, dilation of the pupil of the eye and inhibition of peristalsis and salivation. Parasympathetic overactivity is manifested in reverse fashion, e.g., flushing instead of pallor and increased appetite instead of inhibition of digestive functions. In some neurotics sympathetic overactivity is predominant, and in some parasympathetic overactivity is predominant.

Third, Funkenstein et al. (1951) found that after an injection of Mecholyl, anxious individuals manifest a drop in systolic blood pressure. Physiologists have suggested that this response is due to a diminished state of excitability in the hypothalamus. The individual who habitually responds to stress by anger, on the other hand, rather than by neurotic anxiety, has been reported to show an increase of blood pressure in response to Mecholyl and is believed to have an excitable hypothalamus.

It must be stressed that the deviations in nervous system activity of neurotics—as manifested by EEG patterns, autonomic indicators and response to Mecholyl—may be concomitants or consequences of neurosis rather than its determinants. It is an open question whether a predisposition to neurosis may result from a particular type of nervous functioning.

Psychological Determinants

Freud distinguished between psychoneuroses and "actual" neuroses. The latter, he believed, were due to a biological imbalance between sexual excitation and sexual satisfaction. For example, he believed that neurasthenic fatigue was due to sexual overexcitement and inadequate gratification consequent on excessive masturbation. It has sometimes been hypothesized that anxiety states also have a direct sexual basis.

The large majority of psychologists have disagreed with Freud's distinction and have concluded that *all neuroses are psychoneuroses,* i.e., the most important etiological determinants of all neuroses are psychological. Sexual imbalance may disturb the organism, but the imbalance is accompanied by guilt (or anxiety) and it is the latter which is most important in the etiology of neurosis. The biological imbalance does not act directly but is mediated by psychological variables. Guilt over masturbation or the emotional problems that initially lead to excessive masturbation are more crucial than masturbation itself.

The psychological bases of neuroses—habits of strong defensiveness, repressed hostility, a dependent need for affection, a conviction of inferiority and guilt, and an anxious, indiscriminate expectation of punishment—are molded by repeated childhood experiences. The parents of neurotics tend to be undemonstrative toward each other and their children. They may rebuff the child's need for affection and his primitive efforts to express it. Hostility is also inhibited, either through harsh retribution or guilt-producing moralizing. Masturbation and other childhood expressions of sexuality are likely to be met by dire threats. Attempts to reduce aggressive and sexual drives are punished physically, or by violent outbursts of parental temper or—most frequently—by indirect measures (Greenfield, 1959). The child is made to feel that he has hurt his father or mother, that he is not as good as other children and that no one will love him. His parents wish him, above all else, to be a credit to them; a great deal of emphasis is therefore put on achievement, and the nonachieving child is criticized and nagged.

One or both parents may be overprotective instead of rejecting. They may try too hard to protect the child against physical illness and common physical dangers, they may overgratify many of his needs and at the same time be overconcerned that he avoid temptation. It may then appear to the child that he lives in a dangerous, fearful world; he can trust no one but his parents. In many instances a parent gives verbal assurances of safety—for example, that there is no need to fear thunderstorms or the dark—but nullifies his protective words by the apprehension in his manner and the frequency with which he finds it necessary to reassure the child. The parent's concern with trivialities makes it clear that he is really trying to reassure himself. Overprotection also implies overcontrol and possessive domination; the child is not given responsibility for making decisions and the opportunity to learn by trial and error. Either rejection or overprotection

may result in anxiety, pervasive inhibitions and an insatiable desire to please others.

The child is frequently warned of vague and undefined dangers, particularly in the area of sexual behavior. It has been established experimentally that uncertainty may provoke as much anxiety as unavoidable, unpleasant experiences. It is therefore not surprising that vagueness and uncertainty about sex should result in frigidity, impotence and other sexual difficulties.

The childhood of a neurotic is often marked by parental refusal to give sexual information or, alternatively, by detailed explanations beyond the child's interest or comprehension. It would be erroneous, however, to assume that all non-neurotics are given adequate sexual information. In fact, a study by Landis (1940) revealed that normal women received no more sexual information in childhood than a comparison group of neurotic women. But sexual ignorance affected the two groups differently: the neurotics reacted to their first sexual experiences with surprise, shock and disgust, and could not adjust afterward to the sexual demands made on them. On the other hand, the normal group, perhaps because of a generally positive attitude toward people stemming from good relations with their parents, were less shocked and better able to adjust. It should be noted that Landis' investigation was carried out some decades ago; in the ensuing period sexual information has become generally more available and it may be that today only a child from a deviant cultural background or home would remain completely ignorant of sex. In any event, neurotic patients who were children in earlier decades have so frequently had a history of sexual ignorance and maladjustment that Freud, among others, concluded that neurosis was impossible in the individual who had a normal sex life.

Parental inconsistency—from one occasion to another, and also between the two parents on the same occasions—is a common feature of the neurotic's background. The mother may be domineering and the father weak, or the mother passive and the father authoritarian. As between the two parents, there has been considerable speculation whether the early relationship with the mother or the father is the more significant. Since the mother is the primary agent of socialization during the preschool years, it has generally been assumed that her behavior is more likely to affect the child. However, people tend to marry partners with equivalent emotional maturity so that psychological disturbance in one parent is often accompanied by psychological disturbance in the other. Moreover, there has been an increasing tendency in recent years to recognize that the father's behavior toward the mother has strong effects on the child.

An important factor in the causation of neurosis is identification. Like other parents, neurotics reinforce behaviors similar to their own and thus increase the likelihood that their children will adopt their attitudes and reactions. Since these include anxiety, ambivalence, guilt and hostility turned inward, the child of a neurotic parent incorporates into himself a parental image with which he cannot be at peace; he introjects a troublesome foreign body, so to speak. Neurotic patients frequently criticize their parents, yet feel compelled to repeat their parents' behavior. An important reason why one child of neurotic parents becomes neurotic and another does not seems to be a difference in the depth and breadth of their identifications. These, in turn, may depend on biological factors and on specific pleasurable and distressing experiences with parents.

Neurotic parents differ from each other in just which behaviors they become concerned about and reward or punish. One child may be most strongly rewarded or punished for overeating, another for illness, a third for being fearful, a fourth for resistance to toilet training, a fifth for attempts to be independent and a sixth for exploratory sexual behaviors. Since many of these behaviors are components of pregenital sexual stages, it follows that parental reactions affect the strength of pregenital fixations. It will be recalled that under stress a person is likely to regress to the stage at which his fixations had been strongest. Psychoanalytic theory hypothesizes that a different set of fixations and regressions is associated with each neurosis. It follows from these considerations that parental reinforcement of specific childhood behaviors may affect not only *whether* the child develops a neurotic reaction but also *which* neurotic reaction he will manifest.

A final psychological determinant of neurosis is loss of a parent in childhood. In a study of hospitalized neurotics, Gregory (1959) found that by age 10 a slightly higher proportion of neurotic patients had lost their fathers by death than in a comparable sample of the general population. A similar excess of paternal deaths during the first 10 years of the patients' childhoods was recorded by Norton (1952); also, a large number of patients had lost their fathers early due to parental discord and separation. Combining death and separation, 13 per cent had lost their fathers but only 6 per cent their mothers by age 10. Loss of the mother and loss of both parents seem to precede schizophrenia and antisocial behavior, respectively, rather than neurosis.

A methodological comment is in order before leaving the topic of the psychological determinants of neurosis. Our knowledge of parental behavior and other psychological variables in the childhood of neurotics is largely based on patients' retrospections; these are subject to both deliberate and unconscious distortions. The consistency of patients' retrospections with theory, and also with experimental evidence on the effects of stress, leads us to have some confidence in their statements, despite distortions. But to be certain of the later effects of childhood experiences, it would be necessary to conduct more objective investigations than are presently available. Careful observations of parent-child interactions, particularly between foster parents and foster children so as to eliminate the effect of hereditary mechanisms, and correlation of these observations with evaluations made in adulthood, are needed to establish the etiology of neurosis on a firm basis.

Sociocultural Determinants

The frequency and form of neurotic symptoms vary considerably in different cultures, social classes and time periods. Many observers have felt that our culture fosters anxiety and neurotic competitiveness and frustrates the very needs it stimulates. The effect of culture on neurosis is clearest for obsession-compulsion and conversion reactions. Obsession-compulsion seems to be on the increase, apparently as a reflection of such cultural forces as emphasis on competitive success and the guilt felt when this is not attained fast enough. Over the past several decades, on the other hand, conversion reactions have decreased in western society, most likely because more liberal sexual mores and patterns of child rearing have led to a decrease in sexual repressions. Changes in the kinds of conversion symptoms that occur have also been observed: in the latter part of the nineteenth century, hysterics often manifested gross motor symptoms such as convulsions, whereas today they tend to have "quieter" symptoms such as vague pains and various other sensory difficulties. It is noteworthy that gross motor hysteria has frequently been observed during the past few decades as an acute stress reaction among soldiers from under-developed countries. Since the primary problem of these individuals would appear to be self-preservation rather than sexuality, it follows that hardship—physical and economic—as well as sexual conflicts lead to conversion reactions. A finding of Hollingshead and Redlich (1958) is consistent with this conclusion: although the incidence of neurosis (all types combined) was roughly similar for all five socioeconomic classes, hysterical reactions were virtually absent in the upper three classes but were present in the two lowest and most deprived classes. Obsession-compulsion, on the other hand, occurs fairly often in upper socioeconomic groups of our society but is almost unknown in most primitive tribes, except in the form of institutionalized obsessive rituals shared by the entire tribe. In summary, the frequency of conversion symptoms is negatively correlated with both the sophistication of a society and the class level within the society, whereas the frequency of obsessive-compulsive symptoms is positively correlated with the same variables.

The other neurotic reactions are also related to sociocultural variables. For example, Hollingshead and Redlich found considerable neurotic depression at upper levels and a strong tendency to anxiety at the middle level. Undoubtedly there is great variation in neurotic depression, anxiety and phobias from culture to culture, but no adequate data are available to substantiate this conjecture.

TREATMENT AND PROGNOSIS

Each of the neurotic reaction types may be treated by somatic measures or by various forms of psychotherapy, and each involves somewhat different therapeutic problems.

Anxiety reaction patients are readily helped by sedatives or minor tranquilizers. In addition, they are usually motivated enough to be good candidates for either brief or extensive psychotherapy.

The symptoms of many conversion patients can be removed by suggestion or hypnosis; the "faith cures" of physical ailments at various shrines are examples of the effects of suggestion on conversion hysterics. The effects of suggestion are sometimes short-lived, however, because of the phenomenon of "transfers

and equivalences," i.e., a bodily symptom disappears but then reappears in an equivalent form in another organ. A hand weakness may be succeeded by a leg difficulty, a visual symptom by generalized pain and so forth. It was partly because of the danger of this phenomenon that Freud felt symptoms should be removed only by restoring to the patient's consciousness the repressed memories that gave rise to the symptoms, for insight was presumed to undercut the possibility of symptom recurrence. On the other hand, purely symptomatic treatment sometimes has permanent effects, particularly when combined with removal of the individual from an emotionally stressful situation.

Dissociation symptoms are helped by hypnosis or Pentothal interviews. As in conversion, intensive psychotherapy may be needed for long-lasting results.

In the treatment of phobias it is sometimes a problem to get a patient who is afraid of the outdoors, elevators or tall buildings to the therapist's office. However, the patient may be able to overcome these phobic reactions just enough to begin therapy, especially if a relative accompanies him. Sometimes phobias become temporarily worse rather than better as the patient ventilates his problems; sometimes, like any other habit patterns, phobias are too ingrained to be modified by therapy.

The obsessive patient presents some unique therapeutic problems. He tends to be resistive, to intellectualize his therapy, to doubt the therapist and to argue with him. His defenses may take the form of calmly discussing psychodynamics in a textbook fashion instead of expressing affect; it is as if somebody else were being treated. In such a case the therapist's job is to cut through the defenses and get the patient to verbalize his impulses, especially his hostility, so that therapy will not come to a standstill in endless intellectual discussions. The compulsive patient who acts out his antisocial impulses is even more difficult to work with, for he acts instead of facing his problems. If the therapist can get him to inhibit his antisocial compulsions long enough to begin analyzing their motivations, he may be able to help the patient.

Depressive patients are best treated by a combination of physical therapies, in combination with psychotherapy when the depression is severe and unresponsive to psychotherapy alone. Mood-elevating drugs may be needed to help motivate the person, even to get him to come to the psychotherapist's office. In extreme cases where suicide is likely, electric shock therapy is often used. Neither psychotherapy, nor medication nor electroconvulsive therapy is of much help when the depression is a reaction to a continuing, intolerable environment. In such cases the sensible procedure is to attempt to modify the environment or encourage the patient to make needed changes insofar as is possible. The depressive with severe hypochondriasis is particularly difficult to treat. Such persons resist recognizing that their problems are not physical since such an insight would challenge a whole way of life.

In general, neurosis responds more favorably to psychotherapy or some form of long-term therapy, such as psychoanalysis, than do conduct disorders or functional psychoses. Among the specific symptomatic reactions, anxiety reaction patients have an especially favorable prognosis, perhaps because their anxiety has not yet given way to stable, hardened defenses. Fenichel (1945) felt that the accessibility of neurotics to psychoanalysis was greatest for anxiety and phobic reactions; less for compulsive and conversion reactions, and still less for neurotic depressions. There is also wide individual variation in prognosis within each of these reaction types. In general the prognosis is better: the more recent and rapid the onset of the neurosis, the more stable the patient's personality prior to the neurotic breakdown, the more important the causal role of external stress rather than endogenous factors, and the more the patient tries to combat the neurosis. However, motivation for change is so important and so difficult to measure that even patients whose prognosis is judged to be poor sometimes improve dramatically in therapy.

causal factors within the body

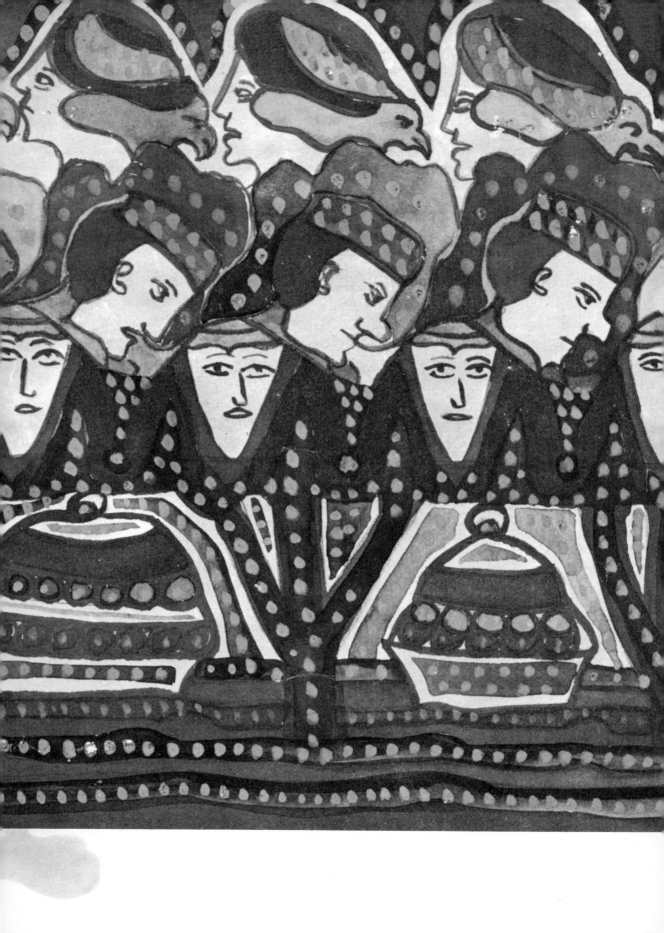

As you ought not to attempt to cure the eyes without the head, or the head without the body, so neither ought you to attempt to cure the body without the soul. And this . . . is the reason why the cure of many diseases is unknown to the physicians of Hellas, because they disregard the whole, which ought to be studied also, for the part can never be well unless the whole is well.

Plato, *Charmides*

PSYCHOPHYSIOLOGIC DISORDERS

Emotional reactions are accompanied by changes in respiration, circulation, digestion and other physiological processes. In a state of intense fear, the individual becomes pale, breathes irregularly and suffers from a dry mouth due to the inhibition of salivation. His appetite vanishes, his digestive processes slow down and he may feel an urge to urinate and defecate. Frequently, his hands and feet become cold and his heart pounds violently. In a state of anger, a number of these changes are also present, but the total pattern of physiological responses differs from the pattern in fear (see Fig. 10–1). In grief, the individual is short of breath, sighs and has choking sensations; as in fear, his skin is pale and his appetite poor and he may feel weak and completely devoid of energy. He does not respond to many stimuli that ordinarily elicit responses, as if his stimulus threshold had increased.

In the normal individual, intense fear, anger or grief is relatively brief in duration, and physiological accompaniments are also brief. However, in an individual who is chronically or frequently at the mercy of an intense and disturbing emotion, exaggerated physiological reactions are

likely to occur for long periods of time. The result is a psychophysiologic disorder, that is, a pathological change of emotional origin in the structure or function of an organ.

An important component of the emotional reactions that culminate in psychophysiologic disorders is conflict. Experiments using hypnosis have clearly and dramatically shown that temporary emotional conflict can produce physiological changes. Wolberg (1947) hypnotized three subjects and created a conflict in each by the suggestion that on awakening he would find a chocolate bar and want to eat it, but would know that to do so would be "wrong." One subject reacted to the induced conflict by not seeing the bar, as if he had a neurotic conversion blindness; a second subject became tense, dizzy and pale, as in a neurotic anxiety reaction; and a third ate the bar with gusto and then suffered a gastrointestinal upset and vomited, as if a small psychophysiologic reaction had been induced by the conflict between appetite and guilt.

Psychophysiologic disorders overlap other disorders, particularly neuroses. Lidz (1959) goes so far as to state, "Most persons suffering

169

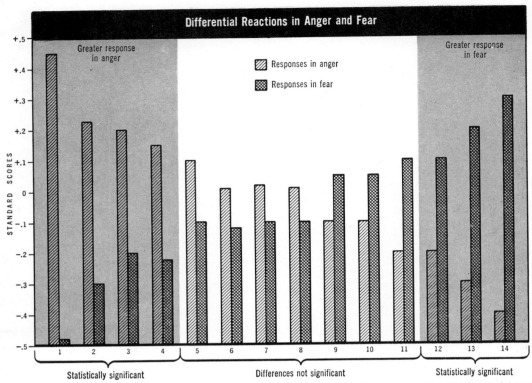

Figure 10–1. *"Physiological responses in anger and fear. The chart plots changes from the normal (zero) level for 14 indicators all simultaneously recorded. The indicators are numbered to correspond to the numbers at the base of the chart. 1, Galvanic skin responses (increases in number); 2, heart rate decreases; 3, muscle tension increases; 4, diastolic blood pressure rises; 5, face temperature decreases; 6, heart stroke volume decreases; 7, heart stroke volume increases; 8, hand temperature decreases; 9, systolic blood pressure increases; 10, face temperature increases; 11, heart rate increases; 12, muscle tension peaks; 13, skin conductance increases; 14, respiration rate increases."* (From Hilgard, E. R. 1957. Introduction to Psychology. 2nd Ed. Harcourt, Brace and Company.)

from neuroses, including the transitory neurotic symptoms that occur in most lives, also suffer from some physiologic dysfunction that gives rise to somatic complaints." The intimate tie between a neurosis and a psychophysiologic disorder is indicated by the fact that the latter has often been designated a "somatization reaction," a term implying that it is a neurotic reaction in the same general class as anxiety reaction, conversion reaction, phobic reaction and so forth. Psychoanalysis has often employed the term "organ neurosis" for psychophysiologic reaction, again implying that it is basically neurotic.

The term *psychosomatic disorders* has frequently been used instead of psychophysiologic disorders. However, "psychosomatic" has also come to mean a holistic orientation toward medicine and psychiatry in general, so that in one sense all disorders may be designated as psychosomatic, i.e., they all have psychological aspects. In tuberculosis, recovery may be notice-

ably retarded if the patient becomes anxious and tense. More cavities have been reported in the teeth of neurotics than in non-neurotic controls (possibly because neurotics are more afraid to visit a dentist). Anxiety may sometimes precipitate a common cold, perhaps because the nasal passages become dry in a state of anxiety. These and numerous other observations have led many physicians to believe that depression and anxiety retard recovery in *any* physical disease and may even make recovery impossible. From a physiological point of view, the mechanisms that obstruct recovery are obscure. A possible factor is an alternation of adrenal functioning in depression or anxiety; adrenal changes, in turn, may lead to diminished resistance to the inroads of the disease process. A diagnosis of psychophysiologic disorder is typically used to refer to a narrower set of phenomena than these broad psychosomatic aspects of disease in general.

Psychophysiologic disorders are characterized

by physical symptoms that are caused by emotional factors. Usually a single organ system which is controlled by the autonomic nervous system is involved. While the physiological changes involved are those that normally accompany specific emotional states, the changes are more intense and more sustained. The individual may or may not be consciously aware of his emotional state. Psychophysiologic disorders are sometimes difficult to distinguish from conversion neuroses. Indeed, some experts question whether such distinctions are of any practical significance. In both disorders the patient is suffering from poorly handled emotional conflicts and experiences relief as a consequence of increased awareness and mastery of such conflicts. However, other experts point out the differing roles played by anxiety in the two types of disorders and tend to support the contention that they are different entities. While there are exceptions, the following general rules have been used in distinguishing between conversion and psychophysiologic disorders: (1) Psychophysiologic disorders involve organs innervated by the autonomic nervous system and thus not under full voluntary control. Conversion symptoms typically involve the cerebrospinal nervous system and are hence subject to voluntary control or perception. This distinction may be breaking down since recent experiments have demonstrated that persons can voluntarily change such behaviors as heart rate and the production of alpha brain waves. (2) Psychophysiologic disorders are typically accompanied by a high anxiety state while the conversion neurotic's symptoms seem to protect him against subjective distress. (3) Psychophysiologic reactions seem to result from the prolonged effect of natural reactions to emotional stress whereas conversion reactions often appear to result from an unconscious, symbolic expression of emotional conflicts. (4) Psychophysiologic reactions may result in structural changes which can be life-threatening whereas such changes are quite rare in conversion disorders.

The first indication of a psychophysiologic disorder is usually a physical symptom such as pain, vomiting, diarrhea or difficulty in breathing. If the symptom causes enough distress, the individual is likely to seek medical help. However, even a physician who is particularly sensitive to the presence of psychopathology is unlikely in most cases to find an obvious psychological abnormality. The typical psychophysiologic patient appears to be quite rational although he is strongly preoccupied with bodily functions. As in neurotic reactions, he shows no impairment of intellectual functioning or memory and no evidence of hallucinations or delusions. He is likely to reject the suggestion that he has emotional difficulties. Sometimes the physician can perceive a covariation in the patient's life between the onset of symptoms and the occurrence of unusually strong stress, but the covariation is not always obvious. The patient may evidence some anxiety or depression or his mood may seem normal. The question of whether psychophysiologic patients manifest any distinguishing personality traits will be discussed later.

THE AUTONOMIC NERVOUS SYSTEM

The link between emotions and the viscera is the autonomic nervous system. This system consists entirely of efferent, or motor, nerves. It has two main divisions: the sympathetic branch which emerges from the middle segment of the spinal cord and the parasympathetic, or craniosacral system, which emerges from both the brain stem and the lower segment of the spinal cord. (See Fig. 10–2.) The nerve cells of the sympathetic fibers are located in ganglia (groups of cells) outside the spine; several different organs are innervated from each ganglion. The nerve cells of the parasympathetic system are located close to or in the organs themselves. The parasympathetic system acts with more precision and less diffuseness than the sympathetic system. Parasympathetic and sympathetic nerve fibers are distributed to the same organs—the heart, lungs, stomach, pancreas, rectum, bladder, genitalia and so forth.

The two sets of nerve fibers act antagonistically. Stimulation of the sympathetic nervous system produces effects similar to the injection of Adrenalin or epinephrine into the blood stream. An increase occurs in heart rate, blood pressure, rate of breathing and blood flow to the muscles of the limbs; a decrease occurs in the activity of the digestive system and in the blood flow to the intestines, skin and brain. These effects prepare the organism for the *emergency action of fighting or fleeing in situations of danger.* Stimulation of the parasympathetic system has opposite effects to those just detailed; parasympathetic activity tends to occur when the organism can relax safely, digest its food or sleep. Essentially, parasympathetic activity maintains bodily homeostasis.

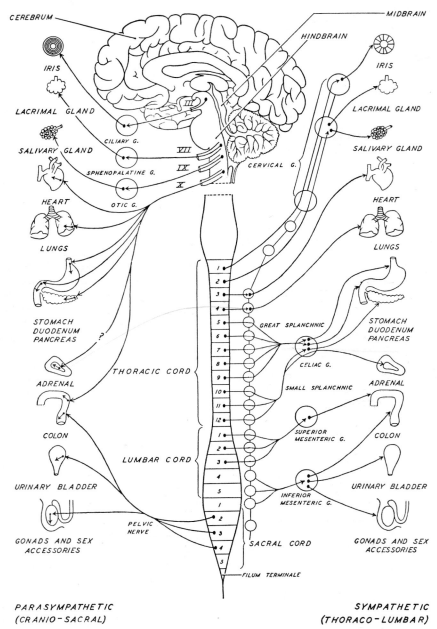

Figure 10–2. A diagram of the autonomic nervous system. The parasympathetic division is shown on the left, the sympathetic division on the right. Roman numerals refer to cranial nerves. (From Turner, C. D., and Bagnara, J. T. 1971. General Endocrinology. 5th Ed. Philadelphia, W. B. Saunders Co.)

The sympathetic and parasympathetic systems are controlled by centers in the hypothalamus of the brain in such a way that under ordinary circumstances the effects of the two systems are kept in approximate balance. In psychophysiologic disorders this balance fails; either sympathetic or parasympathetic activity becomes predominant and floods the circulatory, respiratory or other organ system.

The dangers that bring about autonomic and visceral overactivity in psychophysiologic reactions are usually internal and psychological. Inappropriately, the autonomic nervous system acts as if the dangers were external and physical. A reaction such as increased blood pressure is useful when there is an external physical danger, but it is maladaptive when the "danger" is an unacceptable impulse.

The *specific processes* by which the autonomic nervous system produces psychophysiologic disorders are fairly well known for some reactions but only poorly for others. For example, in neurodermatitis (a skin inflammation of emotional origin) it is not known whether the mechanism consists of sympathetic or parasympathetic overactivity, underactivity, or some combination of these. It will be recalled that in the stress reaction described by Selye sympathetic overactivity is followed by sympathetic exhaustion and underactivity. Over the years the functioning of an emotionally troubled individual may shift progressively toward excessive activity or exhausted inactivity. Alternatively, in some chronic emotional states the parasympathetic branch may be underactive or overactive over long time periods. There is a further complication: while one system is overactive or underactive the other cannot remain constant. Intense sympathetic activity in an emergency reaction is closely followed by an attempt of the parasympathetic system to redress the balance of available bodily energy; similarly, excessive parasympathetic activity is followed by a sympathetic attempt to restore balance. However, these attempts may not be successful. The autonomic system is an extremely complex and delicate mechanism which can break down in many different ways.

THE MAJOR PSYCHOPHYSIOLOGIC DISORDERS

The classification system of the American Psychiatric Association lists 10 categories of psychophysiologic disorders. We shall discuss

and illustrate six of them and touch briefly on the other four. It must be emphasized at the outset that emotional factors are not the only significant causes of the disorders to be described. High blood pressure, for example, may be primarily of emotional origin in one individual, a result of physical disease in another, and due to both factors in a third. Asthma may result from emotional stress, from an allergy (hypersensitivity of tissues to a physical or chemical agent) or from both allergy and stress, with the latter exacerbating the former.

Cardiovascular Reaction

This category includes many cases of hypertension (high blood pressure), migraine (headache accompanied by spasms of the cranial arteries) and other vasomotor disturbances. The causes of *hypertension* may be physical, e.g., kidney disorders, or they may be emotional or unknown; when the origin is emotional or unknown the reaction is termed essential hypertension. *Migraine* is caused by sympathetically innervated contraction, followed by dilation, of blood vessels in the brain. The pain usually occurs on one side of the head but in some cases the pain occurs on both sides or shifts from side to side. In one-sided migraine only the artery on that side has spasms. The particular type of pain varies from patient to patient: it may be dull, throbbing, hammering, pressing or viselike. The patient experiences nausea as well as pain, hence migraine is often called "sick" or "bilious" headache. The attack rarely lasts more than 24 hours and is often much briefer. Many professional observers have noted that migraine patients display tendencies toward compulsive fussiness, anxious conformity and hostility controlled by the defense mechanisms of repression and denial. It has been estimated that in 50 to 80 per cent of cases, migraine appears in successive generations, most often mother and daughter, and almost as often mother and son. The patient described in the following paragraphs, whose mother also suffered from the disorder, was basically a withdrawn and depressed neurotic whose migraine headaches were closely related to her emotional difficulties:

The patient, a married woman aged 46, was admitted to a psychiatric ward with a 40-year history of migraine headaches. Her headaches had increased in frequency and severity over the preceding 10 years and finally incapacitated her so that she was forced to leave her job. She was unable to manage her household or sleep and was so acutely miserable that she spoke of suicide. She overreacted to noise and other physical stimuli and stayed in bed, the doors shut and the blinds pulled.

The patient had had a great deal of medical attention and had been given a tremendous variety of drugs only one of which had appreciably reduced the intensity of the headaches. Recently even this drug had become completely ineffective. All medical and neurological examinations were negative. The patient denied having any emotional problems and maintained that she was the happiest wife there ever was, except for the headaches. In interview she kept repeating, "I have a wonderful husband and children. I have no problems." This statement was in sharp contrast with her appearance and with the actual facts.

The patient reported that she was the third of nine children born to a quiet, peaceable father and a mother who was troubled by chronic migraine headaches from shortly after marriage until menopause. When her mother had a headache, "Father would do anything for her. I would care for her also because I had a taste of what it was like." The patient's headaches, beginning at age six, had forced her to stay home from school on an average of one day a month. She was quite bright, however, and graduated from high school third in her class. Her parents had not approved of many of her friends; they greatly restricted her social life and did not allow her to go out on dates until graduation from high school.

The patient first reported that she had been married only once but later admitted that her first husband had been convicted of robbery and sent to a reformatory before the birth of their first child. The patient returned to live with her parents, went to work and eventually obtained a divorce.

When she was 27 she met a man 16 years older than she who claimed to be a minister. Marriage to a minister seemed ideal and she married him against the advice of her parents. Very quickly she learned that he was not a minister and had not even attended high school. Moreover, he was extremely jealous and possessive; he sold their home and bought a farm so that he could keep her away from other men. She was crushed by his deceit and irrational jealousy but could not bring herself to admit that she had made another mistake. Her husband knew nothing about farming, lost money, and soon had to sell the farm and return to town. Out of jealousy, he sometimes refused to call a doctor when she was ill.

Several years after their marriage the patient learned that her husband had been married previously; he told her that he had divorced his first wife because of infidelity.

The patient was completely frigid but there were eight pregnancies through the years, terminating in five spontaneous abortions and the birth of three children. After a menopause at age 40, she was discouraged to find that her headaches did not diminish as her mother's had, but increased in frequency and

intensity. As her headaches became worse, her husband began to be much more considerate of her; for example, he permitted her to work as a nurse's aide although he was still troubled by the thought that she would meet other men.

Some time before she was hospitalized, the patient learned from her husband's sister that his first wife had divorced him because of his paranoid jealousy. Then the patient's hostility toward her husband became very strong, but she felt trapped in a marriage from which she saw no acceptable escape. Her headaches worsened; her husband became solicitous and attentive to her every whim. She could not continue to feel angry with him when he was so kind, and her hostility was transformed into guilt and depression. Concomitantly the headaches increased even more and she was finally hospitalized.

② **Respiratory Disorders**   MOST COMMON

The two most common psychophysiologic respiratory reactions are hyperventilation and asthma. Some cases of hay fever and sinusitis may also be psychophysiologic. *Hyperventilation* is "overbreathing;" it consists of episodes of fairly deep breathing with the mouth open or fast, shallow panting. It is most likely to occur when the patient experiences anxiety or anger, and it is associated with excessive activity of the sympathetic nervous system.

Asthma, like hyperventilation, occurs in episodic attacks. In psychophysiologic cases of asthma the muscles in the walls of the bronchi (tubes in the lungs) contract because of relative underactivity of the sympathetic system or relative overactivity of the parasympathetic system. As a result of the bronchial spasm, the patient cannot get enough air and he pants, wheezes and experiences a terrifying feeling of suffocation. An injection of Adrenalin to stimulate sympathetic activity relieves the asthmatic attack. In allergic cases, the bronchial spasm is caused by irritation in the lungs due to ragweed or other substances. Some patients have asthmatic attacks only when the ragweed count is high, some only when they are emotionally upset during the ragweed season and some at any time when they are emotionally upset.

Many observers have noted a high frequency of depression and anxiety in asthmatic patients and also a particular family constellation. Asthma frequency occurs in children, especially boys, who have a dominant mother and a passive father. A number of clinicians, impressed by the dependency and the extreme suppressed rage found in many asthmatics, have speculated that

Most vulnerable organs are always attacked + if you have a disorder - it will be there -

such a disorder is linked to a longstanding ambivalence toward the mother. Strong needs for succorance, support, and warmth stand in contrast to the unexpressed anger at her domineering, critical attitude. The child wants love but is afraid to ask, and he wants to express his anger but is afraid of the consequences if he dares to do so. This insolvable problem results in a chronic state of arousal which eventually leads to the bronchial spasm.

Knapp and Nemetz (1960) studied 406 asthmatic attacks in nine patients receiving psychotherapy. One-third of the attacks were preceded by feelings of anger or anxiety and in 45 per cent there were feelings of depression. The antecedent events that gave rise to the anger and anxiety consisted of a threatened loss of some person (27 per cent), a threat to the ego (7 per cent), or a loss of some impersonal substance (10 per cent). These results suggest that the threat of losing something or somebody—not necessarily the mother—is an important precipitant. Consciously, the patient may not be aware so much of a threatened loss of self-esteem or a love object as he is aware of being faced with a difficult situation with which he wishes he did not have to contend. Grace and Graham (1952) reported interviews with seven asthmatics in which the essential conscious attitude preceding attacks was the desire to have nothing to do with an unpleasant situation which had arisen. Typical statements were: "I didn't want to have anything to do with it," "I wanted to blot it all out," and "I wanted to go to bed and pull the sheets over my head." These studies are suggestive but involve few patients and do not exclude other kinds of explanations.

The following case illustrates the role of anger and anxiety in asthma. The patient's personality characteristics and some of her past history were similar to those of the migraine patient described in the preceding section.

The patient was a 34-year-old married woman who had been suffering from increasingly severe and frequent asthmatic attacks over the preceding 12 years. Her maternal grandmother and one maternal aunt had also suffered from the disorder. The patient stated that she was allergic to several fruits and vegetables, but medical tests had not confirmed her statement. It was observed that her attacks tended to be precipitated and aggravated by emotional stress.

She had been the eldest of eight children. Her mother was a dominant and aggressive woman who had been pregnant with her when she married and consequently felt resentment toward her while favoring the younger children. The father was a conscientious man, well liked by everyone but rather passive and ineffectual at home. The patient described her mother as a moody, critical "martyr type" who imposed high standards of behavior on all the family members. During childhood the patient was given a great deal of responsibility in caring for the younger children and as an adolescent was frequently forced to miss social activities in order to help at home. However, she seemed to accept her position in the family and never expressed anger.

In her junior year in high school she became pregnant and was forced to leave school and marry. Pregnancy was always stressful for her and the first attack of asthma occurred soon after the birth of her second child. The attacks became more frequent and severe in subsequent pregnancies and finally she underwent sterilization to free herself of this particular source of stress. However, two years earlier she had become aware that her husband was having an affair with another woman. She was upset but never confronted him with her knowledge. Instead of becoming openly angry, she punished him by denying him sexual relations which she had, in fact, feared since her first pregnancy. His infidelity soon ceased, but she continued to punish him sexually for three years. He then sustained a minor injury in an automobile accident, felt unable to work and left his job. She was sorry for him and resumed sexual relations. At the same time she went to work in order to supplement the family income. Her earnings were insufficient and she became increasingly worried about their financial situation. She began to feel generally depressed and fatigued but unable to sleep. Her appetite decreased and her asthma worsened. Although her husband manufactured a variety of reasons for not working, she repressed her resentment toward him. Finally, after 18 months of increasing misery she sought help.

Gastrointestinal Disorders

Of all the psychophysiologic disorders, gastrointestinal reactions have been investigated most thoroughly. The major gastrointestinal difficulties of emotional origin are peptic ulcer, ulcerative colitis and anorexia nervosa.

Peptic Ulcer. An ulcer is a crater-like area of destroyed tissue on any of the external or internal surfaces of the body. A peptic ulcer is an area of destruction in the mucous membrane that lines the stomach or duodenum. (The duodenum is the first part of the small intestine proximal to the stomach.) Peptic ulcer is caused by the overproduction and secretion of hydrochloric acid and pepsin, an enzyme which digests food, or by the inability of the mucous membrane to resist the corrosive effects of acid secretion even when the acid output is not excessive. It has been demonstrated experimentally (Kirsner, 1961) that pain can be induced in an ulcer patient by instilling hydrochloric acid and can be promptly relieved by neutralizing the acid. Typically, an ulcer patient begins to feel uncomfortable about two hours after eating, for the acid continues to be secreted when his stomach is empty just as it does when his stomach contains food. The patient reports a burning, boring or gnawing sensation in the upper abdomen. If he has a snack, the pain usually ceases. In many patients the pain is worst at night, several hours after the last meal of the day.

Emotional states are closely related to physiological processes in the stomach. Wolf and Wolff (1942, 1947) were able to observe directly the stomach of a patient whose esophagus had been badly burned and closed with scar tissue. In order to feed him it was necessary to make surgical opening into the stomach through the abdominal wall. In states of fear and sadness the mucous membrane of his stomach could be seen to pale and, at the same time, gastric secretion and peristalsis (contractions in the alimentary canal which move food downward to the stomach) diminished. In anger, his mucous membrane blushed and swelled, secretion and stomach contractions increased, and the membrane was judged to be vulnerable to injury and ulcer development.

Peptic ulcers have been reported with high frequency in persons who have a conflict between the infantile need for affection and care, on the one hand, and the mature need for accomplishment, independence and self-sufficiency, on the other. Such an individual may present a façade of hard-driving independence overlying a "soft" inner core of suppressed or repressed dependency. His dependency is then expressed in parasympathetic overactivity and consequent gastric secretion, as if he had a constant need to be fed. It has been speculated that such an expression of dependency may be based on an association established in childhood between love and digestive processes, between parent-child affection and being fed. However, not all ulcer patients are overtly self-sufficient and hard driving, for some are outwardly dependent in a demanding and often angry fashion. It has been speculated that in such cases dependency is also frustrated, but by external circumstances rather than repression. In an ulcer patient of this type the gastrointestinal system reenacts an infantile association

between anger and food, between crying angrily when hungry and being fed. In the peptic ulcer case described in the following paragraphs the etiology was quite complex and consisted of emotional stress, frustration of strong ambition, angry resentment and also excessive use of alcohol.

The patient was the fourth of five boys. His father was an unsuccessful farmer whom the patient had disliked from an early age on and never respected. His mother, to whom he felt much closer, was nervous, frail and had numerous bodily complaints which the family physician regarded as 90 per cent emotional. Nevertheless, she criticized and dominated her husband and nagged her sons into striving for the success that their father had never achieved.

Poverty and a small physical stature contributed to making the patient feel inferior to other children, but he compensated by striving for academic achievement. He was very intelligent and although he worked in a store during noon hours, after school and on Saturdays, he was at the top of his classes. He completed college and two years of law school in evening classes. In World War II he rose from private to captain. At the age of 24 he married and subsequently became the father of three children.

He was as ambitious and hard driving in his career as he had been in school and in the Army. He began to work for a large company at the age of 21 and over the ensuing 25 years rose to a senior executive position. He felt personally responsible for much of the company's growth and expansion. He was away from home traveling on company business a great deal, worked evenings and weekends, ate irregularly, and for 15 years never took a vacation with his family. But after reaching a high position he began to feel that his talents—which were considerable but which he undoubtedly overvalued—and his dedication were neither appreciated nor adequately rewarded. His future seemed bleak, with little opportunity for future advancement financially or in prestige. Every morning he felt sick over the prospect of another day's exhausting demands and inadequate rewards. However, he did not express his feelings of frustration and resentment while at work but became increasingly irritable at home. He also began to drink and smoke very heavily. At this point he developed stomach ulcers. Sedative medication reduced his pain but he continued to drink and become increasingly depressed. An added blow occurred when his eldest daughter married after graduation from high school instead of going on to college; his heart had been set on seeing all his children obtain college degrees. He became extremely unreliable on the job, often failing to keep business appointments, and finally was dropped by the company for alcoholism and unreliability.

Shortly thereafter he was referred for psychiatric treatment. He was angry, tense, tremulous and depressed. As a consequence of losing his position, he was confronted with the necessity of reevaluating his goals and patterns of behavior. He was treated in psychotherapy and by minor tranquilizers and his tension and depression diminished. Being an intelligent man, he was able to acquire insight rapidly, his compulsive ambition decreased, he cut down on smoking and drinking, and his ulcer symptoms receded. He took a less demanding position with another company and during a two year follow-up period there was no recurrence of the ulcers and alcoholism.

Colitis. Colitis is an inflammation of the colon (large intestine) usually accompanied by diarrhea. Associated with it there may be spasm of the walls of the colon or destruction of its surface; the latter is known as *ulcerative colitis*. Patients with colitis often impress hospital personnel as being childish, demanding and jealous of other patients, much like anal-sadistic children. One interpretation of colitis, consistent with this personality pattern, is that it stems from an unconscious rage reaction that is inhibited from direct expression. In an investigation by Engel (1956) it was reported that colitis patients often have headaches when they behave assertively; on the other hand, when they behave in a nonassertive and helpless fashion the headaches vanish but the colitis itself is exacerbated. In the following case, immaturity, anger and hostility played an important role.

The patient, the third of four children born to a tense and overprotective mother, was six years younger than the second child and 12 years older than the fourth one. Not surprisingly, this unusual position in the family resulted in extreme dependence on her parents even after the youngest child was born. Her father was a conscientious and hard working man who had been treated for both asthma and stomach ulcers. The patient remarked, "He looks grouchy but he isn't that way."

As an adolescent in high school she was sexually ignorant and feared she might be pregnant after an episode of petting with a boy of whom she was very fond. A feeling of nausea seemed to confirm her fears. She went on a vacation with her family; when they returned she found that her boy friend was out of town and her diarrhea started. A few weeks later he returned but terminated their relationship. She denied any conscious anger but felt grief. Her diarrhea persisted. Some months later the young man married a girl after she became pregnant. The patient knew the other girl but disliked her and could not understand why she had been preferred. However, the patient again denied hostility and consciously grieved that she herself had not been the one to become pregnant. Her diarrhea increased.

At the age of 18 she married a young man who operated a small restaurant and was away from home 15 hours a day, seven days a week. The patient spent most of her time alone or visiting her family. She became pregnant and again her diarrhea became worse and required medical attention; by the time the baby was born the couple owed a thousand dollars for medical and hospital expenses. She also found it extremely difficult to meet the demands of her child and, in addition, was afraid of further pregnancies but did not use contraceptives for religious reasons. She complained of severe pain on intercourse and avoided it as much as possible. She had been completely unprepared for all these problems. Two months after her child was born, at age 19, she was admitted to a hospital. By this time she was having 10 to 15 watery bowel movements a day and had lost more than 15 pounds during one year. The colon was ulcerated and there was some rectal bleeding. It was suggested that she receive medical and psychotherapeutic treatment, but she accepted the former and rejected the latter. Although she stated that she missed her parents more than her husband and baby, she adamantly denied having emotional problems. Intensive sedation and other medical measures brought her diarrhea under control, but she was unchanged psychologically. On discharge from the hospital it was felt that she was as vulnerable to stress as ever.

Anorexia Nervosa. Anorexia is loss of appetite; *anorexia nervosa* is loss of appetite for emotional reasons. It is much more frequent in women than men. The patient reports that food disgusts her or that she is afraid of choking on it or of vomiting after eating. In a number of cases the disgust reaction is so strong that vomiting does in fact occur. Anorexia nervosa varies in severity; the more severe cases are characterized by weight loss to the point of emaciation and also by cessation of menstruation, poor circulation and often a drop in body temperature. Sometimes the disorder clears up spontaneously and the patient begins to eat again, but sometimes it has a fatal outcome.

Some anorexia patients manifest a distortion of reality close to that found in schizophrenia. They withdraw, are generally uncooperative and cannot be "reached" in psychotherapy. Others have an essentially neurotic personality. A number of investigators consider anorexia nervosa to be a neurotic conversion reaction, despite the role played by the autonomic nervous system. Whether occurring in a neurotic or in a schizoid individual, anorexia nervosa is often related to sexual events in the patient's life history—the onset of puberty, guilt felt in connection with sexual activity or fantasy, and so forth. The motivation of the disorder is often a fear of sexual maturity; self-starvation may be an attempt to remain undeveloped, flat-chested and unfeminine.

Young anorexia patients often will openly express their pleasure in being a child and their desire to remain a favored daughter rather than a grown woman. It is common for symptoms to begin following a weight-reducing diet. For example, a 14-year-old boy began dieting after his basketball coach told him he was too fat. His weight continued to decrease even after he resumed eating normally. Food now made him sick and he routinely vomited after any food intake. He was eventually hospitalized because of severe weight loss and resulting physical concomitants. He reported himself to be his mother's favorite "little boy," was distressed over the fact that he was getting too big to sit on her lap, and was openly distressed over the fact that he would soon be grown. "I would like to be twelve or thirteen forever."

Another motivation, deeply unconscious, is an association of food with impregnation, so that fear of eating represents a fear of becoming pregnant. Such primitive or infantile associations typically arise in girls with a very repressive upbringing. Having little or no sexual information but seeing their mother's abdomen growing, they may assume that the baby is in the stomach and comes from eating some foods. In fact, such beliefs are common in many children but are corrected by added information with maturity. In some persons such childhood ideas are never expressed and corrected and the false belief continues well into adolescence, albeit at an unconscious level.

Still a third element is a continuation of childhood negativism bred by parental worry over the child's health and nourishment. Children quickly learn to refuse to eat in opposition to parents who are overconcerned about diet. Anorexia in adult life may be an extension of this pattern.

Genitourinary Reaction

Since the genitourinary organs are innervated autonomically, emotional difficulties are often important causes of such symptoms as painful or excessively frequent urination, menstrual disturbances, impotence and frigidity. Urinary frequency is one of the more common physiologic symptoms of anxiety. Dysmenorrhea, or painful menstruation, may have an autonomic as well as either a structural or neurotic basis; patients

with dysmenorrhea often have a low threshold for pain. Amenorrhea, or failure to menstruate for several months, may result from various bodily illnesses, and also has been suspected of being a bodily defense against sexuality or a symbolic expression of the wish for pregnancy; either of the latter interpretations implies that fundamentally the symptom is similar to a conversion reaction.

Impotence may be relative or absolute and may be expressed in many different ways. The individual may be potent only with prostitutes or with women whom he holds in contempt. He may be impotent when drunk or, paradoxically, potent only when drunk, i.e., when his guilt over the expression of sexuality is inoperative. Erection may not occur at all or may be partial and inadequate. In another pattern, erection is adequate but the individual does not experience pleasure in intercourse. Most frequent of all male sexual disturbances is premature ejaculation (ejaculatio praecox); in some cases it occurs before intercourse begins. Since the sympathetic system inhibits sexual activity and the parasympathetic system promotes it, failure of erection results from either sympathetic overactivity or parasympathetic underactivity. In ejaculatio praecox, the parasympathetic system is overactive.

The ability to achieve and maintain an erection is closely tied to the male's sexual identity and to his sense of competence, self-worth and adequacy. Because it is so central to the individual's identity, it is extremely vulnerable to real or fantasied loss of esteem. Psychologically, the male is much more vulnerable as a sexual being than the female since the male cannot fake the sex act or have the experience of bringing pleasure through intercourse to his partner if he cannot attain an erection. His failure is readily apparent in a way that is not true for females. In a culture which places a high premium on sexual attractiveness and performance any failure to meet the image of an adequate male only helps to create more anxiety. In fact, pressure to perform, which is effected through the sympathetic nervous system, is antagonistic to the very performance which is desired.

Disturbances in sexual potency may arise from many sources but anxiety is the keynote. The individual may have a great deal of guilt concerning sex, and difficulty in accepting the sexual aspects of his being. Such attitudes may or may not be conscious. Often a person is unaware of any guilt or anxiety concerning sex but is simply prevented from stimulating his guilt by his inability to achieve an erection.

Often such difficulties arise in males because of a combination of factors surrounding the first attempt at intercourse: high level of anticipation, fear of not performing adequately, an inexperienced partner, and poorly selected surroundings. Under such conditions poor performance is quite likely but the failure is often taken as an index of inadequacy and creates more pressure for subsequent attempts. In other instances, the male has been quite adequate in the past but because of a combination of factors such as extreme fatigue, intoxication, extreme ambivalence or poorly recognized anger toward his partner, or the like, he finds himself to be temporarily sexually inadequate. Latent fears of inadequacy are likely to be stimulated by even a single failure and initiate a self-defeating cycle. In fact, some occasional erectile difficulty is quite common and is accepted by mature people without panic.

It is common in married males with impotence complaints to find that both partners contribute to the pressure to perform, and this tends to perpetuate the cycle. The wife fears being left unsatisfied and in her frustration may belittle or criticize her partner. The husband may feel on the spot and watch himself closely to see whether he will be able to follow through. Such attitudes preclude the relaxation essential to sexual arousal. Sometimes the sexual problems in a marriage signal the presence of other marital difficulties. For example, a married lawyer who was impotent complained that his wife was extremely demanding and critical. She seemed never to need his advice, to make important decisions without taking his wishes into account, and to be critical of his work. The wife, on the other hand, complained of her husband's tendency to withhold affection, of his fear of making decisions, and of his waiting for her to do everything. Each of them was right. The wife did have trouble in being passive and not being in control of everything, and her husband did have difficulty in openly expressing himself and in accepting responsibility for his own actions. The sexual difficulty was a manifestation of their broader problems with each other. The wife was unreceptive to sex on any of the husband's terms while the husband's response was his typical passive withdrawal. He was not angry, as he saw it—he simply could not get an erection and it was not his fault that this inability happened to make his wife extremely angry.

In the following case guilt over sex, a feeling of inadequacy, and poorly integrated hostility are seen to intertwine as causal factors.*

A man of twenty-nine, after one month of marriage, came for treatment for premature ejaculation. No other symptoms were evident. He was the third of a family of five. None of the children had been given sexual information and, in fact, the subject was strictly taboo at all times. The mother of the patient was overly religious and although she attended to the ordinary tasks of life she taught her children that religion came before everything else. According to her teaching there were only two important things in life—work and worshipping God. Demonstrations of affection were frowned upon. She kept the patient at arm's length and, in addition, always discouraged his friendships with girls. In spite of this he had numerous sexual fantasies about women. He wished they would surrender themselves to him for sexual pleasure yet he was sure none of them wanted to do so. When he first attempted to kiss a girl he was in great anxiety lest she become angry and scold him. He always expected women to repulse and reproach him. On the one hand he was profoundly grateful to women who would love him and at the same time unconsciously quite hostile to them for the attitude of denial which he felt they all held toward him. When he married he was apprehensive as to whether he could function sexually or not. He was not entirely surprised at his symptom of premature ejaculation. He said, "I can't believe my wife really wants to give herself to me. It seems that I am asking too much. I want sexual pleasure to last longer both for myself and for her but I can't control it."

Inquiry into his daily life revealed that he had always been sensitive to the attentions of both men and women. He craved love and friendship and was easily cast down if disapproved of in any way. He remembered that whenever anyone had shown him much praise or affection, or had given him a present, he would cry. "I was always so ashamed of that. As I grew older and people expected me to be strong emotionally I would be weak. I was ashamed of myself for crying then as I am now about this symptom."

As the treatment interviews went on, the patient more and more related his lack of emotional control in social situations to his lack of ejaculatory control. He said, "When I go the movies and the hero finally gets what he wants, I cry. I want my wife to give me her body for my pleasure. When she does so I release semen too quickly just as I have always released tears too quickly. It seems to me that I can't stand to get what I want without losing control of myself."

At this point the patient brought out hostility toward his mother. "If my mother had only given me more love and led me to expect more, instead of con-

---

*Reprinted by permission from Weiss, E. and English, O. S. 1949. Psychosomatic Medicine. 2nd Ed. Philadelphia, W. B. Saunders Co., pp. 601–602.

stantly preaching and making such an ascetic of me! I am inadequate in making love and I cannot make my wife happy. Perhaps I don't want to, in so far as she represents my mother, but at least I must try to accept pleasure for myself and then maybe I'll be able to give it to her."

After the conscious expression of hostility to his mother he was better able to express his feelings without loss of emotional control. At the same time his ability to maintain erection without ejaculation increased to an entirely satisfactory point.

Frigidity in women, like impotence in men, has many degrees. It ranges from a mild disinterest in sexual relations, to sexual interest without orgasm, to aversion accompanied by an involuntary spasm of the vaginal musculature. Again, as in impotence, anxiety, guilt and hostility may play a role. In many of the cases previously described, frigidity was present as a concomitant of neurotic anxiety. A frigid woman may fear injury by the male or pregnancy. She may feel guilty over her own sexual feelings. Or she may feel hostile to her husband for any of a variety of reasons. As more and more emphasis comes to be placed on adequate sexual performance and having an orgasm with every occasion of intercourse, the female falls subject to the same external pressures which have plagued males over the years.

Other Psychophysiologic Reactions

In addition to the reactions we have discussed—cardiovascular, respiratory, gastrointestinal and genitourinary—several others are generally listed under this classification. *Endocrine reaction* is a glandular disorder such as hyperthyroidism (excessive activity of the thyroid gland) which results from emotional stress. Many hyperthyroid patients are emotionally disturbed for years prior to the onset of the glandular difficulty. Denial of dependence, ambivalence to the mother, sibling rivalry and overcompensatory attempts at domination of others have all been reported in a number of hyperthyroid patients. Loss of the mother is a frequent precipitant. With the onset of the condition, the patient typically manifests irritability, excitability, impatience and explosive rage.

Hemic and lymphatic reaction includes psychophysiologic disorders of the blood and lymph systems, for example, anemia due to emotional and autonomic dysfunction. However, there is no direct evidence to indicate that emotion can play a significant role in anemia or other blood and lymph disorders. The validity

of the category is therefore doubtful. Of course, emotional distress may lead to poor dietary habits and malnutrition which in turn may produce anemia; however, this is an indirect pattern of causation.

Included among psychophysiologic skin disorders are neurodermatitis (inflammation of the skin of emotional origin), some cases of eczema, and hives. Klaber (1960) compared neurodermatitis patients with a control group who had skin diseases of nonemotional origin. On psychological tests the neurodermatitis patients were judged to be the more hostile of the two groups, although outwardly they appeared calm and controlled. Apparently they expended considerable energy keeping hostility in check. In the following case of neurodermatitis it can be seen that hostility and its proper expression was a central problem.*

The patient, a 46-year-old retired policeman, was seen with the chief complaint of a skin rash. The onset of his dermatitis occurred 25 years previously when, shortly after his marriage, he noted the gradual appearance of a diffuse scaling eruption of the scalp. Some time later he developed redness and scaling in the groin, and a more or less generalized eruption, especially around his neck, knees, and elbows. The rash was intensely pruritic [itchy] and the patient frequently scratched until he bled. Two years prior to admission, the eruption became generalized. No relief was obtained from a multitude of medications.

The patient was the second of six children. His father was described as a strict disciplinarian. The mother was described as a warm, understanding person who was affectionate with the children but showed little love toward her husband. The patient's older brother had retired 10 years previously following an acute psychotic episode. The other four siblings appeared to be in good health.

The patient remembered that he was never able to express anger and never disobeyed his father's detailed instructions. As an adolescent the patient was a shy, sensitive boy who was self-conscious and avoided social relationships with girls. There were exaggerated guilt feelings over masturbation. When confronted with social situations that were threatening he would turn to drinking. He stated, "I had a terrific inferiority complex and liquor helped me to overcome it."

Since a civil service position offered a secure position and pension he joined the police force at the suggestion of his father. When 20 years of age he married in the hope of getting away from home. From the first there was marital difficulty and he began to drink a quart of liquor daily.

Fourteen years before psychiatric consultation the

---

*Abbreviated by permission from Kolb, L. C., 1968. Noyes' Modern Clinical Psychiatry. 7th Ed. Philadelphia, W. B. Saunders Co., pp. 440–442.

patient, during a riot, was struck on the head and sustained a concussion. He became tremulous and complained of extreme nervousness. His alcoholic intake increased in an effort to alleviate the pruritus, his anxiety and the constant fear that he was about to die. He was discharged from the police force with a pension and the diagnosis of post-traumatic psychoneurosis.

During the subsequent two years he separated from his wife and child, lost contact with his family and lived with an alcoholic woman. Eight years prior to this consultation and following the death of his female companion he was warned by a physician that if he continued drinking he would probably not survive another year. He discontinued drinking, was reconciled with his wife and his dermatitis cleared. He returned to work as a law clerk, attended church regularly and, in his own words, "became a model citizen." He maintained a rigid routine involving difficult hours of work. He dressed meticulously and attempted to do a perfect job at the office.

During the past two years his rash again became generalized and intensely pruritic. When seen in psychiatric consultation he appeared as a well groomed, neatly attired, middle-aged man, alert and accurate, who spoke of his past experiences with obvious embarrassment. His memory was good, and he was well oriented with average intelligence. During consultation he scratched freely. He volunteered that scratching usually brought him great relief and, at times, a satisfaction not unlike that of sexual pleasure. When psychotherapy was suggested he quickly agreed.

During the first two interviews he discussed the present fear of his father and the avoidance of situations which would bring him in contact with him. His wife frequently accused him of being a coward because of this but he could not admit his fear to her. He described his wife as a stubborn, outspoken woman who was usually the disciplinarian with his 17-year-old boy. When he attempted to punish his son his wife became outraged and pointed out to him how good it was of both of them to accept him back eight years ago. He nevertheless denied that there was friction in the household and stated that, in many ways, they were an ideal family. His son had recently been arrested on a minor charge and it was suggested to the patient that perhaps he was failing as a father by not setting limits for the son.

During the third visit it was noted that there was no improvement in the skin condition. He stated early in the interview, "I followed your advice and asserted myself with the boy but was careful not to become angry." His wife had been angry with him but he pacified her by taking her out for a drive. He admitted that he dare not express anger toward her for fear she would leave him. Scratching was frequent, especially when his fear of expressing anger was discussed. His wife insisted upon knowing what was going on in therapy. He was told that it was not necessary to tell her and he appeared to have considerable anxiety over this.

At work he was accused by a colleague of being a

perfectionist; he admitted being angry at this criticism. When it was suggested that he deal more directly with the problems confronting him at work and at home, he scratched and talked of his extreme loneliness.

At the fourth interview his skin condition was much worse and he was unable to attend work. He had purchased two suits of clothing without consulting his wife who usually accompanied him. He made some rather feeble attempts to tell his wife that he preferred shopping without her but felt that it was unsuccessful. He turned to the interviewer and asked, "Doc, tell me, what do you do when you become angry?" There was a fantasy of telling off a co-worker and he remarked that recently he felt resentful and angry, wondering if his increased scratching was related to this.

At the time of the sixth interview his skin remained unchanged. He expressed his fear of losing control of his anger and appeared more aware of his current problems. He talked of his helplessness and became angry with the interviewer for not being of more help to him.

With the seventh interview his skin looked considerably better. He had informed his wife that he was the boss around the house and, following a minor altercation with his son, had told him that he was "not yet dry around the ears." He appeared surprised that his wife was "snapping to," and that his son was spending more time around the house.

In the ninth week his skin improved remarkably. He related an incident with pride in which, when his wife refused to prepare breakfast for him, he had advised her that she had better behave herself, ordered her to the bedroom, and had intercourse with her. That evening he took her to the movies and noted that she was affectionate. He remarked that during the previous week he had been able to tell his employer that too much of the work fell on him and that this should be changed.

Treatment was terminated [and] the patient was seen in dermatology clinic two months later. His skin had cleared completely except for a small area of dermatitis behind the knees. He was feeling well, had no difficulty sleeping, required no medication and was much satisfied with the changes in his relations with his family and employers.

In *musculoskeletal* reactions the individual experiences pain localized in the bones or voluntary muscles of the back, the head or the rest of the body. Arthritis, inflammation of a joint, is also classified as a musculoskeletal psychophysiologic reaction when it has emotional origins. The bones and voluntary muscles are primarily innervated by the cerebrospinal rather than the autonomic system, but the autonomic system can cause pain in the bones or muscles by reducing the blood supply.

Finally, *psychophysiologic disorders of organs of special sense* include symptoms localized in the eye, ear or other sensory organs, e.g., chronic inflammation of eyelid membranes (conjunctivitis) due to emotional factors. However, it is typically so difficult to separate such reactions from conversion disorders with sensory symptoms that the category is not particularly useful.

THE CAUSATION OF PSYCHOPHYSIOLOGIC DISORDERS

Heredity

There is a considerable amount of evidence to indicate that heredity is important in psychophysiologic reactions. The brothers of ulcer patients are approximately twice as likely to have ulcers as comparable members of the general population. In one study the comparable frequencies were 11.5 vs. 5.5 per cent. Increased frequencies have also been reported for close relatives of patients with asthma, hypertension, migraine and hyperthyroidism. These increased frequencies appear to be specific for the single type of reaction involved; e.g., there is evidence to show that relatives of asthma patients have increased frequencies for asthma but not for migraine or other reactions. It seems unlikely that the tendency for specific psychophysiologic reactions to run in families can be entirely explained as the result of common learning experiences and identification with parents which are so important in the etiology of neurotic reactions, for autonomic nervous system functioning is believed to be less affected by these variables than the cerebrospinal system. Learning experiences or identification also appears to be inadequate as an explanation for the fact that 60 per cent of epileptic individuals have a migrainous heredity, in contrast to fewer than 20 per cent of nonepileptics. Further, persons in blood group O—determined by heredity—are 40 per cent more likely than those belonging to other blood groups to have duodenal ulcers.

A predisposition to high blood pressure has a genetic component that is attributable to multiple minor genes (Roberts, 1959) in the same manner as other continuously graded characteristics such as height, weight or intelligence. Figure 10–3 shows the distribution of blood pressure in a sample of the general population and among the relatives of persons with low or high blood pressure. The tendency for hypertension to run in families is very clear in the distributions.

In hyperthyroidism, the underlying genetic factor is apparently recessive. If a dominant gene or genes were involved, the proportion of hyperthyroid siblings of hyperthyroid patients would be identical with the proportion of hyperthyroid mothers of patients. For a recessive gene, the expected proportions are 25 per cent for siblings and almost zero for mothers; the proportions obtained in genetic studies of hyperthyroidism are close to the expected ones.

Apart from the hereditary components in specific psychophysiologic disorders, there appears to be a hereditary factor in general autonomic reactivity. Vandenberg (1962) studied the reactions of monozygotic and dizygotic twins who were free of psychophysiologic or other identifiable disorders. His results indicated a significant hereditary component in cardiac and respiratory responses to stressful startle stimuli. The implication is that a predisposition to general autonomic and visceral overactivity in response to external stress may be inherited.

Other Biological Determinants

The psychophysiologic disorders have sometimes been termed "disorders of adaptation," i.e., disorders in which there is failure to adapt to stress. Stomach ulcers, for example, have been produced in both animals and humans as a response to extensive skin burns, brain injury, drastic surgery in various parts of the body, cardiac insufficiency or other biological assaults on the organism. Under experimental conditions, exposure of animals to a variety of biological noxious agents has produced hypertension and degenerative changes in the heart, kidneys and joints. Improper diet, smoking and alcohol hasten the development of ulcers in humans and slow down recovery. It is believed that physique is also relevant: peptic ulcers often occur in ectomorphic individuals. Among women, ulcers occur much less frequently before the menopause than after it. Consequently, it has been speculated that a protective hormonal mechanism is active during the years of fertility.

The ratio of males to females is very different for different psychophysiologic reactions. Men more frequently have ulcers and neurodermatitis. Women more frequently have hypertension, migraine, rheumatoid arthritis and hyperthyroidism. The disparity is so great in some reactions—e.g., for hyperthyroidism a ratio of

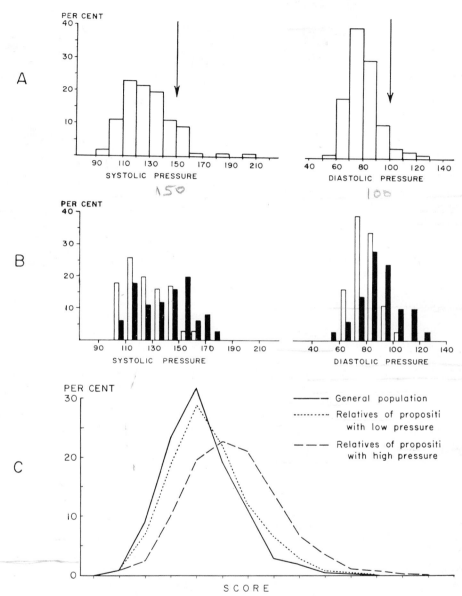

Figure 10–3. Arterial blood pressures. A, Sample of 227 women, 30 to 39 years of age. The arrows point to the systolic and diastolic pressures that are often chosen to separate groups with normal and high blood pressure. B, Forty-six female relatives of propositi with low pressures (light columns represent controls), as compared with 41 female relatives of propositi with high pressures (dark columns represent hypertensives); 30 to 39 years of age. C, Frequency distributions of diastolic pressures for 867 persons from the general population, 371 relatives of controls and 1062 relatives of hypertensives; males and females, 10 to 79 years of age. The curves are adjusted for age and sex, because different age groups as well as both sexes have different mean pressures. (After Hamilton, Pickering, Roberts and Sowry. 1954. Clin. Sci. 13:273–304.)

eight females to each male has been reported—that it seems overwhelmingly likely that biological factors are involved in addition to the differential experiences of males and females. However, a caution is in order: at the present time peptic ulcers occur much more often in men than in women, but the reverse was true two generations ago.

Psychological Determinants

The Problem of Specificity vs. Generality. A crucial issue for the understanding of psychophysiologic reactions is that of specificity vs. generality. We have already mentioned that heredity seems to operate both as a specific predisposition to various reactions and as a general predisposition to autonomic overactivity as such. It is particularly with reference to psychological determinants, however, that the problem of a specific vs. a general causal pattern has arisen and been discussed by various investigators.

A number of students of the question have speculated that each reaction is symbolic of a specific unconscious conflict, is precipitated by a specific stress and occurs in a patient with specific personality characteristics that result from a specific set of early experiences. But others have felt that all the reactions have the same meaning, precipitants, personality constellation and childhood background. Representative of the specificity hypothesis is the interpretation of asthma as a "strangled cry for help and forgiveness" which is precipitated by the threat of estrangement from a dominant mother in a personality that tends to ambivalence and depression as a result of childhood frustration at the hands of the mother. Colitis in female patients has been attributed to a constellation consisting of rejection of femininity, conflict between conformity and rebellion, and a tendency to obsessive brooding. Essential hypertension has been ascribed to anger against a dominant parent which is inhibited in favor of overt submission; the anger and inhibition can, of course, be displaced to substitute figures. Ulcers have been attributed to overriding ambition and an unconscious equation of food with love.

Psychoanalysts have frequently gone even further in the direction of specificity and have hypothesized that psychophysiologic disorders, like conversion symptoms, constitute an "organ language," an expression of unconscious con-

flicts in the "language of the body." Difficulty in swallowing food has been interpreted by analysts as evidence of something "unpalatable" in the person's life situation; nausea is inability to "stomach" something unpleasant; vomiting is rejection; asthmatic difficulties symbolize the existence of a load on one's chest; pain in the shoulder or arm indicates an inhibited impulse to strike out aggressively; and neurodermatitic itching is a somatic expression of the saying, "he gets under my skin." Ruesch (1946) has formulated the role of symbolism in psychophysiologic disorders as a regressive use of body language in an individual whose ability to communicate verbally is defective. A psychophysiologic reaction is an attempt to say something, but it says it in an infantile fashion.

It is difficult to test hypotheses dealing with specificity of symbolic meaning, but there is some evidence for specificity in personality traits. The purported association of ulcers and dependency, for example, is consistent with clinical impressions from Rorschach testing that ulcer patients more than others manifest ungratified dependency needs. Ulcer patients often improve considerably with no treatment other than bed rest, as if the regimen of being cared for satisfied their dependency. Intensive observations of individual cases are also often corroborative. For example, a patient with a chronic peptic ulcer was unusually aggressive, self-sufficient and "crusty" on the surface. As a hobby he painted and used only the softest, most delicate pastel shades in his canvasses; his pictures, like his ulcer, served to express the "soft" inhibited part of his personality. Some evidence and observations also exist to support the specific constellations that have been suggested for the other reactions, i.e., conformity problems in colitis, anger in hypertension and so forth.

But there is also evidence to support an opposite point of view. Buck and Hobbs (1959) studied the frequency of psychophysiologic cardiovascular, gastrointestinal and musculoskeletal disorders, as well as allergic disorders and neuroses, in 187 patients over a five-year period. On the hypothesis that each of the five disorders has a specific, *independent* constellation, one can calculate the number of persons who could be expected to have reactions falling into any two of the categories simultaneously, e.g., both cardiovascular and gastrointestinal, or both cardiovascular and musculoskeletal. (There are ten such possible pairs for five categories.) The investigators found a greater than expected number of individuals with a pair of disorders in six of the ten possible pairs. The implication of the finding is that psychophysiologic reactions are not completely specific and independent, but are somewhat diffuse; the individual with a psychophysiologic disorder is likely to be vulnerable to another one also (or to be allergic or neurotic). It follows, therefore, that the personality constellations in psychologic reactions cannot be completely specific.

A second argument against specificity is that even if a given personality constellation is predominant in a given reaction, it is not the only constellation found in the reaction. Some asthma patients are passive but cheerful and some are depressed; not all ulcer patients are ambitious executives.

A third argument for generality is that a single psychological factor—repressed hostility—is quite often found in a variety of reactions. In the cases of migraine, asthma, neurodermatitis, peptic ulcer, ulcerative colitis, and anorexia, presented earlier in this chapter, repressed hostility was present. Depression was also repeatedly present and it has long been known that a major source of depression is inhibited hostility. It should be noted that a patient with a high enough level of hostility can repress a considerable amount and still appear overtly hostile.

Anxiety is another general factor often reported in various psychophysiologic reactions. Evidence for the importance of anxiety comes from a study by Franks et al. (1959). Sixty-seven psychotics who were also suffering from various psychophysiologic symptoms were subjected to lobotomies or related forms of psychosurgery; the result was a notable decrease of the psychophysiologic symptoms. Similarly, it has been observed that other means of relieving anxiety and tension, such as tranquilizers, frequently result in diminution of psychophysiologic symptoms.

Still another argument is that laboratory investigation has at times failed to confirm behavioral predictions based on specificity. Reasoning from traditional formations of specific personality factors in psychophysiologic disorders, it may be deduced that in a situation involving an insoluble problem, ulcer patients should be persistent and optimistic about finding a solution, whereas colitis patients should be pessimistic and less persistent. Ulcer patients should stress the importance of their own efforts to solve the problem; colitis patients should tend to project blame for their failures externally.

Mednick, Garner and Stone (1959) tested these predictions and found no significant differences between the two groups. Of course, it is possible that the laboratory situation does not tap differences that exist between the two groups in real life.

An alternative to the hypothesis of psychological specificity is the hypothesis of *somatic vulnerability*. This hypothesis asserts that as a response to stress the autonomically unstable organism breaks down in its weakest organ. The ulcer patient does not differ from the asthma patient in motives and traits, but his stomach is weaker than his lungs. Organ weakness may be due to heredity, constitution or life experiences. For example, the gastrointestinal system may be congenitally weak or may have been weakened by poor meals or alcoholism. Illness may also make an organ vulnerable; it has been suspected that whooping cough increases the probability of later asthma and that childhood digestive disturbances precede ulcers.

Hypotheses involving both specificity and generality have also been proposed. Alexander, in various publications, and Alexander and French (1948) have theorized that a conflict between dependency and self-sufficiency is a general factor present in all psychophysiologic disorders, but that the specific fashion in which the individual attempts to solve this conflict influences the kind of disorder he develops. Specificity thus resides not in symbolic functioning but in the emotion and the type of autonomic activity attendant on the particular mode of conflict solution. For example, a regressive search for an infantile type of dependency gratification is accompanied by parasympathetic activity and therefore by ulcers, colitis or asthma, but not migraine, hypertension or arthritis. (*Precisely* which of these the individual develops is affected by organ vulnerability.) On the other hand, if the individual seeks to solve his basic conflict by a compensatory self-sufficiency, sympathetic overactivity occurs and causes migraine, hypertension, arthritis or similar disorders. The gastrointestinal patient tends to oral "parasitic receptiveness," presumably for biological reasons. When this tendency is thwarted by internal conflict or external circumstances, he becomes oral-aggressive instead of receptive and adopts a narcissistic façade of optimism, strength and exaggerated helpfulness in order to cover his unconscious, parasitic dependence on others. Hypertension, on the other hand, occurs in patients whose vasomotor, kidney or endocrine system is predisposed to instability and who, in addition to this somatic predisposition, fear retaliation for their aggressive tendencies and at the same time wish to be cared for in a passive-receptive fashion. Their dependent longing arouses feelings of inferiority and reactivates inhibited hostility, thus leading in circular fashion to even greater fear of retaliation and concomitant sympathetic activity. The difference between the ulcer and hypertensive patients does not reside in the nature of their basic conflicts but in the autonomic activity accompanying the emotions they experience as they attempt to solve the same conflict by diverse means, as well as in organ vulnerability.

The comprehensiveness and flexibility of Alexander's approach and its consistency with much clinical evidence make it very appealing. It should also be noted that an emphasis on the conflict between dependency and self-sufficiency in various psychophysiologic reactions is quite consistent with our earlier emphasis on repressed hostility. Both the expression of infantile dependency and the repression of dependency are likely to be associated with repression of the hostile and angry components of personality.

Predisposing Childhood Experiences. The early history of psychophysiologic patients frequently indicates persistent or recurrent stress. Excessive parental anxiety and concern, overprotection, restriction of activities, deprivation of affection and pressures toward conformity are frequent background factors. In general, the childhood experiences that contribute to psychophysiologic reactions are those that promote anxiety. It is the impression of many observers that the dominant parent is very often the mother and that the relationship between the child and the mother tends to be more pathological than between the child and the father. The father is apt to contribute to the child's faulty adaptation by ineffectuality rather than by harsh and rigid domination, although the latter also occurs.

There is also a widespread impression, based on clinical experience, that the childhood of psychophysiologic patients is marked by an inadequate opportunity to interact with other children of both sexes. They are only children, or their nearest siblings are several years older or younger, or their siblings are all of the same sex, or their interactions are restricted by overprotective or dominating parents. However, these impressions have not been tested statistically on an adequate scale.

The school-adjustment history is often one of conformity and scholastic competitiveness. Conformity and striving for scholastic success frequently are followed by intensive occupational striving and upward socioeconomic mobility. This is not the only contributing pattern, however. In the past, a number of psychophysiologic disorders have been more frequently diagnosed in members of the upper socioeconomic classes and have been regarded as the price of success and prominence. But more recently it has become increasingly apparent that undiagnosed and untreated cases are very common among those of lower socioeconomic status whose lives embody many chronic frustrations.

Psychophysiologic disorders are encountered more frequently among single, widowed or divorced persons than among the married population of equivalent ages. There is often a history of guilt over premarital sexual experience. After marriage, marked sexual inhibitions are frequent even in patients whose primary symptoms are not impotence or frigidity. A vicious cycle is often set up when sexual distaste is evidenced by either marriage partner, for sexual conflict contributes to general marital discord which in turn aggravates the patient's emotional conflict, sexual difficulties and other symptoms. Persistent marital discord also contributes to a perpetuation of similar problems among the children.

Precipitating Psychological Events. A variety of stress situations may act as precipitants. Sexual impotence, for example, may be precipitated by reminders of childhood fears, by lack of privacy in crowded living conditions, by impatience on the part of the sexual partner or by numerous other internal and external events.

To take another disorder as an illustration, peptic ulcer may be precipitated by any type of psychological stress. Earlier, we described an experiment in which Brady (1958) produced ulcers in "executive" monkeys by prolonged, stressful vigilance combined with the necessity for appropriate action to avoid unpleasant stimulation. An important study by Weiner et al. (1957) indicates that in humans neither biological predisposition, nor personality constellation, nor precipitating stress is ordinarily sufficient to produce duodenal ulcers, but rather a combination of all three factors is necessary. The investigators obtained measurements of the gastric secretory activity of the stomach in 2073 Army inductees. From this sample they selected 63 men with very high gastric secretions and 57 men with very low secretions. Each of the subjects was given a battery of personality tests and a radiological examination of the gastrointestinal tract before being sent to basic training. Four men showed evidence of ulcers. After 8 to 16 weeks of basic training—a stressful experience for most men—the subjects were reexamined and five more men were found to have developed duodenal ulcers. All nine were in the group with high gastric secretion. Evaluation of the personality data revealed that seven of the nine had major unresolved conflicts centering about dependency and oral gratification. The investigators concluded that neither a high rate of gastric secretion nor a specific psychodynamic constellation is likely to be independently responsible for the development of most peptic ulcers, but that jointly they constitute the essential determinants for the occurrence of ulcers in stress situations.

Sociocultural Determinants

Primitive cultures in which ulcers are unknown have been reported by observers. In some cultures impotence and frigidity are unknown; on the other hand, in those primitive or advanced cultures in which sexual taboos are pervasive and rigid, both frigidity and impotence occur.

Within a single culture, sociocultural factors such as poverty, unemployment and the severe psychological frustrations associated with these conditions have deleterious effects on the organism, including the autonomic system. Of course, associated physical factors such as poor diet interact with frustration. It was mentioned previously that a higher frequency of psychophysiologic disorders have been reported in disorganized than in better organized societies.

Most dramatic of all the evidences for sociocultural causation is a fact previously cited—the change in the sex-ratio of ulcers. In the nineteenth century, ulcers were apparently more common in women; by the 1930's it was estimated that there were as many as 12 male patients for every female. More recently, the frequency for women has been increasing. A speculative explanation sometimes offered is that in recent decades the dominance of the male in the family has decreased while freedom for women has increased. The true explanation is undoubtedly more complex than this, however. Halliday (1948) reported that in the year 1900 perforated peptic ulcers (ulcers that have penetrated the wall of the stomach or intestine) had been most frequent in younger women and second most frequent in older men. By 1930, peptic ulcers were very much more frequent in younger men and second in frequency among older women. To explain these results solely in terms of sociocultural causation, one must make the very questionable assumption that the burden of frustration has not only shifted from women to men but secondarily also to younger rather than older men and to older rather than younger women.

U.S. Army statistics on peptic ulcers in the two world wars have provided data that introduce an additional complication. From the first to the second war duodenal ulcers almost doubled but stomach ulcers decreased about 35 per cent. A possible implication, consistent with certain physiological findings, is that duodenal ulcers may be more responsive to emotional and sociocultural factors, whereas stomach ulcers may be more responsive to purely physical causes. Diet and other physical factors were better in the second than the first war.

TREATMENT

Successful treatment of abnormality, unlike effective prevention, need bear little or no relation to the causation of abnormality. Regardless of the psychological factors in causation—disturbed interpersonal relationships, conflict, frustration and deprivation—severe bodily pathology requires medical and sometimes surgical treatment. Symptomatic medical treatment of psychophysiologic disorders involves a variety of therapeutic procedures such as drugs and special diets. If an ulcer of the stomach or colon bleeds sufficiently, the patient requires a transfusion, and if an ulcer perforates the wall of the stomach into the abdominal cavity, it requires prompt surgical repair. Ulcers that cannot be controlled by medical treatment may lead to other severe complications; to prevent these it is sometimes necessary to remove part of the stomach or colon. Sympathectomy, the extensive severing of certain sympathetic fibers, is a drastic surgical procedure that has sometimes been used to bring hypertension or other sympathetically caused disorders under control.

In most instances, attempts should be made to improve the patient's life situation by modifying his environment so as to reduce daily stress. Short-term supportive psychotherapy may also relieve anxiety and symptoms and may lead to at least temporary improvement in the life situation. It may be very difficult to decide whether to undertake long-term psychotherapy in the hope of preventing future symptomatology. Although many psychophysiologic patients are good candidates for uncovering therapy, it is also true that a number are poorly motivated for change and resist it. Genuine psychotherapy cannot start so long as the patient insists that his troubles are purely physical and denies that he is unhappy or dissatisfied. Once the patient verbalizes his unhappiness, the therapist may help him realize that his physical symptoms are not the sole reasons for his misery.

The goal of uncovering therapy with psychophysiologic patients is primarily to help them gain insight into their emotional conflicts. A good relationship between patient and therapist is obviously crucial. The therapist must guard against frightening the patient by pushing him into acquisition of insights before he is ready. It should be noted that it is unnecessary and often impossible for the patient to gain understanding of the precise connections between his conflicts and symptoms. Insight into conflicts as such may be very helpful even when their connections with symptoms are ignored.

The evidence for the effectiveness of psychotherapy in treating psychophysiologic disorders is inconclusive. However, the results suggest that, in conjunction with proper medical treatment, psychotherapy is effective at least in decreasing the individual's vulnerability to subsequent stress. An example of the studies supporting this view is provided by O'Connor et al. (1964). These authors studied 57 ulcerative colitis patients who were seen regularly by a psychotherapist after their illness was diagnosed. Compared with a control group of 57 ulcerative colitis patients who were not given psychotherapy, the treated group showed a marked and sustained improvement in various physiological criteria while the control group remained unchanged.

11
AFFECTIVE DISORDERS

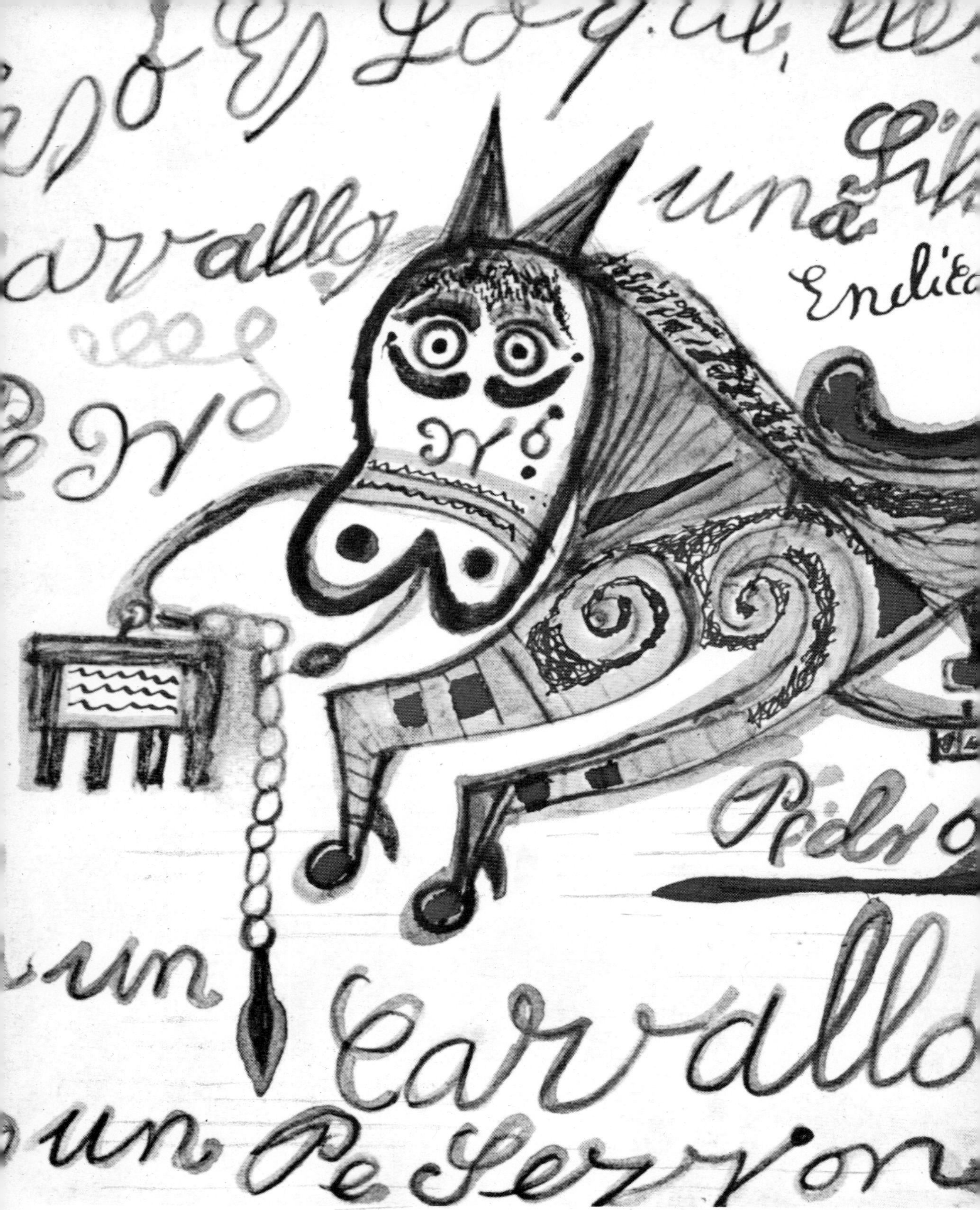

I'll change my state with any wretch,
Thou canst from gaol or dunghill fetch;
My pain's past cure, another hell,
I may not in this torment dwell!
Now desperate I hate my life,
Lend me a halter or a knife;
All my griefs to this are jolly,
Naught so damn'd as melancholy.

Robert Burton, *The Anatomy of Melancholy*

AFFECTIVE DISORDERS

The most conspicuous feature of affective disorders is a marked deviation in mood from the normal which is manifested as either depression or euphoria. The severely depressed individual views the world with extreme pessimism and is deeply convinced that he and others are evil. The euphoric individual is unrealistically optimistic, feels that he and others are wonderful, and elatedly anticipates a rosy future.

Affective disorders are less common than schizophrenia among mental hospital admissions, but are by no means rare. In 1968, of all first admissions to U.S. mental hospitals, 4.0 per cent were diagnosed as psychotic depressive reaction, manic-depressive reaction or involutional psychotic reaction. (In the last group a majority of the patients are predominantly depressed and a minority are predominantly paranoid.) The percentage of resident patients with the same disorders was 6.0. However, many affectively disturbed individuals are never hospitalized or even evaluated in clinics or private practice. An investigation of manic-depression in Sweden, for example, concluded that the number of diagnosed patients was only one-seventh the total number of manic-depres-

sives in the general population (Larsson and Sjögren, 1954).

A number of depressed or euphorically manic individuals—but by no means all—also have secondary disturbances of perception, cognitive functioning and overt behavior which are manifested in hallucinations, delusions and suicidal or homicidal tendencies. In an affective disorder, secondary disturbances are consistent with the patient's prevailing mood; in schizophrenia, by contrast, the patient's thinking, perception and overt behavior are often quite inconsistent with his mood as well as with each other. In consequence, affectively disordered patients appear less disorganized than schizophrenics.

Individuals who do not evidence hallucinations, delusions or other secondary symptoms but only a mood deviation are nevertheless often considered psychotic rather than neurotic. The justification for the label "psychotic" in such cases is that euphoria or depression, *when sufficiently intense*, constitutes a break with reality. The manic individual overvalues his abilities, intelligence, power or charm to the point of absurdity. He makes impossible plans

[margin handwritten: MANIC / DEPP.]

and promises, and his behavior is not influenced by the reactions of others. The psychotically depressed person has a hopeless feeling that nothing can possibly make him feel better; in defiance of the fact that he has improved after past episodes of depression, he is convinced that this time he will *not* improve. Associated with this hopelessness is a perception of himself so negative that it constitutes a delusion. Rado (1928) comments as follows:

> The most striking feature in the picture displayed by the symptoms of depressive conditions is the fall in self-esteem and self-satisfaction. The depressive neurotic for the most part attempts to conceal this disturbance; in melancholia it finds clamorous expression in the patients' delusional self-accusations and self-aspersions, which we call "the delusion" of moral inferiority.

THE PROBLEM OF CLASSIFICATION

Attempts to classify affective disorders into subtypes have a long history. Two of the four basic temperaments recognized by the Greeks were the melancholic and the sanguine, or optimistic. As long ago as the first century A.D., Aretaeus speculated that manic excitement and melancholia or depression were really one disorder. In the nineteenth century, a number of French physicians went a step further by reporting observations of alternating attacks of depression and excitement in the same individual. In 1854, Falret described such alternations as "la folie circulaire" (circular insanity) or "folie à double forme" (insanity in a double guise). In 1899, Kraepelin coined the term manic-depressive psychosis. The implication of Falret's and Kraepelin's terms is that mania and depression constitute a single entity, that is, they are characterized by an identical pathological process that is different from the pathology found in other syndromes.

At first blush it is not at all apparent how two such opposite mood deviations as depression and excited euphoria can be classified under one heading. The fact that mania and depression alternate cyclically is not quite sufficient justification, for only a minority of affectively disturbed patients manifest this circularity. Manic-depressives can be divided into three groups. The largest number suffer from recurrent attacks of depression only and never evidence mania; the next largest number suffer from repeated manic attacks only; and in the smallest number there is a history of true "circular in-

sanity." (There are also some cases in which manic and depressive symptoms occur simultaneously.) However, there is a strong reason to believe that mania and depression, whether alternating or not, share a common dynamic substructure. Mania, in fact, may be viewed as *a defense against depression* by a "flight into reality." The manic uses reality as a distraction from his emotional problems. Rado (1961) remarks, "Elation is for the organism a calamitous way of cutting short the agony of depression." The depressive withdraws his psychic energy or libido from the external world and directs it entirely toward himself; the manic feverishly plunges into external reality in order to deny internal reality.

Various systems of classification have described a number of affective disturbances other than manic-depression. The boundaries separating them are often vague; how many affective disorders should be differentiated is a matter of dispute. The diagnostic manual of the American Psychiatric Association includes only one other, involutional melancholia, as one of the affective disorders. Involutional melancholia is defined as occurring in the involutional period of life in a patient with no previous history of mania or depression. Some involutional patients are primarily characterized by paranoid ideas, but in most the symptom constellation consists of severe, agitated depression, worry, insomnia, guilt and hypochondria or somatic delusions. This disorder is distinguished from manic-depressive illness by the absence of previous episodes; from schizophrenia by a primary disorder of mood rather than thought, and from other depressive reactions by the fact that the depression is frequently unrelated to any external loss.

Psychotic depressive reactions are not included as one of the affective psychoses in spite of the fact that they are primarily a disorder of affect. In a psychotic depressive reaction there is no history of either repeated depression or marked, cyclothymic mood swings, and there is likely to be an environmental precipitant. Manic-depressive reaction, on the other hand, is defined as a disorder that tends to recur (as mania or depression or both) and also to be independent of exogenous precipitation; it is presumed to be a reaction to an internal rather than an external state of affairs. *[handwritten: recur + internal]*

However, it is actually quite common for the manic or depressive phase of a recurrent manic-depressive psychosis to develop immediately after an obvious precipitating stress. Further-

[margin handwritten notes: APA / 1 manic / 4; ① ; ② ; NB ; parts of middle age / w 3 min pow ; D I F F E R S ; a) b) c)]

[bottom handwritten notes:]
1) depressed - depressed
2) MANIC - MANIC
3) MANIC - depressive - (Women higher) 45 - later than others - 33

[bottom right handwritten: environmental - outside the body]

more, it is often very difficult to distinguish a psychotic depressive reaction in an older individual from an involutional reaction. For these reasons the separate category termed "psychotic depressive reaction" is very unreliable and we shall not use it.

A problem in classification arises from the fact that depression or excitement can occur as the secondary feature of a disorder that is basically not affective. For example, brain damage causes both primary symptoms of intellectual impairment and secondary symptoms that are due to the release of hitherto latent personality characteristics; among the latter may be tendencies to depression or excitement that were kept under control prior to the occurrence of the brain damage. Secondary depression or excitement may also be associated with sociopathic personality, paranoid or schizophrenic reactions or any of the syndromes that are discussed in subsequent chapters. When affective and schizophrenic symptoms occur simultaneously, the diagnosis of schizo-affective reaction may be made with the implication that the patient's basic disorder is schizophrenic rather than affective.

MANIC-DEPRESSIVE ILLNESS

Manic-depressive reaction occurs much more often in women than men; data for the United States and Sweden indicate that more than 60 per cent of manic-depressives are female. In consequence, it has been speculated that a hormonal factor may be present in the etiology of the disorder. Depressive or manic episodes sometimes occur during pregnancy or immediately after childbirth. (An emotional disturbance occurring after childbirth is a *postpartum reaction*. Only a minority of postpartum reactions are affective; the rest are neurotic, psychophysiologic, schizophrenic, paranoid or organic.)

The average age at first admission for manic-depressive illness in 1968 was 44 years, almost 12 years older than the average schizophrenic patient at first admission. A larger percentage of manic-depressives than schizophrenics are married. The difference in marital status has at least two sources. First, the older manic-depressive is more likely to have married than the younger schizophrenic. Second, manic-depressives are believed to be more extraverted and less withdrawn than schizophrenics.

More than 10 per cent of manic-depressives

are heavy drinkers, for the most part as a consequence rather than a cause of their difficulties. The depressive drinks to feel better and the manic drinks as an expression of his euphoric state.

Any combination of mania and depression may occur, e.g., a single episode of either, repeated attacks of either with lucid intervals (remissions) between the attacks, a regular alternation of the two, a completely irregular sequence of manic and depressive episodes, or a simultaneous mixture of the two. A manic-depressive mixture usually consists of excitement and overactivity accompanying morbid ideas and a despairing mood. In another and very rare mixture, the patient is in a state of maniacal stupor that consists of an elated mood and, simultaneously, a seemingly depressive lack of motor activity. In more than 70 per cent of all cases the first attack is depressive.

The average interval between attacks in cases marked by recurrence or alternation has been reported in various studies as somewhere between three and ten years. The duration of a single attack of either mania or depression may vary from a few hours to a lifetime; for *untreated* depression, the average was formerly recorded as about one and one-half years, and for *untreated* mania it was four to six months. In recent years, patients with severe affective disorders have rarely gone untreated and the average duration of attacks has decreased markedly. The briefer the attack, the less likely the patient is to manifest any deterioration of personality. With advancing age, patients display a tendency toward longer attacks, shorter remissions and, among manics, personality deterioration.

The rate of readmission to mental hospitals is high in manic-depression. Rennie (1942) followed up 208 cases of manic-depression for over 30 years after hospital admission. During this period only 21 per cent had a single attack, 79 per cent had at least two attacks, 63 per cent at least three and 45 per cent at least four.

Depressive Episodes

A number of observers have distinguished three degrees of increasing severity of depression. From least to most severe the three have been termed simple depression, acute depression and depressive stupor. These three states are not separated by sharp boundaries but shade into each other.

Simple Depression. In this degree of depression the individual is somewhat retarded or somewhat anxious, upset and agitated. Involutional melancholics are almost invariably characterized by the agitated type of depression, whereas some manic-depressives in a depressed phase are retarded and some agitated. The individual feels guilty and discouraged. He is likely to talk in a monotone, with little variation in pitch, rhythm or volume. Except when there is also an organic brain syndrome, his intellect, memory and orientation are not impaired. He has no illusions or hallucinations. It is not uncommon for the individual to "fight" a simple depression, whereas in the more severe acute and stuporous depressions he gives up the struggle. A simple depression is more likely to be treated on an outpatient basis than to lead to hospitalization; often it is not treated at all.

The following Thematic Apperception Test (TAT) stories were told by an intelligent, 40-year-old married woman suffering from a simple depression in which marital difficulties played an important part. In both stories she attempted to resist her depression and overcome it by the mechanism of denial.

The TAT picture shows a young woman standing with downcast head, one hand covering her face and the other resting on a door.

Pt. This is a peculiar picture, it is not . . . not . . . (*one minute pause*). This woman is very definitely sad or shocked. The blackness behind her must be grief. She has turned her back to it. She has started through the open door, away from this grief. (*Patient puts the picture away, at arm's length.*) She is resting or stopping to compose herself. And I would say that this woman would be a better woman if . . . because her back is definitely to all this grief and sadness, behind her. I like these lines here. (*Patient points to the door frame.*) She is holding onto it as if she wanted to . . . I don't know . . . support herself. Well, she stops, but I am sure she will go forward beyond this blackness. She did not take just the handle to hold on to or the door frame.

Ex. [Examiner]. Tell me more about her. Remember you are to make a complete story.

Pt. As long as I said black on one side and light on the other, she is going on to more joy and very little grief.

Ex. Is she married?

Pt. (*20 second pause.*) Well, you are supposed to put yourself into this, or are you. . . . In some respects I can see myself here. Yes, she is married. (*Patient puts the card away.*)

The second picture consists of a woman's head against a man's shoulder.

Pt. The dark background signifies grief or sadness. These two people are unemotional but very passive, no tears. Contented in sharing of this grief. I am sure they will accept the results of this grief, the cause of whatever it was. . . .

Ex. Who are they?

Pt. I would say this is a father and mother or a husband and wife.

Acute Depression. The most severe forms of acute depression, as well as stuporous depression, are seen less frequently today than a few decades ago, due, in part, to earlier recognition and more effective treatment. In an acute depression, the patient has an emotional reaction variously described as disconsolate, dejected, despondent or desperate. Any minor frustration can cause an exacerbation of this reaction. Two patterns of motor activity occur. In one, the patient sits or stands in a dejected attitude, preoccupied with his inner misery and indifferent to his appearance and surroundings. In the other, he paces the floor or wanders aimlessly and agitatedly, wringing his hands or even tearing his hair or clothing. The patient's face is haggard and drawn and the creases in the upper eyelid are accentuated. Many acute depressives weep a great deal. They tend not to initiate conversations. They answer questions after lengthy pauses, in very few words and in a low, monotonous voice, as if they had very little energy for thinking or talking. The acute depressive's manner of speech may cause him to appear intellectually impaired, but his replies to questions are rational though brief. His outlook is gloomy and morbid, and he complains of feeling tired, listless, lacking in energy and "run down" or "dragged out." He shows little initiative and cannot become interested in activities that he previously enjoyed.

Frequently, depressives complain of various cognitive deficiencies, such as poor concentration, difficulty in remembering and decreased mental alertness. However, the person's estimation of his cognitive abilities may be unrealistic because of his depressed state. Friedman (1964) gave 33 cognitive, perceptual and psychomotor tests to 55 severely depressed persons. Compared to a control group matched for age, sex, education and vocabulary score, the depressed group performed more poorly on only 3 of 82 test scores. Thus the actual ability to perform during severe depression is not consistent with the patient's unrealistically low image of himself.

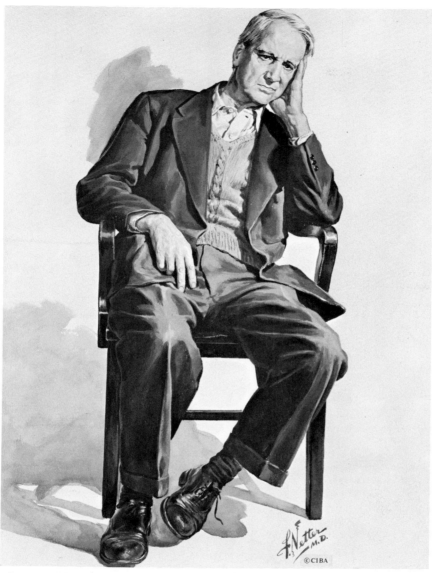

Figure 11-1. *Retarded depression. (Illustration developed by Frank H. Netter, M.D., in collaboration with Frank J. Ayd, Jr., M.D. Copyright Clinical Symposia published by CIBA Pharmaceutical Company, Summit, N.J.)*

Acutely depressed patients suffer from insomnia. They have difficulty falling asleep and when they do they soon awake. For many patients, depression is more severe in the morning than at any other time. Loss of appetite, loss of weight and constipation are common. Sexual desire tends to diminish and the patient is likely to become frigid or impotent. In women it is not uncommon for menstruation to cease during a depressive episode and to resume spontaneously on recovery. A depressed individual is apt to be unduly sensitive to minor pains and to be hypochondriacal about minor disturbances in his physical functioning. In fact the depression is sometimes completely masked by physical complaints. Jones and Hall (1963), after studying 200 cases of severe depression, found that the chief emphasis in presenting complaints was on physical symptoms, and in a considerable proportion of cases the patient failed to mention his depressed mood. In some very severe cases, hypochondria becomes the basis

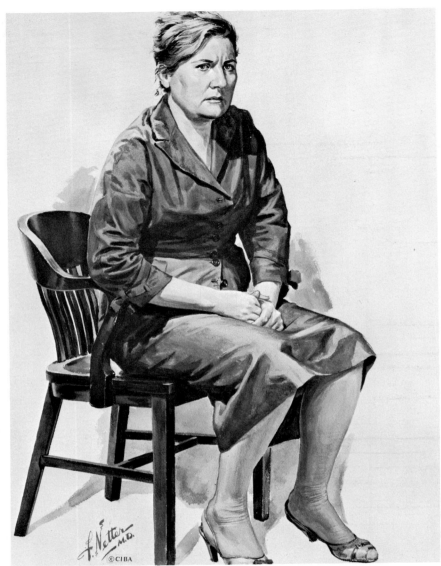

Figure 11-2. *Agitated depression. (Illustration developed by Frank H. Netter, M.D., in collaboration with Frank J. Ayd, Jr., M.D. Copyright Clinical Symposia published by CIBA Pharmaceutical Company, Summit, N.J.)*

NB

of somatic delusions, and the patient believes that his stomach has turned to stone or his liver has been taken away, and so forth.

Just as an acutely depressed person is sensitive to physical pain, so he is sensitive to psychic pain resulting from the harsh judgments of his conscience. He has a pervasive feeling of guilt and is preoccupied with remorse for his past mistakes, even if they were the most trivial of misdemeanors. He is extremely intropunitive and continually condemns himself without ade-

quate cause: One can almost hear a severe depressive say to himself, "I have failed all my life, I am a failure now, and I am sure to fail again." The three parts of this statement reflect remorse, a feeling of worthlessness and a feeling of hopelessness. In his despair, he may feel that the world would be a better place if he were to commit suicide. About 75 per cent of depressives have suicidal ideas and at least 10 to 15 per cent actually attempt to carry them out (Arieti, 1959).

Depression and Suicide. It is a popular misconception that people who speak of committing suicide do not carry out their threats. In a study of 134 suicides, Robins et al. (1959) found that 68 per cent had expressed suicidal ideas and 38 per cent had specifically stated that they intended to kill themselves. Pokorny (1960) reported that 31 of 44 patients who committed suicide had made previous threats or actual suicidal attempts. Four out of five persons who kill themselves have attempted to do so at least once previously. Suicidal persons frequently convey their intentions through their behavior, actions or actual expressions of intent. Many leave notes to be discovered prior to the anticipated attempt. It is a grave mistake to dismiss such gestures as mere bids for attention. This may sometimes be true, but the need for affection, interest and concern is often intense and without them death may be chosen as the solution. Spiegel and Newringer (1963) studied actual and fake suicide notes and concluded that genuine notes were less explicit in expressing suicidal intention, contained fewer suicide synonyms, had more instruction to the reader and were more disorganized than fake notes.

Studies (e.g., Norris, 1959) of various diagnostic categories indicate that the highest frequency of suicide occurs among patients with diagnoses of manic-depressive psychosis and schizophrenia. Retrospective evaluations of successful suicides indicate a high frequency of manic-depression (depressed phase), involutional reaction and schizo-affective reaction, whereas persons who have unsuccessfully attempted suicide are more likely to be neurotics or sociopaths. It is generally assumed in our society that persons who commit suicide or make serious attempts to kill themselves are depressed to a psychotic degree, whether or not they have shown previous symptoms. Hirsh (1960) remarks: "Whether precipitate or calculatedly deliberate, there is an overwhelming body of evidence to suggest that the suicide is rarely a rational being eliminating himself for thoroughly valid reasons. More often than not, he is emotionally and often physically ill." Of the 134 suicides studied by Robins et al. (1959), 101 were diagnosed retrospectively as suffering from specific psychiatric disorders; 25 others were considered to be disturbed psychiatrically, although specific diagnoses could not be made; 5 were suffering from terminal medical illnesses without concomitant psychiatric disorders; and only 3 were apparently well clinically. James and Levin (1964) estimated that the annual incidence of suicide among former mental patients in Australia is over 4 times as high for men and nearly 9 times as high for women in this group as in the rest of the population.

It is widely recognized that a severely depressed person is a suicidal risk, but it is less often realized that other persons may also be endangered. Depressed persons sometimes take the lives of family members prior to taking their own. Sometimes a suicide pact is involved, but more often the depressed individual becomes convinced that life is as hopeless for his family as for himself, and he kills them in the conscious belief that he is doing them a favor, with no insight into the hostility that is involved.

Acutely depressed persons sometimes complain of depersonalization and unreality feelings. Kraines (1957) reports the following verbatim comments by a 44-year-old depressed businessman:*

I don't recognize my body. The other day, I lay in bed, and I actually felt petrified. My head feels like wood. When I strike my head, it seems feelingless—I have to feel myself to know it's me. I have no illusions, but everything seems so unreal. In the beginning, I had different sensations go through my head but now it's a blank. It feels like a vacuum. Sometimes in bed, I raise my leg and look at it. Yes, it's me, but it doesn't seem like me. . . . At times, I wish I had some anxiety, so that at least I could "feel" something that was normal. It may seem funny to you, but I am happy when I sneeze; it's something real. I'm even envious of people who have headaches, because those are real. . . .

Only my dreams seem real to me. I dream of business deals, of people I meet, and they seem real to me, in my dreams—so it seems when I awake—but when I'm awake the real world seems unreal. . . .

I look at people and they seem so small, so insignificant. I went to church and people were like shriveled-up little creatures. And I couldn't pray as I used to, with fervor. Now my prayers are just the repetition of words; I have no feeling in them. . . . Then at times, my brother-in-law looks so large and powerful to me, because he can get up in the morning and go to work, and all I can do is lie there in bed, and feel like wood. When I try to have intercourse with my wife, she seems so immense, so big and strong, and I feel so weak and puny. [The patient was 6 ft. tall and weighed 210 lb.—his wife, 5 ft. 2 in., weighed 122 lb.] The world seems so big, and the people so small.

Acute depressives suffer from delusional distortions of reality. Characteristically, the delusions consist of false self-accusation, a con-

---

*From Kraines, S. H., 1957. Mental Depressions and Their Treatment. New York, The Macmillan Co., p. 234.

self ceased to exist

viction of worthlessness, and nihilism, the belief that the self and external reality have ceased to exist. These delusions are usually not accompanied by illusions and hallucinations. Prior to World War II, about 30 per cent of manic-depressives were reported to manifest illusions and hallucinations, but more recently the tendency has been to diagnose such patients as schizo-affective.

Depressive Stupor. This is the most severe degree of depression, and occurs in only a minority of cases. It can be forestalled by treatment. The untreated, stuporous patient is unresponsive and motionless for long periods of time and usually requires tube feeding. The following case notes describe a depressive stupor:

> The patient lies in bed hardly moving. He does not talk and does not look at anyone passing by his bed. His facial expression is empty and unchanging. He is thin and pale and he looks physically ill. He refuses to eat and has to be fed by stomach tube. He cannot control urination or defecation. Occasionally he mutters a few words like "Sin . . . sinners . . . hell," apparently preoccupied completely by thoughts of sin and punishment. We are quite sure he does not know where he is—he may believe he is in hell.

In any degree of depression, from simple to stuporous, anger is also likely to be present, although often unconsciously. Anger is of great importance in the dynamics of depression, for the most widely accepted interpretation is that depression is retroflexed rage, i.e., rage that is turned back upon the self when it cannot be expressed against the outward source of frustration or the love object that has been lost. Rado (1928) has theorized that depression is "a great despairing cry for love"; the cry is an angry as well as a pleading one. Sometimes, however, the depressed individual expresses hostility both inwardly and outwardly.

intro-punitive

Manic Episodes

H ypomania
A cute
D elirious

Manic behavior, like depression, may be arbitrarily subdivided into three degrees: hypomania, acute mania and delirious mania.

Hypomania. This degree of mania is relatively mild. The individual feels friendly, zestful, self-confident and energetic. He is full of ideas, monopolizes conversations and eagerly undertakes extra tasks. He describes himself as sitting on top of the world. However, he is not merely euphoric and high-spirited, for he may also behave foolishly and impulsively. For example, he may be sexually promiscuous during a hypomanic episode and later, after remission of the episode, may recall his behavior with considerable guilt and remorse. Hypomania also differs from genuine good humor in that a trivial frustration may be excessively irritating or may plunge the individual into depression. Like simple depressives, many hypomaniacs receive no treatment.

Acute Mania. This degree of manic behavior is marked by elation, exaltation, accelerated thought and speech, and motor excitement. The patient is gay and animated, supremely happy and full of witticisms. He is likely to have delusions of grandeur which involve unrealistic ideas of power, wealth, strength, beauty or intellectual brilliance. He is friendly and genial, but with increasing psychomotor activity he is apt to become sarcastic, irritable, vulgar, aggressive and even assaultive. He cannot cooperate with others, is insensitive to their feelings and insists on having his own way. While the prevailing emotional tone is one of elation, there is usually considerable emotional fluctuation, and in some patients there are repeated episodes of weeping or other evidences of depression.

The acute manic is heedless of the consequences of his behavior. He may spend money recklessly, get into fights or become sexually promiscuous. He behaves as if liberated from the pressures of conscience. In contrast to the depressive, he is insensitive to both bodily and psychic pain. One of the authors has seen a manic patient walk around a hospital ward singing happily during an attack of acute appendicitis, which was undoubtedly painful, and with a temperature of 104° (in surgery the appendix was found to have perforated).

In acute mania the patient is likely to be careless of his appearance or to overdress decoratively. He may talk so much that he becomes hoarse or loses his voice. He is continually stimulated by new thoughts and by the external environment. It is usually possible to hold his attention long enough for him to answer questions or, at least, to start doing so. However, he frequently manifests a flight of ideas to tangentially related topics. He tends to make puns, to associate by rhyming and—in extreme cases—to associate by sounds (clang associations) rather than by ideas. It is rare, however, for a manic's associations to be as disconnected and fragmented as are those of severely disorganized schizophrenics.

The following description of manic behavior in a 54-year-old patient, taken from Kolb, is typical:*

At ages 35, 41, and 47, the patient suffered from depressed episodes, each attack being from four to six months in duration. In January he became restless and talkative. Early in February he began to send checks to friends, sometimes even to strangers who, he said, might be in need. Ten days later he was sent home from the office where he was employed with the explanation that he was becoming overwrought. A few days after his suspension from work he was admitted to a private institution for mental disorders where he pretended to commit suicide by mercury poisoning. He then drew a skull and cross bones on the wall of his room. After three weeks he was taken home, but a few days later he was committed to a public institution where he bustled about the ward, giving the impression that he had important business to which he must attend.

Occasionally he would be seen lying on a bench, pretending to sleep, but in a few minutes he resumed his usual activity. He talked quickly, loudly, and nearly constantly. He was interested in everything and everyone around him. He talked familiarly to patients, attendants, nurses, and physicians. He took a fancy to the woman physician on duty in the admission building, calling her by her first name and annoying her with letters and with his familiar, ill-mannered, and obtrusive attentions. On his arrival he gave five dollars to one patient and one dollar to another. He made many comments and asked many questions about other patients and promised that he would secure their discharge. He interfered with their affairs and soon received a blow on the jaw from one patient and a black eye from another. He wrote letters demanding his release, also letters to friends describing in a circumstantial, inaccurate, and facetious way conditions in the hospital. His letters were interlarded with trite Latin phrases. He drew caricatures of the physicians and nurses and wrote music on toilet paper. He drew pictures on his arms; on one occasion he secured a bottle of mercurochrome and painted the face of another manic patient. When permitted to play the ward piano, he played piece after piece without stopping, improvising a great deal. A doctor rarely passed through the ward without being called by the patient, who would slap the physician on the back or shake hands effusively and talk until the door closed. At times during an interview his voice became tremulous, tears came to his eyes, and he sobbed audibly with his face buried in his arms. A moment later, however, he was laughing—a manifestation of the bipolarity of emotion so markedly illustrated in this disease.

Delirious Mania. This stage is reached by relatively few patients, and is marked by a

furious excitement. The patient shouts and laughs constantly. His tempo of speech is too fast to be understood, he tears his clothes and upsets furniture, and he has delusions of both persecution and grandeur. His memory and orientation are impaired during the attack and he is likely to experience vivid hallucinations.

In the case described in the following paragraphs, a tragic and acutely traumatic event precipitated an episode of acute mania. This was soon followed by severe depression and two suicidal attempts, the second of which was unfortunately successful.

The patient was the eldest of four children in a family with no history of psychopathology or disturbed interpersonal relationships. She grew up in average economic circumstances and was apparently a happy, sociable child. At the age of 17 she left school, worked until the age of 23 and then married. Her school and work records were both uneventful. Her husband, a farmer nine years older than she, was described as calm and stable. The couple had three children and were relatively prosperous. The patient was highly regarded by her family and friends and was characterized by them as talkative and carefree. At times she seemed overly excitable and became very angry with the children, but her husband could always calm her down; still she manifested neither pathological euphoria nor depression prior to the onset of her disorder at the age of 38. The onset occurred as follows:

The patient and her husband were driving with several other people to attend a plowing contest. Riding in the back seat, she complained of feeling car-sick and her husband suggested that they change places and she drive. She drove until a warning signal at a railroad crossing indicated an approaching train. She stopped, but the car behind failed to see the signal, ran into her car and pushed it onto the tracks. Her car stalled and she was unable to start it. At the last moment she yelled for everyone to jump out. Her husband and his sister, both in the back seat, were unable to get out in time. The sister-in-law eventually recovered but her husband was killed instantly.

For a day or two after the accident the patient seemed numb and in a state of shock. However, by the time of the funeral she appeared to have recovered her spontaneity and two days later suddenly became quite euphoric. She stated that her husband was far happier with the angels than with her. She bought a new car and drove it so recklessly that friends and neighbors became concerned. She bought a tractor and truck, new clothes, an electric blanket, new beds for her family, a new furnace and insulation for her house. She bought a freezer for her sister and beds for a neighbor. When asked how she could pay for everything she said she was going to get $100,000 from the man who had pushed her car onto the tracks. For the next several days she was talkative, laughed a

---

*From Kolb, L. C., 1968. Noyes' Modern Clinical Psychiatry, 7th Ed. Philadelphia, W. B. Saunders Co., p. 340.

great deal, told crude jokes, called herself the ''Merry Widow,'' acted self-importantly and uninhibitedly called people to account. She phoned people at such unusual hours as 5 A.M. to come visit her or to suggest that she visit them. She lost control of her temper and threw a butcher knife at one of her children. She struck a three-year-old nephew and then promised to take out a large life insurance policy on the child because he did not cry. She was too busy to eat properly and too active to sleep at night. Two weeks after the death of her husband, her relatives, puzzled by her potentially dangerous behavior, had her committed to a hospital.

On arrival she was vivacious and animated but very angry at being hospitalized. She drew up a list of people whom she planned to sue and another of people to whom she intended to give a thousand dollars each. She wrote a letter to tell a female friend that she was stupid and was not to visit her again; another to a bachelor whom she had decided to marry; and another to the son of a patient to tell him his mother was not being looked after properly. She told a staff psychiatrist: ''If you send me out of here I'll give you a thousand dollars. You understand I can sue you for anything. I'm not mental and I won't stay here. My children need me. My mother will be frantic. You will have to drive me home. People don't know why I am so happy after my husband died. They can't understand that I have got religion to help me now, whereas others haven't. I've got to get out so that I can plant bulbs on my husband's grave. I don't want anyone else to do it for me. You're a doctor, I can tell you the real reasons for all this. I want to get married again and I want to get everything straightened up before I do. Once you've been married you need the security of marriage. I've gotten well rested now and I'll be able to carry on at home.''

Tranquilizing medication and electric shock therapy resulted in a remission of symptoms sufficient for the patient to be discharged from the hospital after three months. Within ten days she was back in the hospital following a suicidal attempt by an overdose of sleeping pills. She had become depressed over her actions while in the manic state. In the hospital she oscillated between depression and euphoria for several months. After six months her mood stabilized for several weeks and she was again permitted to go home.

Litigation concerning the accident was still pending. Her financial situation deteriorated and she was forced to put up the farm for sale. Her depression returned in a severe form. Early one morning, thirteen months after the death of her husband, she parked her car on a railroad crossing and sat in it until a train came and killed her. The manner in which she chose to commit suicide was obviously an attempt to expiate the guilt she still felt over her husband's death.

INVOLUTIONAL MELANCHOLIA

As mentioned previously, this disorder occurs in the involutional period of life and is charac-

terized by tension, anxiety, agitation and pronounced insomnia. Extreme guilt is typical, as are somatic preoccupations, either of which can reach delusional proportions. There is an absence of previous episodes and, while the patient may be delusional, he fails to show the impairment of thought and association which characterize the schizophrenic.

Involutional melancholia is three times as frequent in women as in men. Its frequency has been increasing in recent decades, perhaps because of the increasing longevity of the general population.

The involutional period is generally considered to range from 40 to 55 years of age in women and 50 to 65 in men. In both sexes the involutional period is characterized by a number of potentially stressful biological and psychological changes. In women, the menopause may bring with it a feeling of uselessness, and the decline in physical attractiveness may lower self-esteem. In men, a loss of self-esteem may result from occupational frustrations or a diminution of sexual potency. Both sexes usually experience a decline in health, strength and intellectual capability, particularly in intellectual tasks that require speed. Women may feel superfluous after their children have grown up and left home, and men after retirement. Involutional melancholics typically have no hobbies or outside interests to absorb them when their major occupations are no longer available. Fear of death is common in the involutional period; the individual may be oppressed by the thought that time is short, that he has achieved little and can no longer look forward to future achievement. The involutional period calls for new adjustments if the individual is to avoid psychological disorder, but he may be too rigid and compulsive to change. He feels that he has failed, is overcome by an intropunitive conviction that he must have deserved to fail, and sinks into a depression. The more rigid, narrow and intropunitive the pre-illness personality of an involutional melancholic, the less likely the patient is to recover fully.

The following case illustrates some aspects of involutional melancholia:

A 53-year-old woman was admitted to a state hospital after several weeks of worry over financial difficulties and loss of ability to eat and sleep. She paced about restlessly day and night, convinced that she had done something dreadful. Efforts by relatives to talk her out of this delusion failed.

The patient was the fourth of six children. Her father had been subject to episodes of mild depression, but there was no history of severe psychopathology in the family. She grew up in marginal economic circumstances and married a farmer at the age of 19. When she was 39 her husband developed tuberculosis which gradually worsened. For three years prior to her breakdown he had been in a sanatorium while she remained home with two sons who successfully worked the farm.

The patient's older son described her as over-conscientious and a meticulous housekeeper who hated dirt and disorder. Her only interests were home and church. On the very morning of her admission to the hospital she was up at 6 o'clock to cook breakfast for her sons. She always found something to worry about and for as long as her sons could remember she had had episodes lasting a few days at a time in which she felt low in spirits, but she had never had a major attack of depression.

In the hospital she was completely careless of her appearance. Her hair and clothing were untidy and she used no cosmetics. She paced about restlessly or sat motionless in an attitude of dejection. Her facial expression was one of constant misery and she periodically moaned. From time to time she wrung her hands, pulled her fingers, examined her nails and picked and scratched at her clothing. She frequently failed to respond to questions about herself, her family, the time and the place. At other times she answered, "I don't know" and then remarked, "Something went wrong with my head. I don't seem to remember at all. I can't tell you what. There is something wrong with my head. I don't remember."

Within a few days her confusion disappeared, indicating that she did not have brain damage. She began to answer questions appropriately, but her dejection and the delusion that her family was in financial straits persisted. "I just realized what I have done," she said. "I did something I shouldn't have. I made the boys lose the place on account of my worrying. I guess it's too late to do anything about it now." She felt she was worthless and that the future was completely bleak and hopeless.

The patient was given 12 ECT's. A marked improvement in mood and activity level resulted and she was able to return to the farm three months after admission. Follow-up interviews during the next two years indicated no recurrence of symptoms.

THE CAUSATION OF AFFECTIVE DISORDERS

Heredity

The results of a number of twin studies of manic-depression are summarized in Table 11–1. The estimates of concordance have varied from 57 to 100 per cent for monozygotic twins and from 15 to 38 per cent for dizygotic twins. The index of heritability (H) computed from these figures as a measure of the significance of heredity in determining predisposition to manic-depressive psychosis varies from 39 per cent (Slater's data) to 100 per cent (Kallmann's data). Slater's study is based on a very small sample. In the studies based on larger samples, H varies from 60 to 100 per cent. We may conclude from the data that a genetic factor is present in manic-depression, but its precise importance is obscured by variation in the results as well as methodological flaws inherent in most twin studies.

Estimates by various investigators of the frequency of manic-depressive psychosis among relatives of manic-depressive patients are shown in Table 11–2. The estimates vary markedly within each class of relatives, but the average estimate for each class is sizable.

For involutional melancholia, the major findings come from a study by Kallmann (1950)

TABLE 11–1. Estimated Concordance Rates in Monozygotic and Dizygotic Co-twins of Manic-depressive Twins

Investigator	Apparent Zygosity of Twins	Number of Pairs	Estimated Concordance Rate (Per Cent)	Heritability
Rosanoff et al., 1935	MZ	23	70	0.64
	DZ	67	16	
Luxenburger, 1942 (cited by Gedda, 1951)	MZ	56	84	0.81
	DZ	83	15	
Kallmann, 1953	MZ	27	100*	1.00
	DZ	58	26*	
Slater, 1953	MZ	8	57*	0.39
	DZ	30	29*	
Da Fonseca, 1959	MZ	21	75	0.60
	DZ	39	38	

*Corrected for age.
Modified after Shields, J., and Slater, E. Heredity and psychological abnormality. In Eysenck, H. J. (Editor). 1960. Handbook of Abnormal Psychology. London, Pitman Medical Publishing Co., p. 326.

TABLE 11–2. Expectancy (Per Cent) of Manic-Depressive Disorders Among Relatives of Manic-Depressive Probands

Investigator	Parents	Sibs	Children
Banse, 1929	10.8	18.1	
Röll and Entres 1936	13.0		10.7
Slater, 1938	15.5		15.2
Strömgren, 1938	7.5	10.7	
Sjögren, 1948	7.0	3.6	
Kallmann, 1950	23.4	23.0	
		26.3*	
Stenstedt, 1952	7.4	12.3	9.4

*Dizygotic twins.
Modified after Shields, J., and Slater, E. Heredity and psychological abnormality. *In* Eysenck, H. J. (Editor). 1960. Handbook of Abnormal Psychology. London, Pitman Medical Publishing Co., p. 306.

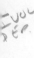

of 29 pairs of monozygotic twins and 67 pairs of dizygotic twins. The concordance rate among monozygotic twins was 61 per cent and among dizygotic twins 6 per cent. These figures yield a heritable component (H) of 58 per cent. Kallmann also reported that 6 per cent of both the parents and siblings of affected individuals suffered from involutional psychoses. A striking finding was that fewer than 1 per cent of the involutional patients' parents and siblings had a history of manic-depressive psychoses, but more than 4 per cent were schizophrenic. Kallmann therefore concluded that melancholia is genetically related to schizophrenia rather than manic-depression. In our present state of knowledge, however, this conclusion must be regarded as speculative.

In summary, the twin and family data for affective disorders constitute strong evidence for some form of hereditary predisposition. In some of the studies, the concordance rates for twins and the observed frequencies for siblings and parents are higher than the corresponding figures for the twin and family studies of schizophrenia. However, in genetic studies of schizophrenia the samples have been larger and the results more consistent than in the studies of the affective disorders. It is therefore doubtful whether a stronger case for hereditary predisposition can be made for the affective disorders than for schizophrenia.

Other Biological Determinants

A great variety of bodily dysfunctions may act as precipitating stresses and lead to the development of affective disorders. The expression "seeing things through jaundiced eyes" implies that jaundice is accompanied by depression; in actual fact, depression is frequently associated with jaundice, mononucleosis and various other physical disorders. In postpartum depression, hormonal changes as well as physical exhaustion may play a role. It should be added that psychological factors such as resentment of the responsibilities involved in motherhood are at least as important as the biological factors. Hormonal changes associated with the menopause have also been suspected of being important in the development of involutional reactions. At times, illness and other physical stresses result in euphoria, apparently as a defense against depression. For example, manic attacks have been observed to occur immediately after the onset of bodily disorders such as blindness or cancer.

The mechanism by which bodily dysfunctions precipitate affective disorders may be primarily biological or primarily psychological; that is, the disorder may result from the disturbed physiology itself or from the emotional impact of loss of health, loss of earning power or anticipation of death. In practice, psychological stress is nearly always the more important factor. It is known, however, that apparently for biological reasons excessive doses of certain hormones (cortisone from the adrenal cortex and adrenocorticotropic hormone [ACTH] from the pituitary gland) and of some sedative and tranquilizing drugs result in affective disturbances. A fascinating account of a manic episode precipitated by cortisone was written by Roueché (1954) under the title "Ten Feet Tall." However, even these agents do not invariably produce an affective disorder for individual predisposition has a considerable influence.

Attempts to demonstrate a constitutional predisposition to affective disorders date back more than two thousand years. Burton's *Anatomy of Melancholy* refers to Democritus' dissection of various animals in the hope that he would find evidence of the bile which he assumed was responsible for his own melancholy temperament. Kretschmer associated a pyknic physique with manic-depression; Sheldon correlates the endomorphic component with a tendency to affective symptomatology.

A variety of physiological correlates of affective disorders have also been reported in recent years. Unfortunately, the studies on which these reports are based tend to have little or no connection with each other and therefore do not provide a basis for a consistent theory. To cite a few of the studies, Funkenstein (1954) reported that depression is associated with excessive section of epinephrine (produced in the adrenal glands), whereas externally directed anger is associated with the secretion of norepinephrine (a somewhat different substance also produced in the adrenal glands). Of course, this finding is correlational rather than causal. Shagass (1957) reported that following intermittent stimulation by light flashes and also following the administration of an intravenous sedative drug, changes occurred in the EEG of depressed persons but not in nondepressed controls. The implication is that in some unknown manner depressives are biologically different from nondepressives. Kaplan (1960) presented evidence that both visual sensitivity to color stimuli and the after-images of color differ in depressed patients and normals. Kaplan's results imply that vision in depressives is not adequately regulated by the nervous system; possibly other functions are also poorly regulated in depressives.

An interesting correlational study by Shinfuku et al. (1959) investigated the body changes associated with the mood swings of a manic-depressive patient over a five-year period. The patient, a woman in her fifties, had a regular 21-day cycle of manic overactivity alternating with depressive stupor. The manic phase was characterized by excessive urination, deficiency of a type of cells in the blood known as eosinophil cells, low blood pressure, and a high level of the female hormone known as estrogen. In contrast, the depressive phase was characterized by diminished urination, an excess of eosinophil cells, high blood pressure and a low estrogen level. In both the manic and depressed phases there was an excess of cholesterol in the blood, but it was much higher in the depressed phase.

Studies and observations such as those just reported are representative of the biological investigations of affective disorders. As yet it has not been possible to combine them into a consistent and meaningful structure.

Psychological Determinants

Three psychoanalysts—Sigmund Freud, Karl Abraham and Sandor Rado—have contributed a great deal toward understanding the psychology of manic-depression. Freud (1917) analyzed the self-reproaches of depressed patients and found that they made sense if the name of an ambivalently regarded person was substituted for the patient's own name. The depressed individual says, "I am evil because I am a liar," but he means, "X is evil because he is a liar" or "I am angry with X because he lied to me." In other words, the depressive *introjects* an ambivalently loved person who is the true focus of the anger that he expresses against himself.

The mechanism of introjection is evident in a case report by Nemiah (1961) of a 37-year-old unmarried female patient who had become extremely dependent on a kindly and supportive psychiatrist. Unfortunately the psychiatrist had to move permanently to another city. The patient reacted with panic, loneliness, depression and desperation. The intensity of her introjection is manifest in the following words:

> Sometimes I start crying. I call for Dr. Jones and then I feel as though he's real near to me . . . close to me . . . beside me . . . almost as though he's right inside me. This is what I feel. . . . It's as though when I call him, I get ahold of him and that he won't run away from me again. . . . I get closer to him and I really cry it out and I feel as if I've got him so close—right inside. (To demonstrate, the patient grabbed at an imaginary object in front of her and pulled it toward her, pressing her clenched fists vigorously against her sternum.) These are the thoughts that are really coming to me as we talk, because I don't know how to feel or express it. . . . But it's like I've finally caught him again . . . as if I'd brought him back to me.

Freud also stressed the fact that the depressive has a dominant and punitive superego, for the source of his reproaches against the introjected figure is his own superego. The ego of the manic-depressive, like that of the neurotic, lacks the strength to cope with the pressures of his own moral standards.

Abraham (1927) provided clinical evidence to support Freud's conception of introjection in manic-depression. For example, he described a patient who delusively accused herself of being a thief after her father had been arrested for theft. She had loved him, but his arrest had estranged her from him psychologically as well as physically. She thereupon introjected his image and began to experience delusional self-reproaches. Abraham also went further than Freud with the dynamics of manic-depression and hypothesized that behind every adult depression there was a forgotten childhood depression. Furthermore, all depressives were basically oral individuals who needed more love and affection than they received. Abraham thought that the source of this fundamental orality was constitutional.

Rado's approach (1954) emphasizes the hostility behind the patient's guilty reproaches. His theory is well expressed in the following quotation:*

We interpret it [depression] as a particular form of emergency dyscontrol. The patient has suffered a severe loss, or in any case, behaves as if he has suffered one. His emotional reaction to this actual or presumed emergency is overwhelming and threatens to destroy his capacity for adaptive control. At first he is torn between coercive rage and guilty fear, which drive him in opposite directions. Then his mounting guilty fear gains the upper hand. It splits his defeated coercive rage into two unequal parts that undergo different vicissitudes. The smaller part—the stubborn core—is forced underground. There it remains what it was, coercive rage directed against the environment. The larger part of defeated rage escapes repression because its flexibility permits its assimilation to the now prevailing pattern of guilty fear. This portion of defeated rage is turned against the patient himself and is vented in remorseful bouts of self-reproach. Though such self-punishment from retroflexed rage is excruciatingly painful, the patient's remorse is but a facade. Beneath this facade he has utmost contempt for himself because of his inability to live up to his expectations. Bitter with wounded pride, he thus punishes himself—not in contrition—but for his failure to gain his coercive ends. This deeply hidden meaning of self-punishment from retroflexed rage makes mockery of the patient's remorse and reveals the real root of his sense of unworthiness.

The emotional storm deprives the patient of his capacity for mature life performance. Subjectively, he is reduced from a self-reliant adult to a frightened and helpless child. The patient's adaptive degradation—a consequence of his loss of self-confidence—is our decisive clue to the understanding of his depressive spell. He senses in the present emergency a threat of starvation and responds to it by reproducing the hungry infant's cry for his mother's help. But the patient's situation, as compared with that of the hungry infant, is complicated by his guilty fear. Excessive guilty fear, heightened by retroflexed rage, forces him into expiation. Thus, it is by means of punishing himself that he hopes to regain his mother, her loving care, and above all, her feeding breast. . . .

A large range of *psychological precipitants* may trigger this reaction of remorse and rage, or there may be no identifiable precipitant at all. Kraepelin (1921) cites the case of a woman who became depressed three times in her life—

after the deaths of her husband, dog and dove. Obviously, her predisposition to depression was so strong that the mildest of precipitants had as much effect as the most severe. Travis (1933) studied 70 patients with manic-depressive psychoses and found that the precipitating factors fell into seven main categories: marital maladjustment; death in the family; childbirth; physical condition; economic stress; antagonism toward parents; and illness in the family. In a more recent study, Bruhn (1962) compared the histories of 91 persons who attempted suicide with those of 91 nonsuicidal psychiatric outpatients. In the year immediately prior to the study, there was a greater prevalence of absence or death of a family member, unemployment of the family breadwinner, residential mobility and marital disharmony among the suicidal patients than among the controls. Of course, marital disharmony may be a symptom or effect of affective disorder as well as a cause; during a manic episode, for example, an individual may make an impulsive decision regarding marriage or divorce, or his spouse may initiate divorce proceedings because of his behavior.

Among the *predisposing psychological determinants* of affective disorders is oral deprivation. As mentioned earlier, oral deprivation in infancy has been linked to adult pessimism, clinging dependence and impatience. Goldman-Eisler (1953) reported that lateness of weaning correlated negatively with ratings of pessimism in later life. *later the weaning the higher the pessam*

A parent is a potential source of a child's later depression, both as a source of oral deprivation and as a superego model. Rado (1928) theorized that depression is in part an unconscious attempt to win love and forgiveness from the parents (i.e., from the introjected image of the parents in the patient's superego). The superego reproduces the punishments received in childhood and the patient behaves as if he anticipates being punished by his parents again. His self-punishment is an effort to earn parental (superego) forgiveness.

Parental deprivation in childhood is another important predisposing variable. Brown (1961) presented statistical evidence that early loss by death of both father and mother was much more frequent for depressed patients than for nonpsychiatric control groups. Forty-one per cent of depressive patients had lost a parent before the age of 15 as compared with fewer than 20 per cent of the controls. The effect of parental deprivation was interpreted by Brown,

---

*Reprinted by permission from Rado, S. 1954. Hedonic control, action-self and the depressive spell. *In* Hoch, P. H., and Zubin, J. (Editors). Depression. New York, Grune & Stratton, Inc.

Epps and McGlashan (1961) as follows: "Our hypothesis is that a child can be sensitized by situations of loss of love and emotional deprivation so that he breaks down in various ways in later life when faced with subsequent situations of loss and rejection." In the study of suicidal and nonsuicidal patients referred to earlier, Bruhn found a higher frequency of parental deprivation in childhood among the individuals who later attempted suicide. Forty-two per cent of the attempted suicides came from homes broken by the loss of one or both parents before the patient was 15 years old, as compared to 25 per cent for the nonsuicidal controls. Further, in the year immediately preceding the study, a prolonged absence or death in the family occurred in 66 per cent of the subgroup of attempted suicides who came from broken homes, as compared with 22 per cent among nonsuicidal patients from broken homes. The data thus suggest that a traumatic experience of loss in childhood and a repetition of the loss years later contribute heavily to suicidal attempts. Early deprivation makes the individual vulnerable to later loss.

Cohen et al. (1954) intensively investigated the family backgrounds of 12 manic-depressive patients and reported that the families had been set apart from their environments by one or another factor such as minority status, economic difficulties or aberrant behavior in a member of the family. The families attempted to counteract the resultant social isolation by placing a high premium on conformity and making a prodigious effort to raise their economic positions. As a result of these pressures and strivings, the status of the family was given prime importance and individual family members became merely instruments for achieving prestige. The need for winning prestige was usually inculcated by the mother. She tended to be the dominant parent and was regarded by the children as strong and reliable but cold and unlovable. By contrast, the father was perceived as weak but lovable. The mother blamed the father for the family's social failure and he accepted the blame; the children found themselves in the dilemma of believing that they should strive for the goals set by the disliked mother and avoid becoming like the loved father. The mother had found the complete dependency of the infant in his first year pleasurable, but she turned harsh and punitive as the child became increasingly independent and rebellious. Further, as a child the manic-depressive patient was likely to have occupied a special position in the family as the eldest or only son, or as the sibling who worked the hardest. He was envied by his siblings but was unaware of the envy and he sacrificed his personal desires for the sake of the family. He became lonely, isolated and predisposed to depression because he was not valued for his own sake.

Since these conclusions were based on only 12 patients with no control group, Gibson (1958) used a technique that differed from that of the previous study to investigate the 12 patients a second time, and, in addition, to study a group of manic-depressives with a control group of schizophrenics. In general, his results were consistent with those of the previous study: the two manic-depressive groups were very similar to each other in family background and differed from the schizophrenics in having been subjected to greater family pressure toward acquisition of prestige and, also, to a greater degree of sibling envy. The mothers of manic-depressives were more reliable than the fathers, a family constellation not true for schizophrenics. (In one major respect the second study did not bear out the first: the prestige strivings of the second manic-depressive group did not emerge from social isolation but from the personality makeup of the parents.) However, Gibson's study suffered from a serious methodological weakness: he obtained the additional manic-depressive group by taking 120 consecutive hospital admissions diagnosed manic-depressive and then eliminating all but 27 of them on the grounds that for the rejected patients the diagnosis was not certain enough or reliable information concerning family background was not available. The likelihood of selective bias in eliminating patients on so large a scale is very strong. Further studies are needed in which the danger of bias in selection will be avoided.

Support for some of Gibson's conclusions, nevertheless, seems to be provided in a study by Becker (1960) and another by Becker, Spielberger and Parker (1963). The first study found that manic-depressives, as compared to nonpsychiatric controls, are more ambitious, more authoritarian and more prone to believe that both parent-child and husband-wife relationships should be autocratic. The second study found that manic-depressives exceed neurotic depressives and schizophrenics on the same variables. (The latter two groups, in turn, had higher scores on the variables than nonpatients.) The results were consistent with the belief that manic-depressives emphasize prestige striving and are characterized by strong and rigid superegos formed by introjection of parental attitudes.

Clinical impressions indicate that the childhood interpersonal relationships of manic-depressives are almost invariably disturbed, *but the disturbance is not consistent from patient to patient.* In many cases maternal deprivation and pressures to conformity are present, as stressed in Cohen's study. In others, a warm and satisfactory relationship with both parents is interrupted by the loss of a parent, usually the father. In still others, the father is absent much of the time or is psychologically distant and cold. (The latter, however, appears more frequently in the background of schizophrenic patients.) Alternatively, the father may have episodes of depression in which he is incapacitated and inaccessible; there are many cases in which relationships with parents show a marked fluctuation associated with parental mood swings.

Apart from relationships with parents, it is the impression of most clinicians that the manic-depressive's childhood is marked by activity, extraversion and cyclothymic mood swings. However, this childhood portrait is not invariable. In fact, a study by Kohn and Clausen (1955) had a surprising outcome: as high a proportion of manic-depressives as schizophrenics were found to have been socially isolated in early adolescence. In both groups the proportion of isolates was close to one-third; for a normal control group it was almost zero. These results are not consistent with the prevalent assumption that in their younger years manic-depressives are invariably extraverted and schizophrenics are predominantly introverted and isolated. For the results to be consistent with this assumption, the proportion of isolates among manic-depressives should have been close to zero and the proportion among schizophrenics should have been well over one half. Kohn and Clausen suggest that a crucial variable in some cases of *both* manic-depression and schizophrenia is a feeling of alienation from one's peers which may or may not lead to social isolation.

In contrast to manic-depressives, the prepsychotic personality of involutional melancholics is commonly believed to be marked by shyness and introversion, and also by obsessive and perfectionistic concern over adherence to standards of conscience. There is a dearth of objective data to support this belief, but it is consistent with many clinical impressions.

Sociocultural Determinants

It is generally agreed that suicide, which, as we have seen, is closely related to affective disorders, is less frequent among primitive tribes than among civilized communities. However, it should be recognized that death may be self-induced even when it results from behavior not ordinarily considered suicidal. An individual in a primitive culture who runs amok and attacks others has turned his aggression outward rather than inward, yet he is effectively committing suicide, since he knows that the inevitable consequence for him is death at the hands of the tribe. Within nonprimitive cultures, closed communities—e.g., the Hutterites—have a very low frequency of suicide. The more open the culture, the higher the suicide rate. In Figure 11–3 the suicide rates for selected countries of western civilization are presented.

In our own society, suicide and homicide both increase in times of economic distress and unemployment, and both are committed far more often by males than females, but the relation between suicide and homicide is inverse with respect to a number of other variables. Suicide is more frequent in peace than in war, among whites than nonwhites, among older persons than younger, in higher socioeconomic levels than lower, and among persons with high rather than low I.Q.'s. Homicide is more often committed in war time, by nonwhites and individuals who are young, low in socioeconomic level, and low in I.Q. Finally for males, the suicide rate increases progressively throughout life, reaching its peak in the very oldest age group, but for females it reaches a peak at 45 to 65 and then declines. It is clear from these data that sociocultural and biological factors both influence suicide and presumably also the affective disorders correlated with suicide.

Sociocultural factors such as family living patterns, job stability and ethnic group membership have been causally related to the incidence of suicide and depression. Tuckman and Connor (1962), after the study of 100 consecutive attempted suicides by persons under the age of 18, concluded that family disorganization and delinquency were often related to suicide attempts by adolescents and children. After studying cases of 103 white male suicides between the ages of 20 and 60, Breed (1963) found

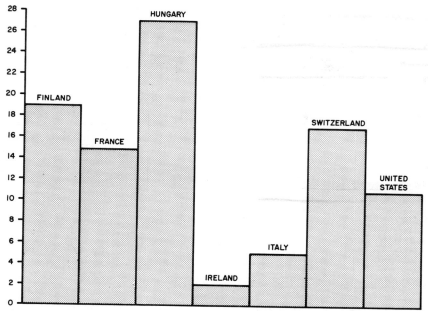

Figure 11–3. *Suicide rates per 100,000 persons for selected countries of western civilization.*

a very high incidence of downward work mobility, reduced income and unemployment. Those social factors which contribute to family disruptions and work interference are thus clearly related to the incidence of suicide, and further study is needed to define more precisely the nature of the factors involved.

Apart from the data for suicide, the importance of sociocultural factors in affective disorders is reflected in studies comparing different time periods, cross-cultural studies and studies of single sociocultural variables. There has apparently been a decrease of severe forms of manic-depression in the United States over the last few decades. The decrease undoubtedly reflects both increased usage of the diagnostic label "schizo-affective" and the trend toward earlier and more effective treatment, but it may also be a consequence of cultural changes. Arieti (1959) has speculated that an inner-directed culture—with its stress on duty, hard work, and guilt as a penalty for failure—conduces to manic-depression, whereas an outer-directed culture conduces to other difficulties. If this hypothesis is correct, the decrease in manic-depression is explainable as a consequence of the progressive shift in our culture from inner- to outer-directedness.

Cross-cultural studies have reported high frequencies of manic-depression in Mediterranean countries, Ireland and the Fiji Islands, and low frequencies in Oriental countries where Buddhism and Hinduism prevail. (In the latter countries, schizophrenia seems to be frequent.) For the year 1959, the first-admission rates for manic-depression were twice as high in Italy as in the United States, but the rates for schizophrenia were twice as high in the United States as in Italy. Of course, first-admission rates are subject to many influences other than true incidence, but it is the impression of professional persons who have an intimate knowledge of mental disorders in the two countries that the *difference* in rates corresponds to a real difference in incidence.

There is at least one striking exception to the generalization that suicide and affective disorders are correlated: although the Hutterites have a low frequency of suicide, they have a higher frequency of depression than any of nine other groups with whom they were compared in a study by Eaton and Weil (1955). The investigators attributed the depressive tendency of the Hutterites to the emphasis of their value system on duty, guilt, and internalized rather than externalized aggression.

Studies of single sociocultural variables have reported higher frequencies of manic-depression among Negroes than whites, immigrants than native-born, and populations defeated in war than victorious populations. Unemployment is a

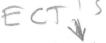

precipitating factor, just as in suicide. During the economically depressed year of 1933 in New York State, loss of employment or financial worth was an apparent precipitant for 26 per cent of first admissions diagnosed manic-depressive but for only 10 per cent of first admissions diagnosed schizophrenic. In contrast with the clear-cut relation of manic-depression to minority status, outcome of war and unemployment, it is not certain how the disorder is related to neighborhood disorganization and socioeconomic membership. Faris and Dunham (1939) found that manic-depressive psychoses were randomly distributed across well-organized and disorganized neighborhoods, in contrast with the concentration of schizophrenia in disorganized neighborhoods. Some subsequent studies have suggested that the frequency of manic-depressive psychoses is positively correlated with socioeconomic status, in direct contrast with schizophrenia. However, Hollingshead and Redlich (1958) reported a higher frequency of affective *neuroses* in the upper classes and of affective *psychoses* in the lower classes. Further research on socioeconomic variables and manic-depression is needed to clarify the issue.

TREATMENT AND PROGNOSIS

The treatment of affective disorders may be directed toward remission of a current episode or prevention of future recurrences. It may consist of drug therapy, other somatic therapies, psychotherapy and milieu therapy (environmental manipulation).

Chlorpromazine and other tranquilizing drugs that have been found effective in the treatment of schizophrenia are ineffective for most depressive patients or may even accentuate their symptoms. The psychomotor overactivity of the manic, on the other hand, is considerably reduced by tranquilizers. A number of antidepressive drugs have been developed that hold considerable promise, particularly for retarded depressives. The drugs diminish apathy and apparently speed remissions. Among the most widely used of these drugs are Tofranil, Elavil and Parnate. In the agitated type of depression, a combination of tranquilizing and anti-depressive drugs is sometimes useful.

Many psychiatrists consider electroconvulsive therapy to be the most consistently effective method of treatment for producing remission in psychotic depression, either of the manic-

depressive or the involutional variety. Approximately 90 per cent of severe depressives improve dramatically in less than one month of ECT. Usually six to twelve treatments are administered over a period of two to four weeks. Manic episodes may also be shortened by ECT, but the manic patient is likely to require a longer series of treatments than the depressive, and many manics who improve during treatments relapse immediately afterwards. In some hospitals, ECT is used only when an affective disorder has proved resistant to drugs; in others it is preferred to drugs.

As usually employed, drugs and ECT bring about remission of symptoms but do not diminish future recurrences. For the latter purpose, long-term medication, maintenance ECT, and psychotherapy are sometimes employed. In long-term medication drugs are administered to the patient on an outpatient basis after he is discharged from the hospital. Maintenance ECT consists of one treatment per week or even as few as one per month after remission; the widely spaced treatments tend to maintain the patient's functioning at an improved level. Obviously, the success of either long-term medication or maintenance ECT depends on the patient's continuing cooperation.

Psychotherapy is usually considered the ideal method of diminishing the probability of recurrence, but a great many affective patients are not amenable to intensive psychotherapy. During a depression of psychotic proportions the patient cannot be "reached": he does not communicate well and his anxiety level is too high for him to benefit from a therapeutic relationship. Similarly, intensive psychotherapy during a manic episode is likely to be ineffective; as threatening material is uncovered, the patient's anxiety may be increased and he is likely to defend himself by becoming more manic than ever. Because of these difficulties, it is often best to undertake psychotherapy only after remission of the more acute symptoms. In addition, attempts are sometimes made in the quiescent phase to improve the patient's environment by removing external causes that exacerbate his disturbance.

For the majority of manic-depressives and involutional psychotics, little or no attempt is made in current clinical practice to modify the emotional basis of their disturbances and thus reduce the likelihood of recurrence. They are treated by one or another means intended solely to bring about a remission. Not many years ago no method was known to produce rapid remis-

TABLE 11–3. Suicide Rate per 1000 Population Among 3800 Attempted Suicides, by High- and Low-Risk Categories of Risk-Related Factors*

Factor	High-Risk Category	Suicide Rate	Low-Risk Category	Suicide Rate
Age	45 years of age and older	24.0	Under 45 years of age	9.4
Sex	Male	19.9	Female	9.2
Race	White	14.3	Nonwhite	8.7
Marital status	Separated, divorced, widowed	12.5	Single, married	8.6
Living Arrangements	Alone	48.4	With others	10.1
Employment status	Unemployed, retired	16.8	Employed	14.3
Physical health	Poor (acute or chronic condition in the 6-month period preceding the attempt	14.0	Good	12.4
Mental condition	Nervous or mental disorder, mood or behavioral symptoms including alcoholism	19.1	Presumably normal, including brief situational reactions	7.2
Medical care (within 6 months)	Yes	16.4	No	10.8
Method	Hanging, firearms, jumping, drowning	28.4	Cutting or piercing, gas or carbon monoxide, poison, combination of other methods, other	12.0
Season	Warm months (April–September)	14.2	Cold months (October–March)	10.9
Time of day	6:00 AM–5:59 PM	15.1	6:00 PM–5:59 AM	10.5
Where attempt was made	Own or someone's home	14.3	Other type of premises, outdoors	11.9
Time interval between attempt and discovery	Almost immediately, reported by person making attempt	10.9	Later	7.2
Intent to kill (self-report)	No	14.5	Yes	8.5
Suicide note	Yes	16.7	No	12.3
Previous attempt or threat	Yes	25.2	No	11.0

*Reproduced by permission from Tuckman, J. and Youngman, W. 1968. A scale for assessing suicide risks of attempted suicides. J. Clin. Psychol. 24:17–19.

sions. Today we have largely solved this problem but not that of preventing recurrences.

Suicide Prevention. It has been increasingly recognized in recent years that many suicides can be prevented. Appreciation of this fact has led to the establishment of a national Center for Studies of Suicide Prevention whose mission is to catalyze suicide prevention activities in this country. In 1968 there were 40 functioning, local suicide prevention centers in 17 states. These centers operate on the assumption that many persons who are contemplating suicide remain ambivalent about the actual act until almost the final moment. If given an easy opportunity to discuss their problem with a skilled listener, many will take advantage of it and be dissuaded from killing themselves.

The typical suicide prevention center is staffed by mental health professionals plus a number of carefully selected and trained lay volunteers to help man the telephones. The number is generally listed with other emergency numbers in the telephone book and is also widely known by persons in emergency-prone situations, such as telephone operators, police and the like. Calls may be made by the suicidal patient or by friends or relatives.

The person taking the call attempts to establish rapport quickly, to focus on the patient's desire to live rather than on his hopeless despair, to evaluate the seriousness of the risk posed and to make appropriate immediate referral for more sustained help. Research has shown that suicide potential can be determined rather quickly even from information obtained in a friendly, accepting telephone conversation. Table 11–3 lists those factors associated with higher and lower risk. Thus, a call from a 48-year-old single, white male with a history of previous suicide attempts and a loaded pistol in his possession constitutes a much greater risk than a call from a young married woman who feels discouraged and thinks vaguely of ending it all but has no definite plans. After evaluating the risk, the stress the caller is under, his life style, and whether or not he has a definite plan, the staff member attempts to intervene, to offer some hope, and to try to reestablish a source of continued emotional support through appropriate referral.

It is not known how effective such centers are in an absolute sense. The largest suicide prevention center, which is in Los Angeles, receives calls from more than 500 persons per month. Of these calls fully 99 per cent are sincere appeals for help. One third of the callers are people who are distressed but far from an actual suicide attempt. However, at least 10 per cent of all calls are made by persons moderately to seriously suicidal, and of these one in six is on the verge of death.

Some suicidal persons are dissuaded from making an attempt after a single phone call. Others respond to the renewed interest and attention of friends and relatives whom they had perceived as uncaring. For the majority, counseling, psychotherapy or hospitalization may be required.

The widespread acceptance and utilization of suicide prevention centers make this movement one of the more significant innovations which modern society has devised to meet the challenge of emotional breakdown.

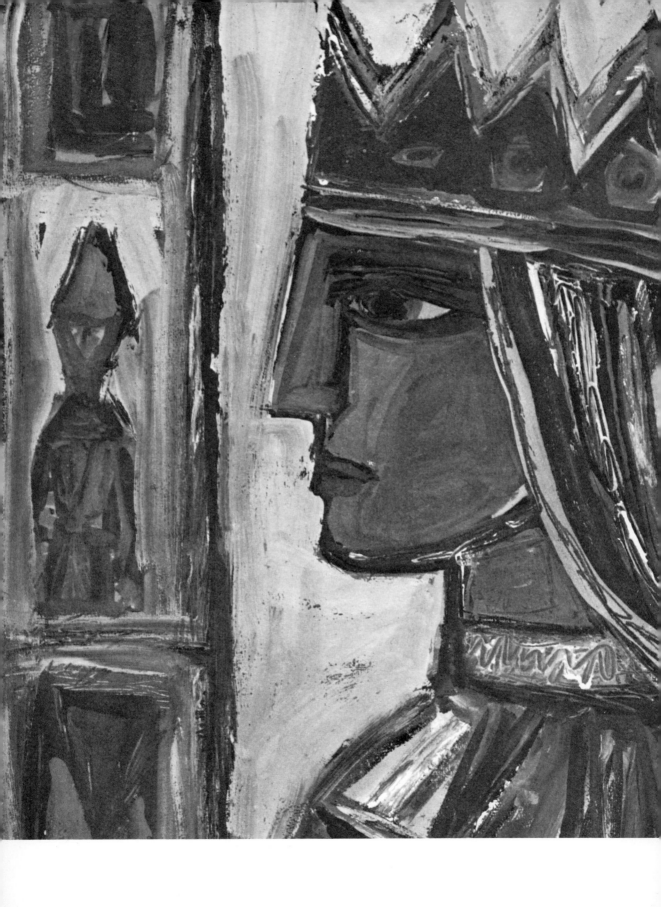

Babylon in all its desolation is a sight not so awful
as that of the human mind in ruins.

Scrope Davies, *Letters to Thomas Raikes* 12

SCHIZOPHRENIA

— apathic withdraw

Stoneface, lability lacking, inappropriate affect, ambivalence, cognitive slippage.

1 % of pop
1890 — 1st
48% — resident patients
2/3 of Males — single

MOREL
KRAEPLIN

Among psychiatric disorders, schizophrenia is one of the most interesting, yet baffling. It is manifested in a bewildering variety of subtypes and an ever greater variety of symptoms within most of the subtypes. A tremendous amount of research has led to many explanatory hypotheses, yet the ultimate nature and causation of schizophrenia still remain matters of dispute.

The frequency of schizophrenia is relatively high. Current estimates indicate that in the United States and a number of European countries the lifetime expectancy of schizophrenia is approximately 1 per cent of the general population. In all public hospitals in the United States in 1968, 18.0 per cent of first admissions and 48.8 per cent of resident patients were diagnozed schizophrenic reaction. The total number of schizophrenic resident patients was 165,837. The resident rate is more than twice the first-admission rate because, *on the average,* schizophrenia is a chronic, long-lasting disorder. The median age of the first admissions was 33.4 years; for the resident patients it was 50.3. Males and females are equally vulnerable. The rates for single and divorced persons are far higher than for married persons, especially for males: roughly two-thirds of male schizophrenics are single at the time of first admission to a hospital.

The term "schizophrenia" is a comparatively recent one. In 1860, the Belgian psychiatrist Morel reported a case of progressive deterioration of intellect and personality in a 14-year-old boy. The boy had been an excellent student, previously, but seemed to have become stupid. He forgot what he had learned, withdrew into himself and was preoccupied with morbid fantasies. Morel coined the term *démence précoce* (premature dementia, i.e., dementia occurring at an unexpectedly early age) to describe the pathological process. Over the ensuing three decades, the terms *dementia paranoides* (paranoid dementia), *hebephrenia* and *catatonia* were introduced by various investigators to designate different forms of gross disorganization of personality. In 1896, the German psychiatrist Kraepelin introduced the term *dementia praecox,* the equivalent of Morel's démence précoce, to include paranoid dementia, hebephrenia and catatonia; later he also included the subcategory of *dementia praecox simplex* (simple dementia).

deterioration — young — occurred early in youth.

THE PRIMARY SYMPTOMS OF SCHIZOPHRENIA

Kraepelin considered the common denominators of the four syndromes to be early onset and progression to permanent and irrecoverable dementia. However, the Swiss psychiatrist Eugen Bleuler (1911) pointed out that in many cases neither early onset nor irrecoverable intellectual deterioration occurred, so that the terms "dementia" and "praecox" were both inaccurate. It is now known that onset of the

213

[handwritten: 15–45]
[handwritten: BLEULER]
[handwritten: Shitz can occur anytime not just (praecot) young.]

reaction may occur anywhere from childhood to later middle age; in the majority of cases the age of onset is between 15 and 45. Bleuler coined the term schizophrenia to embrace Kraepelin's four dementia praecox syndromes.

Literally, schizophrenia means "splitting of the mind." It is a popular misconception that schizophrenia consists of a split or multiple personality; in actual fact, multiple personality is a rare manifestation of a neurotic dissociative reaction. The schizophrenic's split is not among alternative personalities but among the various psychological processes within the personality. Bleuler felt that in all four major subdivisions of schizophrenia—*simple, paranoid, catatonic* and *hebephrenic*—the split was manifested in four primary symptoms: (1) loosening of thought associations, (2) autistic withdrawal into a private world of preoccupation with the self, (3) ambivalence toward the environment and (4) inappropriateness of affect.

Many modern experts have disputed the existence of Bleuler's primary symptoms in all schizophrenics and have proposed defining the entity according to different dimensions. Some of these proposals will be discussed subsequently. Nevertheless, the so-called "four A's" are still considered by many to be the cardinal features of schizophrenia, and are still preserved in the standard nomenclature. Usually certain secondary symptoms are also found. The following discussion of the primary symptoms draws heavily on Bleuler's original formulations, since his work provided the basis for the current diagnostic categories and since it is his ideas that are coming under heavy attack by recent investigators, who consider schizophrenia to be not one but several distinct disorders.

Loosening of Associations

To a normal individual, the schizophrenic's thinking often seems bizarre and unpredictable. In one of his early writings, Jung commented: "If a man could walk and talk in his dreams his total behavior would be in no way different from that of a patient with schizophrenia." Although Jung's statement exaggerates, it expresses the unreal and fantasy-like character of schizophrenic thinking with its lack of control and direction. Meehl (1962) describes this type of thinking by the apt phrase "cognitive slippage." The patient sometimes appears to

employ mere fragments of ideas and concepts. He stops in the middle of a thought or blocks in passing from one thought to another or suddenly jumps to an irrelevant idea in the midst of a train of thought. He may combine two unrelated ideas or manifest a poverty of thinking by which he repeats a few simple ideas over and over, to the exclusion of others.

Schizophrenic thinking has been termed *paralogical,* that is, it manifests logical fallacies. Vigotsky (1934) analyzed the thinking of schizophrenics and concluded that in paralogical fashion they tend to identify objects on the basis of identical predicates so that two objects with a common property may be perceived as the same. This is illustrated by the following case:

The girl friend of a schizophrenic patient became pregnant by another man and informed the patient of her pregnancy without mentioning the other man. The patient and the girl had not had intercourse. He concluded that the conception was immaculate, she was the Virgin Mary and he, God. The paralogical structure of his delusion was (1) conception was immaculate for the Virgin Mary; (2) conception was immaculate for his girl friend; (3) the Virgin Mary and his girl must therefore be one and the same; similarly, God and he were the same.

Logical errors such as these are promoted partly by the intellectual inefficiency attendant on the schizophrenic's high level of anxiety, but mostly by his defensive need to avoid certain aspects of reality. The patient just cited had an overriding need to deny that an emotional and sexual relation could possibly exist between his girl friend and another man.

To a greater or lesser extent, the schizophrenic manifests distortions of concept formation. In a fashion somewhat reminiscent of children, mental defectives and individuals with organic brain damage, he has difficulty with abstract concepts. His thinking tends to the concrete and literal. Bleuler cites the example of a patient who was asked, "Is something weighing heavily on your mind?" The patient responded, "Yes. Iron is heavy." The following interpretations of proverbs by different schizophrenic patients illustrate concrete thinking:

A rolling stone gathers no moss:
Response 1: It won't grow any grass.
Response 2: The stone keeps rolling endlessly.

People in glass houses shouldn't throw stones:
Because they'd break the glass.

When the cat's away, the mice will play:
There's nobody to watch the kittens, I mean the mice.

[handwritten at bottom: OVERINCLUSIVENESS— overgeneraliz]

A new broom sweeps clean.
No, it doesn't because the bristles are stiff.

Schizophrenic thinking is sometimes marked by a bizarre and "peculiar" quality rather than concrete imagery. For example, a patient reported that when he was a high-school student he could not make up his mind whether to arrange his books by topic or author; he therefore arranged them by the colors of the spectrum. Bleuler reports the definition of "hay" given by a schizophrenic patient: "a means of maintenance of the cow." The schizophrenic's thinking sometimes appears peculiar because it is overinclusive (Cameron, 1938); that is, the patient is unable to preserve conceptual boundaries so that distantly associated or even totally irrelevant ideas become essential parts of the concept. As a consequence, his thought becomes vague and imprecise. Asked to interpret the proverb, "Still waters run deep," a patient's distant and vague response was, "How deep is the ocean." Overinclusion, vagueness and bizarre expressions often are accompanied by a stilted and pompous manner of expression. The following letter from a hospitalized paranoid schizophrenic to a psychologist on the staff is illustrative. (Spelling and punctuation are unchanged.)

Celestial Bond ass.   Universal American Mills
annum abstracts   Fiscal Progress
            Imperial Scroll

Dear ----,

    It certainly has been an inspiration to have your hand in the enlightenment of the long sought social Debut. The fine things usually present a seemingly inarticulate outlay that requires full time, just to live down, but with your friendship to go with it, I've found a satisfactory schedule & a progressive Par in Modern Cosmopolitan Progress, in every desirable way, essential to peace & Secureity. After I rehabilitate, I may study piano music and I may find further cultivation & refinement on the associated conditions & provisions when little things stick, in the real story in Unity. until that time, Conservation will be the alternative, I don't care to make an influid dedication & disipate time, sentiment & vitality that could be utilized to a civil advantage, eventually in unity & Health. Citizenship looks like a blessing even in an elementary capacity in christ but without christ in any capacity, Interdependence may be vanity and I appreciate your acceptance. liveing with the year around responsibility in Justice is a futile looking job as it is. about the other letter, The car salesman might say Martin was the subject of concern & there might be 1001 cases in 1001 different lights in the 100% Imperial aspect.

                      Love
                      Jr.

On a Christmas card to the psychologist the same patient wrote:

    I am priviledged to write & associate with you in ways. I have a brother that looks quite a bit like you and similaritys in character are crudely the same. I never knew what it meant to have freindship like that until the last log of the old book closed in the fullfillment of the WAR #II dispensational reafirmation, after War II. & it was the #1 conditions that inspired my interest in C.B.A. that was about the same but not quite such an old story. about all I knew about any of it was the (concords & strains) of occasional that rose me up to myself once in a while. Certification in desolation & Innosence & chastity. after last slaudye. I don't feel runtly in spite of LIMITations. I do have this & that. Persent Productive the advent. it'll mean a golden success to me & an encoureagement to others.

                      associated #

    Parenthetically, it may be mentioned that the patient was emotionally and sexually attracted to the psychologist.

    The schizophrenic's speech sometimes darts from idea to idea in a fragmented and disconnected manner. Cameron reports a schizophrenic's response to the question, "Why are you in the hospital?"[*]

    I'm a cut donator, donated by double sacrifice. I get two days for every one. That's known as double sacrifice; in other words, standard cut donator. You know, we considered it. He couldn't have anything for the cut, or for these patients. All of them are double sacrifice because it's unlawful for it to be donated any more. (Well, what do you do here?) I do what is known as the double criminal treatment. Something that he badly wanted, he gets that, and seven days' criminal protection. That's all he gets, and the rest I do for my friend. (Who is the other person that gets all this?) That's the way the asylum cut is donated. (But who is the other person?) He's a criminal. He gets so much. He gets twenty years' criminal treatment, would make forty years; and he gets seven days' criminal protection and that makes fourteen days. That's all he gets. (And what are you?) What is known as cut donator Christ. None of them couldn't be able to have anything; so it has to be true works or prove true to have anything, too. He gets two days, and that twenty years makes forty years. He loses by causing. He's what is known as a murder. He causes that. He's a murder by cause because he causes that. He can't get anything else. A double sacrifice is what is known as where murder turns, turns the friend into a cut donator and that's what makes a daughter-son. (A daughter-son?) Effeminate. A turned Christ. The criminal is a birth murder because he makes him a double. He gets two days' work for every day's work.

---

[*]From Cameron, N. 1947. The Psychology of Behavior Disorders. Boston, Houghton Mifflin Co., pp. 466–467.

... (What is 'a birth murder'?) A birth murder is a murder that turns a cut donator Christ into a double daughter-son. He's turned effeminate and weak. He makes him a double by making him weak. He gets two days' work for every one day's work because after he's made a double, he gets twice as much as it is. He's considered worth twice that much more. He has to be sacrificed to be a double.

The schizophrenic may become fascinated by the sound of words to the exclusion of their sense. Sometimes he coins words (neologisms). Often these are combinations of two or more words that express a personalized meaning not readily understood by others. A schizophrenic patient wrote, "The religionation of the actionation is joy awoy." (The neologisms of schizophrenics are sometimes reminiscent of Lewis Carroll's classic verses beginning "'Twas brillig, and the slithy toves . . .'" in *Through the Looking Glass and What Alice Found There*.) See also Figure 12–1.

The looseness, distorted logic, fragmentation, concreteness and overinclusiveness of schizophrenic thinking are examples of that form of mental activity which Freud labeled *primary process*. Primary process thinking is characterized by a tolerance for immediate discharge of impulses without regard to logic or the demands of the environment. (In contrast, *secondary process* refers to thinking controlled by logic, environmental demands and anticipated future consequences.) The primary process is uninhibited and uncontrolled. It makes free use of analogy, allusion, displacement, condensation and symbolic representation. Because his behavior is largely characterized by primary process thinking, the schizophrenic has sometimes been described as an individual who wears his unconscious on his sleeve.

Autistic Withdrawal

A relatively mild schizophrenic has a tenuous and unstable relation to reality. A severely disturbed schizophrenic may go further; he may break completely with reality and withdraw into a world of his own. He is preoccupied with an encapsulated world inhabited by his own wishes, fears, persecutory ideas and fantasies. Affect, thinking, speech and overt behavior are dominated by his inner life. The aspects of external reality that filter through to him are misinterpreted and distorted. Another person's smile may be interpreted as a sneer, or a harsh comment as a sign of secret approval.

Bleuler cites the case of a schizophrenic woman who made a rag doll which she called the child of her imaginary lover. When he left on a trip she decided to send "the child" after him and inquired of the police whether it should be sent as luggage or on a passenger ticket. Another patient, asked if he had been in a hospital before, made the autistic reply, "No, but unjustly."

Responses to proverbs may indicate autistic, highly personal interpretations. In the following responses, concrete thinking is present as in the examples cited earlier, but there is an additional element of idiosyncratic distortion of the stimulus.

A rolling stone gathers no moss:
A person could answer that better if they were a stone.

People in glass houses shouldn't throw stones:
Response 1: You shouldn't throw stones at people.
Response 2: You shouldn't throw stones through windows—that's what I've been trying to avoid doing.

When the cat's away, the mice will play:
If the father is away, things get harmed, too.

Ambivalence

Schizophrenics are ambivalent toward themselves and others. They have a deep mistrust of people, even those for whom they feel affection. A severely ill schizophrenic may strip off his clothes in front of other people while berating himself for his immodesty, or he may rapidly alternate between laughing and crying. Sometimes he seems to laugh and cry simultaneously. A wholehearted emotional response, free of contradiction, is difficult for him.

Inappropriateness of Affect

Schizophrenic distortions of affect take many forms. The patient may sit with an expressionless face, indicating neither pleasure nor pain and seemingly indifferent to what happens to him. On the other hand, affect is in some cases excessively labile and the patient overreacts and jumps from mood to mood. His affect may also be out of keeping with reality or with his own thoughts. Told that his wife has recovered from an illness, a schizophrenic may respond, "That's good," while his tone of voice indicates sadness rather than joy. Conversely, disturbing news may be accepted with a blissful smile or laughter.

NB.

JUNG—"Dreams" close to skitz.

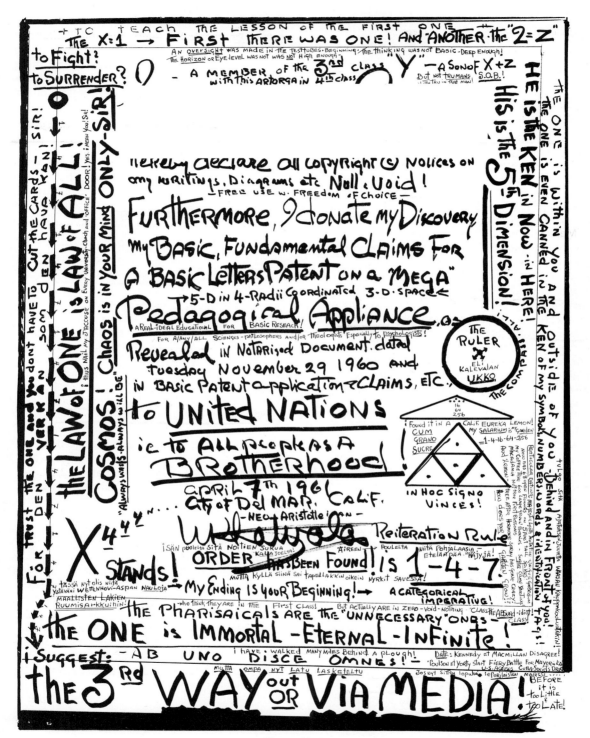

Figure 12–1.

Schizophrenic affect is insufficiently regulated by social standards. Some patients relate past misdeeds—real or fanciful—with no sign of shame, or use very obscene language, or masturbate openly and unconcernedly.

Other Primary Symptoms

Meehl (1962) has proposed a somewhat related set of primary symptoms which are more firmly based on recent research findings and increased neurological sophistication. Instead of loosened associations, Meehl proposes the term *cognitive slippage* so as to include those associative difficulties and minor cognitive errors found in mildly disfunctioning individuals who do not usually come to the attention of a mental health expert. Meehl's other cardinal features of schizophrenia are *interpersonal aversiveness, anhedonia* and *ambivalence*. The latter is used in the same sense as in Bleuler's conceptions. Interpersonal aversiveness refers to the schizophrenic's "social fear, distrust, expectation of rejection, and conviction of his own unlovability" which, Meehl says, "cannot be matched in its depth, pervasity, and resistance to corrective experience by any other diagnostic group." Anhedonia is a term originally coined by Rado (1956) to refer to the schizophrenic's marked deficit in the capacity for pleasure or enjoyment. It is different from the low mood of the depressive in that it is described subjectively as more of a flatness than a lowering of mood. Patients often describe it as a sensation of grayness, sameness, or lack of response to normally enjoyable activities. Asked if he enjoyed a party, the patient may reply that there was lots of music, that the food was exotic and that everyone said they enjoyed themselves. He seems to reason that the party was enjoyable since all the objective indicators point in that direction. He does not say, "It was great! I had the time of my life!"

Meehl's conceptualizations are intimately linked to his theory of the etiology of schizophrenia. It is his opinion that schizophrenia should be thought of as the outcome of inherited personality traits interacting with certain types of environmental pressures. In this view, what is inherited is believed to be a neurological integrative defect which invariably results in a personality characterized by the primary signs listed above. However, for the majority of such persons the cognitive slippage, anhedonia and other features remain un-

potentiated and relatively mild in their effect on the total personality. A minority of such predisposed persons, on the other hand, are subjected to such severe environmental stresses (such as a disturbed mother) that they develop clinical schizophrenia. The appeal of this theory lies in its suggestiveness for future research and in its integration of information from biological, genetic and psychological points of view.

THE SECONDARY SYMPTOMS OF SCHIZOPHRENIA

In addition to the primary symptoms just discussed, the schizophrenic may manifest some of the following secondary symptoms, which vary widely among the different diagnostic types and among the patients within each type. *Hallucinations* are common and may involve any sense modality. Most frequently they are auditory; the patient hears "voices" of imaginary persons, or persons who are real but absent or silent. These may talk to or about him. The voices may threaten and curse, criticize, warn or command him. While he is eating, he may hear a voice saying, "You ought to starve," or, "It [the food] will kill you." Alternatively, a voice may order him to eat or not to eat, or it may describe his behavior; for example, it may repeat, "You're eating, you're eating."

Visual hallucinations, sometimes called "visions" by patients, are less common than auditory but occur in the earlier and more acute phases of schizophrenia. The patient may see vague images, threatening figures, or angels and devils. Taste, smell and tactile hallucinations occur fairly often. The patient may perceive a peculiar taste in his food, usually associated with a delusory belief that someone is trying to poison him. He may smell a foul odor, attribute it to his own body, and interpret it to mean that he is sexually evil and foul. Patients may feel unwarranted pain, cold, heat, electric currents, delicate touches or any other variety of sensation. Sexual hallucinations are fairly common: for example, a patient may feel peculiar sensations in his genitals and interpret them as evidence of unwelcome interference by some external agency.

The schizophrenic's *delusions* are autistic expressions of his needs and fears and may be based on his hallucinatory experiences. By definition, they are gross distortions of reality. They tend to be unsystematized and chaotic, lacking in unity and internally contradictory.

The schizophrenic's delusions thus indicate the presence of a thought disorder, but they are secondary symptoms since a thought disorder may occur without delusions.

All types of delusions occur in schizophrenia—reference, active influence, passive influence, persecution, grandeur, and somatic, or hypochondriacal. In patients who are depressed, as well as schizophrenic, delusions of self-accusation, worthlessness and helplessness may also be found. In a delusion of reference, the patient may believe that the content of books and newspapers or the gestures, words and actions of other people refer to him. Bleuler cites the example of a child passing in front of a patient whereupon the patient feels he must protest, "I am not the father of this child." A schizophrenic university student believed that the major purpose of the university was to conduct an elaborate experiment in which she was the sole subject. The faculty chose courses to test their effect on her and during lectures various "judges," masquerading as students, recorded her reactions. The courses that she did not attend were offered in order to disguise the existence of the experiment.

In persecutory delusions it is very common for a patient to believe that all his misfortunes are the work of a nameless group, often designated as "they." He may have no understanding of exactly how "they" operate or he may construct elaborate theories of "their" mode of operation which involve secret messages, spies, radio, television, computers or other mechanisms. Belief in persecution by specific individuals is also widespread. For example, a female schizophrenic may accuse a hospital physician of having raped her, but, at the same time, denying, not surprisingly, any conscious erotic attraction to the object of her delusion.

Somatic delusions tend to be hypochondriacal. The patient may believe that all his strength has been drained out of him by a secret process, that he has a tumor in his head, that his bones are water, that his genitals are gone, or that only his head is alive and the rest of him is dead.

The following letter was written by a woman with persecutory, somatic and sexual delusions, and addressed to a television station. (Spelling and punctuation are unchanged.)

Dear Sir,

This is not my shape or face Mary _____ has given me her glass eye and she has my noise. Bob Hope. Crooked mouth Peter Lin Hayes, has given me his lop sided shoulder. & terrible mans figure. He sold his shape to Mr. Albright, I want my own things

Frances _____, Pinky tongue. She has my noise.

Cathy Crosby has most of my things I want them. I have little Reds Kork leg, from the _____ Hotel he lives most of the time & a few other bad features I cant mention he gave me. I guess knowing him you must know what it is.

Dolores _____ club finger & two other fingers she had smashed in a defense plant Ruth _____ one finger she had off in a defense plant.

Peggy _____ or Hildegard has my hands & has gave me her large lump in the back of the neck & her large head.

Ida _____

Jeanette _____ has my eyes & hair & other things so make her give them back. I don't want these things any more the Contest is over.

I want my own things back & also my daughter.

Dr. _____ has Patricia & I want her back immediately Im going to the police. I know all her markings & I have all hers & my pictures with my attorney. Patricia took 3 screen test I have proof for these things I took one also.

Distortions of memory sometimes occur in schizophrenia. The patient manifests an amnesic gap or unexpected accuracy for some long past event that had great emotional importance for him. Sometimes memory is falsified rather than lost. For example, a patient repeatedly requests that he be transferred to another ward and afterward insists that it was the doctor who wanted him transferred.

A variety of disorders occur in the realm of speech, in addition to those that indicate disturbances of thinking. The patient may be mute or excessively talkative (logorrhea) or manifest verbigeration (the monotonous repetition of words or sentences). Some patients talk only in monosyllables with no intonation. In others, speech is very vehement, abnormally loud and excited. The catatonic may manifest echolalia (the repetition of words said to him).

Motor disturbances occur, particularly in catatonics. The patient may be stuporous or overactive, or may manifest a cataleptic muscle rigidity and fixity of posture. In rare cases, waxy flexibility occurs. A patient may grimace or repeatedly perform mechanical, automatic gestures. Echopraxia, the imitation of another's movements, is occasionally encountered as is negativism which, in a sense, is the opposite of echopraxia since the compulsive imitation of the latter indicates heightened suggestibility. Sometimes negativism is a response to hallucinated voices commanding the patient to do the reverse of what he is supposed to do.

Schizophrenics show an impairment of role-taking and empathy. They cannot easily put themselves in the place of others. Their communication difficulties largely stem from an inability to imagine and anticipate others' reactions. Helfand (1956) had a group of chronic schizophrenics and a group of normals read the autobiography of a nonpsychotic individual. The subjects were asked to predict his responses to a series of test items covering attitudes to his parents and siblings, courtship, marriage, sex, education and vocation. The normals' predictions were significantly more accurate than those of the chronic schizophrenics. (A striking finding was that another group of schizophrenics who were well on the way toward recovery were *superior* to the normals in their predictions.) Apparently the predictions of the normals were based on a standard conception of a conventional, "generalized other," whereas the chronic schizophrenics lacked a universally shared frame of reference on which to base their judgments.

The schizophrenic suffers from *anhedonia,* an impaired capacity to experience pleasure. His interactions with others are fearful and his sexual responsiveness tends to be rudimentary and joyless. He has difficulty in feeling affection, eliciting it from others, and reciprocating when it is offered.

Associated with anhedonia is a *pervasive and easily aroused anxiety.* It is difficult for the patient to tolerate his almost constant state of anxiety. As a defense, he may seek to ward off all emotion and therefore appear cold and over-intellectualized. If he cannot defend himself, he is flooded by feelings of anxiety and other unpleasant affects, particularly in the earlier stages of schizophrenia. A number of theorists have felt that the schizophrenic's anhedonia and intense anxiety are more crucial than the thinking disturbance stressed by Bleuler. On this basis, anxiety is as fundamental a component of schizophrenia as of the neuroses; the difference is that the neurotic's anxiety does not lead to disorganized thinking and a divorce from reality.

The schizophrenic often has a strong craving for *protection* and *dependency.* Precisely because he experiences little pleasure and much fear, he may make frequent but awkward attempts to be approved or shielded. However, because of his ambivalence and disorganization it is difficult for him to express his dependency needs in an acceptable manner. Consequently, he behaves like a very anxious child and attacks the very people whose affection he desperately wants.

Both the primary and secondary symptoms

just described are *regressive,* that is, indicative of a lower level of functioning than is characteristic of the mature adult. The schizophrenic's relations to other persons, sexuality, emotionality and cognitive behavior are infantile. However, although schizophrenia is regressive, it is not a literal return to childhood, for the behavior of the normal child is in most respects quite different from that of the adult schizophrenic. The symptoms of schizophrenia evidence a *distortion* of infantile modes of behavior. A number of the secondary symptoms are *restitutional* as well as regressive; that is, they represent the patient's misguided attempts to regain a lost reality. The schizophrenic's delusions, hallucinations and catatonic motor behavior may be viewed as desperate, immature and inappropriate attempts to reestablish a lost relationship with the world.

In view of his peculiar relation to reality, it is not surprising that the schizophrenic shows a *defect in sustained activity* toward a goal, even prior to breakdown. His life history often reveals a lack of continuity with frequent shifting from job to job and residence to residence. Frequently, he is an under-achiever as a student and employee.

A recurrent question in discussions of schizophrenia is whether *progressive intellectual deterioration* inevitably occurs. The overt behavior of many schizophrenics seems to indicate a continuous intellectual loss; some, however, manifest an alternation of higher and lower levels of intellectual functioning, and still others stabilize at some level without further decline. A schizophrenic's emotional and motivational difficulties may bring about test performances far below capacity and prevent an accurate assessment of his "true" intellectual capacity. Paralogical thinking may also interfere with adequate use of intellect. For example, a nurse may smile at an intelligent but sexually disturbed schizophrenic who, in paralogical fashion, equates her with her smile, smiles back, and then makes the absurd claim that he has had sexual relations with her. A number of patients improve intellectually as they improve emotionally. It must be concluded that although intellectual deterioration does occur, it is neither inevitable nor irreversible.

Schizophrenic Stages

The course of schizophrenia is variable. It runs the gamut from an acute attack which lasts a few hours, days or months, to chronic, life-long illness. Among chronic patients, some stabilize at a certain stage and thereafter show little change in symptomatology, whereas others manifest a continuous disintegration of personality. The *typical* chronic schizophrenic goes through a series of stages. In the first—the breakdown—he experiences anxiety and panic; he is confused by the strange things that are happening to him. In the beginning he may manifest only relatively subtle signs of disturbance, such as a variety of hypochondriacal complaints, but soon delusions and hallucinations appear and proliferate, and he becomes still more confused. Many patients in this stage are unsure whether the voices they hear are real, and they ask the opinion of others. In this early stage it is difficult to classify patients into any of the major types of schizophrenia, for the symptoms range widely across the different types.

However, the patient soon enters a second stage in which he "accepts" his symptoms and settles into them. He is less upset by them and no longer doubts that they are real. His symptoms for the most part begin to conform to one or the other of the major types and he is classifiable as paranoid, catatonic, hebephrenic or simple.

Eventually, many of his symptoms may disappear and he enters a third stage in which he is again difficult to classify. In this stage, the patient is sometimes referred to as a "burned out" schizophrenic, for he is more likely to manifest profound apathy and flat affect than anxiety and excitement. Along with apathy there may be a regression to a very primitive level of functioning in which he stuffs his mouth with food, talks childishly and illogically, and appears indifferent to his surroundings.

THE MAJOR TYPES OF SCHIZOPHRENIA

Kraepelin's four major types—simple, hebephrenic, catatonic and paranoid—as well as a number of other types are all used in current clinical practice. However, during the past few decades, changes in diagnostic emphasis and the advent of intensive and early therapy have resulted in certain shifts in diagnostic frequency. Patients are less often categorized as simple or hebephrenic than formerly and more often as paranoid, acute, chronic undifferentiated, schizo-affective, childhood or residual types.

Chronic catatonics have become rare because ECT is effective in dispelling catatonic stupor and tranquilizers effectively subdue catatonic excitement in new patients. However, acute, brief catatonic reactions remain very frequent. About 40 per cent of hospitalized schizophrenics are paranoid, and the other 60 per cent are distributed over all other categories. The following description of the separate schizophrenic reactions emphasizes the differences among them rather than their common features.

Simple Schizophrenia

The simple schizophrenic is usually described in such terms as careless, lacking in initiative, shy, withdrawn, apathetic, preoccupied, colorless and "shut-in." The patient manifests poor attention, few external interests and an impoverishment of human relationships. He hardly talks with other people. He may display irritability, but other affects are minimal or absent. The sexual drive is weak or vanishes. He neglects his personal appearance and cleanliness. He may seem grouchy, but except for an occasional and explosive lack of control he tends to be unaggressive. In the rare instances in which he does attempt to become involved in relation with others, he is ineffectual. For example, he may become dependent on someone who dislikes being depended on and rejects him; as a result he becomes moody and even more withdrawn. The simple schizophrenic usually does *not* manifest delusions or hallucinations. If he experiences an occasional hallucination, he is likely to deny it. As time passes, however, he gives increasing evidence of disorganized thinking and impaired intellectual functioning.

The onset tends to be early and insidious and the course chronic, particularly when untreated. Among hospitalized patients, the diagnosis is relatively infrequent since many simple schizophrenics remain at home under family care. Sometimes they work at very simple, routine jobs, or become prostitutes (with a low sexual drive), vagrants or petty criminals. Simple schizophrenics are inevitably under-achievers. Family members are upset by the "do-nothing" traits of a simple schizophrenic and urge him to "snap out of it," but their exhortations are useless because he does not share the values of society.

The patient described in the following paragraphs illustrates many of the features of simple schizophrenia:

An unmarried woman was admitted to a state hospital at the age of 28. Her mother and sister reported that during the previous five years she had gradually become inactive and withdrawn. She refused to go outdoors and spent much of her time lying in bed. She became very careless of her appearance, often did not answer questions that were put to her, and sometimes talked aloud to herself. Occasionally she would become very tense, her face would turn red and she would bite herself on the arm.

The patient came from a family characterized by isolation and social nonparticipation. She was the third of four children, none of whom had married when she was hospitalized. Her mother was 38 and her father 44 when she was born. The parents had few friends. The mother was quiet, inactive and overcontrolled. The father had been incapacitated by a neurological disorder for five years prior to the patient's hospitalization.

The patient had been sickly as a child. She attended school until the age of 18, stayed home with her mother until she was 21 and left to work as a stenographer. After one year she returned home where she remained until hospitalized. For a brief period during adolescence, she had been fairly active in girls' clubs, but she had never had a boy friend or been out on a date.

On arrival in the hospital she was unattractive and appeared unconcerned. Her clothes hung loosely, she wore no makeup and her behavior was self-effacing. Her voice was colorless and flat. She lacked insight into her condition. "I really don't know why they sent me here," she said, "I know I have a bad heart, but otherwise I don't know." Asked how her heart bothered her, she replied, "Just weakness. I just haven't as much life in me as most people have." Her perception of her mother, a markedly quiet and passive person, was very ambivalent and idiosyncratic. "I guess mother and I don't get along as well as we might," she stated. "She tells people everything she knows. She can't seem to sit down. She's on the go all the time."

In the hospital the patient was completely disinterested in war activities. She never became excited or otherwise evidenced affect and never initiated interactions with other patients. In group therapy she was an apathetic nonparticipant with nothing to say. She seemed to be devoid of ideas, yet an intelligence test revealed an I.Q. of 110; she was autistically preoccupied rather than mentally defective. On the Rorschach ink blots she manifested strong feelings of insignificance and inferiority.

Hebephrenic Schizophrenia

A number of hebephrenic schizophrenics become idiosyncratically preoccupied in youth with trivia or grandiose, philosophical issues. With time, they deteriorate to a lower level of behavior than schizophrenics of other types. However, they are more active than simple schizophrenics. Their preoccupation with fantasies and divorce from reality results in grimaces, mannerisms, strange gestures, empty giggling, incoherent babbling and neologisms, quick and impulsive actions which are sometimes assaultive, and bizarre appearance. The patient may have a silly, fixed smile for lengthy periods as if he had abandoned his internal struggles. He may regress to a very infantile level, and in some cases there is smearing of excrement. The patient may hear voices vividly and obscenely accusing him of sexual immorality or complimenting him for fancied achievements. Transient, poorly systematized delusions, often very bizarre, occur; e.g., "I am 950 years old." Somatic delusions, in which the patient believes that part of his body has been altered or stolen, are common, as are grandiose religious delusions.

The symptoms of the following patient were typical, but the precipitation of her hebephrenic disintegration by a single traumatic event was unusual. A long-standing Oedipal attachment to her father was brought to a head by the traumatic event.

The patient was hospitalized at the age of 18. During the preceding year there had been a gradual disintegration of personality, evidenced by inappropriate laughing and giggling, bizarre conversation and failure in school.

She was the eldest of four children, having a brother and two sisters. Her mother stated that the patient felt loved and wanted by her parents and was her father's favorite. The patient's school work was good and she had many friends until a traumatic event occurred when she was 17. Her father, who had been drinking excessively, attempted to rape her next younger sister. The attempt was interrupted by the youngest sister who reported it to the patient; in turn, the patient reported it to her mother who called the police. The father was jailed for three weeks and then released. He was not permitted to return to his family and went to work in another city.

The patient's illness began soon after the father's departure. As described by the patient's mother, "She started to worry about a year ago. My husband left and she began to think about him all the time. She used to talk funny—funny things like she would hear an airplane and stand on the kitchen table looking at the ceiling. She would look out of the kitchen window at children who were playing at school about a mile away and ask if the other children could see her. She would stay away from school and wouldn't help with the housework but stood outside staring at nothing.

She would say, "I don't know whether I am a boy or a girl. Do you think I will ever get married and have a baby?' And she would say to me, 'You are staying young and I am growing old.'"

The sexual content of the patient's disturbance was intermixed with rivalry toward her mother as well as emotional dependence on her father. After he had been forced to live away from home, she went to see him but when she arrived he had left the city. She then started to complain of a cramp in her stomach and began to cry and laugh alternately. She would fall to the bathroom floor for no apparent reason. She stopped eating and had to be fed with a spoon.

In the hospital, the patient, in a remarkable description of schizophrenic confusion, said, "Things don't work right in my mind the way they should and I know it definitely. It seems to me lately that whenever I read or write, well that is the whole question, it affects my mind. I sort of . . . I don't know what you call it, but when I think of one thing, I don't take it the way I should at the time. My mind seems to wander at the time—I don't hit the right target at the right time. I am all someplace else. I feel as if it is crossing and then coming down . . ."; at this point, the patient waved a finger over her head several times.

When her mother visited her in the hospital, the patient said, "Go on home, you make me worse," and she angrily threw things on the floor. She called her mother and aunt obscene names while laughing and crying. She often grimaced, ran up and down the ward—frequently chasing after male hospital personnel—and was sometimes disheveled and sometimes ornately overdressed.

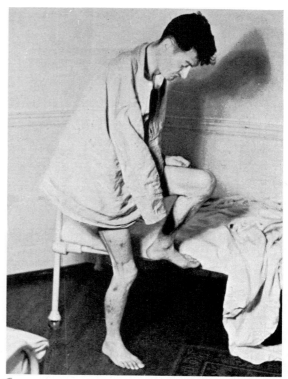

Figure 12–2. "Posturing of catatonic patient aged thirty-two. Remained in this position for more than fifteen minutes. Hits out when disturbed." (Reprinted by permission from Clinical Psychiatry by Mayer-Gross, Slater and Roth, Cassell: London, 1960.)

Catatonic Schizophrenia

The motor disturbances of the catatonic type are expressed in either generalized inhibition (mutism, motor retardation, stupor) or excessive activity and excitement. A catatonic patient may have repeated episodes of stupor without excitement or excitement without stupor, or he may dramatically and unpredictably swing from one extreme to the other. Although the pattern of motor activity has some similarity to that observed in manic-depression, the specific motor symptoms of the catatonic have some unique features. For example, the patient may sit and rock his body backward and forward for hours on end or he may manifest any of the symptoms described earlier—muscular rigidity, the posturing found in waxy flexibility, echopraxia, echolalia and negativism. The pupils of the eyes may show irregular contraction and dilation, or the eyelids may be tightly closed. Although unresponsive to external stimuli, the patient may be acutely aware of events and conversations in his vicinity, and he may be able to report them

accurately months later. In the excited state, he becomes extremely agitated and destructive. He is likely to destroy furniture, tear his clothes, assault others, or injure and mutilate himself. The catatonic may also, like the hebephrenic, regress to such behaviors as smearing feces.

In addition to motor symptoms, the catatonic displays typical schizophrenic thinking and affect. While either stuporous or excited, he experiences vivid fantasies, fears and hallucinations. He has delusions that are sometimes of a cosmic nature, e.g., "The world will come to an end if I move."

In many cases the onset is sudden. With early treatment the prognosis is good, especially for cases with a sudden onset. Prior to the discovery of modern methods of treatment, catatonics sometimes underwent spontaneous remissions, but others became chronically stuporous or died of exhaustion in a state of excitement.

In the following case report, reprinted with some abbreviations from Arieti (1961), the pa-

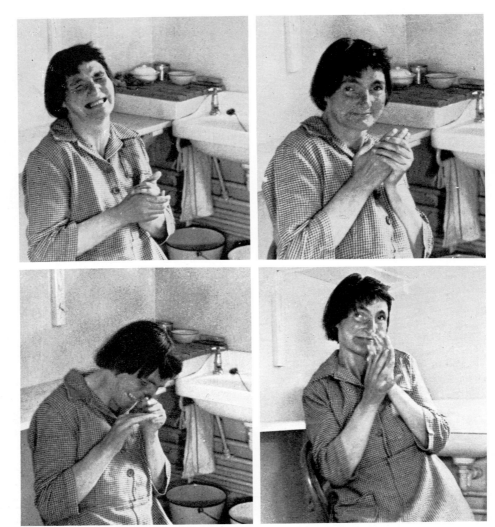

Figure 12-3. *"Grimacing and posturing in a woman of forty-four with chronic catatonic schizophrenia. She is subject to outbursts of inane incongruous laughter, aggressive behaviour and stereotyped movement in response to auditory hallucinations." (Reprinted by permission from Clinical Psychiatry by Mayer-Gross, Slater and Roth, Cassell: London, 1960.)*

tient had a far higher socioeconomic and educational level than is usual for catatonics. (A high level is more common among paranoid schizophrenics.) His intellect and education made it possible for him to reconstruct the development and some of the dynamics of his illness in rich detail.*

John is an intelligent professional man in his thirties, Catholic, who was referred to me because of

his rapidly increasing anxiety—anxiety which reminded him of the one he experienced about ten years previously, when he developed a full catatonic episode. Wanting to prevent a recurrence of the event, he sought treatment.

The following is . . . a brief history of the patient and a description and interpretation of his catatonic episode as it was reconstructed and analyzed during the treatment.

The patient is one of four children. The father is described as a bad husband, an adventurer who, although a good provider, always caused trouble and home instability. The mother is a somewhat inadequate person, distant from the patient. John was raised more or less by a maternal aunt who lived in the family and acted as a housekeeper.

*Abbreviated by permission from Arieti, S. 1961. Volition and value: a study based on catatonic schizophrenia. Compr. Psychiat. 2:74–82.

Early childhood memories are mostly unpleasant for John. He recollects attacks of anxiety going back to his early childhood. He also remembers how he needed to cling to his aunt; how painful it always was to separate from her. The aunt also had the habit of undressing in his presence, causing him mixed feelings of sexual excitement and guilt. Between 9 and 10 there was an attempted homosexual relation with his best friend. During the prepuberal period he remembers his desire to look at pictures of naked women, and how occasionally he would surreptitiously borrow some pornographic books or magazines from his father's collection and look at them. Fleeting homosexual desires would also occur occasionally. . . . Among the things that he remembers from his early life are also obsessive preoccupations with feces of animals and excretions in general of human beings. He had a special admiration for horses, because "They excreted such beautiful feces coming from such statuesque bodies."

In spite of all these circumstances, John managed to grow more or less adequately, was not too disturbed by the death of his aunt, and did well in school. There were practically no dates with girls until much later in life. After puberty he became very interested in religion, especially in order to find a method to control his sexual impulses. Anything connected with sex was evil and had to be eliminated. This attitude was in a certain way the opposite of that of one of his sisters who was leading a very promiscuous life. John considered the possibility of becoming a monk several times; however, he was discouraged from doing so by a priest he had consulted. When he finished college at the age of 20, he decided to make a complete attempt to remove sex from his life. He also decided to go for a rest and summer vacation at a farm for young men where he would cut trees, enjoy the country, and be far way from the temptations of the city. On this farm, however, he soon became anxious and depressed. He found out that he resented the other fellows more and more. They were rough boys. They used profane language. He felt as if he were going to pieces progressively. He remembers that one night he was saying to himself, "I cannot stand it any more. Why am I in this way, so anxious for no reason? I have done no wrong in my whole life. Perhaps I should become a priest or get married." When he was feeling very badly he would console himself by thinking that perhaps what he was experiencing was in accordance with the will of God.

Obsessions and compulsions acquired more and more prominence. The campers had to go chopping wood. This practice became an ordeal for John because he was possessed by doubts. He would think, for instance: "Maybe I should not cut this tree because it is too small. Next year it will be bigger. But if I don't cut this tree another fellow will. Maybe it is better if he cuts it, or maybe that I do so." As he expressed himself, he found himself, "doubting and doubting his doubts, and doubting the doubting of his doubts." It was an overwhelming, spreading anxiety. The anxiety gradually extended to every act he had to perform. He was literally possessed by intense terror. One day, while he was in this predicament, he observed another phenomenon which he could not understand. There was a discrepancy between the act he wanted to perform and the action that he really carried out. For instance, when he was undressing he wanted to drop a shoe, and instead he dropped a big log; he wanted to put something in a drawer and instead he threw a stone away. However, there was a similarity between the act that he had wanted and anticipated and the act he actually performed. The same phenomenon appeared in talking. He would utter words, which were not the ones he meant to say, but related to them. Later, however, his actions became more and more disconnected. He was mentally lucid and able to perceive what was happening but he realized he had no control over his actions. He thought he could commit crimes, even kill somebody and became even more afraid. He was saying to himself: "I don't want to be damned in this world as well as in the other. I am trying to be good and I can't. It is not fair. I may kill somebody when I want a piece of bread." At other times he had different feelings. He felt as if some movement or action he would make could produce disaster not only to himself but to the whole camp. By not acting or moving he was protecting the whole group. He felt that he had become his brother's keeper.

Fear soon became connected with any possible movement. The fear was so intense as to actually inhibit any movement. He was almost literally petrified. To use his own words, he "saw himself solidifying, assuming statuesque positions." However, he was not always in this condition. As a matter of fact, the following day he could move again and go to chop wood. He had one purpose in mind: to kill himself. He remembers that he was very capable of observing himself, and of deciding that it would be better for him to die than to commit crimes. He climbed a big tree and jumped down in an attempt to kill himself but received only minor contusions. The other men, who ran to help him, realized that he was mentally ill, and he was soon sent to a psychiatric hospital. . . . In the hospital he found that he could not move at all. He was like a statue of stone.

There were some actions, however, which could escape this otherwise complete immobility: the actions needed for the purpose of committing suicide. In fact he was sure that he had to die to avoid the terror of becoming a murderer. He had to kill himself before that could happen.

During his hospitalization, John made 71 suicidal attempts. Although he was generally in a state of catatonia he would occasionally make impulsive acts such as tearing his straight jacket to pieces and making a rope of it to hang himself. Another time he broke a dish in order to cut the veins of his wrist. Other times he swallowed stones. He was always put under restraint after a suicidal attempt. He remembers, however, understanding everything that was going on. As a matter of fact, his acuity in devising methods for committing suicide seemed sharpened.

When I questioned him further about this long series of suicidal attempts, John added that the most drastic attempts were actually the first ten or twelve. Only these could really have killed him. Later, the suicidal attempts were not very dangerous. He performed such acts as swallowing a small object or inflicting a small injury on himself with a sharp object. When I asked him whether he knew why he had to repeat these token suicidal attempts, he gave me two reasons. The first was to relieve his feeling of guilt and fulfill his duty of preventing himself from committing crimes. But the second reason, which he discovered during the present treatment, is even stranger. To commit suicide was the only act which he could perform, the only act which would go beyond the barrier of immobility. Thus, to commit suicide was to live; the only act of life left to him.

The patient was given a course of electric shock treatment. . . . He improved for about two weeks, but then he relapsed into catatonic stupor interrupted only by additional suicidal attempts. While he was in stupor he remembered a young psychiatrist saying to a nurse, "Poor fellow, so young and so sick. He will continue to deteriorate for the rest of his life." After five or six months of hospitalization his catatonic state became somewhat less rigid and he was able to walk and to utter a few words. At this time he had noticed that a new doctor seemed to take some interest in him. One day this doctor told him, "You want to kill yourself. Isn't there anything at all in life that you want?" With great effort the patient mumbled, "Eat, to eat." In fact, he really was hungry as his immobility prevented him from eating properly, and he was inefficiently spoon fed. The doctor took him to the patients' cafeteria and told him, "You may eat anything you want." John immediately grabbed a large quantity of food and ate in a ravenous manner. . . . From that day on John lived only for the sake of eating. He gained about sixty pounds in a few weeks. When I asked him if he ate so much because he was really hungry, he said, "No, that was only at the beginning. The pleasure in eating consisted partially in grabbing food and putting it into my mouth. . . ."

John continued to improve and in a few months he was able to leave the hospital. He was able to make a satisfactory adjustment, to work, and later to go to a professional school and obtain his Ph.D. degree. On the whole he has managed fairly well until shortly before he decided to come for psychoanalytic treatment.

In his discussion of John's symptoms and dynamics, Arieti makes the following comments, here somewhat abridged:

. . . It is obvious that John underwent an overpowering increase in anxiety when he went to the camp and was exposed to close homosexual stimulation. His early interpersonal relations had subjected him to great instability and insecurity and had made him very vulnerable to many sources of anxiety. This anxiety, however, retained a propensity to be aroused by or be channeled in the pattern of sexual stimulation and inhibition. His personality defenses and cultural background made the situation worse. John was not . . . deprived of that part of the self called social self, conscience or superego; nor could he go against his cultural-religious background as his philandering father and promiscuous sister. Sex was evil for him, and homosexuality much more so. As a matter of fact, homosexual desires were not even permitted to become fully conscious.

When he was about to be overwhelmed by the anxiety, he at first resorted to some of the defenses commonly found in precatatonics. He found refuge in religious feelings. God or religion gave him the order of eliminating sex from his life and of becoming a monk. This may be considered a form of autohypnosis, but . . . hypnosis and autohypnosis do not work well with catatonics. He resorted, then, to obsessive-compulsive mechanisms. The anxiety which presumably was at first connected with any action that had something to do with sexual feelings became extended to practically every action. . . . Every action became loaded with a sense of responsibility. Every willed movement came to be seen not as a function but as a moral issue. Every motion was not considered as a fact but as a value. This primitive generalization of his responsibility extended to what he could cause to the whole community. By moving he could produce havoc not only to himself but to the whole camp. His feelings were reminiscent of the feelings of cosmic power or negative omnipotence experienced by other catatonics who believe that by acting they may cause the destruction of the universe. . . .

To protect himself at first, John resorted to obsessive thinking and compulsions, as, for instance, when he was cutting trees. But even this defense was not sufficient to dam his anxiety; as a matter of fact, it made the situation worse and gave rise to other symptoms. The first one was the unrelatedness between the act, as anticipated and willed, and the action which followed. But, and this is a point of great importance, at first the actions were not completely unrelated from their anticipation. They were analogic. In other words, two actions, like dropping a shoe and dropping a log, had become psychologically equivalent, i.e., they were identified just because they were similar or had something in common. . . .

. . . In most patients the symptomatology proceeds rapidly to following stages, e.g., the stage where the actions are completely unrelated to the will, as in catatonic excitement, or the stage in which the actions are all eliminated, as in catatonic stupor. The catatonic excitement may be the result of two facts. In some cases the patient senses that he is sinking into stupor because he is afraid to act and tries to prevent this occurrence by becoming overactive and submerging himself in a rapid sequence of aimless acts. In other instances the opposite is true and the patient acts, but his actions are so unrelated to the conceived or willed actions as to result in a real

sudden & short *age is older*

movement-salad, the motor equivalent of word-salad. The patient then has no other resort but to sink into the immobility of the stupor.

In many cases the barrier of immobility is not completely closed. In a very selective way it may allow passage to actions of obedience to the will of others or to some special actions of the patient himself.

In the case of John the actions necessary for the suicidal attempts were allowed to go through. . . . What is of particular interest in our case is the fact that the suicidal act eventually became for John the only act of living. It is not possible here to examine in greater detail the therapeutic effect of the encounter of John with the doctor in the hospital. Important is the fact that the doctor gave John permission to eat as much as he wanted. Thus the only previously possible act (of killing oneself) was replaced with one of the most primitive acts of life, nourishing oneself. . . .

Paranoid Schizophrenia

The paranoid schizophrenic is usually less disturbed in appearance and overt behavior than the hebephrenic or catatonic. Consistent with his delusions, the paranoid is likely to be suspicious, serious, unsmiling and intense. He may have a hostile, glaring expression and be argumentative or assaultive, but is likely to deny that he is hostile and to employ the mechanism of projection to conclude that everyone else is hostile, while he is not. However, as his personality deteriorates with time, a paranoid schizophrenic tends to become quiet, withdrawn and apathetic rather than aggressive. He may also regress and begin to hoard valueless objects, engage in stereotyped ritual acts or show other evidences of infantilism.

The paranoid schizophrenic manifests autistic or paralogical thinking with delusions of reference, influence, persecution or grandeur. The delusions are poorly systematized, internally illogical and changeable over time, and they are accompanied by vivid auditory hallucinations. The patient's life is controlled by his delusions and hallucinations instead of by reality; inevitably his behavior is erratic and his judgment poor. Early in the course of the disorder his delusions and hallucinations tend to be fairly straightforward projections of his drives and anxieties. Later on, however, it may be impossible to understand the meaning of his delusions and hallucinations, for these change as if they had a life of their own: as they become more all-embracing they also become more disorganized and fragmented.

NB

changes ↑

The average age of onset is slightly higher than for the previously described forms of schizophrenia. When the onset of symptoms is acute, there are often obvious precipitating stresses and the response to treatment tends to be favorable. On the other hand, when paranoid schizophrenia develops gradually in an isolated and hypersensitive individual, with no evidence of external precipitating stresses, the psychosis is much more likely to become permanent.

The following case of paranoid schizophrenia is noteworthy for the patient's delusions of grandeur and their transparent motivations:

A 30-year-old college instructor was hospitalized soon after claiming that he was "a pope" and demanding that he be treated accordingly. "I've been made a pope and left to shift for myself," he complained. On inquiry, it became apparent that his delusions had begun two years earlier while he was a graduate student in a major university. He had been studying hard and living a life of social isolation in a desperate and unsuccessful attempt to earn a Ph.D. degree. One day he experienced "a delicious cold feeling inside" followed by a feeling that everything inside him was aflame, as if his heart had "opened up." This ecstatic feeling lasted for about six hours and he regarded it as the most wonderful experience of his life. He interpreted it as a religious call and for some months considered entering a seminary.

Meanwhile he became aware that he was being singled out for additional and special attentions. An airplane flew over his apartment several times and he decided that he was being buzzed. Grandiose ideas of reference appeared and he thought he heard strangers on the street making remarks such as "There goes the big shot" and "There goes number one." (It will later become clear that to him "the big shot" and "number one" signified his father.) He applied for a number of teaching positions but was accepted at only two colleges which he regarded as inferior; he concluded that his correspondence was being censored and that he was being discriminated against unjustly.

In spite of his paranoid ideation, his intellectual performance was unimpaired and his abnormality was not recognized so that he was able to teach for more than a year. One day, however, he thought he recognized a nun in a teaching order as someone he had known a few years earlier and had regarded as very attractive. She was "too beautiful to have her talents covered by the robes of her order." He perceived her as a victim of circumstances like himself, condemned to "teach in the sticks." He did not speak to her but began to ponder how he might have her released from her vows so that he could marry her. He felt that she was being guarded very closely to prevent him from doing so. He decided that he was a pope who had the power to grant her a dispensation from her vows, and that their marriage would follow. His behavior now became increasingly bizarre. During the last few weeks before admission to the hospital, his delusions of grandeur changed rapidly and assumed various forms. He telephoned the President of the United States, giving the name of a fictitious ambassador; he wrote to a general in Washington, signing the letter with the name of a fictitious general:

"This morning the secretary very rudely handed me some routine University matters as if to say, tend to your knitting or we'll get rid of you. Also, she has consistently refused to handle my typing, causing me to handle the entire burden myself. I can no longer bear the brunt of this despicable treatment. I think the secretary ought to be fired.

"General, I have been subject to the most unspeakable treatment in a community I have been earnestly trying to defend. I have appealed to Admiral _____ [his father's name] but he has left me entirely to my own resources, causing much hardship and crippling the operation of the entire Strategic Command.

"What are the services coming to, if her own officers are muzzled and fear to speak out in defense of each other?

Sincerely yours,
General_____, Commandant
_____ Command.''

He also wrote to his father:

"I cannot welcome back to this community a person who will not defend his own flesh and blood as an individual upon whose shoulders has been laid the highest title in Christiandom. You had definite knowledge of this whole matter last summer and you did nothing. How foolish can a person be! I refuse to accept your correspondence or phone calls unless you address me by my proper title."

He had no insight into his illness. On admission to the hospital he was serious and unsmiling and his manner was stiff and formal. The interviewing psychiatrist characterized him as conscientious, ambitious and "intense." Asked what three wishes he would make if he could have anything he wanted, he replied with firmness and some bitterness:

"1. To get married to a girl who is a nun.
"2. People are calling me pope, and I'd rather have training to be that than remain a college instructor.
"3. I'm not so awfully hard to please—so long as I have a responsible position and am supported in this. One of the things that galls me is that I haven't got a doctorate—I've got more than enough credits piled up but I have not been permitted to register."

The patient was the eldest of five children. He was named after his father, a research scientist with an international reputation at a major university, and was expected to follow in his father's footsteps. In spite of his scientific accomplishments, the father had never acquired a Ph.D. degree and constantly exhorted the patient to earn the degree. The father was narcissistic and demanding; the mother, by comparison, was inconspicuous. She was "the wife of the great man";

she referred to herself as "Mrs. _____" and did not use her own first name.

The patient described his father as engrossed in his work and criticized him for neglecting his family and religion; the mother, like the patient, was religious. The patient admired his father's professional ability but felt that he "always kept his world to himself and never drew others into it." He stated that his mother cheerfully performed many tasks that his father should have done. The only criticism he made of his mother was that she took no part in community activities; he identified strongly with her and his social isolation apparently was related to hers.

As an infant, the patient had feeding difficulties which were attributed to a faulty metabolism of carbohydrates. Frequent measurements of his blood-sugar level were made throughout his childhood. During his first two years he was subject to "nervous spells" every few weeks. He would wake from a sound sleep and scream in violent terror. His parents claimed that he began to speak at seven months and learned to read in his third year. At five, he had an attack of vomiting which lasted for three days; following this, he developed twitches around the mouth and eyes and tremors in the hands. His muscular coordination remained poor and he was nine years old before he could tie his shoelaces. He stuttered, lacked energy, and failed to establish satisfactory relationships with other children.

His parents regarded him as exceptionally well behaved and encouraged him in intellectual pursuits, so that by the age of 12 he was an excellent chess player and had read widely. At school, however, he was scolded and punished for restless, uncontrollable movements and then punished again for attempting to control his restlessness by sitting on his hands. His parents stated that in response to this treatment, he developed a "persecution complex" and on occasion came home from school completely shaken and exhausted. His feelings of persecution were reinforced by the mother's references to his teachers as "nasty" and her belief that it was all their fault. The father was convinced that the boy's problems were all due to low blood sugar, and he continued to have extensive blood-sugar tests undertaken and attempted to ward off the attacks of nervousness by controlling the boy's diet. Neither the father nor mother realized that the interpersonal relations within the family were disturbed and that they all needed help.

In adolescence, the patient was a choir boy and developed deep religious convictions. He was a studious, shy, reserved, overconforming intellectual who desperately wanted to achieve distinction and did not know how to get along with members of his own or the opposite sex.

After high school he attended the university where his father taught. He graduated cum laude and enrolled in an outstanding graduate school on a scholarship. He received little financial support from his father and had to live with his grandfather at a considerable distance from the university. In his first semester, he studied extremely hard and obtained an

A average, but then broke down and was hospitalized with an acute schizophrenic reaction. After a brief course of electroconvulsive treatments, he reintegrated rapidly (i.e., he returned to his pre-breakdown level of functioning). He then worked as a clerk and machine operator for nearly a year and at 24 was drafted into the Army despite his earlier breakdown. In the Army he was assigned to duties as a clerk typist, but he had an additional brief psychotic episode and was discharged before the end of the normal service period. He recommenced his graduate studies for the next two years; at the end of this period the religious revelation and delusions described earlier began.

In the hospital he was treated by tranquilizing drugs and intensive psychotherapy for some months, but his delusional convictions remained unchanged. It was therefore decided to treat him by ECT; after 20 treatments he improved but then rapidly relapsed and expressed delusions of being God, the devil, a brigadier general and, once again, a pope. He was then treated by regressive shock therapy, receiving 30 further ECT's in less than two weeks. This procedure resulted in a state of profound confusion, along with disappearance of his delusions. On recovery from the confusional state he was again tranquilized and also treated by supportive psychotherapy. He now recognized that his former beliefs were unrealistic and he was discharged after deciding that he would abandon his long struggle for a doctorate. Despite his illness and the drastic treatment, his intellectual performance was still in the very superior range and he planned to return to college teaching.

OTHER SCHIZOPHRENIC TYPES

Other types of schizophrenia will be discussed more briefly. *Acute schizophrenia* and *chronic undifferentiated schizophrenia* both show a wide variety of symptoms that do not conform to any of the four major types but cut across them. In an acute schizophrenic episode the person is likely to be confused and perplexed by what is happening to him, for he is in a state of cognitive and emotional turmoil. A chronic undifferentiated schizophrenic, on the other hand, tends to "settle down" with his disorder and manifests considerable apathy.

The *schizo-affective type* is characterized by a combination of schizophrenic thinking and motor behavior with an affective disorder, either euphoric or depressed. The most common form of schizo-affective reaction is a combination of paranoid schizophrenia with severe depression. Over a period of time, the intensity of the affective symptoms is likely to fluctuate, whereas the schizophrenic symptoms, if not arrested or reversed by treatment, are apt to become progressively more severe.

Childhood schizophrenia has its onset at any time prior to the age of 15 and may assume any of the forms already outlined. A schizophrenic child may fail to learn to talk and may show other evidences of intellectual subnormality. The result may be a mistaken diagnosis of mental deficiency. Alternatively, the schizophrenic child may have severe anxiety attacks and manifest a lack of emotional proportion. His ego is too weak for adequate control, and he is too passive, or too explosive, or too insistent on pursuing a single trivial interest to the exclusion of other activities. Childhood schizophrenia is discussed more fully in a later chapter on the disorders of childhood.

The term *residual schizophrenia* is sometimes applied to patients who have improved sufficiently after one or another schizophrenic reaction to be able to get along in the community but who still show residual disturbances of affect, thought or outward behavior.

Latent schizophrenia is the category used to describe patients who have some clear-cut symptoms of schizophrenia but no history of an actual schizophrenic episode. Disorders sometimes characterized as borderline schizophrenia, pseudo-neurotic schizophrenia and pseudo-psychopathic schizophrenia are included.

The term *pseudo-neurotic schizophrenia* has become increasingly popular since Hoch and Polatin (1949) pointed out that many apparently neurotic patients are subsequently found to manifest clear-cut evidences of a schizophrenic thought disorder. The patient manifests excessive and diffuse anxiety ("pan-anxiety") which pervades all areas of his life. He is also likely to display the symptoms of several neurotic subtypes simultaneously—conversions, obsessions, phobias and so forth. Beneath this outward appearance of a severe, mixed neurosis is a latent or incipient psychosis.

Parallel to pseudo-neurotic schizophrenia is the concept of *pseudo-psychopathic schizophrenia,* a term introduced by Dunaif and Hoch (1955) to describe patients in whom schizophrenic traits are initially masked by delinquent or antisocial behavior. The patient's antisocial behavior often involves him in sexual deviations; a characteristic of many schizophrenics is a chaotic, disorganized kind of sexuality.

ARE THERE TWO BASIC TYPES OF SCHIZOPHRENIA?

Schizophrenic patients are sometimes categorized into one of two classes which cut across all the major and minor types just described. Some investigators distinguish between *nuclear* and *peripheral* schizophrenics, others between *process* and *reactive* schizophrenics, and others between *poor premorbid* and *good premorbid* schizophrenics. (Nuclear vs. peripheral, process vs. reactive, and poor vs. good premorbid are similar but not identical pairs of concepts.)

Nuclear schizophrenia refers to those forms of the disorder in which patients have an early and insidious onset of symptoms, a poor prepsychotic personality and a poor prognosis. *Peripheral schizophrenia* is characterized by a later and more acute onset, a more adequate prepsychotic personality and a tendency to spontaneous remission or favorable response to treatment. Simple and hebephrenic schizophrenics are more likely to be nuclear, whereas catatonics and paranoids are more likely to be peripheral.

A dichotomy based on prepsychotic personality, rapidity of onset, and prognosis has most often been discussed in the psychological literature under the headings of process vs. reactive schizophrenia. *Process schizophrenia* is defined as the type that occurs in socially inadequate persons, beginning with a gradual onset and having a poor prognosis. A number of theorists have viewed process schizophrenia as the "true" form of schizophrenia and have postulated an endogenous, biological basis for it. *Reactive schizophrenia,* on the other hand, occurs as a response to stress in more adequate individuals, with an acute onset and a favorable prognosis. It is characterized by a lesser degree of regression than process schizophrenia and has often been viewed as "schizophreniform," i.e., schizophrenic in its form but not in its fundamental nature. Reactive schizophrenics are less likely than process schizophrenics to have had school difficulties in childhood and also are less likely to have had pathological siblings or to have manifested strong introversion. In adolescence, they are more likely to display heterosexual interests. Reactive schizophrenia has been theorized to have an environmental, functional etiology. Tutko and Spence (1962) found that on a sorting task a group of process schizophrenics, *like brain injured individuals,* could not generalize enough to name a common property of related objects. By contrast, reactive schizophrenics tended to designate a common property that was too broad, vague or idiosyncratic. King (1958) found that the level of autonomic responsiveness was lower in process than reactive

schizophrenics. Nevertheless, the hypothesis that one kind of schizophrenia has a biological etiology and the other a psychological etiology does not have a solid enough basis at the present time to be more than speculative.

The distinction between *good vs. poor adjustment in the premorbid stage*—i.e., adequacy vs. inadequacy of the patient's functioning prior to his illness—has been stressed by Garmezy and Rodnick (1959). Empirical study indicates that patients with poor premorbid adjustment have poorer prognoses, more disturbed relationships with their mothers, and greater sensitivity to social censure than good premorbid patients. The Phillips Scale (1953)—a set of items that cover the patient's social history—is usually used to differentiate poor from good premorbid schizophrenics. In the group with poor social relations in the pre-illness stage, the mothers tend to be dominant and the fathers submissive, whereas the reverse is true for the good premorbid group. These and related findings are reviewed in more detail in the following section on etiology. An important feature of distinguishing between good and poor premorbid schizophrenics is that in many respects patients can be classified in more detail than by gross symptomatology. A poor premorbid paranoid schizophrenic may behave more like a poor premorbid simple schizophrenic than like a good premorbid paranoid schizophrenic.

An important study of good and poor premorbid adjustment is that of Zigler and Phillips (1962). The case histories of 806 patients—schizophrenics, manic-depressives, psychoneurotics and character disorder patients—were examined to test two hypotheses: (1) within a schizophrenic population patients who exhibit a relatively good level of premorbid social competence are likely to turn against themselves, whereas patients who exhibit poor social competence are likely to avoid others or turn against them and simultaneously to be self-indulgent; (2) the hypothesis just specified holds for other disorders as well as for schizophrenia. Both hypotheses were confirmed. The investigators concluded that the dimension of social maturity and competence is fundamental for all forms of psychopathology.

CAUSATION AND DYNAMICS

The etiology of schizophrenia, like that of other disorders, is multiple. There are biological, psychological and sociocultural factors. The specific nature of these factors and their mode of interaction vary from patient to patient.

Heredity

The evidence that is reviewed in this section points strongly to the existence of a genetic predisposition to schizophrenia, although neither its exact importance nor its mode of transmission is known with certainty. It is also unclear whether a genetic predisposition is a *necessary* cause of schizophrenia—in which case an individual subjected to a rejecting mother, an isolated childhood or traumatic later life experiences will not develop the disorder if he is not genetically predisposed—schizophrenia can develop if *either* the genetic predisposition *or* some other combination of causes is strong enough. A few theorists, such as Kallmann, believe that heredity is not merely a necessary cause, but actually a sufficient one.

The evidence itself is complex. First, it has long been known that a much greater frequency of schizophrenia occurs among the relatives of schizophrenic patients than among the general population. However, high intrafamilial concentrations may be due not to heredity but to direct nongenetic transmission from one affected individual to another, or to a common and undesirable environment.

Second, there have been eleven major studies of schizophrenia in twins. The results of these studies are summarized in Table 12–1. In all studies a much higher frequency of schizophrenia was found among monozygotic than dizygotic co-twins. The concordance rates (percentage of cases in which both twins were schizophrenic) are much more consistent with each other than the concordance rates reported in twin studies of manic-depression. The index of heritability shown in the last column of the table indicates a sizable hereditary contribution.

It is possible that some forms of schizophrenia are predominantly determined by heredity and some by environmental factors. Rosenthal (1959) examined the case histories of monozygotic twins that had previously been published by Slater (1953) and found a history of schizophrenia in one or more family members of approximately 60 per cent of the families of the concordant twin pairs, in contrast with an almost total absence of schizophrenia in the families of discordant twin pairs. Rosenthal concluded that two broad types of schizophrenia were differentiated by this method of analysis: in one, the genetic contribution was considerable; in the other, the genetic contribution was absent or minimal. An additional finding, consistent with the distinction between process and reactive schizophrenics discussed earlier, was that

TABLE 12–1. Estimated Concordance Rates in Monozygotic and Dizygotic Co-twins of Schizophrenics

Investigator, Country and Year	Apparent Zygosity of Twins	Number of Pairs	Estimated Concordance Rate (Per cent)	Heritability $H = \dfrac{CMZ - CDZ}{100 - CDZ}$
Luxenburger, Germany, 1928	MZ	17	67	
	DZ	33	0	0.67
Rosanoff, United States, 1934	MZ	41	67	
	DZ	101	10	0.63
Essen-Moller, Sweden, 1941	MZ	7	71	
	DZ	24	17	0.65
Slater, England, 1953	MZ	41	76	
	DZ	115	14	0.72
Kallmann, United States, 1953	MZ	268	86	
	DZ	685	15	0.84
Inouye, Japan, 1961	MZ	55	76	
	DZ	17	22	0.69
Tienari, Finland, 1963	MZ	16	0	
	DZ	21	10	minus 0.11
Harvald and Hauge, Denmark, 1965	MZ	7	29	
	DZ	59	5	0.25
Kringlen, Norway, 1966	MZ	50	28	
	DZ	175	7	0.23
Gottesman and Shields, England, 1966	MZ	24	42	
	DZ	33	9	0.36
Cohen, Allen, Pollin and Hoffer United States, 1971	MZ	81	23	
	DZ	113	5	0.19

concordant twins tended to have an earlier age of onset, a less competent prepsychotic personality, and a poorer outcome than discordant male twins.

The study by Inouye (1961) listed in Table 12–1 led to a similar conclusion. Inouye divided the patients who belonged to monozygotic pairs into subgroups based on severity and duration of illness. In a chronic subgroup, 74 per cent of the co-twins also were schizophrenic, but in a subgroup characterized by brief duration of illness, the concordance rate was only 39 per cent. The implication is that severe, chronic schizophrenia is more a function of heredity than less severe and protracted forms of the disorder, a conclusion supported by the work of Gottesman and Shields (1966). Heston compared the psychosocial adjustment of 47 adults born to schizophrenic mothers with 50 control adults, where all subjects had been separated from their natural mothers from the first few days of life. A significant excess of both schizophrenic and sociopathic personality disorders were found among the offspring of schizophrenics, in comparison with the offspring of normal adults. The offspring of schizophrenic mothers included five with schizophrenia, four with mental deficiency, nine with sociopathic personality, and 13 with neurotic personality disorders. The offspring of the normal controls (also separated from their natural mothers) included none with schizophrenia or mental deficiency, two with sociopathic personality, and seven with neurotic personality disorders. The results are suggestive of both specific and nonspecific hereditary transmission, but require verification from further foster child studies.

The mode of genetic transmission has been investigated by comparing the observed frequencies of schizophrenia in various classes of relatives of patients with the frequencies that would be expected if schizophrenia were transmitted by a single dominant gene and with the frequencies to be expected for transmission by a pair of recessive genes. Gregory (1960) made such a comparison and concluded that the observed frequencies are lower than would be expected for simple recessive inheritance and much lower than expected for inheritance via a single dominant gene. The observed frequencies are more nearly consistent with a hypothesis of polygenic transmission. One of the implications of a polygenic mode of transmission is that schizophrenia could not be rapidly reduced by eugenic control as it theoretically

could be if the mode of transmission were by a single dominant gene. Gregory's conclusion concerning a polygenic theory of schizophrenia is highly consistent with the theoretical formulations of Gottesman and Shields (1969).

From a genetic point of view it is interesting to note that the probability of schizophrenia correlates negatively with intelligence and socioeconomic status. Follow-up studies of intellectually superior school children indicate a low frequency of schizophrenia among them in later life. Since intelligence has a strong genetic component and is associated with socioeconomic status, the high frequency of schizophrenia in lower socioeconomic groups may be due to a genetic component that affects both intelligence and predisposition to schizophrenia. The high rate of maternal mortality known to occur during the early childhood of schizophrenics may also have a genetic basis since resistance to bodily disease—like intelligence —appears to have a hereditary, polygenic component. Resistance to bodily disease is also positively correlated with socioeconomic status. However, there is an alternative, nongenetic explanation of the negative correlations between schizophrenia and intelligence, socioeconomic status and resistance to disease: socioeconomic deprivation may conduce simultaneously to a lower intellectual level, physical illness and schizophrenic disturbance.

Other Biological Factors

Variations in somatotype, immaturity of body structure and brain tissue degeneration have all been studied as possible factors in schizophrenia. A number of investigators have reported positive results.

Wittman, Sheldon and Katz (1948) found a positive correlation between predominantly ectomorphic body build and hebephrenic-like behavior, and between mesomorphic body build and paranoid behavior. Rees (1960) reported that schizophrenics were smaller in stature than normal and tended to be leptomorphic (asthenic) in body type. Doust (1952a) found that schizophrenics, as well as other psychiatric patients, were less mature in bodily development than normals. Incomplete development of the heart and circulatory system in catatonics and hebephrenics has been reported by a number of investigators. It has also been reported that the cutaneous capillaries of schizophrenics show such deviations from the normal as reduction in number, lack of uniformity in size, various bizarre shapes, rate of blood flow both faster and slower than normal, and frequent hemorrhages. In cases of chronic schizophrenia, some investigators have reported finding destroyed brain tissue, particularly in the frontal area.

However, these findings are methodologically suspect. Capillary and heart peculiarities may be due to environmental conditions or physical disease; brain tissue destruction seems to be no more frequent in chronic schizophrenia than in control groups *of the same age*; and the reported correlations of physique and schizophrenia need to be replicated before they can be accepted as fact. Neither definite proof nor disproof of a constitutional defect or bodily predisposition in schizophrenia has yet been offered.

In the area of biological function, as apart from structure, investigators have suggested that schizophrenia may be precipitated by a number of infectious agents. Most frequently cited has been the bacillus causing tuberculosis; rates of tuberculosis among schizophrenics have been quite high. However, a possible explanation is that a patient may inherit a susceptibility to the two disorders, rather than one disorder precipitating the other. Still another possibility is that schizophrenics, particularly those in crowded state hospitals, have been exposed to tuberculosis more than other persons.

Doust (1952b) found that the medical histories of schizophrenic patients included significantly more illnesses than the histories of normals, neurotics or patients with psychopathic personalities. Particularly common were musculoskeletal and cardiovascular diseases. One hypothesis is that schizophrenics are congenitally defective in the ability to develop immunity on exposure to physical disease.

Long-term investigations of catatonic patients have shown changes in basal metabolic rate and biochemical variables that correlate with appearance and disappearance of symptoms. In many schizophrenics, adrenal functioning appears to be disturbed, and some investigators have also reported thyroid underactivity. Blood pressure in schizophrenics is lower on the average than in normals. Of course, these findings are correlational rather than causal. However, Heath and his associates (1957) reported the extraction of a substance, presumably a protein, from the blood serum of schizophrenics which, when injected into nor-

mal subjects, was capable of reproducing such symptoms as depersonalization and difficulties in thinking. Heath termed this substance "taraxein." A number of investigators in the United States have been unable to reproduce his results, but Swedish and Russian scientists have reported experimental verification. If further corroborated, the findings would point strongly to a biological factor in schizophrenia.

Beckett et al. (1960) reported in schizophrenics, correlations between disturbances in ability to mobilize energy and severity of symptoms. Schizophrenics apparently have difficulty in converting glucose into energy, and, as a result, are unable to cope with stress. The schizophrenic's withdrawal from reality may thus have a biochemical basis. Beckett reported that patients who were severely incapacitated, as judged by clinical observations of overt behavior, were more defective in the mobilization of energy than less severely incapacitated patients. Some chronic schizophrenic patients, on the other hand, evidenced a continual overproduction of biologic energy that was apparently related to aggressive outbursts. Again, however, the correlations are compatible with causation but do not necessarily imply it.

The precipitation of psychotic behavior by sleep deprivation, sensory isolation, and the administration of hallucinogenic drugs has been extensively studied. Luby et al. (1962) reported that prolonged sleep deprivation in normals resulted in disturbed carbohydrate metabolism and the production of a blood serum substance believed to be similar to that found in naturally occurring schizophrenics. Furthermore, when schizophrenic patients were deprived of sleep, their symptoms were accentuated. However, sensory isolation, which produces hallucinations and delusions in some normal subjects, was better tolerated by schizophrenics than by normal controls. A possible implication may be that schizophrenic withdrawal serves the adaptive function of reducing an overload of incoming stimulation. Withdrawal may be a form of learned and self-imposed sensory isolation; the schizophrenic, so to speak, may *need* to withdraw.

In summary, a variety of structural and biochemical deviations have been linked to schizophrenia. As yet, however, no consistent and clear evidence of causality has emerged. It is perilous to deduce causality from the occurrence of differences between normals and schizophrenics. Horwitt (1956) makes the point that since schizophrenics are in a state of emotional stress, comparing them with normals on physiological variables is like comparing soldiers on the battlefield with persons in a relaxed condition. Physiology affects response to stress, but emotional stress also affects physiology.

An additional difficulty of the biological investigations is that schizophrenics are in many respects more heterogeneous than normals. Body temperature, rate of blood circulation, basal metabolic rate and many other measures have a greater range among schizophrenics than normals. Consequently, for a given biological characteristic, a number of schizophrenics will fall below most normals and a number will fall above them. The mean found for a schizophrenic group in a particular study may therefore depend more on the particular type of schizophrenic patient studied than on the intrinsic nature of schizophrenia.

Dynamics and Psychological Determinants

The schizophrenic is an individual with an ego that has broken down and retreated from reality. Freud (1924) characterized the difference between neurosis and psychosis as the difference between "the ego [that] remains true to its allegiance to the outer world and endeavors to subjugate the id, or . . . allows itself to be overwhelmed by the id and thus torn away from reality." An equivalent formulation is that a psychotic—particularly a schizophrenic—regresses to a greater degree of narcissism and a more infantile state of psychosexual development than does a neurotic.

Psychoanalysts, following the guidelines established by Freud, have stressed regression as a basic mechanism of schizophrenia. The patient behaves as if he is reliving infantile conflicts. His hallucinations, according to psychoanalytic theory, are projected images of his parents; his delusions represent primitive and unconscious impulses; and his paralogical thinking stems from a childish tendency to magical and irrational thinking. The specific psychological etiology of this regression has been the focus of much speculation and empirical study. A widespread point of view is that expressed by Arieti (1960):

All cases which have been studied psychoanalytically by various authors have demonstrated, without variation, severe and early psychological maladjustment, poor family relations, unhappy childhood, severe conflicts, and a paucity of adequate defenses. Severe and badly compensated conflict seems a necessary antecedent to schizophrenia.

An important component and possible cause of the schizophrenic's maladjustment is social isolation. The human ego seems to need constant social stimulation in order to remain separate from the id, that is, to avoid regression to a state in which the individual is ruled by primary process thinking. Barthell and Holmes (1968) examined yearbook senior summaries of high school graduates who later became schizophrenic. It was found that those persons who were later diagnosed as schizophrenic had participated in significantly fewer activities in high school than their normal controls. In the absence of social interaction, the individual narcissistically directs his libido inward instead of outward, loses the frame of reference provided by social reality, and suffers a disruption of learned, adaptive habits. A schizophrenic may withdraw from social interaction because of innate tendencies—for example, an innately high level of anxiety—or because of environmental circumstances, or both. Many theorists feel that schizophrenic withdrawal represents an avoidance of threatening interpersonal relationships, criticism and failure. To quote Schilder (1939): "It is as if the schizophrenic would say, 'This fully differentiated world of yours is much too difficult and dangerous and therefore I content myself with a more primitive world.'" It should be added that a feeling of threat may also directly hinder discrimination and differentiation between different aspects of the outer world and between reality and inner fantasy. Fromm-Reichmann (1950) attributed the schizophrenic's aloofness to a desire to avoid the rebuffs that he had experienced in childhood, and that he had come to feel were inevitable.

Harlow (1962) found that young monkeys who are deprived of contact with mothers and peers display gross behavioral abnormalities when they are fully grown, including heterosexual avoidance and catatonic-like symptoms. A similar deprivation of social relationships in children may be a crucial predisposing factor in schizophrenia. Social isolation from peers may, of course, be the outcome of influences by parents who are themselves socially isolated and perceive interpersonal relationships as unrewarding and dangerous.

In many cases the childhood of schizophrenics is marked by "good" behavior and overconformity to social standards rather than overt withdrawal. However, such an outward façade may conceal emotional withdrawal, as the child may behave in an exemplary manner in order to avoid struggle and active interaction with others. Kohn and Clausen (1955) found that one-third of the schizophrenic patients whom they studied had a history of social isolation in adolescence, a far larger percentage than in normals. The other two-thirds did not, but it is likely that many of them *felt* socially alienated while interacting with others superficially and "correctly." They may have been isolated in a psychological, but not physical, sense. A feeling of social alienation tends to be accompanied by social awkwardness and self-consciousness, inhibition of impulses and avoidance of adult social responsibilities. It will be remembered that approximately two-thirds of male schizophrenics are unmarried.

Accompanying his physical or emotional isolation, the schizophrenic displays excessive fantasy, the substitution of an unrealistic world for the threatening real one and the projection of sexual and aggressive impulses, as well as the blame for his difficulties, onto others. Schizophrenic withdrawal, fantasy and projection are *defensive*. It is only a step from these defenses to delusions; ultimately, delusions are also defensive.

Considerable experimental study has demonstrated that the basis of the schizophrenic's withdrawal is the strength of his *aversive motivation*. When rewarded for making discriminations in a complex learning task, schizophrenics perform as competently as normals, but under conditions of punishment or criticism performance is more impaired than for normals (Garmezy, 1952). Garmezy and Rodnick (1959) and a number of their students have hypothesized that the schizophrenic with a poor premorbid adjustment is much more controlled by aversive motivation than the schizophrenic with a good premorbid adjustment. The latter still has adaptive, nonaversive potentialities and hence a good prognosis; the poor premorbid patient, on the other hand, is aversive to friends, marriage, community activities or any other social involvement. Experimental results have partially supported this hypothesis. In an experimental situation in which subjects first guessed what an individual in a picture would do and then were told that their guesses were wrong, poor premorbids reversed their guesses more often than good premorbids or normals. Dunn (1954) found that poor premorbids had no particular

difficulty in a visual discrimination task in which pictorial materials were used as stimuli, except when the pictured scene was that of a mother scolding a child. Presumably, the performance of the poor premorbid patient was disrupted by a spread of aversiveness from his actual childhood relationship with his mother to the experimental stimulus.

Aversive motivation in schizophrenia has been studied in relation to other variables also. For example, Feffer (1961) hypothesized that pathologically concrete thinking in schizophrenia represents an avoidance response to affective stimuli, i.e., that some of the schizophrenic's thought difficulties result from aversive motivation. To test this hypothesis, Feffer constructed a figure-ground situation in which the locus of the affective stimuli (emotionally upsetting words) was sometimes in the figure and sometimes in the ground. The stimuli were presented on a tachistoscope. It was found that schizophrenics who were strongly marked by concrete thinking tended to avoid the affective words by concentrating on the ground when the affective words were in the figure, and on the figure when the affective words were in the ground. Normals, as well as a group of schizophrenics not characterized by concrete thinking, did not avoid the affective stimuli. Extrapolating from these results, it may be inferred that the schizophrenic whose thinking is concrete may be *afraid* to use adequately broad, abstract categories. Like social isolation, concrete thinking may be governed by aversive motivation.

The aversive motivation of a schizophrenic may have a neurological basis. The cortical "punishment centers" of a schizophrenic may be stimulated more than in a normal individual. It is also possible that the neurological functioning of a poor premorbid schizophrenic differs from that of a good premorbid. Alternatively, early childhood experiences rather than neurological factors may be responsible for variations in the strength of aversive motivation.

A note of caution must be added with respect to the postulated aversive motivation of schizophrenics. Fontana et al. (1967) failed to find any differential response to censure among good and poor premorbid schizophrenics and normals. Klein et al. (1967) found that both schizophrenics and normals had a faster reaction time in response to mild verbal censure than in response to praise. Perhaps the schizophrenic's aversive response to censure is operative only in situations which are more directly reminiscent of the original family learning context and where censure has no informational value with respect to task performance.

A schizophrenic episode *may be precipitated by a specific trauma or may progress imperceptibly out of a schizoid personality* with no identifiable precipitating cause. In the latter event, the development of schizophrenia parallels the development of a symptom neurosis from a neurotic personality. (Of course, a combination of a schizoid personality and an identifiable precipitant may also occur.) A common precipitant is a new situation with which the patient cannot cope—the arousal of sexual or other conflicts by marriage, the responsibility of parenthood, a transfer to a new job in which the individual feels threatened, enforced interaction with a person who resembles a threatening childhood figure and so forth. The new situation overwhelms a brittle ego and the individual's psychotic tendencies break out openly.

Jenkins (1950) describes the schizoid personality as follows:*

Its essence seems to be a lack of attention to and of reactivity to the nonverbal cues to feeling and thinking for which one normally watches. In social relations the normally reacting person is not only listening to words; he watches expression, movement, gesture. He picks up cues from intonation, stress, action, choice of words. He is alert to reversals of meaning implied by a tone of sarcasm or irony. He is alive to many impressions, the sources of which he could describe or analyze only very imperfectly, if at all. Typically he will describe the results of these observations in terms of his sensing feelings rather than in terms of describing actions. "She seemed pleased underneath it all." "His laughter seemed forced." "He was very controlled, but you felt he was angry."

The schizoid manner is recognized by the normal person and is described in feeling language, typically without clear perception of what brings about the impression. "He seemed to be in another world." "You felt he might as well have been on Mars." "It was as though we were talking through a glass wall." "Somehow you felt he wasn't really there." "He didn't seem to feel I existed."

The schizoid personality is also characterized by oversensitivity, an unstable alternation of inhibited behavior and impulsiveness, an absence of interests and a paucity of techniques for obtaining satisfaction in the real world. The schizoid youngster is typically an underachiever. As compared to other children who have been referred to guidance clinics, he is

*From Jenkins, R. 1950. Nature of the schizophrenic process. A.M.A. Arch. Neurol. & Psychiat., *64*:243–262.

likely to be intellectually superior but scholastically retarded. Furthermore, Jenkins and Glickman (1946) found that the performance I.Q. of the schizoid child was 10 or more points below his verbal I.Q. Thus the practical component of his intelligence is relatively low and he is easily frustrated.

In a study of a large number of hospitalized schizophrenics, Schofield and Balian (1959) found that as compared to physically ill subjects, the schizophrenics' early histories were characterized by a significantly higher incidence of poor relationships with parents, poor attitudes to school and poor school achievement. Schizophrenics also had little occupational success and satisfaction. They manifested more social withdrawal, a lack of adeptness and poise in social situations, narrow interests, limited aspirations, vagueness in life plans and a lack of initiative. These characteristics are all consistent with the general concept of the schizoid personality. A word of caution is needed, however: on all characteristics there was considerable overlap of the physically ill and schizophrenic groups. For example, narrowness of interests was noted in 20.7 per cent of the physically ill and 35.2 per cent of the schizophrenic patients. The difference is highly significant statistically, yet most schizophrenics as well as most physically ill subjects had some breadth of interests. A schizoid personality characterizes a substantial number of persons who later become schizophrenic, but far from all; it also characterizes a smaller but definite number of persons who never develop schizophrenia. Perhaps the life experiences of the latter group are psychologically favorable enough to prevent breakdown.

We have repeatedly hinted at the importance of *poor family relationships* in the causation of schizophrenia. Few aspects of schizophrenia have been more studied than family relationships and attitudes. Sullivan (1953) hypothesized that schizophrenia is an indirect outcome of parent-child relationships in which the child is not permitted to establish patterns of response that will serve to eliminate anxiety. The anxious child misinterprets interpersonal situations (parataxic distortions, to use Sullivan's term), eventually loses the consensual validation of social reality and withdraws into an autistic world. Kasanin, Knight and Sage (1934) examined 45 case histories of schizophrenics and reported that maternal overprotection or rejection was present in 60 per cent. Despert (1942) reported that the mothers of schizophrenic children were aggressive, overanxious, oversolicitous and often strongly ambivalent. Tietze (1949) described the mothers of 25 schizophrenics as perfectionistic, self-righteous and dominating, most often in a subtle way. Gerard and Siegel (1950) studied the family background of 71 male schizophrenics and concluded that the parents were immature, had a poor marital relationship and often overprotected the child. Reichard and Tillman (1950) emphasized the dominating, egocentric and manipulative role of the mother. They perceived her as unable to form a proper respect for the child's need to be himself and unable to accept him in his own right. Reports such as these have led to the concept of the "schizophrenogenic mother," a term that embodies the hypothesis that the mother is the main cause or genesis of the child's later psychotic breakdown.

Mark (1953) administered an attitude survey to 100 mothers of male schizophrenics and a control group of 100 mothers of normals. A large number of items differentiated the two groups at a statistically significant level. The mothers of schizophrenics believed in restrictive control of children. They were perfectionistic, upset by children's sexual impulses, and both excessively devoted and coolly detached. They conceived of themselves as self-sacrificing martyrs. The following items are representative of many others in the study; on each, a larger proportion of mothers of schizophrenics than controls were in agreement with the statement.

Children should be taken to and from school until the age of eight just to make sure there are no accidents.

A mother should make it her business to know everything her children are thinking.

If children are quiet for a little while a mother should immediately find out what they are thinking about.

Children should not annoy parents with their unimportant problems.

A devoted mother has no time for social life.

Playing too much with a child will spoil him.

A parent must never make mistakes in front of the child.

A mother has to suffer much and say little.

Children who take part in sex play become sex criminals when they grow up.

Answering questions about sex is embarrassing and unnecessary.

It is all right for a mother to sleep with a child because it gives him a feeling of being loved and wanted.

Spanking a child does more good than harm.

There's little thanks or pleasure in raising children.

Some children are just naturally bad.

A good mother should shelter her child from life's little difficulties.

Every parent has a favorite child.

It is better for children to play at home than to visit other children.

A study by McGhie (1961) led to the conclusion that the schizophrenic's mother has remarkable capacity for denying the patient's early difficulties. "Not only does she distort reality in projecting the cause of the patient's abnormal reactions outside of him, but she also accepts, approves and actively encourages the deviant features in his development. Her influence on the patient is almost specifically designed effectively to cripple the child's attempts to reach an independent and stable level of adjustment." In McGhie's interviews with schizophrenics' mothers, some striking findings emerged concerning their own early history. They tended to report an unhappy early home life which was often disrupted by parental loss. As children, they had been unhappy, insecure and unable to make good contact with others. As they grew up, they remained somewhat isolated socially. Psychologically, they rejected their femininity. Their marriages were predestined to failure by their unsolved problems.

Several investigators have focused attention on the childhood relationship between the schizophrenic and his father and also on the relationship between the parents. Lidz and Lidz (1949) studied the clinical histories of 50 schizophrenic patients and found that fewer than 10 per cent came from well integrated homes in which both parents were reasonably stable. "In our data it is apparent that the paternal influences are noxious as frequently as the maternal," they concluded. Further, "The study of the histories of these patients impresses . . . that one patient after another was subjected to a piling up of adverse intrafamilial forces that were major factors in moulding the misshapen personality, and which repeatedly interfered with the patient's attempts at maturation in a most discouraging fashion." Lidz and Fleck (1960) reviewed the results of subsequent intensive analyses of schizophrenics' families. Among the characteristics noted for the typical mother were an imperviousness to what the child sought to convey, combined with an inordinate intrusiveness, a confusion of the child's needs with her own due to projection, and a disparity between what she said and what she really demanded of the child. The investigators found that the fathers *impenetrable*

NORMALS

were disturbed as often and as much as the mothers. The fathers were often very insecure in their masculinity and needed constant admiration and attention to bolster their self-esteem. A quality of imperviousness to the feelings and sensitivities of others epitomized many of the fathers as well as the mothers. Lidz and Fleck pointed out that a father may exert an adverse influence on a child either directly or through the relationship with the mother. Frequently the relationships between mother and father were characterized by "marital schism," a condition of severe and chronic discord. Each partner was disillusioned with the other: the husband saw the wife as disregarding his own best interests and failing as a mother, and the wife was disappointed in the husband's failure to be the strong father figure she had hoped for. In numerous other instances there was a condition of "marital skew" in which the dominant parent manifested serious psychological disturbance which was accepted or shared by the other parent.

In a more recent study, Fleck, Lidz and Cornelison (1963) compared the parent-child relationships of male and female schizophrenics and found that the males often came from skewed families with passive, ineffectual fathers and disturbed, engulfing mothers. Schizophrenic girls, on the other hand, typically grew up in families with weak, emotionally distant mothers and narcissistic fathers who were often somewhat paranoid; the fathers disparaged women but were seductive toward their daughters. It is obvious that these family constellations are made to order for the production of severe disturbances in psychosexual identification.

An important study by Kohn and Clausen (1956) investigated schizophrenics' and normals' *perceptions* of their parents. Both male and female schizophrenics more often than normals perceived their mothers as having played a major role in the family decision processes. The patients regarded their mothers as strict, dominant and restrictive of their freedom; more often than normals, they felt that paternal authority was weak. Among the normals, the females felt that they were controlled by their mothers, but the males did not; schizophrenic males thus perceived their mothers much as did normal females.

A finding of great interest in Kohn and Clausen's study is that the proportion of schizophrenics perceiving the mother as the principal authority figure is independent of social class. Among normals, on the other hand, the mother

independent of SES

tends to be seen as the principal authority in lower classes only; in the upper groups, the father is perceived as the principal authority. Hence schizophrenic patients, including those with an upper class origin, manifest attitudes characteristic of lower socioeconomic groups. This finding may conceivably hold a clue to explain the high incidence of schizophrenia at low socioeconomic levels.

An additional finding was that those female schizophrenics who perceived themselves as dominated by their mothers felt emotionally closer to their weak fathers, whereas the male patients felt closer to their domineering mothers. As in the previously cited study by Fleck, Lidz and Cornelison, both male and female patients appear to have acquired a confused and undesirable set of psychosexual identifications with the "wrong" parent. It should be noted that since Kohn and Clausen investigated perceptions of parents, but not parents' actual behavior, we cannot be sure that the perceptions were accurate. But whether accurate or distorted, a schizophrenic's perceptions are part of his disorder and may also be a causal factor in generating it.

Bowen and his associates (1959) intensively studied a small number of families with a schizophrenic child and found that the mother and father were separated by a barrier strong enough to be termed an "emotional divorce." The patient's function was that of an unsuccessful mediator in a war. The parental war often led to the formation of a twosome between mother and child from which the father was excluded, usually by his own volition.

Garmezy and Rodnick (1959) reviewed the results of studies relating differences between good and poor premorbid schizophrenics to differences in family organization. In one study, patients were asked to answer child-rearing attitude scales as they believed their mothers and fathers would have answered when the latter were growing up. Poor premorbid patients ascribed more deviant attitudes to both parents than good premorbids or normal controls. Poor premorbid patients tended to perceive their mothers as more dominant and their fathers as less dominant than did good premorbids. Normals indicated a pattern of shared authority with very little conflict between parents. These results were substantiated by a study in which Farina (1960) used a structured situational test consisting of hypothetical problem situations, e.g., "Your 12-year-old son gets home from school. He throws his books down, telling you what you have been teaching him is wrong and that he is not going to listen to you any more." The responses of the parents, indicating what they believed they would do in 12 such problem situations, pointed to maternal dominance in the families of poor premorbid schizophrenics and paternal dominance in the families of the good premorbids. Apparently the failure of a father to provide an adequately masculine role model contributes to the malignancy of the disorder.

Bateson et al. (1956) advanced the concept of the "double bind" as a pattern of communication that provokes schizophrenic behaviors by directing to the individual a pair of messages that are closely related but sharply incongruent with each other. It is not easy for the patient to perceive this lack of congruence and he cannot respond effectively. The messages influence him toward responses that are incompatible with each other; he is damned if he does and damned if he doesn't. A mother may tell her daughter, "Have some cake. I baked it especially for you," (implying, "You'll hurt my feelings if you don't"). Immediately afterward the mother remarks, "You're overweight," (implying, "I don't approve of people who are overweight. You shouldn't have eaten it"). When the mother of a schizophrenic daughter asked what she was doing, the patient replied that she was finishing a letter to her fiancé so it would catch the last mail. The mother nagged and scolded the daughter into helping with the dishes and as a result the daughter was unable to finish the letter in time; the mother remarked, "You don't really like him very much, do you?" A young man who later became schizophrenic regularly sent his pay check while in the Army to his mother. Their understanding was that she would use part for her living expenses and save the rest so that he could attend college after discharge. When he asked for his share, she told him she had spent it all and added, "A good boy wouldn't ask for it," putting him in the impossible position of having to give up his due or be a "bad boy." The double bind obviously operates to generate anxiety and painful conflict.

The following verbatim letter to a hospitalized schizophrenic and its double-bind interpretation are quoted from Weakland and Fry.* (The patient's mother and father were divorced. The father had remarried and the

___

*From Weakland, J. H., and Fry, W. F. 1962. Letters of mothers of schizophrenics, Amer. J. Orthopsychiat., 32:604–623. Copyright, The American Orthopsychiatric Association, Inc. Reproduced by permission.

parents visited the patient separately. The "Clem" referred to in the letter was the patient's husband, reportedly sadistic to her. He did not visit her in the hospital.)

Dear Janet
Just a few lines again
I talked to your Dad on the phone and he said you dident answer his letter. You better write to him.
I want to have you visit me one of these days & maybe you can visit him too.
And by the way you havent written to me. (You did call me.)
And you know Janet I don't like to even think of Clem it seems to remind me of trouble. Id rather just not think of him.
And dont you let the cigarette habit get stronger than you are.
Sometimes these habits have a way of doing that.
When I get a chance Ill get you a Carton.
But too much smoking is bad business.
I want so much too have you visit me as soon as possible, so be good and write to me.
Your Dad said you dident answer his letter so maybe you ought to, but dont tell him I told you.
Well I better close now. Hope I can visit you soon.
Lots & Lots of Love.

Mother

Weakland and Fry comment as follows on the letter:

The letter begins with self-deprecation, "Just a few lines again," which also may 1) reflect deprecatively on the recipient as not worth more, and 2) make any strong impact it might have difficult to attribute to the communication. That is, since it is "just a few lines," if the patient should be upset on reading it one implication is that this outcome reflects something wrong with the patient rather than with the letter or its author.

Next, mother benevolently minds the patient's business in telling her to write her father, although the parents are divorced and avoid meeting. Similar influence is continued in the suggestion about possibly visiting father. Coupled to this is an expression of a wish that Janet might visit her, the mother. This looks positive, but may be difficult for the patient. In the first place, the statements about visiting father and visiting mother are closely juxtaposed and similar in phrasing, but very different fundamentally: One is a controlling suggestion concerning another person, the other expresses a wish of the writer; moreover, the people involved in the similarity are at odds with each other. This combination of similarity and difference is confusing in itself. Second, the apparent invitation to visit mother is vague and casual, an indefinite "one of these days" statement. Seen in context, with the recipient a daughter confined in a mental hospital, this casualness must to some extent convey a raising of hopes but treating them lightly, brushing the patient off again. Even this

feeble overture toward contact is immediately followed by an underplayed ("and by the way") reproach
("You haven't written me"), and then another reversal
("You did call me"), with this also underplayed by
being put in parentheses. The mother next reminds
the patient of her own estranged husband; this appears as a gratuitous recalling of this painful topic to
the daughter's mind while saying, "I'd rather just not
think of him."

After this brief but comprehensive handling of
family relationships, the mother turns to the bad habit
of smoking. She cautions her daughter, imputing a
weakness or inability to take charge of her own
smoking, though Janet is a grown married woman. Yet
this as a personal accusation is obscured by the impersonal phrasing concretizing the "cigarette habit"
and its influence. Then, having indirectly told Janet
"Don't smoke so much," she promises to send a
whole carton of cigarettes. And the gift offer, like the
visit offer, is casual—"When I get the chance."
Again, though, she disqualifies this offer by "too much
smoking is bad business."

The letter then returns to the family themes. Again a
completely indefinite hope about a visit home is held
out, followed abruptly by an implied condition for
such a visit—"so be good and write me." The more
complete message here then appears to be "I want
to see you if you behave as I like." Yet this is uncertain too; the original statement is so inexplicit that
nothing is even testable. There is also a further development on controlling the relationship of Janet and
her father ("You ought to answer his letter" again)
plus suggested conspiracy to conceal the mother's
influence ("don't tell him I told you"). The letter is
then terminated by unspecific, indefinite positive—
"Hope I can visit you soon," and "Lots and lots of
love."

This detailed recital of incongruent alternations:
yes-only-no, do-only-don't, come-yet-wait—which
may not be visible to the patient because of the
vagueness and generality in the letter, its "played-
down" nature, and its over-all framing as benevolent—provides recurrent exemplification of
messages fitting our double-bind concept.

Clinical evidence indicates that many schizophrenics are the recipients of double-bind communications in childhood and later. However,
thus far research evidence has failed to show
that double-bind communication is more
likely to lead to schizophrenia than to other
forms of psychological disturbance (Schuham,
1967). For example, the individual could respond by rebellion and sociopathic, instead of
schizophrenic, behavior. Furthermore, normal
persons also receive many double-bind communications but take them in stride, whereas a
schizophrenic is made anxious. A schizophrenic is also likely to perceive a double bind
in situations in which others do not. Finally, it

should be realized that a parent may in some
cases direct a double-bind message to a
schizophrenic offspring precisely because the
latter is schizophrenic and therefore difficult to
communicate with. In general, deviant parental
attitudes and overt behaviors—like deviant
patterns of communication—may result from
psychopathology in children as well as cause it.
Often a vicious circle is set up; as Arieti (1959)
puts it: "It is a two-way stream, a reverberation
of anxiety from the parent to the child and
from the child to the parent."

Sociocultural Determinants

Schizophrenia occurs in every country and
culture, but its symptoms are not universal. In
primitive cultures, schizophrenics are likely to
believe that they have been bewitched or
poisoned. The case history of a paranoid with a
delusion of malignant witchcraft is presented in
the next chapter. In more advanced cultures
they often believe that they are being persecuted
by complex mechanical or electronic devices.
In a review of mental illness in primitive
societies, Benedict and Jacks (1954) concluded that more schizophrenics in these
settings are of the "nuclear" type (early and
insidious onset, premorbid schizoid personality,
poor prognosis) and fewer of the more intact,
"peripheral" type than in nonprimitive societies.
Furthermore, homicidal behavior accompanied
by confused excitement was reported to be frequent among the primitive groups but depressive
symptoms were comparatively infrequent. Benedict and Jacks therefore suggested that in a
primitive culture the psychotic individual tends
to direct his hostility outward, whereas in
western society he is more likely to direct it
inward.

A number of investigators have suggested
that changes in the frequency and symptoms of
schizophrenia over long time periods are attributable to cultural factors. First admissions of
schizophrenics have increased rapidly in the
past several decades in the United States, but a
large part of this increase consists of relatively
mild cases. Nowadays, fewer patients than
formerly are seen in a continuous state of
excitement and with extremely vivid, in-
cessant hallucinations. The trend away from the
more excited kind of symptoms must be
attributed largely to early diagnosis and treatment, but such sociocultural factors as wide-

spread education and the increasing emphasis on getting along with other people may also have played a role.

Within our culture, relatively high rates for schizophrenia have been found among the foreign-born (particularly recent immigrants), Negroes and persons of low education and low socioeconomic level of occupational status. High rates also characterize urban rather than rural areas. However, data from both Britain and the United States have shown that when schizophrenics are classified according to their fathers' social statuses, all classes are represented proportionally. This suggests that premorbid symptoms of schizophrenia lead to downward social drift (Hollingshead and Redlich, 1958; Goldberg and Morrison, 1963). Within urban areas, first-admission rates have been repeatedly shown to be highest in neighborhoods marked by social disorganization. For example, Gerard and Houston (1953) analyzed the distribution of schizophrenia in Worcester, Massachusetts, and found that it was most frequent in disorganized neighborhoods where single, separated and divorced men tended to live. The findings were supported in other investigations, including a study of Bristol, England, by Hare (1956). The excess of schizophrenia in areas where unmarried men are concentrated is explainable by the hypothesis that individuals with personality difficulties tend to drift toward the more disorganized areas of a city. However, an alternative and more cogent explanation is that community disorganization and individual alienation from the family are direct causes of schizophrenia.

In their extensive study of social class and mental illness, Hollingshead and Redlich (1958) found that the overall prevalence of schizophrenia (as estimated by number of patients in treatment or receiving custodial care) was inversely related to the social class of the patient. In the lowest class the rate was eight times larger than in the highest. The incidence of newly diagnosed cases of schizophrenia showed a similar, although less marked, inverse relationship: In the lowest class, incidence over a six-month period was 2.5 times greater than in the highest. Hollingshead and Redlich concluded that the excess at the lower levels was a product of undesirable life conditions and that the greater tendency to chronicity among members of the lower classes was related to the poorer quality of the psychiatric treatment they received.

TREATMENT

The sooner a schizophrenic is treated, the better. His chances of recovery diminish steadily as the disorder progresses and if he is not discharged within the first year of hospitalization the probability that he will be discharged at any later time is less than 50 per cent.

Somatic treatments, such as electric shock and tranquilizers, are among the most frequently used techniques with schizophrenics. A minority of experts prefer psychotherapy, but they too advocate somatic treatment for patients when psychotherapy is not available (i.e., in the majority of cases), or when it has failed, or when patients are too withdrawn to be reached by psychotherapy.

In the 1940's, insulin coma treatment was generally accepted as the best somatic procedure for schizophrenics. A commission on New York State hospital problems in 1944, comparing the outcome for 1128 patients who had received insulin coma therapy with the outcome for 897 matched control patients, found that 80 per cent of the insulin-treated patients had left the hospital but only 59 per cent of the controls. The treated patients had an average hospital stay four months shorter than the untreated group. However, follow-up studies indicated later relapses in as many as 50 per cent of the discharged patients who had been treated by insulin and lower relapse rates for the controls. A possible reason for the high rate of relapse among the insulin-treated patients is that they may have been discharged too soon because of the hospital personnel's faith in the treatment. In any event, the long-range superiority of insulin was very minor. The best one can hope for with insulin treatment is a lasting recovery rate of only 40 to 50 per cent. Among the varieties of schizophrenic reaction, catatonics respond best to insulin and paranoids next best.

Because of the difficulties and risks of insulin coma therapy, a number of psychiatrists came to prefer ECT. However, although ECT is helpful in controlling the symptoms of catatonic stupor or excitement, it is otherwise unimpressive with schizophrenics. In a study by Rees (1960), patients treated by insulin, ECT or electronarcosis were compared with untreated patients. Only the insulin group showed much better results. Within a few years, however, insulin treatment had been almost wholly superseded by tranquilizers.

Psychosurgery has rarely been performed on schizophrenics unless all other available forms of treatment have failed. Most often it has been used with chronic, regressed patients judged to be hopeless. As might be expected, the results have been poorer with schizophrenia than with severe obsessive-compulsive disorders or involutional melancholia. However, a number of studies have indicated that a considerable proportion of even chronic schizophrenics can be returned to the community after psychosurgery and as many as one-fourth can become self-supporting.

Since the advent of chlorpromazine in 1953 and the great variety of tranquilizing drugs which subsequently became available, there has been a therapeutic revolution in the treatment of schizophrenia. Insulin coma therapy and psychosurgery have been completely discontinued in many hospitals and are used only infrequently in others. Initially the tranquilizing drugs were found to be most helpful for the control of excessive psychomotor activity and aggressive behavior, but soon it was discovered that they also reduced hallucinations, delusions, irrational thinking, disorganized speech, anxiety and inappropriate affect. Efforts to develop energizing drugs to stimulate chronically inactive and apathetic schizophrenics have so far been much less successful.

Over the last few decades a great many schizophrenics have been treated in individual and group psychotherapy. The basis of psychotherapy with a schizophrenic is the hypothesis that he "is not happy with his withdrawal, as some psychiatrists used to believe, and he is ready to resume interpersonal relations, provided he finds a person he trusts, a person who is capable of removing that suspiciousness and distrust which originated with the first interpersonal relations" (Arieti, 1959). The therapist must be kind and understanding; the schizophrenic, even more than the neurotic, must not feel rejected by the therapist. However, while agreeing on the importance of this point, therapists who work with schizophrenics disagree on many others. Some psychotherapists feel that the schizophrenic should be treated as a mature adult even when he behaves in an infantile fashion and that it may be wise to adopt a reserved attitude with him. Other therapists deliberately assume the role of a powerful but loving mother or father in order to substitute for the benevolent parent that the patient never had.

Whichever approach is taken, it is important to trust and like the patient and not fear him.

The schizophrenic may be afraid of being hurt by the therapist—as he has been hurt in other relationships—and may therefore attack before he is attacked. The therapist must be able to tolerate this hostility without fear and without counter-hostility. Obviously, not all therapists can do this; many are highly skilled in the treatment of neurotics but inadequate with schizophrenics. It is also important not to rush the patient nor intrude on him. Especially in the early stages of treatment, the therapist must avoid questioning the schizophrenic. Some therapists feel that it is wise to talk about neutral topics frequently in order to desensitize the patient and lower his anxiety level. Others think long periods of silence are desirable. In the beginning stages of therapy with severely disturbed schizophrenics, a number of therapists have experimented with daily sessions in which the therapist and patient merely sit and perhaps smoke a cigarette together. In a variation of this approach, the therapist may regularly bring presents such as articles of food to the patient until the latter begins to trust him enough to talk.

It is essential to be honest with the patient. If the latter is incoherent, it is pointless or even harmful for the therapist to pretend he understands. If the patient asks whether his behavior is "crazy," he must be given an honest answer. Again, not all therapists find this easy to do.

It is even more difficult to avoid challenging the patient's delusions and hallucinations. Telling the patient that these are unreal is useless, for to him they are real enough. Furthermore, challenging a patient with persecutory delusions merely confirms his belief that he is being persecuted. Nor should the therapist "agree" with the delusions. He must steer a difficult middle course in which he accepts them as experiences that are real to the patient, must try sympathetically to understand them, and nevertheless must avoid being "for" or "against" them. If the patient says, "Everyone is against me," a therapeutic response is rarely "No, they aren't" or "Yes, they are," but rather, "What do you mean by everyone?" or "How are they against you?" Of course, the patient's response to such a question must be followed up, and the therapist may find himself deeply enmeshed in the patient's world.

The couch is usually avoided, even when the therapist subscribes to a psychoanalytic point of view, for the patient needs to be kept close to reality and away from the fantasy world that is encouraged by lying on a psychoanalytic couch.

The therapist also keeps the patient in touch with reality by insisting that appointments be kept punctually. A number of therapists believe that schizophrenics need guidance, control and support more than insight, and they concentrate on helping patients regulate their lives to conform with reality. Increased insight, in fact, may hurt rather than help, as it involves a danger of arousing conflicts more strongly than ever. In a sense, the psychotic patient needs socially sanctioned repressions more than the lifting of repressions. Grayson and Olinger (1957) demonstrated the importance of a correct understanding of reality in a study of 45 hospitalized patients, 24 of whom were schizophrenic. The patients were asked to answer the items of the Minnesota Multiphasic Personality Inventory "the way a typical well-adjusted person on the outside would do." The schizophrenics who were able to simulate normal profiles successfully were more likely to improve enough to leave the hospital than were those less successful in simulating normalcy. The members of the improved group, in essence, were better able to understand and adopt the role of a normal individual than those in the unimproved group.

There are certain dangers in psychotherapy with a schizophrenic. His conflicts may be aroused too strongly for his weakened ego to tolerate. He may bog down in a fruitless analysis of his inner life instead of learning to cope with external life. One of the arguments for group rather than individual therapy with schizophrenics is that the other group members check on each patient's attitude and fantasies and provide him with a kind of external reality which may be a useful prelude to social reality outside of therapy.

Finally, milieu therapy in the hospital, involving group therapeutic activities and the open hospital concept, is playing an increasingly important part in treatment. In an interesting study, Murray and Cohen (1959) compared the social structure in a hospital ward employing milieu and group therapy and a ward primarily employing somatic therapy. In the milieu-oriented ward, the interactions among the patients were more complex and the patients often made "reciprocal choices" of each other: if patient A had a positive attitude toward patient B, the latter was likely to reciprocate it. In addition, it was found that the introduction of milieu therapy into locked wards with very ill patients led to an increase in social interaction.

With the advent of the community mental health movement in this country, more alternatives to hospitalization have become available for meeting the needs of the schizophrenic. Increasingly patients are seen locally on an outpatient basis instead of being sent away to a hospital for a long duration and thus increasing their alienation from the community. Hospitalization is frequently unnecessary or is employed only until the patient is over the acute phase. The centers make available supportive services such as some psychotherapy, drug supervision, and meaningful activities with other members of the community. The clinics may also provide after-care services to patients who have been hospitalized for longer periods of time. While data are still scarce, such programs appear to be having some success and provide a viable alternative to long-term hospital confinement. Orlinsky, and D'Elia (1964) found that only 25.7 per cent of 1336 schizophrenic patients who attended an after-care clinic following discharge were rehospitalized within 12 months. On the other hand, 45.5 per cent of 769 schizophrenics who could not attend such a clinic had to be rehospitalized within a year of discharge.

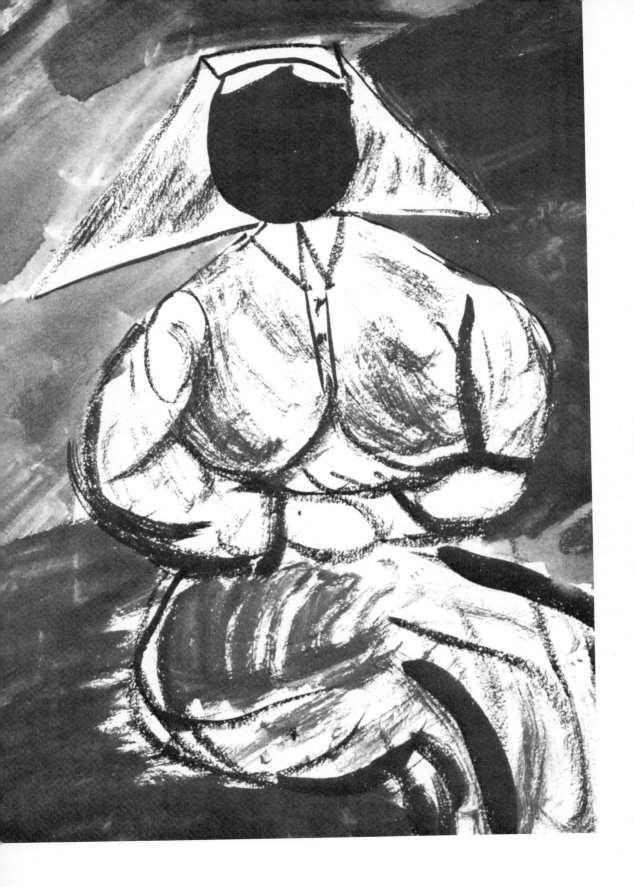

Trifles light as air
Are to the jealous confirmations strong
As proofs of holy writ. . . .

William Shakespeare, *Othello*

PARANOID STATES

"DEGREE"

very stern { DELUSIONS - SYSTEMATIZED - CONSISTENT
BETTER INT. FUNCTIONS

The term "paranoia" antedates Hippocrates. As used by the early Greeks, it meant little more than insanity. The term reappeared during the eighteenth century as a name for disorders that were characterized by delusions and delirium. By the nineteenth century, it was used for a variety of disorders until Kraepelin, in 1893, distinguished paranoia from paraphrenia (a European equivalent of the terms paranoid reactions or paranoid states) and paranoid dementia praecox (paranoid schizophrenia).

Paranoid states are similar to paranoid schizophrenia in many respects and somewhat different in others. Like paranoid schizophrenia, a paranoid state is characterized by delusions, but the delusions are more systematized and closely interrelated than in paranoid schizophrenia. In addition, in paranoid states, intellectual functioning is better preserved and emotional and social responses are more appropriate. Thus, while the paranoid state patient is organized better and fragmented less than a schizophrenic, the difference is but a matter of degree.

The two major types of paranoid states are paranoia and involutional paranoid states. Paranoia is quite rare and is marked by the gradual development of an elaborate delusion which is often based on the misinterpretation of some actual event. While the false belief and its elaboration may be based on some actual

event the interpretation is highly idiosyncratic. The fact that such paranoid systems serve a purpose in the emotional life of the subject is readily seen in the resistance which meets any attempts to expose its irrational underpinnings. Involutional paranoid states occur in the involutional period of life and are characterized by a well-formed delusional system without the conspicuous thought disorder which marks the schizophrenic.

Most authorities question the utility of the paranoid state diagnosis and maintain that it is merely a variant of either paranoid schizophrenia or paranoid personality. The argument for a separate entity turns on the fact that some persons develop elaborate paranoid systems in the absence of any of the deterioration in thought, behavior or mood which characterize the schizophrenias, the affective psychoses, or even many of the personality disorders. While the paranoid delusion may be quite bizarre, it is nevertheless tightly reasoned, and the subject is rational and normal in other areas of living. To clinicians and investigators in the United States such distinctions seem more a matter of degree than of kind, and the diagnosis has been used less and less over the last decade.

The onset of a paranoid state usually occurs later than paranoid schizophrenia. The median age of first admissions diagnosed as paranoid state was 49.4 and the median age of resident

i) PARA
2 INVOLUTIONAL

Grandiose = MEGALOMANIA
Persecution to grandiose

paranoids was 65.9, in United States' mental hospitals in 1968. More women than men develop the reactions. Although only 0.5 per cent of first admissions to United States' mental hospitals in 1959 and 1.2 per cent of resident patients were diagnosed paranoid state, the figures underestimate by far the frequency of the disorder in the population. When a paranoid becomes aware that people consider his beliefs "crazy," he may cover up and deny them and so escape detection.

CHARACTERISTICS

Paranoids tend to be egocentric and narcissistic. They deny their own hostility and use the mechanism of projection excessively. They are sensitive, introverted, mistrustful of others, jealous and suspicious. For example, a paranoid patient with a very high I.Q. responded to the sentence completion test item, "You can trust people who . . ." by changing it to "You can trust people? Who?" Some paranoids are very authoritarian and ethnocentric and may adhere to extremist political and social views (Rosen, 1949). At a deeper level, they have strong but unconscious feelings of inferiority that are masked by a grandiose superiority or rationalized by persecutory delusions. Many paranoids have a history of occupational or marital failures and the projection of blame for the failures becomes part of their delusions.

INFERIOR

A paranoid's conversation is likely to center almost exclusively on his delusional preoccupations. One individual, for example, was convinced that he was the rightful owner of a baseball stadium and spoke of nothing but "*my* ball park" and "*my* team." Over a period of 20 years he spent all the money he could spare in fruitless litigation against the legal owners.

CENTER ON DELUSION

Often a paranoid displays the mechanism of "the self-fulfilling prophecy," that is, behaving in a manner to elicit complementary behavior that confirms his expectations. For example, he "prophesies" that a stranger will be against him and, therefore, curtly repulses the stranger's advances; the stranger becomes hostile, consequently, and thus confirms the prophecy made by the paranoid. This confirmation also increases the probability that the paranoid will be surly toward the next stranger. Of course, the same mechanism is seen less dramatically in the submissive neurotic who elicits dominating behavior from others, or in the extraverted, friendly individual who expects others to meet his overtures with equal friendliness and usually turns out to be correct.

APPLAUD

AUTHOR TIARLAN

EITHER - OR

THE VARIETIES OF PARANOID DELUSIONS

The delusions of the paranoid resemble those of the paranoid schizophrenic. They fall into four types: delusions of grandeur, delusions of influence and persecution, erotic delusions in which the individual fears sexual attack by others, and delusions of jealousy.

Grandiose delusions of power, wealth or self-importance tend to be particularly persistent and unmodifiable, perhaps because they distort reality so greatly that they become immune to the corrective influence of day-by-day reality experiences. A grandiose delusion is sometimes referred to as *megalomania*.

Delusions of persecution are based on a "pseudocommunity" (Cameron, 1947), an imaginary organization which the patient perceives composed of real or imagined persons united for the purpose of carrying out some action against him. Once such beliefs have crystallized, there are two logical courses of action: the patient may seek to protect himself by escape and withdrawal or he may attempt to retaliate by assault or litigation. Male paranoids are more likely to be assaultive than females. The following case illustrates retaliatory paranoid behavior which took the form of attempted murder.

A 75-year-old man, separated from his wife for 40 years, had been living in a run-down shack with a number of chickens, dogs and cats. He had always been eccentric, suspicious and irascible. For 20 years he had been trying to get elected to the City Council and one year stood for election as mayor. He felt that the taxpayers were not getting a fair deal and claimed that many of the councilors were crooked. During the preceding 10 years he had been arrested 12 times, charged with gambling, leaving his animals at large, assault and possession of an unregistered revolver. For years he had believed that the wife of a neighbor was a witch who made small animals come to him. Finally, he shot her and was then hospitalized.

The patient had been born in Italy of illiterate parents and had had little schooling. As a child he had frequently been ill. He had a history of street fighting in which one eye had been permanently injured and part of an ear lost. In his twenties he spent three years working on a railroad in Germany and then returned to Italy. At 27 he married, emigrated and subsequently had four children. He reported that he eventually became upset by his wife's nagging and left his family to establish residence in the shack.

In the hospital he appeared to have auditory hallucinations and talked out loud when no one was near. He believed that when he was a child he and his

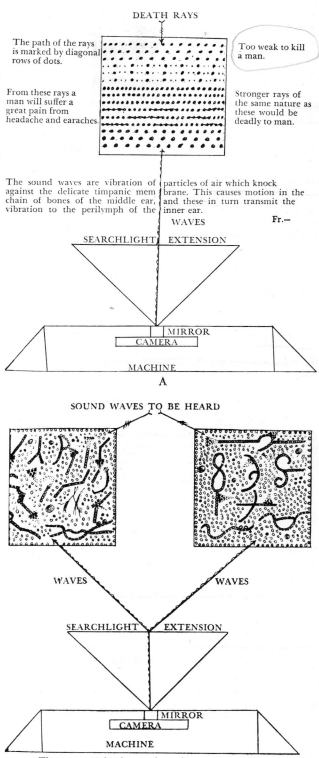

Figure 13–1. "'An influencing machine.' A forty-year-old paranoiac drew these diagrams of a mysterious 'machine' which, he claimed retrospectively, his 'enemies' had been using since his birth to read and control his thoughts and feelings, govern his actions through 'hip-not-ism' and 'electronic waves,' cause him to entertain evil sexual and other forbidden desires, and suffer trances, illnesses, or, if they finally willed it, eventual death. The patient's persecutors were vaguely and variously identified as secret police, 'astrologers,' or supernatural cosmic agents possessed of an omnipotent influence called 'Sumna Loqui' (the 'highest word'?) but presumably jealous of his own great powers. These delusions evidently served a number of purposes: they replaced feelings of failure and deep inadequacy with fantasies of vicarious self-aggrandizement; they projected his erotic, homosexual and destructive impulses onto others and thus relieved him of responsibility for any counter-action he might take, and, less directly, they made it necessary for him to regress, in effect, to the custodial safety of a psychiatric hospital. The fixity of the patient's basic delusional formations is symbolized by the fact that, although the patient drew many diagrams of this machine, the ground plan of the construction was always the same and the object it influenced varied within narrow limits (compare A and B)." (Material courtesy of Adrian H. Vander Veer, M.D., from Masserman, J. H. 1961. Principles of Dynamic Psychiatry. 2nd Ed. Philadelphia, W. B. Saunders Co.)

DEATH RAYS

The path of the rays is marked by diagonal rows of dots.

Too weak to kill a man.

From these rays a man will suffer a great pain from headache and earaches.

Stronger rays of the same nature as these would be deadly to man.

The sound waves are vibration of particles of air which knock against the delicate timpanic membrane. This causes motion in the chain of bones of the middle ear, and these in turn transmit the vibration to the perilymph of the inner ear.

WAVES   Fr.—

SEARCHLIGHT EXTENSION

MIRROR
CAMERA
MACHINE

A

SOUND WAVES TO BE HEARD

WAVES   WAVES

SEARCHLIGHT EXTENSION

MIRROR
CAMERA
MACHINE

These rays can be thrown almost in any color, such as red, dark red, blue and silver.

B

mother had been confronted by a witch who had brought about the death of two children in the neighborhood. (Belief in witchcraft was common enough in the culture in which he grew up. However, his paranoid personality resulted in his clinging to the belief when he migrated to another culture with which it was incompatible.) He claimed that his mother stood her ground and extracted a promise from the witch that no harm would befall her family for seven generations. He reported that when he was working in Germany he met another witch who criticized his behavior and annoyed him persistently. The third witch he encountered was the neighbor's wife. He claimed she had been annoying him for five years and that she frequently visited him disguised as wind, smoke, misty colors or an animal. He stated that she and other witches tried to kill children on Wednesday and Friday nights and that she had been poisoning his liquor. On one occasion he slashed at the wind with his knife and was gratified to see his neighbor's wife limping the following day.

Despite his age, there was no disorientation, impairment of memory or other sign of brain disorder, and there was little indication of schizophrenic disorganization or deterioration. Basically, he suffered from a paranoid reaction with persecutory delusions. In view of his longstanding psychological disturbance and his homicidal retaliation against "persecutors," he was kept in the hospital for permanent custodial care.

The following newspaper account, modified slightly to disguise names and places, describes the seclusive and litigious behavior of an unmarried woman who died at the age of 72 and left an estate of $106,000.

She was known as the eccentric victim of a persecution complex, and was popularly but erroneously supposed to have been a lawyer, or at least to have received formal training in the law.

A successful business woman before she succumbed to her obsession, she undertook her own study of legal matters when, in the 1920's, lawyers refused to act in her behalf. She attempted to bring so many suits that the Legislature passed the Vexatious Proceedings Act to control her passion for litigation. Under this act, she, or any other person to whom it was applied, could only bring court actions with the permission of a Supreme Court judge. The act has since been applied to only two other persons.

Despite her familiarity with legal processes, Miss_____ left no will that can be found by the administrators of her estate. Her estate, when it has been probated, will be divided among her six surviving brothers and sisters.

As a young woman, Miss _____ had run a prosperous fuel business. In her declining years she lived frugally in the isolation of her home, which had been barricaded against her imagined persecutors. Although she spent little on her own comfort, she dispatched a voluminous correspondence of letters and telegrams to public figures in Canada and the United States.

As a result of an action she brought against the postal authorities, there was no postal delivery to her home; she had complained that persons unknown were reading her mail; the post office held her mail for her. A large bagful of letters and circulars was sorted in the process of winding up her estate.

3 *Erotic delusions* are often clear-cut projections of the patient's own erotic impulses: the patient unconsciously *wishes* to be attacked sexually.

4 *Delusions of jealousy and infidelity* are quite common. The individual believes that his marital partner is unfaithful and his belief is bolstered by any and every little incident—an expression of interest by the spouse in a person of the opposite sex, the way a stranger looks at the spouse and so forth. A paranoid with a delusion of infidelity may be said to have developed a *selective reactive sensitivity,* i.e., he is oversensitive to selected cues and ignores others. The following case illustrates this mechanism.

An intelligent, well-educated, 37-year-old woman was referred for psychiatric evaluation when she became convinced that people were talking about her and her relationship with her husband. She had no symptoms of schizophrenia, but she believed that her husband was having an affair with another woman. The husband and other persons in the small town where they lived repeatedly assured her that her belief had no basis in fact. Temporarily she would be reassured, but soon she would find further "evidence" to support her doubts and fears and her delusional conviction would return. In her first evaluative interview she was obviously unsure whether her suspicions were founded on fact:

"I thought someone was talking about me and I let it become an obsession. It's never happened before—if someone has disapproved of me before, I've never let it bother me—I'd go my own way if I knew it was right. We've had a bad year—a lot of illness in my husband's family—his father died last fall and his mother was taken to a hospital right afterward with a recurrence of cancer. She was in the hospital two months and was never the same again mentally. We were remodeling the business and there were so many pressures—I was involved in so many civic affairs and practically never saw my husband. I felt very insecure—I felt I wasn't satisfying my husband although I was bending over backwards. He has never given me cause for jealousy, but I got it in my mind that his secretary was talking about me—she was always laughing when I saw her. My husband and I went on a trip this spring and when we got back I got it in my head that he must be stepping out on me and he says he isn't but I just can't get it out of my mind. The more I sit at home, the more I think about it. I thought the secretary and others were talking about his stepping out on me. Then there were some little incidents. When a certain woman's name came up, and there was a pause in conversation, people looked at me and I thought everything seemed to fit together. We went to a party one night and this woman was there and she gave me an odd look—my interpretation of the look was, 'Do you or don't you know?' When my husband joined us she got up and walked away. I felt that something was the matter with our relationship. It just happened very innocently—the first time was after our return from the trip when this woman's name came up—she was supposed to be on a committee—and the others stopped talking. I felt my husband was talking about her more than he ever had and was driving past her place more than he ever had. This last year we have had our problems and I felt I wasn't satisfying my husband—I wasn't doing anything as well as he wanted. I'd just draw into myself and let him make all the decisions. When I speak up and tell him what I want, he doesn't want to do it that way." Asked if there had been any change in their sexual relationship, she replied, "No, except that I thought he was paying more attention to me—more than he needed or wanted to. He was making love to me more often than he ever had, and I didn't feel it was spontaneous—as though he thought I expected him to do it that way." This reaction is characteristic of paranoids; the husband would have been guilty in the patient's eyes if he had ignored her and he was equally guilty when he did not ignore her.

The most crucial predisposing event of her childhood was the divorce of her parents when she was three years old. She was the youngest of six children, with a large age difference between her and the next older child. The divorce was followed by years of adverse relationships and experiences and she grew up in economic and emotional insecurity. Her main childhood relationship was with her hostile, demanding mother. "Mother worked awfully hard bringing up us kids and she was rather bitter and I can remember her telling me many times how horrible men were. And she was very suspicious of me in high school. She was strict with me and suspicious of where I'd been and it used to bother me. She accused me of smoking and I'd never even tried it. She'd often accuse me of things I hadn't thought of doing, I always used to excuse her because she had a hard life, but it hurt me. Money bothered me—there just wasn't any extra—and I still have that feeling now. We had the necessities of food and clothing, but mother made my dresses too big—she was very practical—I had to go without toys and party dresses. I didn't blame her, but it always bothered me that I didn't have a father. In the sixth grade we copied a poem about father and made a booklet that we were supposed to take home to father. I took it home to my eldest brother and everyone in the family laughed at me—it hurt me and I ran to my room and cried. My four brothers teased me a lot and everybody told me what to do. I was never sure whether I would be able

to do something—whether there would be enough money. The other girls were all so free and easy—I felt better when I started earning money baby sitting in high school, but I remember saving money for material for a dress and my mother made it, but all the same she complained about it—she did that lots of times when things that seemed important to me—she made me feel constantly guilty. I've been wondering why I'm so inhibited and don't speak up when I disagree. I don't remember being terribly unhappy as a child, but there were a lot of people who expected me to do things a certain way—I've always tried to be a good girl and I want people to like me."

After graduation from college, the patient married a well-to-do businessman. They both regarded their sexual relationship as satisfactory although the patient had known nothing about sex until she was a high-school senior. "I wondered if mother was frigid—she wasn't demonstrative—she always kept her feelings to herself. She never touched the children, never told me anything about sex or menstruation."

The main difficulties in the patient's married life were related to her feelings of insecurity and alienation from other people. When she and her husband moved to a new city where he became prominent in the community, she had difficulty making new friends and was reluctant to entertain business acquaintances or members of his family as often as he wished. Her reluctance precipitated a violent quarrel in the heat of which he remarked, "Maybe we should get a divorce." The patient reported, "That really upset me. I think from that time on I was very, very worried about our relationship—the mention of divorce. I've felt very insecure—worried that anything I might do might be the wrong thing." Apparently the idea of divorce reawakened her childhood problems and threatened the loss of whatever security she had gained in their marriage. Neither of them mentioned divorce again, but she began to believe he was unfaithful. The delusion "explained" why he wished to divorce her and assured her that it was not her fault, for he was sexually guilty and therefore hated her unjustifiably.

In the hospital she was treated by one of the phenothiazine drugs and psychotherapy. Interviews were also held with her husband. Within two weeks she was discharged, but continued to take medication; a follow-up for several months revealed no recurrence of her paranoid ideation and an improvement in their relationship. The treatment was effective because she had been caught before her paranoid delusions had become crystallized.

Folie à Deux

Two persons who live together for a lengthy period and have a close emotional relationship may come to share a psychosis. The technical term for such a situation is *folie à deux*, which can be translated as "double insanity." The psychosis shared by the two persons usually involves delusions. Sometimes one member of the pair is highly suggestible and completely dominated by the other, and sometimes neither partner is especially dominant. Gralnick (1942) reviewed 109 pairs of folie à deux recorded in the literature and reported that 40 consisted of two sisters, 26 of husband and wife, 24 of mother and child, 11 of two brothers, 6 of brother and sister, and 2 of father and child. It is noteworthy that folie à deux rarely involves two men but quite often is shared by two women. In the following example, the delusions of an only daughter were adopted by her elderly mother.

The daughter was 28 years old and the mother 65 at the time of their admission to a mental hospital from the women's jail of a large city in Canada. Both they and the girl's father had been born abroad and had come to Canada when the daughter was a child. They were quite poor and neither mother nor daughter had much education. Six months before their admission to the hospital, the father was admitted to an old people's home. Even before this, the mother and daughter had worked, eaten and slept together for many years.

On arrival at the hospital, the daughter stated that six years previously she had developed a nasal obstruction and a plastic surgeon in the United States had performed an operation on her nose. Soon after, she was involved in an automobile accident on her way to the doctor's office and was thrown against the windshield of the car. She complained that ever since she suffered from excruciating pains in her nose, face and neck. She had attempted to sue the doctor for half a million dollars but no lawyer would take the case. Subsequently, she and her mother entered the doctor's house and refused to leave until he paid. They were arrested, jailed and deported to Canada. On five occasions after this the two entered the United States and attempted to sue the doctor. Finally, the United States immigration officer in Canada refused to issue visas to them. They decided that the doctor was paying the immigration officer to keep them out of the United States and therefore tried to collect the half million dollars from the immigration officer. For several weeks they waited in his office every day until they were arrested and taken to jail from which they were transferred to the hospital.

In addition to her primary delusions, the daughter reported that she and her mother had a great deal of trouble in rooming houses during the preceding months because other people were after their money. The mother told exactly the same story as the daughter and felt that all of the daughter's claims were well founded. She was very anxious for the daughter to marry and looked forward to living with her and the hypothetical son-in-law, but she believed that it would be impossible for the girl to find a husband unless her nose was healed. Both wished to be released as soon as possible in order to return to the United States and collect their money from the doctor.

Shortly after admission, they were separated from each other for three months while the daughter underwent an intensive program of ECT and insulin coma treatment. Initially, her delusional system changed and she began to believe that the doctor wished to pay her the half million dollars but was being prevented from doing so by her relatives. Soon, however, she reverted to her former beliefs and thereafter these remained unshakable. During the period of separation, the mother first became severely depressed and then, as often happens with separation in folie à deux, lost her faith in the daughter's delusional system. Nevertheless, she could not accept the fact that her daughter was ill and remained anxious for the two of them to leave the hospital. When treatment of the daughter was terminated as useless she was reunited with her mother and they remained inseparable companions in a chronic ward of the hospital.

CAUSATION AND DYNAMICS

Since paranoid states and paranoid schizophrenia differ primarily in degree, the etiological factors that are important to schizophrenia may be assumed to have some influence on paranoid states also. A number of investigations, however, have been concerned solely with paranoid states. The results of investigations of heredity factors have been unimpressive. For example, Miller (1941, 1942) reviewed the histories of 400 hospitalized psychotic patients with marked paranoid trends and found that although 11 per cent were descendants of persons known to have suffered from a psychiatric disorder, there was evidence of specifically paranoid illness in the ancestry of only 2 per cent. Other biological factors such as physique and metabolism also have been demonstrated not to play a causal role in paranoid states.

The main contributions to our understanding of the psychodynamics of paranoid psychoses were made by Freud. He formulated the concept of projection in 1896, and applied it to psychosis. In 1911, he analyzed the memoirs of Dr. Schreber, a judge who had partially recovered from paranoid schizophrenia and then had described his subjective experiences and delusions in an autobiography. Schreber believed that he had a special relation to God and a mission to redeem the world and restore it to a state of bliss. He could only accomplish this, however, if he were first transformed from a

Kid

man into a woman. His internal organs, he believed, had been destroyed, but divine rays had restored them. A great number of "female nerves" had passed into his body and from these he expected a new race of man to be born. His body was being used sexually by God. Schreber's delusional system lends itself to an interpretation in terms of a denied and projected homosexual drive; Freud made this interpretation in an ingenious and closely reasoned argument and then extrapolated the interpretation into a classic formulation of the genesis of paranoid psychoses.

Essentially, Freud's theory asserts that a paranoid delusion is a consequence of repressed and projected homosexuality. The sequence of internal events can be formulated as follows: the individual starts with the thought, "I love a man." He then denies what he has asserted and, by a mechanism of reaction-formation, transforms it into its opposite, "I do not love him—I hate him." However, if the hostility in this statement is unacceptable, it is projected, resulting in the delusion of persecution, "He hates me." An alternative mechanism consists of denying homosexual impulses by asserting, "I do not love him—I love her." Projection then changes this into "She loves me," and the result is an erotic delusion. In a third variant, the formula is, "I don't love him—she loves him," giving rise to delusions and suspicions of jealousy. Finally, a fourth possibility consists of the assertion, "I do not love him—in fact, I do not love anyone but myself." The result is grandiose megalomania.

In clinical practice, paranoids often show evidence of homosexual impulses. A number of analysts have followed Freud and postulated that *all* paranoid states in men and women result from homosexual problems. However, many clinicians and investigators, while conceding that homosexuality is often relevant, have stressed that guilt over hostile, heterosexual, or other impulses may equally well result in paranoid projection. A delusion of jealousy in a hostile paranoid woman may conform to the formula, "I hate my husband. I reject him sexually," followed by "I do not hate him. I love him, but he is unfaithful to me. It is he who rejects me." Similarly, a paranoid woman with erotic delusions of sexual assault may in effect be saying, "I am attracted to men other than my husband," followed by, "I do not want sexual relations with anyone but my husband, but someone is trying to seduce me."

The intense hostility that is so common in paranoids apparently develops from childhood. There is reason to believe that, as children, paranoids tend to be aloof, suspicious and stubborn. These traits constitute a preparanoid personality in the same way that the schizoid personality is preschizophrenic. They are likely to emerge from a restrictive and authoritarian family atmosphere in which the child feels more pressure than it can handle comfortably.

Some of the sociocultural factors in paranoid reactions were illuminated in a study by Kay and Roth (1961). They studied 99 patients aged 60 years and over who were suffering from paraphrenia and had been admitted to a Swedish and a British mental hospital. Both groups showed a predominance of females over males in a ratio of approximately 7 to 1 and an excess of unmarried patients among both sexes. In contrast with comparable patients suffering from affective disorders, significantly more paraphrenics were living alone and had no friends at the time they became ill. It has been conjectured by some observers that the paranoid's tendency not to marry reflects latent homosexual trends.

An intensive study by Weinstein (1962) of 148 patients in the Virgin Islands demonstrated the close relation of delusions to cultural factors. The inhabitants of the Virgin Islands fall into relatively clear ethnic and cultural groups. Among those of British extraction there is a heavy emphasis on religion in everyday living; a large percentage of the patients from this group had religious delusions. The French inhabitants have a double standard of sexual morality for men and women; French patients frequently had sexual delusions. Among the native islanders, on the other hand, there is considerable sexual equality between men and women, with many of the women working outside the home; sexual delusions were few in this group. The native islanders dislike farming, whereas a group of immigrants from the British island of Tortola are peasant proprietors; native islanders had few delusions involving land, whereas the Tortola patients had many delusions of land being stolen from them. The French tend to value their children for the contribution they can make to economic welfare; very few French patients had delusions involving children. The natives idealize children and value them as a source of emotional gratification; a considerable number of native patients had delusions involving children.

In England, Lucas et al. (1962) studied the relations between the content of delusions and

H SES
L SES

the variables of age, sex and social familial characteristics. Delusions with religious or supernatural content were more frequent in persons of high social status and in the unmarried. Grandiose delusions were also more frequent at higher social levels and tended to occur in eldest rather than youngest siblings, whereas delusions of inferiority were more common at lower social levels and among youngest siblings. Persecutory delusions increased in frequency with increasing age of onset and were more common in youngest siblings. Sexual delusions occurred much more often in women than men and were more frequent in the married than single persons. A close analysis of these results will reveal that they "make sense": supernaturalism and grandiosity go with higher social positions where the individual is likely to have had experiences of power; it seems reasonable that delusions of inferiority should be associated with lower social status and the least powerful family position; it is equally reasonable that feelings of persecution should increase with age and, like inferiority feelings, be associated with position as a youngest sibling; and similarly for the other results of the study.

Several investigators have noted a high frequency of paranoid states among displaced persons from Eastern European countries who subsequently immigrated to the United States, Canada and Australia. Concepts such as "the persecutory delusions of lingually isolated persons" and "aliens' paranoid reactions" have been used in the psychiatric literature. Displaced persons are displaced horizontally to a new country with a new language and vertically to a lower socioeconomic level. They are exposed to loneliness and adaptational stresses which may precipitate paranoid states.

TREATMENT

cut nerves that connect frontal lobe + thalamus

The treatment of paranoid states is very similar to that of paranoid schizophrenia. Drug therapy, ECT, occasionally lobotomy, individual and group psychotherapy, and environmental manipulation have all been used. Unfortunately, the prospects of changing the delusional system of an intact paranoid and producing a remission by any form of therapy are much poorer than for paranoid schizophrenia. Psychotherapy is particularly difficult with a patient enveloped in a systematized delusion. The therapeutic goals —reducing his anxiety and guilt so that it is unnecessary for him to project and distort reality, and helping him to reappraise his relation to reality—are impossible to attain unless the patient comes to trust the therapist. This necessary trust is almost impossible to establish, except for patients with whom psychotherapy begins early in the development of their delusions. For somatic treatment measures also, the likelihood of recovery is considerable only if treatment is undertaken early.

worse for para then
shiz "~

14

DELINQUENCY, CRIME AND ANTISOCIAL PERSONALITY

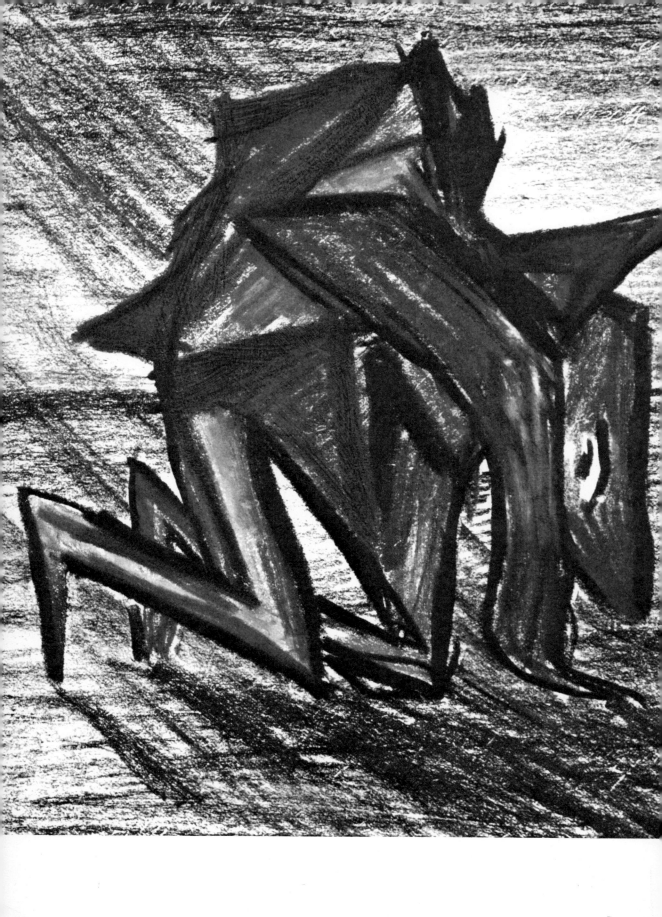

> ...the psychopath is a rebel without a cause, an agitator without a slogan, a revolutionary without a program; in other words, his rebelliousness is aimed to achieve goals satisfactory to himself alone; he is incapable of exertions for the sake of others.
>
> Robert Lindner, *Rebel Without a Cause*

14

DELINQUENCY, CRIME AND ANTISOCIAL PERSONALITY

An infant has no standards of right or wrong. If his "right" responses—as society defines "right"—are reinforced with some consistency while his "wrong" responses are not, he will begin to abandon unacceptable behavior. At first his behavior is controlled by external punishments and rewards, but they are replaced by internalized guilt or self-approval as his superego develops. However, should he fail to develop internalized controls, he will not acquire socially acceptable habits and will become a psychopath or sociopath, or in current parlance, an antisocial personality. McCord and McCord (1956) define the psychopath as "an anti-social, aggressive, highly impulsive person, who feels little or no guilt and is unable to form lasting bonds of affection with other human beings." Emotionally, the adult antisocial personality has some resemblance to the normal two-year-old; indeed, it may be said that everyone begins life as an uninhibited and uncontrolled sociopath.

Sociopathy, like any of the neuroses or psychoses, is a question of degree: an individual displays more or less superego weakness and behaves more or less unacceptably. Even in an intense form, however, antisocial behavior is very widespread. Although the number of hospitalized sociopaths is relatively small, many are in jails and prisons and even more live within the community at large as impostors, confidence men, tricksters, prostitutes or unscrupulous business or professional men. There are sociopathic policemen, politicians, lawyers, physicians and even psychiatrists (see Cleckley's *The Mask of Sanity* for a detailed and fascinating account of a sociopathic psychiatrist who exploited his patients financially and sexually).

The terms "sociopath," "psychopath" and "antisocial personality" are used more or less interchangeably and are closely related to other descriptive terms such as "character disorder," "conduct disorder" or "behavior disorder." At differing times various diagnostic labels have been fashionable in designating patterns of impulsive, antisocial behavior unaccompanied by neurotic anxiety or psychotic misinterpretation of reality. An individual may repetitively engage in a single type of unacceptable behavior— stealing, excessive drinking and so forth—or he may run the gamut of many such behaviors.

It should be understood that crime and delinquency are not psychological or psychiatric terms but are legal terms. A crime is an act prohibited by law or a failure to perform an act that is prescribed by law. It may be either a

255

misdemeanor or minor crime, such as disorderly conduct, or a felony or serious crime, such as robbery, forgery, rape or murder. MacIver (1942) points out that a crime may be committed by a maniac or a genius, a scoundrel or a patriot, a man without scruples or a man who puts his scruples above the law, a reckless exploiter or a man in desperate need. Obviously it is unreasonable to expect that all criminals should have similar personality characteristics.

The term "delinquency," as used in the United States, encompasses an even wider range of behaviors than the term "crime." Delinquencies range all the way from truancy, drinking or smoking in public, or frequent disobedience of parents, to murder. Of the children brought to the attention of the police because of a delinquent act, the majority are not persistent delinquents nor do they become persistent criminals in later life. Nevertheless, there is a close relation between delinquency and crime, for a considerable proportion of adult criminal offenders have records of delinquency. Furthermore, delinquency and crime are closely related to sociopathic personality, for almost all sociopaths frequently break laws, and most *persistent* delinquents or criminals—but not occasional—are sociopaths. In a study of 10,000 men incarcerated in Sing Sing prison in New York (Mental Health in Corrective Institutions, 1941), 66 per cent were categorized as "sociopathic personalities." The remaining 34 per cent were neurotics, psychotics, mental defectives or alcoholics, and some of the last group were undoubtedly also sociopathic.

The term "antisocial personality" was preceded by a number of others that stem from the early nineteenth century. Prichard (1835) introduced the concept of "moral insanity" to designate criminals who manifested an absence of control and ethical sense. A morally insane individual was considered to have an unimpaired intellect but to be, nevertheless, incapable of "conducting himself with decency and propriety." Some decades later the concept of "constitutional psychopathic inferiority" was introduced. It was based on the unproved assumption that a severe type of impulsive, antisocial behavior disorder could only occur if the individual had a constitutional defect of the nervous system. In the first half of the present century the term "psychopathic personality" came into widespread use in the United States and is still frequently employed. A psychopath is defined by the American Psychiatric Associa-

tion as "a person whose behavior is predominantly amoral or antisocial and characterized by impulsive, irresponsible actions satisfying only immediate and narcissistic interests, without concern for obvious and implicit social consequences, accompanied with minimal outward evidence of anxiety or guilt."

Most of these terms and concepts are plagued by a confusion in the criteria used to define them. In part, the concepts are defined by a social criterion but in larger part they are defined negatively, by exclusion: moral insanity and psychopathy designate those social maladjustments that are *not* due to mental defect, neurosis, psychosis and so forth. Such a definition by exclusion tends to result in a "wastepaper basket" category, that is, a loose category which lumps cases that cannot be fitted elsewhere. In an effort to sharpen the category, Cleckley (1955) distinguished a core group of "true" or "primary" psychopathic personalities with the following characteristics, a few of which are negative (e.g., absence of delusions) but most of which are positive and definite. (Cleckley's characteristics are very similar to those currently attributed to the antisocial personality. See Table 14–1.)

1. Superficial charm and good "intelligence." [The quotation marks about the word "intelligence" indicate Cleckley's belief that the psychopath is intelligent only in a superficial sense.]
2. Absence of delusions and other signs of irrational "thinking."
3. Absence of "nervousness" or psychoneurotic manifestations.
4. Unreliability.
5. Untruthfulness and insincerity.
6. Lack of remorse or shame.
7. Inadequately motivated antisocial behavior.
8. Poor judgment and failure to learn by experience.
9. Pathologic egocentricity and incapacity for love.
10. General poverty in major affective reactions.
11. Specific loss of insight.
12. Unresponsiveness in general interpersonal relations.
13. Fantastic and uninviting behavior, with drink and sometimes without.
14. Suicide rarely carried out. [In actual fact, successful suicide does occur among psychopaths. However, the psychopath's suicide is impulsive rather than planned over a long period of time.]
15. Sex life impersonal, trivial and poorly integrated.
16. Failure to follow any life plan.

In the 1950's and 1960's, the standard nomenclature of the American Psychiatric Association made use of the term "sociopath" instead of "psychopath" and attempted to distinguish between several major subgroups: antisocial reactions (impulsive, pleasure-seeking, egocentric, loyal to no group, code or person), dyssocial reactions (capable of loyalty to a predatory or criminal group), sexual deviation, and alcohol and drug addiction. However, sexual deviations and the addictions are very heterogeneous and often result from neurotic or psychotic personality problems rather than sociopathy. They are discussed in later chapters.

Currently, the tendency is to speak of antisocial personality disorders, which are defined largely along the lines proposed by Cleckley. The terms "dyssocial reactions" and "group delinquent reactions" are used to designate those individuals who have acquired the values and behavior of a delinquent group and thus show a rudimentary form of socialization, which is typically missing in antisocial personalities.

Some degree of sociopathy may exist in combination with other disorders. For example,

in pseudo-sociopathic schizophrenia, the individual's schizophrenic traits are initially masked by delinquent or criminal behavior. Sociopathy and paranoid behavior are also often present in the same individual, as are sociopathic and manic behavior.

ANTISOCIAL PERSONALITY DISORDER

In many respects, antisocial sociopathy and neurosis may be considered opposites, with normality situated between them. The typical characteristics of the antisocial personality disorder and the neurotic are contrasted in Table 14–1. Of course, no single individual will manifest all the characteristics of either set, but the closer the fit, the more truly sociopathic or neurotic the individual is. A thread running through many of the sociopathic characteristics is *lack of control*, evidenced by superego defect, impulsiveness and reckless irresponsibility. The

TABLE 14–1. Characteristics of the Typical Antisocial Personality and Neurotic

Antisocial Personality	Neurotic
Predominantly male (approx. 3:1).	Predominantly female (approx. 3:2).
First psychiatric contact in adolescence or as young adult.	First psychiatric contact at any time in adult life.
Concentration in lower socioeconomic classes.	High frequency in all socioeconomic classes, but concentration of treated cases in middle and upper classes.
Defective or absent superego.	Rigid superego.
Minimal or no guilt or depression over serious antisocial behavior.	Frequent guilt and depression over minor or imagined misdeeds.
Uninhibited acting out of impulses, with inability to postpone gratification of future reward. Reckless nonconformity.	Excessive inhibition of sexual or aggressive impulses in anticipation of long-range advantages. Conformity with standards of society.
Amoral, unreliable, irresponsible. Pathological liar, cheat, swindler, thief. May be promiscuous, violent or addicted to alcohol or drugs. Confident and carefree. Indifferent to religion.	Moral, reliable and responsible, but lacking in self-confidence and often indecisive. Religious or conflicted over religion.
No long-range plans or efforts. Freedom from worry or anxiety.	Ambitious plans and striving for future goals. Intangible ideals with much doubt, fear, anxiety and apprehension.
Indifferent to others' opinions except when these frustrate immediate needs.	Insecure and sensitive to criticism. Frequent feelings of inadequacy.
Incapable of true affection. Superficial charm and plausibility used to manipulate others.	Capable of affection and has strong need for affection, but latent or unconscious hostility often interferes with ability to maintain deep relationships.
Transient, uninhibited sexual behavior with wide variety of partners.	Sexual impulses and behavior perceived as dangerous or disgusting. Frigidity or impotence.
Tendency to express hostility directly and violently except when direct expression would interfere with momentary goals.	Hostility not permitted direct expression but may be expressed indirectly or displaced.
Frequent EEG abnormalities.	Autonomic lability.
Tendency to mesomorphic body build.	Tendency to ectomorphic body build (except in conversion reactions).
Frequent history of sociopathy in parents and siblings.	Frequent history of neurosis in parents and siblings.
Parental deprivation, discord, deceit, lack of supervision, occasionally overindulgence.	Parental deprivation, discord, domination.
Association with delinquent peers or siblings.	Restricted relationships with siblings and peers.
Truancy, job instability and nomadism (pathological roaming from place to place). Record of conflict with police or military authorities.	Often high achievement in school and occupation.

sociopath may become involved in promiscuous sexual behavior, heterosexual or other, not because of a strong sex drive but because his lack of control leads to an attitude of "Why not?" He may impulsively assault others when momentarily angry or make an ineffectual suicidal gesture when momentarily depressed. His life is planless and lacks the coherence characteristic of well-controlled persons so that from year to year his residence, occupation, acquaintances (he has no true friends) and sexual partners may change. He is not a calculated criminal but drifts into crime just as he drifts into sexual deviations, alcoholism or drug addiction. He lacks a long-range perspective and cannot project himself into the future.

The sociopath's susceptibility to accidental injury or so-called "accident proneness" reflects his recklessness. The following case is an example:

An impulsive sociopath suffered a dozen "accidents" during adolescence, including being thrown from a horse he had been told not to ride; he received severe injuries on three occasions while fighting with other adolescents, was knifed while fighting with his brother, and injured again when he and his brother "horsed around" with pitchforks.

It is not surprising that sociopaths have a high rate of mortality which results in a lower frequency of sociopathic behavior among older persons. Other causes of the reduced frequency with age are imprisonment and a tendency of some older sociopaths to chronic alcoholism with a concomitant abandonment of other sociopathic behaviors. Still other sociopaths gradually renounce antisocial behavior as they become older, without becoming alcoholics.

The antisocial sociopath fails to profit from social rewards or punishments. This is illustrated by the following case:

A 16-year-old sociopath, whose I.Q. was above average, manifested a repetitive pattern of thefts and burglaries each of which resulted in arrest. One night he noisily broke into a gas station and then went to a hamburger stand across the street where he ordered a hamburger and sat without eating until the police, called by a neighbor who had heard the noise, came and arrested him. On another occasion when his family changed residences he went to the local high school to register. He gave his address to the teacher on duty and then, when she was called to answer the telephone, ran off with her purse. Again, he attempted to rob a store owner who knew him and his family by sight.

Behavior such as this has led to the hypothesis that the antisocial sociopath suffers from a *need*

for punishment although he is not aware of his motive: he offends society in order to be punished. We shall return to this controversial hypothesis at a later point. In any event, an inability to modify behavior as a result of social reinforcement—a defect in social learning—is an important characteristic of the antisocial personality.

The sociopath's defect in social learning is closely related to his low level of anxiety. Lykken (1957) studied a group of individuals who conformed to Cleckley's description of the primary psychopath, and determined that the psychopaths' level of anxiety was too low for efficient conditioning or avoidance learning. As compared to nonsociopathic controls, the psychopaths manifested little anxiety on a questionnaire measure, displayed a lower level of galvanic skin reactivity to a conditioned stimulus associated with electric shock, and were relatively incapable of learning to avoid punished responses in a laboratory learning situation.

The antisocial sociopath cannot sustain intimate relationships with people and is insensitive to them—he cannot "feel" their reactions empathically. If someone becomes attached to him sooner or later he will take advantage of the attachment to exploit the individual. True loyalty is impossible for him. In some sociopaths, social alienation is reflected in appearance, manner and language. Special haircuts, special modes of dress—for instance, the motorcyclist's black leather jacket—and extensive use of slang, frequently indicate sociopathy. Just as often, however, the sociopath hides his attitudes as well as his antisocial history and cannot be so easily identified.

The sociopath is aggressive and extrapunitive. The blame he casts on others is not a paranoid delusional projection but rather a transient expression of hostility. He feels hostile toward his parents, particularly the father, and resentment and rebellion are likely to culminate during adolescence in a complete rupture with his family and in his leaving home. Hostility toward the parents generalizes and spreads so that he is at odds with school authorities and employers. Truancy and job instability are common among sociopaths; their achievements in school and on the job fall below intellectual capacity.

Greenwald (1967) describes the inner feelings of the psychopath as follows:

. . . Can you imagine if you were a Jew and you were suddenly dropped into Nazi Germany surrounded by SS men during the height of the Hitler terror against the Jews: What feelings of morality would you have? What kind of ability would you have to empathize with the people around you? What immediate gratification would you want to postpone? What would there be that you would not be willing to do? This is how the psychopath views the world around him. He believes himself to be surrounded by deadly enemies. His early life experience has usually been such that this estimate is correct. He has grown up in the kind of milieu . . . where he feels surrounded by enemies and therefore has no hopes beyond survival and enjoyment of immediate gratification because everyone is against him anyway.

The sociopath may be extrapunitive even toward his victims. This is illustrated by the following case:

A 35-year-old sociopath with a record of arrests for drunkenness and various sexual transgressions was jailed for having sexual intercourse with a 15-year-old baby sitter. Both he and his wife worked but he said he "did not feel much like working that day" and returned home one hour after reporting for work. In prison, while completing a self-administered paper and pencil test, he carried on a running monologue for the benefit of the examiner. When he came to the item, "I know who is responsible for most of my troubles," he said, "I know who is responsible for my troubles—I am." There was a pause and then he remarked in true sociopathic fashion, "Well—that's not true either. Sometimes they fool you. You just can't tell how old they are."

The sociopath's tolerance of frustration is low and he is quickly bored by almost any sort of sustained and unexciting effort, physical or mental. He rarely displays forethought. He may become depressed when frustrated, but not because of guilt feelings. If depressed, he may threaten to harm himself or others.

When the wife of a middle aged sociopath with a lifelong record of lying and cheating divorced him, he thereupon became depressed and threatened to kill himself or her. They had met when he had been in the military police and she had been a prostitute. Ostensibly in the line of duty, he used to clear all military personnel away from her residence but then returned to spend the night with her. After they married, each continued to be promiscuous, but he became increasingly jealous of her extramarital activities and sometimes beat her. The divorce followed.

Because she refused to return to him, his depression deepened and he again threatened suicide. However, he expressed no guilt or remorse over his past behavior, and when it became evident that she had no intention of returning, his depression cleared up rapidly and he promised to marry another woman with whom he had already started a liaison. (He had no intention of keeping his word.)

By threatening suicide or making a suicidal gesture, a sociopath sometimes succeeds in manipulating the behavior of another person, particularly if the latter believes the threat or gesture to be genuine. For example:

A girl attempted suicide when she was rejected by her boy friend and then made the following statement: "I decided he couldn't do this to me so I tried to talk him out of it but it didn't work. So I thought I'd try to scare him more by trying to commit suicide. I didn't really want to die. I just wanted more or less to scare him, so I took a bunch of tranquilizers and sedatives and aspirin and I meant to tell my roommate what I was doing but I got so sleepy I dropped off. My boy friend says he doesn't feel guilty but he does, and he thinks I did it for him and that I really was trying to kill myself. The situation is now almost the same as it was before, except I've got more of a hold over him." (The hold did not last, however, and he was soon able to escape from the relationship.)

Sociopathy starts early and usually persists a long time. As the sociopath ages, however, he may be less and less able to "get away" with sociopathic behavior. The changes that sometimes occur in a sociopath's life may be illustrated by the history of an individual whose pattern of behavior caught up with him in his forties:

He began drinking at the age of 12, ran way from home at 14 to be a boxer, returned two years later and entered high school, and within six months was forced to drop out of school in order to marry the 21-year-old teacher whom he had made pregnant. The couple remained married for 19 years although the patient was away from home most of the time working as a boxer, wrestler, rodeo rider and animal trainer. He claimed that at various times he had also owned a meat market and been a foreman in an aircraft factory. He described numerous brief extramarital affairs and reported that he spent money freely and drank excessively. His drinking led to brief psychiatric hospitalizations on several occasions. However, his marriage broke up only when his wife divorced him so that she could marry another man.

He obtained a job as an orderly in a psychiatric hospital and soon married a divorced psychiatric aide with two sons. The early years of the marriage were surprisingly stable: two children were born, his drinking ceased, he stayed on the same job and his work was highly regarded. However, the relationship with his wife eventually deteriorated; she began to go out with other men and he resumed his pattern of excessive drinking. While drunk one day, he began to beat her and pushed her down the basement stairs, whereupon one of her sons shot him in the leg. Later, the leg had to be amputated.

He was now 48 years old and his life entered a new and discouraging phase. When he was ready to leave the hospital after surgery his wife and family no longer wanted him home. He could not return to his job as an orderly. He was referred for vocational rehabilitation but refused to accept counseling or retraining. He was then placed in a boarding home where he bitterly complained that he had no money to spend on his children, that he felt miserable and that life was not worth living. He did not accept any responsibility for his difficulties but blamed his wife and various other people. He complained of persistent pain, depression and difficulty in sleeping. Somehow he acquired a large supply of pain-killing, anti-depressive and sedative medications which he took to produce the effects he had previously obtained from alcohol. An overdose of sleeping pills led to his admission to a psychiatric ward where he was found to be moderately depressed; his mood soon improved radically and he was discharged in three weeks. Again he was referred for vocational rehabilitation and a number of job opportunities were explored with him but again he was too poorly motivated to work and returned to the kind of boarding home in which he had been living earlier. His character structure was clearly still sociopathic, but from the time he had become physically incapacitated he felt abandoned and lost. He could no longer pursue his lifelong pattern of impulsive aggression nor could he adopt a normal pattern.

One of the most striking characteristics of the typical sociopath is his charm. He talks well and gives the impression of being alert and clear-headed. He knows how to employ his skills to manipulate other people and how to ingratiate himself by entertaining them with exciting accounts of his exploits. However, his accounts consist of lies as well as real past events, for he is likely to be a *pathological liar,* i.e., to build himself up by telling tall tales in which he plays the central role. His description of events differs markedly from the description given by other people. This is illustrated by the following case:

A 15-year-old sociopath with an I.Q. of 140 and an extraordinary degree of inventiveness and charm was forced by his father, a retired Army sergeant who disciplined the boy harshly, to play a wind instrument in the school orchestra. One day the boy came home from school in tears with the story that while he was waiting for a bus a car had pulled up to the curb before him and a man had stepped out, snatched the horn and driven off with it. Despite countless past lies, the boy's manner and his tears were so convincing that the father and the rest of the family never thought to disbelieve him. The police were called to talk to the boy and as they were leaving he said, "You know, talking to you has helped me remember what the car looked like—it was green." The police dutifully jotted this fact down, patted the boy on the head with compliments for his sharp eye for detail and told him

not to worry. Again they were taking their leave when the boy began to recall, detail by detail, the make and year of the car, the fact that there were two men in it and the appearance of the men. Finally, he suggested that since he had succeeded in dredging up all these details, he might help to apprehend the malefactors by riding around in a squad car with the police.

Unbelievably, his offer was accepted, and for several days he was picked up by a police officer after school to cruise the streets of the town for an hour. Periodically, he would shout, "There they go!" and the officer would turn on the siren and force the designated car to the curb. The boy would look at the occupants and shake his head sadly: "No, that's not them—it looked like them from a distance," and the police car would resume cruising. The adventure ended when the proprietor of a drug store near the bus stop phoned the boy's father to ask if someone would come and pick up the instrument. He said the boy had asked him to keep it "for a little while" but he did not want the responsibility any longer.

In the following case of antisocial behavior, the patient's casual attitude toward his difficulties is very marked. The statement made by the patient's father points up many of the etiological factors in the case: He set a bad example for his son, was amused by his behavior and frequently protected him from the consequences of his actions. The father also displayed strong hostility while the mother had, in all likelihood, encouraged the son to be hostile and rebellious toward the father.

A young man, aged 20, was admitted to a psychiatric hospital on a court order at the instigation of his father. The latter hoped that through hospitalization the son would escape the legal consequences of several traffic violations and arrest for theft of auto-mobile parts. The patient was a mesomorphic, un-smiling and surly individual. He was more withdrawn and less communicative than the typical talkative and joking sociopath and he obviously had some schizoid as well as sociopathic traits. Unlike the behavior of most hospitalized male sociopaths, he paid no attention to the younger female patients on the ward but spent most of his time watching television.

The father—a bluff, hearty mesomorphic business-man—had attempted to have his son hospitalized once before. The patient's own description of the events leading to hospitalization revealed his sociopathic impulsiveness, lack of anxiety, failure to anticipate the consequences of his actions and pattern of self defeat:

"My father put out a warrant for me to be put in the hospital because I was sitting around the house doing nothing—so I got a job then, and was living with some friends in an apartment. I left home about four months ago, and then one day I went home and my folks weren't home, and I talked to a few of my friends and everyone was busy, so I sat watching TV and some friends came and we had a little party and I was sitting out in this girl's car talking. I was behind the wheel—I don't have a license—and followed a friend home three blocks, and on the way the police stopped me. I had had my license suspended for speeding. After the police arrested me and handcuffed me, I ran away to a friend's house and took the handcuffs off—his father had a hacksaw and grinder—and then went out of town for a couple of months and worked in a gas station. Then the police came down and picked me up there and took me to jail for a night, but they found my father had a warrant out to take me to the hospital so they had to take me there."

The patient was the oldest of three boys. The father was a part-time law enforcement officer as well as a successful businessman. He himself often drove far in excess of the speed limit because he could get away with it. The mother was quite anxious and concerned about the boy's behavior. She felt overwhelmed by the father and their three sons and stood by to bail them out of trouble. The father had agreed to take care of the bill for his son's psychiatric evaluation, but although he could easily afford it he failed, in psychopathic fashion, to do so. The mother paid belatedly

A joint interview with the parents revealed that the son had a very long history of aggressive rebellion, stealing, pathological lying and undependability. Despite his schizoid traits, the boy knew how to persuade others to do what he wanted: "The problem started in the first grade of school," stated the father. "He was a nonconformist from the beginning. The teachers would say, 'Take out paper and pencil,' and he would if he felt like it. He skimmed through the first six grades not using his ability. We sent him to a private day school in the seventh grade and he continued the same pattern.

"He has always been skinny and sensitive about this. [The patient was well-built but may have been thin as a child.] He wouldn't swim at the public beach—we'd have to go up a way. I could never work with him. We were at each other's throats all the time. He'd never cooperate. Whatever you did, he'd fight it every inch of the way. He was at the private school for three years and didn't participate in anything. They tried everything—marking him high, no pressure, then pressure, competition with other boys—nothing worked. They asked to have him withdrawn so we put him back in public school and he got into lots of trouble. He just sat there and did nothing—they didn't want him back there any more. He had to repeat grade 11. He was only kept in high school to keep him off the street and he didn't graduate.

"He'd take the car without our permission. He stole hub caps and there were traffic violations. He ran away from home for two, three days with the car. We had him see a psychiatrist and then took him to court. We tried voluntary probation but he didn't keep his appointments. He was uncooperative at home, making life miserable for everybody. When he quit school, we told him he couldn't just sit home so he got a job. Our last dealings at home I couldn't talk to him at all. He lied to me brazenly. I couldn't believe anything he said. We sent him to summer camps but

no one was ever able to change him. He worked for six months and then got into trouble. He won't take a bus. He'll walk several miles rather than ride a bus. When he has a job, it's all right as long as someone picks him up. On his own, he's late or sick and doesn't go.

"At the age of 17 he was in a psychiatric hospital for six weeks. He was incorrigible. He stole a car—I imagine a lot of boys his age do take a car now and then. He took this car and was speeding about 120 miles an hour to escape the police. He knocked one of the tires off the wheel by hitting the center island, but he still drove the car about half a mile trying to get away. They booked him for drunken driving but didn't press charges on stealing the car. I fixed that up with the owner and had it repaired. Through all these escapades—we finally talked to the judge about the question of whether he should go to the reformatory or was he mentally ill—so we put him in the hospital for six weeks. As far as the psychiatrist was concerned at that time, it was a character disorder, which could go one way or the other.

"After leaving the hospital he fooled around in school for another year, then got a job for six months, then got into trouble with other boys stealing batteries and cars. He was in jail a couple of days and lost his job. His accident record was terrible—every time he took a car he'd be picked up. I talked his grandmother into giving him her car for half of what it was worth and he got risk insurance. He promised he wouldn't change the car but in a couple of weeks he did. He had his license taken away from him three times but he continued driving anyway and he got picked up for having a loud muffler. You almost have the impression he's trying to get punished.

"Three things happened at the same time—stealing, driving after his license was suspended, and something else—he was locked up and the fine was $150. We wouldn't pay the fine but his friends pooled their cash and did. He promised the lawyer and judge to go into military service but he didn't. He has never had to face consequences. He just sat home and didn't go into service. It was impossible living with him. He'd do everything to aggravate us, so I gave him $100 to get out of the house and he rented a room. The landlord heard him pacing the floor all night and reported his friends were hoodlums. They had parties and made too much noise, so he had to move. The landlord arranged with him to take a course at vocational school but he only went for a couple of days and then quit. At summer school he'd only go when he could drive the car. He sat home for three months doing nothing. We finally said he was going to go voluntarily for psychiatric help or we'd have him committed. His main job was aggravating his mother. We got the ambulance and he ran away and lived with friends in the neighborhood for six weeks. He came home to wash his clothes. The police had a warrant and told me I was to call them, but I was afraid to.

"Then we went away for a weekend and he got into the house and had a party. He drove a girl home in her car and the police caught him. They handcuffed him and he ran away and went to a friend's house, got rid of the handcuffs and got the friend to take him out of town. He worked in a filling station until a couple of days before the police picked him up there and took him to jail."

The patient was of at least average intelligence and showed no evidence of organic difficulties or psychotic reality distortion. He felt no guilt or remorse over his antisocial behavior. On the MMPI his score on the psychopathic deviate scale was elevated, but all the neurotic and psychotic scales were within the normal range. Since he was not mentally defective or mentally ill, he was returned to the police to stand trial. It was recommended that he be brought into group therapy after the trial.

GROUP DELINQUENCY REACTION OF ADOLESCENCE

Young people who are in the category labeled group delinquency reactions are just as much at odds with society as the antisocial sociopath, but the background and development are different. The group delinquent emerges from an abnormal moral environment, identifies with criminal figures, models himself after them and then adheres to the values of a criminal or predatory group. He is capable of strong loyalty to such a group in contrast to the antisocial sociopath's loyalty to no one. His sociopathy, in short, is an adaptation to a special environment. Adhering to a group as he does, the group delinquent is not as disorganized, impulsive and self-defeating as the antisocial type. His superego is deviant rather than weak. His behavior is controlled, but his goals are unacceptable to society. He does not lack in affective reactions to others, but his affect is distorted and dominated by hostility.

The following excerpts* from a delinquent's own story graphically illustrate the traditions, activities and standards of a delinquent gang and the development of a particular life style. The storyteller's behavior is a clear reflection of the abnormal moral environment in which he grew up.

When I started to play in the alleys around my home I first heard about a bunch of older boys called the "Pirates." My oldest brother was in this gang and so I went around with them. There were about ten boys in this gang and the youngest one was eleven and the oldest one was about fifteen. . . .

---

*Reprinted from The Jack-Roller by C. R. Shaw by permission of The University of Chicago Press. Copyright 1930 by The University of Chicago.

Tony, Sollie, and my brother John were the big guys in the gang. Tony was fifteen and was short and heavy. He was a good fighter and the young guys were afraid of him because he hit them and beat them up. . . . My brother was fifteen and was bigger than Tony and was a good fighter. He could beat any guy in the gang by fighting, so he was a good leader and everybody looked up to him as a big guy. I looked up to him as a big guy and was proud to be his brother. . . .

When I started to hang out with the Pirates I first learned about robbin [sic]. The guys would talk about robbin and stealing and went out on "jobs" every night. When I was eight I started to go out robbin with my brother's gang. We first robbed junk from a junk yard and sometimes from the peddlar. Sometimes we robbed stores. We would go to a store, and while one guy asked to buy something the other guys would rob anything like candy and cigarettes and then run. We did this every day. . . .

The gang had a hangout in an alley and we would meet there every night and smoke and tell stories and plan for robbin. I was little and so I only listened. The big guys talked about going robbin and told stories about girls and sex things. The guys always thought about robbin and bummin from school and sometimes from home. . . .

When I was ten the gang started to robbin stores and homes. We would jimmy the door or window and rob the place. I always stayed outside and gave jiggers. The big guys went in and raided the place. They showed me how to pick locks, jimmy doors, cut glass and use skeleton keys and everything to get into stores and houses. Every guy had to keep everything a secret and not tell anybody or he would be beat up and razzed. The police were enemies and not to be trusted. When we would get caught by the police we had to keep mum and not tell a word even in the third degree.

I looked up to my brother and the other big guys because of their courage and nerve and the way they could rob. They would tell me never to say a word to anybody about our robbin. My mother didn't even know it. Some kids couldn't be in the gang because they would tell everything and some didn't have the nerve to go robbin. The guys with a record were looked up to and admired by the young guys. A stool-pigeon was looked down on and razzed and could not stay in the gang. . . .

The guys stuck together and helped each other out of trouble. They were real good pals and would stick up for each other.

CAUSATION

Heredity and Other Biological Determinants

Very little is known about the role of heredity in the antisocial personality. O'Neal et al. (1962)

compared the parents of 84 males diagnosed as sociopathic with the parents of 166 males in other psychiatric disorders and the parents of 75 males free of obvious psychological disturbance. Table 14–2 shows the percentage of sociopathic personality for the parents in each group. The fathers of the sociopaths were much more likely to be sociopaths than the fathers in the other two groups; the mothers showed some tendency in the same direction. Another finding of the study was that the percentage of cases in which both father and son were sociopaths was the same for those sociopaths who lived with their fathers throughout childhood and for those who had been separated from them in childhood by family break-up. This finding is explainable by the hypothesis that heredity determines sociopathy, but it should be recognized that environmental factors may be as influential in broken homes as in those in which a son can identify directly with a physically present father.

Adult criminality—related to sociopathic personality, it should be remembered, but not identical with it—has been studied by twin investigations. Shields and Slater (1960) combined and analyzed five such studies and reported the concordance rate for criminal behavior among monozygotic twins to be 68 per cent and for dizygotic twins of the same sex, 35 per cent. The index of heritability (H) computed from these rates is $\frac{68-35}{100-35} = 0.51$, suggesting that both hereditary and environmental factors are important in the causation of criminal behavior in adults. For juvenile delinquency, Rosanoff et al. (1941) found concordance rates of 85 per cent in monozygotic twins and 75 per cent in same-sexed dizygotic twins, yielding a value for H of 0.40. Although this is a substantial figure, the concordance rate for nonidentical twins—75 per cent—was so close to the rate for the identical twins that the value of H may be considered an overestimate. (When the concordance

TABLE 14–2. Percentage of Parents Diagnosed as Sociopathic Personality in the Study by O'Neal, Robins and King

	Percentage of Fathers	Percentage of Mothers
84 Sociopaths	51	13
166 Psychiatric patients (nonsociopaths)	33	9
75 Normals	19	4

TABLE 14–3. Incidence of Somatotype Component Dominance

	496 Delinquents (Per Cent)	482 Non-delinquents (Per Cent)
Endomorphic dominance	11.8	15.0
Mesomorphic dominance	60.1	30.7
Ectomorphic dominance	14.4	39.6
Balanced types (No component dominance)	13.5	14.7

Modified from Glueck, S., and Glueck, E. 1956. Physique and Delinquency, New York, Hoeber-Harper.

rates for MZ and DZ twins are both very high, the contribution of environment is necessarily large and the statistic H becomes a poor estimator.)

The frequency of sociopathic behavior is considerably higher among males than females, but it is not clear to what extent this fact reflects inherent biological differences as opposed to differences in learned, sociocultural roles. Similarly, the fact that sociopathy is particularly common in adolescence may point to a biological origin or to the psychological problems of adolescents in our culture. Apart from such speculations, a number of studies have clarified the role of biological determinants other than heredity in delinquency and sociopathy. In a comparison of 496 delinquent boys with 482 nondelinquent controls matched for age, intelligence, national origin and residence in underprivileged neighborhoods, Glueck and Gleuck (1956) found a strong statistical association between delinquency and mesomorphic body build. Table 14–3 summarizes their findings: mesomorphs were twice as frequent (60.1 per cent vs. 30.7 per cent) and ectomorphs less than half as frequent (14.4 vs. 39.6 per cent). Glueck and Glueck concluded that differences in physical and temperamental structure result in different responses to environmental pressures, so that mesomorphs are more likely than other types to respond by aggressive, rebellious delinquency to the environmental deprivation of poor neighborhoods. An interesting implication of this study is its contradiction of the age-old notion that the delinquent or criminal is constitutionally inferior; he seems, rather, to be muscular and energetic.

Stott (1962) analyzed data on delinquency among British boys who were born during World War II. He found that the rates of delinquency were higher for boys born during those war years in which the rates for congenital physical malformation were also high. There are several possible reasons for a high incidence of malformation at birth in wartime. Nutritional deficiencies, inadequate public health services and ingestion of industrial poisons that are used in the manufacture of arms may all play a role. Stott reasoned that the covariation of congenital malformations and delinquency rates must have resulted from prenatal impairment of various organs, including those parts of the nervous system that control behavior. Consistent with this conclusion is the fact that brain disorders are known, in some cases, to result in uncontrolled behavior. Extensive injury to the frontal lobes of the brain, due to tumors, birth injury, later traumatic injury or surgery, often has as one of its results an indifference to social convention. Epilepsy is sometimes accompanied by aggressive antisocial behavior. Encephalitis frequently results in aggressive overactivity and loss of control; "post-encephalitic syndrome" is a recognized psychiatric category.

A number of EEG studies have provided strong evidence of a biological factor in sociopathy. Hill and Watterson (1942) found abnormal EEG patterns in 48 per cent of a large group of psychopaths, and the frequency of these patterns was particularly high for the more aggressive individuals in the sample. Silverman (1944) found EEG peculiarities in 80 per cent of a psychopathic sample. Other investigators have confirmed these findings; in general, the rate of EEG abnormality among sociopaths is reported to be 50 per cent or more. It is possible, however, that many sociopaths with EEG abnormalities are really epileptics who do not have seizures but, instead, manifest an aggressive lack of control. Another limitation of the EEG studies of sociopathy is that disturbed electrical activity of the brain may be a *result* rather than a cause of psychological disturbance. Nevertheless, the cumulative total of the studies of physique, congenital malformation, brain injury and EEG peculiarities points strongly to the likelihood that biological factors are significant contributing causes in some cases of delinquency and sociopathy. In other cases, however, psychological and sociocultural causes seem to be primary.

Psychological Determinants

Anything that leads to a defective moral development, uncontrolled behavior and a shallow affective life can be a cause of sociopathy. Weinberg (1952) pinpoints some of the crucial psychological causes: "The psychopath develops within a matrix of distant and impersonal parent-child relationships, and especially amidst changing and emotionally depriving parent figures." A study by Bandura and Walters (1959) corroborated this formulation. Twenty-six antisocial, adolescent boys and their parents were intensively interviewed, along with a control group of 26 well-socialized adolescents and their parents. The major difference found between the two groups was that one or both parents of the antisocial boys were less affectionate and psychologically nurturant than the control parents. As a consequence, the dependency needs of the antisocial boys were frustrated and they felt rejected, became critical of parental authority—particularly paternal—and expressed aggression directly and without inhibition. Their internal control systems and their aggressions could be kept in check only by external restraints. A study of delinquents from upper socioeconomic groups by Herskovitz, Levine and Spivak (1959) reported results very similar to those of Bandura and Walters. Apparently the emotional deprivation sustained when the child's dependency needs are frustrated produces antisocial aggression in upper as well as lower socioeconomic levels.

The importance of deprivation was also indicated in a study by Silverman (1943). In an investigation of the family histories of 35 criminal psychopaths, he found that one-fourth had been rejected and otherwise emotionally deprived by parents, one-third had been markedly insecure in childhood and one-third gave indications of unresolved Oedipal conflicts.

Deprivation is aggravated by parental separation or loss. Gregory (1959) found a higher frequency of desertion by the father during the childhood of individuals who later became psychopaths than for any other psychiatric disorder. More than 10 per cent had lost *both* parents by the age of 10, a higher figure than for any other psychiatric disorder. Not surprisingly, the frequency of illegitimacy was also highest for the psychopaths. Glueck and Glueck (1950) found that the homes of 60 per cent of a sample of 500 delinquents had been breached by separation, desertion, death or prolonged parental absence, as compared to 34 per cent for a sample of nondelinquents of equivalent age, intelligence, national origin and type of neighborhood (see Table 14–4). For each category in the table—sporadic separation,

TABLE 14–4. Nature of All Breaches in Family Life

Description	Delinquents		Nondelinquents		Difference	P
	Number	Per Cent	Number	Per Cent	Per Cent	
Parents separated sporadically	136	27.2	46	9.2	18.0	<.01
Parents separated or divorced	111	22.2	64	12.8	9.4	<.01
One or both parents died*	100	20.0	68	13.6	6.4	<.01
One or both parents away from home for at least a year†	70	14.0	30	6.0	8.0	<.01
Parents abandoned boy at birth‡	24	4.8	5	1.0	3.8	<.01

Note. Percentages are based on totals of 500.
*Four delinquents and 2 non-delinquents lost both parents.
†Because of criminalism or illness.
‡Parents not married and did not live together after birth of boy either at all or for long.
From Glueck, S., and Glueck, E. 1950. Unraveling Juvenile Delinquency. Cambridge, Mass., Commonwealth Fund and Harvard University Press.

permanent separation or divorce, death, prolonged absence from the home, and abandonment at birth—the difference between the delinquents and nondelinquents was statistically significant. Not shown in the table is an additional and important fact: the first breach in family life had occurred by the age of five for 170 delinquents but only 80 nondelinquents.

Parental separation or loss is particularly likely to breed sociopathy if the child is institutionalized or placed in a foster home. The institutionalized child has no chance to develop primary emotional relationships with parents and, in a desperate, substitute bid for attention, is likely to become directly aggressive and lie or steal.

However, a large number of delinquents and sociopaths do not come from institutions or broken homes but from homes that are physically intact but emotionally disturbed. The parents may provide a poor example; Gregory (1959) found that 15 per cent of the fathers and 5 per cent of the mothers of psychopaths had a history of excessive drinking. These percentages are much higher than for the population at large. The parents may reject the child in the manner already described and make it impossible for him to develop the identification needed for an adequate superego or the empathy needed for close human relationships. If he is not rewarded for desirable behavior, he may accept the values of a delinquent peer group. On the other hand, the parents may overindulge the child, and because he is permitted to express his aggressive and other needs without inhibition, he may develop a very lax superego and become psychopathic. At a deeper level, overindulgence may be a manifestation of rejection by a parent who does not

care enough to control the child, or a reaction-formation to ward off the guilt that would be aroused by conscious recognition of hostility and feelings of rejection toward the child. O'Neal et al. (1962) found that both parental repudiation and inadequate supervision were more frequent in the background of sociopaths than patients with other psychiatric disorders.

The child may also be exposed to an inconsistent alternation between rejection and indulgence, either within his home or in a succession of foster homes or institutions. Fenichel (1945) cites the case of a patient whose pathologically inconsistent father gave him a generous present one moment and took it back the next, or made promises that were never kept. To defend himself, the child learned to take whatever he could as quickly as possible. This pattern became generalized and he began to follow any impulse whatever before it could be prohibited by someone.

In still another pattern, each parent is consistent with himself but not with the other. Most often, this constellation consists of an austere, distant and highly moral father and an indulgent, pleasure-loving mother. The father is likely to be highly respected in the community and contemptuously critical of his children. The mother, on the other hand, may be quietly contemptuous of the father's achievements. The child finds it difficult to identify with the emotionally distant father and aggressively rebels against him and his moral standards; he adopts the mother's indulgent attitudes to excuse his failure to come up to his father's expectations, and learns to deny, conceal or rationalize his inadequacies. He is not without a superego but it is a useless one that does not control his behavior. In a family of this type, the members devote themselves to preserving a "good" façade for the inspection of the outside world. The contradiction between façade and internal family conflicts contributes to the shallowness of the child's affective development and to his perception of the world as a place where one must try to get away with as much as possible.

In countless cases of children who have become promiscuous, irresponsibly reckless or alcoholic, the parents have been moral, valued members of the community—ministers, professors, judges, philanthropists and so forth—who are inconsistent or in conflict. This is illustrated by the following case:

The daughter of a prominent couple, whom the community considered happily married, had a lengthy history of deceit and rebellion. She was attractive and brilliant but a nonachiever and in continual trouble at college because of gross violation of rules. On inquiry, it was learned that the mother had not wanted children, but after some years had yielded to the demands of her husband. The child quickly became the focus of parental conflict, with the mother indulgently protecting her from the supposedly unreasonable demands of the father. When the child developed temper tantrums, there were a few painful scenes in which the father spanked her while the mother watched, wringing her hands and weeping. The father soon abandoned physical attempts to control his daughter and resorted to dire threats of punishment or withdrawal of privileges which he never carried out. He pressed the mother to set simple tasks for the daughter such as tidying her room and helping with the dishes, but the mother preferred to wait on the girl hand and foot. The daughter began to associate with a family that the father considered undesirable and he threatened to make her leave home; nevertheless, when she continued to visit her friends he came without comment to pick her up. The mother smoked, although the father strongly disapproved, and when the daughter started to smoke the mother rewarded her with tête-à-têtes in which they talked and smoked together. Nor was the father as moral as he seemed: he professed respect for the letter of the law but flagrantly disregarded traffic and other regulations that inconvenienced him. Regulations were only for "people who needed them to be kept under control." In short, the daughter was the victim of her parents' private inconsistencies and conflicts.

Sometimes parents sanction and foster unacceptable behavior; Johnson (1959) hypothesized that the antisocial behavior of a child vicariously gratifies the parents' own forbidden impulses. Furthermore, whatever hostile and destructive wishes the parents feel toward the child are gratified by the continuous defeat the child experiences as a result of his sociopathic be-

havior. The parents' attitude is, "Go ahead and do it and see what happens to you!" Kiernan and Porter (1963) have presented data showing that some problem children have behaviors which are almost identical to those displayed by the parents when they were young. While some delinquents appear to be acting out the unconscious desires of their parents, it would be a mistake to assume that such factors apply to all cases.

A number of theorists have speculated that two different types of persons may develop behavior or conduct disorders: the *true, or primary, sociopath* who has a low anxiety level and a defective superego, and the *neurotic sociopath*—paradoxical as this term may seem—who has a high anxiety level which is "acted out" antisocially. In the study previously cited, Lykken (1957) identified a neurotic group of sociopaths who, in contrast to the primary sociopaths, scored significantly *higher* than normal on anxiety measurements. The neurotic sociopath's anxiety mounts and eventually overflows into unacceptable behavior. When his anxiety and guilt become too intense, he attempts to ward them off by the paradoxical procedure of acting out rather than by repression or other intrapersonal defenses. In an episodic fashion he gambles, drinks, behaves promiscuously, steals and hurts people, not because he has no conscience but in a vain effort to keep a too-strong conscience at bay. The ordinary neurotic reproduces his conflicts in fantasy; the neurotic sociopath acts them out upon the environment.

A theoretical approach to sociopathy that is closely related to the concept of the neurotic sociopath holds that *even the primary sociopath has a strong conscience but it is deeply repressed*. Support for this hypothesis comes from clinical observation of the frequency with which sociopaths behave as if they wished to be punished, i.e., as if they were motivated by a completely unconscious but clamorous superego. An example is the case of a sociopath who was questioned by the police when his wife disappeared. He told a very plausible story disclaiming any knowledge of her disappearance, but two weeks later a bloody weapon which he had used to kill her was found in the trunk of his car. His failure to get rid of the weapon was not due to mental deficiency, for his intelligence was well above average.

An implication of the hypothesis that sociopaths have an unconscious need to be punished is that sociopathy is ultimately a defense against neurosis. Were the sociopath to become conscious of his deeply repressed guilt and anxiety, he would feel overwhelmed. As a defense, he keeps *all* affective reactions in check. It is not possible to state with any certainty how many sociopaths are motivated by mechanisms of this type and how many have a genuine superego weakness, but future research may clarify the matter.

Sociocultural Determinants

There have been few studies of the sociocultural determinants of sociopathic personality as such, but many studies have concentrated on the determinants of delinquency and crime. Leighton (1959) reported a higher frequency of antisocial behavior in disorganized as compared to better organized communities in an east coast province of Canada. The same results have been reported in other countries. The rates of delinquency and crime are universally accepted as indices of the degree of disorganization in a community.

The very highest delinquency rates are found among boys resident in the underprivileged areas of large cities. For example, in Shaw and McKay's analysis of delinquency in Chicago (1942), the highest rates for the years 1900 to 1906 occurred in underprivileged areas which, for the most part, were located near the center business district, and the lowest rates were concentrated near the periphery of the city where the residents were relatively well-to-do. Shaw and McKay correlated the rates in the different city areas for 1900 to 1906 with the rates for 1917 to 1923 and also for 1927 to 1933. The first of these correlation coefficients was +.85 and the second was +.61; i.e., in general the high-rate areas remained high and the low-rate areas remained low, despite the fact that the ethnic origins of the residents of the low-rate areas changed markedly in the interim. The investigators concluded that delinquency was best understood as a subcultural tradition in areas inhabited by the lower socioeconomic classes.

Many subsequent studies have confirmed the existence of an association between delinquency and low socioeconomic level. For the city of Baltimore, Lander (1954) reported a correlation between overcrowding and juvenile delinquency of +.73. Substandard housing and delinquency correlated +.69. The average number of years of schooling of the adult population in the different areas of Baltimore correlated —.53 with rates of delinquency; of course, lack of schooling may not be a direct cause of delinquency, but both may reflect low socioeconomic level. (It is also true that average I.Q. is lower in slum than nonslum areas, but *within* a slum area delinquency is not related to I.Q.) The correlation between delinquency and the percentage of foreign-born residents in the various areas of Baltimore was —.16, i.e., there was a slight tendency to a *lower* rate for the foreign-born. In a number of studies, some foreign-born groups have had higher rates of delinquency than the native-born and others have had lower rates. Apparently the relation between national origin and delinquency rate reflects socioeconomic status, for it has been found that *within* a slum neighborhood the differences in rate of delinquency among national groups are small. Socioeconomic status itself influences delinquency via the mediating variable of a breakdown in social organization. Thus, Lander interpreted the data for Baltimore to mean that poverty, poor housing, nearness to the center of the city and other economic and demographic variables were surface manifestations of disorganization: "When the group norms are no longer binding or valid in an area or for a population subgroup, in so far is individual behavior likely to lead to deviant behavior. Delinquency is a function of the stability and acceptance of the group norms with legal sanctions and the consequent effectiveness of the social controls in securing conforming juvenile behavior."

A somewhat different interpretation of delinquency was made by Cohen (1955) who emphasized that lower class children tend to be reared in surroundings that have quite different standards from the middle class standards of the schools they attend. Status frustration and the loss of self-esteem consequent on this discrepancy lead the lower class children to draw together in gangs. The delinquent subculture that is formed by this process rewards those who assault the middle class status system. However, it should be remembered that not all boys from a high delinquency area rebel against the standards of the larger society. Scarpitti et al. (1960) investigated the interesting question of why some boys who live in high delinquency areas remain "good." It was found that the "good" boys came from very stable families, evaluated their home life as satisfactory and liked school and their teachers. As pre-adolescents they formed positive self-images and isolated themselves from the de-linquent gangs which did not share their values.

Still another aspect of sociocultural influence on delinquency is high-lighted in the study of a British mining town by Carter and Jephcott (1952–1954). Delinquency was found to be concentrated in five fairly small areas in the town. Within each area a pair of streets was selected for investigation, one with a high frequency of delinquency and the other a lower frequency. The streets within each pair appeared superficially similar, but intensive observation revealed marked differences among the resident families. The majority of families on the high delinquency streets engaged in domestic violence, street brawling, drunkenness and promiscuity. The children in these families were exposed to adults whose behavior rejected the norms of the wider society and exemplified self-interest and a disregard for the rights of others. The majority of families on the low delinquency streets were proud of their homes and reputations, supervised their children closely and placed a premium on education as a means to social and economic betterment. It would seem that the *family within the community is more important than the community itself* in the causation of antisocial behavior.

Just as not all children in poor communities become delinquent, so delinquency is not restricted to urban, lower class neighborhoods. There is reason to believe that delinquency has been increasing in the suburban middle class in recent years. In a large scale study published in 1963, Hathaway and Monachesi found that the rate for boys from professional families was 25 per cent. This was almost as large as the 30 per cent reported for the families of day laborers. The investigators concluded that delinquency "is a phenomenon almost as significant in suburbia as anywhere. Our fast diminishing rural population is the only remaining low group." It may therefore be that the traditional association between antisocial behavior and community disorganization is weakening.

Palmar et al (1967), after studying 453 British juvenile offenders, concluded: (1) that delinquency was derived evenly from all social classes, (2) that the type of offense varied little from class to class, and (3) that boys and girls differed markedly in both number and type of offenses. While such studies help to prevent the automatic assumption that delinquency and lower socioeconomic class are synonymous,

social factors can never be discounted entirely. Gordon (1967) reviewed some of the frequent experimental and statistical errors found in previous research on the relationship between delinquency and socioeconomic status. He concluded that "when all of these errors are taken into account, it turns out that the association between delinquency and socioeconomic status is unambiguously very strong."

Hollingshead and Redlich found enormous differences between the treatment accorded to unacceptable behavior in different classes:*

The case histories of two compulsively promiscuous adolescent females will be drawn upon to illustrate the differential impact of class status on the way in which lay persons and psychiatrists perceive and appraise similar behavior. Both girls came to the attention of the police at about the same time but under very different circumstances. One came from a core group class I family, the other from a class V family broken by the desertion of the father. The class I girl, after one of her frequent drinking and sexual escapades on a weekend away from an exclusive boarding school, became involved in an automobile accident while drunk. Her family immediately arranged for bail through the influence of a member of an outstanding law firm; a powerful friend telephoned a newspaper contact, and the report of the accident was not published. Within twenty-four hours, the girl was returned to school. In a few weeks the school authorities realized that the girl was pregnant and notified her parents. A psychiatrist was called in for consultation by the parents with the expectation, expressed frankly, that he was to recommend a therapeutic interruption of the pregnancy. He did not see fit to do this and, instead, recommended hospitalization in a psychiatric institution to initiate psychotherapy. The parents, though disappointed that the girl would not have a "therapeutic" abortion, finally consented to hospitalization. In due course, the girl delivered a healthy baby who was placed for adoption. Throughout her stay in the hospital she received intensive psychotherapy and after being discharged continued in treatment with a highly regarded psychoanalyst.

The class V girl was arrested by the police after she was observed having intercourse with four or five sailors from a nearby naval base. At the end of a brief and perfunctory trial, the girl was sentenced to a reform school. After two years there she was paroled as an unpaid domestic. While on parole, she became involved in promiscuous activity, was caught by the police, and sent to the state reformatory for women. She accepted her sentence as deserved "punishment" but created enough disturbance in the reformatory to attract the attention of a guidance officer. This

---

*Reprinted with permission from Hollingshead, A. B., and Redlich, F. C. 1958. Social Class and Mental Illness. New York, John Wiley & Sons, Inc.

official recommended that a psychiatrist be consulted. The psychiatrist who saw her was impressed by her crudeness and inability to communicate with him on most subjects. He was alienated by the fact that she thought masturbation was "bad," whereas intercourse with many men whom she hardly knew was "O.K." The psychiatrist's recommendation was to return the girl to her regular routine because she was not "able to profit from psychotherapy."

A cross-cultural study of crime and delinquency by Bacon, Child and Barry (1963) resulted in some interesting and important findings. In a sample of 48 nonliterate societies widely scattered over Africa, Asia, Oceania and North and South America, the frequency of theft and personal crime were separately correlated with ratings for a number of cultural variables. (By personal crime is meant assault, murder, rape, false accusations and so forth.) Both theft and personal crime occurred significantly more often in societies in which boys were unable to form an identification with the father. For example, there were high frequencies in those societies in which it was customary for a mother and her children to live apart from the father. This finding is consistent with the data cited earlier indicating an association within our own society between sociopathy and paternal absence. The finding was interpreted by Bacon, Child and Barry as a corroboration of a hypothesis that stems from a psychoanalytic point of view: crime in males represents a struggle against a feminine identification. A fuller statement of this hypothesis was made by Rohrer and Edmonson* in their study of the matriarchal households found in the South:

Gang life begins early, more or less contemporaneously with the first years of schooling, and for many men lasts until death. . . . Although each gang is a somewhat distinct group, all of them appear to have a common structure expressing and reinforcing the gang ideology. Thus an organizational form that springs from the little boy's search for a masculinity he cannot find at home becomes first a protest against femininity and then an assertion of hypervirility. On the way it acquires a structuring in which the aspirations and goals of the matriarchy or the middle class are seen as soft, effeminate, and despicable. The gang ideology of masculine independence is formed from these perceptions, and the gang then sees its common enemy not as a class, nor even perhaps as a sex, but as the "feminine principle" in society. The gang member rejects this femininity in every form, and he

*From Rohrer, J. H., and Edmonson, M. S. (Editors). 1960. Eighth Generation: Cultures and Personalities of New Orleans Negroes. New York, Harper & Row, Publishers, Inc.

sees it in women and in effeminate men, in laws and morals and religion, in schools and occupational striving.

To return to Bacon, Child and Barry's cross-cultural investigation, it was also found that theft was more frequent in societies in which a high degree of anxiety was aroused by punishment of irresponsible behavior in childhood. As in our society, the child who feels deprived of affection is more likely to steal. In addition, theft was associated with status differentiation: societies with a high degree of social stratification and control seem to arouse feelings of insecurity and resentment which lead to theft. (It is also possible that the causal arrow points in the opposite direction: a high frequency of theft may necessitate elaborate social controls.) One other outcome of the investigation was the finding that personal crime was widespread in those cultures that were marked by a general adult attitude of mistrust and suspicion.

TREATMENT

There have been occasional reports of successful somatic treatment of psychopaths but none of these treatments appears to hold promise as a treatment of choice. Green et al. (1943) used ECT with 24 psychopaths, each having a minimum of five treatments, and reported that both behavior and the EEG improved in some patients. However, in a few patients the EEG actually changed for the worse.

Treatment has been attempted by various drugs including Dilantin, an anti-convulsant drug frequently used to prevent epileptic seizures. The rationale for the use of Dilantin is that at least 50 per cent of sociopaths and a larger number of epileptics show abnormal EEG patterns. Silverman (1943, 1944) reported that Dilantin resulted in considerable improvement among psychopaths in stabilizing behavior and reducing antisocial trends. Other investigators have reported beneficial results with various sedative drugs. There is always the possibility, however, that patients who improve with these treatment measures are really neurotics or undiagnosed epileptics rather than true sociopaths.

In a study of psychosurgery, Darling and Sanddal (1952) found that 17 of 18 severe psychopaths improved following lobotomies. More than half improved sufficiently to be able to return to the community and function adequately. Of course, lobotomy is as rarely used with sociopaths as with other psychiatric groups.

For many years a great deal of interest has been focused on the psychotherapeutic treatment of sociopaths. It should be clear that there is no such thing as a prescribed set of treatment goals for the delinquent or criminal *per se*. A neurotic criminal needs treatment for his neurosis, not his crime, and a psychotic criminal for his psychosis. The usual therapeutic goals with a sociopath are to help him establish identifications with acceptable models and develop inhibitions, controls and satisfying affective relationships with others. The sociopath makes an interesting patient: he talks well, makes himself liked by the therapist, and quickly learns to give the impression that he is acquiring insight into his disorder. He masters the therapist's vocabulary and sometimes outdoes the latter in use of technical language. He may promise to reform and be "a new person." Yet psychotherapy with sociopaths has not proved to be frequently successful in achieving marked and sustained improvement.

Psychoanalysis has rarely succeeded: in a representative report by Hendrick (1958), of 23 psychopaths accepted for analysis at the Berlin Psychoanalytic Institute, 18 discontinued treatment, four were unimproved and only one was considered improved. Most other psychotherapeutic approaches have also fared poorly. To quote Cleckley (1959): "The general discouragement about our having any regularly successful type of psychotherapy to offer most of these patients seems justified."

The failure of psychotherapy largely stems from the sociopath's lack of therapeutic motivation. The antisocial sociopath has a weak ego and experiences too little conscious anxiety to feel the need for change in his mode of living. (It might be said that in order to modify his behavior it is necessary to make him more neurotic and then treat the neurosis.) Furthermore, he is as unable to establish a genuine emotional relationship with the therapist as with other persons. Sociopaths may also resist treatment because after years of difficulties with authority—parents, teachers, policemen, judges, and reform school and prison personnel—the therapist is perceived as one more representative of authority. To them, he is no different from a "cop," who is not to be trusted. Sometimes a sociopath tests out a therapist by confessing to a crime for which he was never apprehended and then waiting to see if the therapist reports it. The therapist is put in a moral dilemma by such a situation; therapists disagree on the proper course to take.

Some therapists have a more positive attitude toward working with such patients than the previous paragraphs might lead one to expect (Greenwald, 1968; Ellis, 1963). Greenwald finds it difficult to establish a cooperative working relationship with psychopaths and emphasizes the need for the therapist to resist any moralizing about the transgressions of the patient. To Greenwald, the central problem in therapy is the problem of control. He feels that psychopaths often fail to control themselves out of a deep fear that they lack the ability to do so. To counteract this attitude the therapist institutes some controls as a part of the treatment situation, such as asking the patient to refrain from smoking during the therapy sessions. Through the experience of finding himself capable of some controls, the patient comes to alter his questioning of his ability to constrain himself in other areas. Greenwald believes that one of the biggest problems in dealing with such patients is the fact that often the psychopathic behavior masks a psychosis. However, Greenwald feels that "by emphasizing the problems of control, you deal with the underlying problems because, as they control themselves, they can also control the psychotic-like behavior which lies underneath the psychopathy and the self-destructiveness."

Other therapists have had some success in the use of hypnotherapy with psychopathic patients. Probably the most complete and intriguing account of such a course of treatment was that supplied by Linder in his popular book *Rebel Without a Cause*.

Truax, Silber and Wargo (1966) reported a positive effect on delinquent girls who were seen in group psychotherapy. Institutionalized delinquents were seen in group psychotherapy twice a week for three months. The therapists were chosen because of their high degree of empathy and nonpossessive warmth. Compared to a control group of untreated girls from the same institution, those in group therapy were more likely to remain out of the institution after discharge, scored lower on a scale designed to measure delinquency proneness, and had self images which were closer to their concept of their ideal self.

A problem in treating young delinquents

who live at home is that of treating the family. If a parent encourages antisocial behavior, subtly or crudely, treatment of the delinquent is possible only if the parent is also treated or if the two are separated. Most such parents are as resistant to treatment as their offspring, or more so.

A number of observers have suggested that what the sociopath needs is training in special institutions—neither jails nor mental hospitals—with consistent, nonpunitive discipline that forces him to face the consequences of his actions. A program of this type emphasizes close supervision and group rather than individual psychotherapy. Aichhorn (1935) has reported favorable results in retraining antisocial youngsters committed to a training institution. The therapist in the institution acts as an affectionate but strong father-substitute. At first he compensates for the sociopath's lack of love in childhood, but then he begins to make an increasing number of demands on the patient. He is "smarter" than the patient and constantly points out the latter's self-defeating errors in failing to conform to demands. Hopefully, the patient first comes to respond affectionately toward the father-figure and then to admire his cleverness, thus providing the basis for identi-

fication with him and renunciation of antisocial behavior.

A promising approach is that of Jones (1953) who established a "therapeutic community" for 100 patients, some psychopaths and some not, in a British hospital. The patients worked in a shop for several hours a day where they were given vocational training. They were responsible for directing their own social activities and were required to adhere to a set of behavior regulations and to participate in group therapy. In essence, this program consists of creating a small society in which patients learn to live harmoniously. A favorable outcome has been reported for many cases. There is always the possibility, however, that the patients who are helped by either individual or group procedures are really more neurotic than sociopathic.

Nevertheless, with no treatment whatever, sociopaths sometimes abandon their customary mode of behavior as they age. They "burn out" and become better socialized, perhaps because of physiological changes or perhaps because the self-defeating nature of their behavior eventually gets through to them. The therapeutic problem is to encourage and hasten the processes that promote socialization.

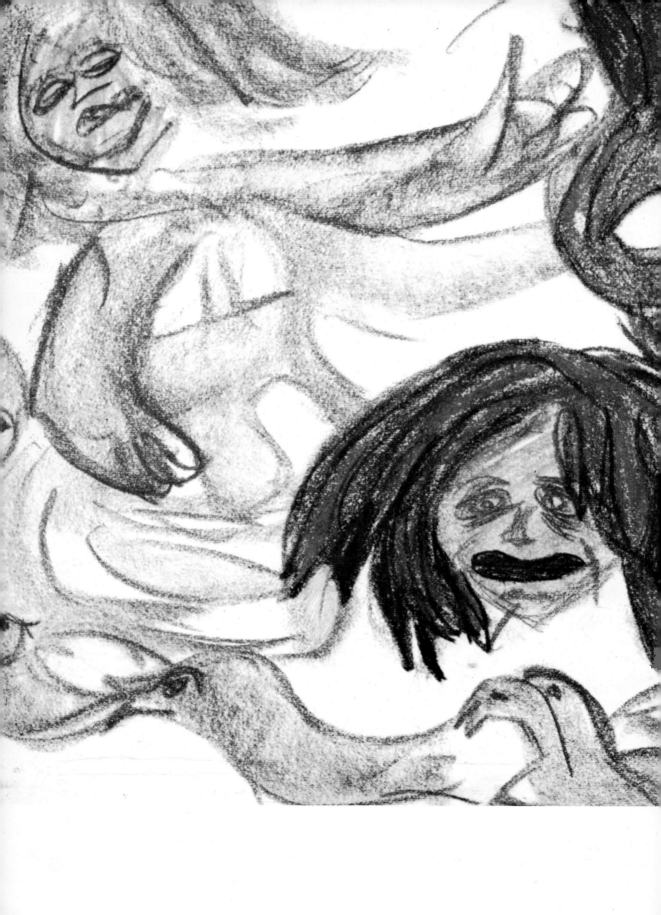

Human sexual behavior is more variable and more easily affected by
learning and social conditioning than is that of any other species. . . .

C. S. Ford and F. A. Beach, *Patterns of Sexual Behavior*

15

SEXUAL DEVIATION

Among the "innumerable peculiarities of the erotic life of human beings"—to borrow a phrase from Freud (1905)—sexual deviation is difficult to distinguish from sexual normality. How does one draw the line between a very strong but normal sexual drive and nymphomania (insatiable impulse to sexual gratification in women) or satyriasis (insatiable impulse to sexual gratification in men), between normal and deviant oral activity, or between aggressively masculine sexual behavior and sadism?

One solution is to substitute the legal concept of a sexual offense for the psychological concept of a sexual deviation. Karpman (1954) defines a sexual offense as ". . . behavior that offends the particular society in which the offender lives. English and American legal codes consider all premarital, extramarital and post-marital intercourse, mouth-genital and anal contacts, whether in or out of marriage, all sexual contacts with animals, and the public exhibition of any kind of sexual activity, as sexual offenses punishable by penalties. Normal sexuality is regarded as heterosexual relations voluntarily practiced in a normal manner by responsible adults not too closely related and married to each other or (possibly) not married at all. All else is taboo."

The definition of a sexual offense is clear, but for psychological and psychiatric purposes it is inadequate. First, it fails to consider motivational and emotional factors. Second, what con-

stitutes an offense in the eyes of Anglo-American law may be permissible under other legal codes. Laws reflect cultures: in some cultures kissing is regarded as perverse behavior; in some, prostitution is an accepted and even highly regarded social institution; and in some, anal intercourse and intercourse with animals are prescribed in tribal initiation rites. Within the United States also, there is wide variability in the law; for example, the penalty for sodomy (ano-genital activity between males) may be imprisonment for 30 days or life, depending on the state in which the act is committed. Glueck (1956) noted that approximately 25 per cent of the Connecticut prison population were sentenced for sexual offenses in contrast with 10 per cent of the New York prison population. The disparity is due solely to the greater severity of penalties for sexual offenses in Connecticut. A third difficulty is that in practice the term "sexual offenders" is applied only to individuals who have been caught and convicted. A far greater number commit offenses but are not apprehended.

From a psychological point of view, a sexual deviation, also termed a *perversion* or *paraphilia*, is best understood as a failure of psychosexual development. The normal individual progresses from diffuse infantile sexuality that consists of oral, anal, autoerotic, homoerotic, exhibitionistic, voyeuristic and other components, to mature sexuality in which these components are sub-

273

ordinated to genital, heterosexual activity that is relatively free of conflict. The sexually deviant individual fails to make this progression. *In our society a failure of development, associated with anxiety and conflict, culminating in a persistent or frequently recurring preference for any form of sexual behavior that is a substitute for, and does not terminate in, genital coitus with an adult of the opposite sex, is a sexual deviation.* Nongenital behavior as a final aim that substitutes for genitality is deviant; nongenital behavior as a foreplay to heterosexual coitus is not deviant, although it may be illegal.

Three points should be noted about the concept of sexual deviation. First, a sexual deviation is relative to the culture, as is a sexual offense. For example, in ancient Greece, homosexuality was not considered a deviation. Second, although most deviations are also sexual offenses, a large number of offenses—for example, extramarital intercourse or nongenital heterosexual foreplay—are not deviations. Third, an important component of the concept of deviation is its stress on *persistence* in habit patterns. The individual who occasionally departs from normal sexual behavior is very different from the persistent deviate.

THE PSYCHOPATHOLOGY OF THE SEXUAL DEVIATE

There are enormous differences in the behavior and personality of sexually deviant persons. Few deviates become involved in more than one kind of deviation; an exception is the high frequency with which voyeurism and exhibitionism are associated. To some extent, the particular type of deviation is associated with particular personality traits. The impotent old man who engages in sexual play with a small child is entirely different from the young sadist who rapes or kills a child.

Within any single deviation there are also wide differences in personality. Many deviant individuals are antisocial personalities; in fact, the term "sexual psychopathy" has often been used loosely to refer to all types of sexual deviation or offense. However, many other sexual deviants are not sociopathic but psychotic or mentally retarded, and even more are neurotic. The term "sexual psychopathy" should therefore be used only for that antisocial minority among persistent deviates whose sexual offenses are potentially dangerous to others.

In any event, a persistent sexual deviate is very unlikely to approximate normality in nonsexual as well as sexual areas. The further his sexual preference is from adult, genital heterosexuality, the more pathological his personality is likely to be and the more reality distortion he is likely to evidence. It should be added, however, that many sexually deviant persons have been extraordinarily creative. Rousseau found normal sexuality repugnant, Swinburne was a sadomasochist, many artists and writers from Michelangelo to Gide have been homosexual, and Mozart wrote pornographic letters.

Some sexual deviates are active, energetic and aggressive, but the majority tend to be shy, reserved, timid and uncomfortable in interpersonal relationships with other adults. The majority are also evasive and noncommunicative; the more deviant the behavior, the greater the tendency to evasion. With amazing frequency, deviates are grossly ignorant and misinformed about sexual functioning. Quite often they are undersexed; the popular stereotype of the oversexed maniac fits very few.

In the more severe forms of deviation, marked signs of either anxiety and depression or apathy and indifference are common. In a number of cases, the individual's conscience is grossly impaired in the sexual area but is otherwise well preserved; a homosexual or exhibitionist may be scrupulously honest, kind and so forth. However, the deviate who is sociopathic or psychotic tends to manifest a generalized deficiency of conscience and impulse control.

The Neurotic

The sexually deviant neurotic is inhibited and often quite prudish. For example, an exhibitionist who was studied intensively by one of the authors had an extremely obsessive and compulsive personality structure, was highly moralistic and condemned all but the most straight-laced behavior. He was deeply ashamed of his exhibitionism but could not control it: whenever his anxiety mounted sufficiently, the urge to exhibit himself became irresistible. He did not smoke or drink, attended church regularly and was completely dependable and honest. Neurotic deviates of this type sometimes manifest frigidity or impotence. Others attempt to compensate for their inhibitions and tensions by periodic flights into promiscuity, but afterward are likely to feel very guilty.

Neurotics rarely become involved in such direct sexual aggression as rape, but the frequency of neurosis is high in homosexuality, voyeurism, exhibitionism, fetishism and the milder degrees of sado-masochism. Brancale, Ellis and Doorbar (1952) reported that 64 per cent of a sample of 300 convicted sex offenders were neurotic. A subgroup of neurotic deviants tends toward hysteria: in general, the full-fledged conversion hysteric represses his pregenital urges whereas the overt deviate is conscious of them, but periodically the hysteric may engage in perverse behavior and periodically the deviate may push his impulses out of consciousness.

The Antisocial Personality

Typically, a sociopathic individual becomes involved in promiscuity and uninhibited sexuality with a variety of partners. Although he prefers partners who consent, he sometimes resorts to force, intimidation or fraud. Consequently, the sociopath more often than other types is charged with seduction or abduction. An otherwise willing female partner may complain that a male sociopath abuses her excessively or tries to tie her to the bed during prolonged periods of sexual indulgence. Adult sociopaths are often attracted to adolescent rather than adult females. Occasionally a male sociopath may become involved in homosexual activity with an adult for financial motives. Homosexual involvement with a child is rare among sociopaths. The more extreme sexual deviations are rarely associated with sociopathic personality but may occur in pseudosociopathic schizophrenia.

The Functional Psychotic

The hypomanic patient frequently becomes involved in promiscuity or, occasionally, in sadistic or assaultive sexual behavior as a concomitant of his euphoric overactivity. In psychotic depression, on the other hand, there is usually a profound inhibition of all sexual responses, with temporary frigidity or impotence. In some depressed patients, feelings of guilt and a desire for punishment lead to masochistic sexual behavior, often rationalized as "mortification of the sinful flesh." In schizophrenic and paranoid reactions, there is often a lifelong denial of heterosexuality, ranging from impotence or frigidity to total inability to establish a meaningful relationship with any other

human being. Many schizophrenics rely exclusively on masturbation for the relief of sexual tensions. Other schizophrenics turn to a variety of deviant practices. Psychoanalysis has postulated that the chaotic sexuality of the schizophrenic is equivalent to the polymorphous (many-formed) perversity attributed to the infant by Freud. In any event, it is widely agreed that the most bizarre forms of sexual offense and deviation, such as extreme sadism or masochism, are indicative of overt schizophrenia.

The Brain-Damaged Individual

A variety of deviations may be precipitated by the onset of organic intellectual impairment and the deterioration of superego controls in such disorders as prolonged alcoholism or senile psychoses. Older men with organic disorders are particularly likely to prefer adolescent or prepubertal girls as sexual objects, often in an incestuous relationship. (In the absence of brain damage, offenses by older men against children and adolescents often are attributable to loss of sexual potency or deterioration of the marital relationship.)

The Mentally Retarded Individual

Intellectual subnormality is not unduly frequent among sexual offenders, although a relatively mild degree of intellectual deficiency is associated with irresponsibility and promiscuity, particularly among females. Many intellectually deficient males do not marry and have no available sexual outlets. Their frustrations may precipitate occasional sexual assaults and more primitive substitutive outlets, such as sexual intercourse with animals. On the whole, society recognizes the sexual behavior of a retarded individual as an understandable manifestation of his limitations and institutionalizes him as a defective instead of prosecuting him as a criminal offender.

Whatever their personality traits and diagnoses, most male deviates have a pervasive fear, often unconscious, of sexual contact with adult females. Hammer and Glueck (1955) reached this conclusion in a study of sex offenders in Sing Sing prison. The investigators analyzed the responses to a Thematic Apperception Test card which depicts a clothed man standing in the foreground and a semi-nude female lying in bed in the background (card 13). The theme of the usual story by normal males includes sexual contact between the two figures, either in a marital or nonmarital setting. However, 93 per cent of the sex offenders rejected a heterosexual theme and expressed hostility to the female figure by telling stories in which she was sick, dying or dead. The investigators felt that the results supported the hypothesis that fear of the adult female inhibits normal sexuality and results in sexual deviations. At a later point we shall return to this hypothesis and the related Freudian hypothesis that the primary determinant of fear of the opposite sex is castration anxiety in men and penis envy in women.

THE MAJOR VARIETIES OF SEXUAL DEVIATION

Sexual behavior varies in (1) the intensity of the drive and the frequency of its gratification; (2) the mode of gratification; (3) the sexual object; and (4) the context within which the drive is aroused and gratified. A category of sexual deviation corresponds to each of these four dimensions.

1. In nymphomania, satyriasis and promiscuity there is excessive sexual activity, with inadequate attention to time, place or object. (Impotence and frigidity, in which sexuality is deficient, were discussed earlier in Chapter 10.)

2. The nature or mode of the sexual act—the "sexual aim of the impulse," in Freud's language—is deviant in masturbation, oro-genital or ano-genital activity, voyeurism, exhibitionism, transvestism (obtaining sexual gratification by wearing clothing appropriate to the opposite sex), sadism and forcible rape, and masochism. Each mode of sexual activity may occur with a variety of different sexual objects. For example, in autoerotic masturbation the individual is his own object (although there are likely to be other objects in fantasy); in mutual masturbation the object may be an adult of the same sex, an adult of the opposite sex, a child and so forth.

3. The object of the sexual act is deviant in homosexuality, fetishism, preference for children, bestiality, incest and so forth.

4. The social and physical contexts are deviant in prostitution.

The most important of these four categories are the second and third, comprising deviations of mode and object. The categories, of course, are not mutually exclusive; for example, in overt homosexuality both the object and the act—most commonly mutual masturbation, oro-genital activity or ano-genital activity—are deviant.

5. The use of pornography is not a sexual deviation unless such materials come to take the place of a live sexual object. Pornography is, however, used frequently by adults in connection with excessive masturbation, or by persons whose primary gratification is voyeuristic. Because pornography is frequently used by persons who are deviate in either the preferred mode or object of sexual gratification, and because there exists so much misunderstanding about the effect of such materials on behavior, a brief discussion of the topic is appropriate here.

We shall now discuss each of the categories in detail.

Excessive Sexual Activity

The typical individual with an insatiable impulse to sexual gratification—satyriasis in men and nymphomania in women—is heterosexually oriented and dominated by genital rather than pregenital urges. Similarly, promiscuity—that is, nonselective sexual intercourse with a variety of partners—tends to be heterosexual and genital. Satyriasis, nymphomania and promiscuity are thus usually free of deviation in mode or in type of sexual object, and technically do not fall entirely within the province of sexual deviations as defined earlier in this chapter. However, satyriasis, nymphomania and promiscuity are often associated with *emotional and motivational deviation.* Promiscuity most frequently comes to public attention when the offender is a young woman involved in transient and casual relations. Often, she comes from a family with little warmth and her behavior is a desperate bid for attention and love. In an alternative pattern, the behavior is a defiant act of protest against a very strict family. Many promiscuous girls have sociopathic traits; in a few, the sexual pattern is a secondary manifestation of schizoid tendencies. Some promiscuous females are very responsive sexually, but a large number are wholly or partially frigid.

The male may engage in a parallel pattern for parallel reasons: to feel wanted and fight nagging fears that he is inadequate, sexually or otherwise, or to revolt against a harsh morality. In both male and female, a motive of hostile revenge may also be present: it has been speculated that the promiscuous male avenges the infantile disappointments he experienced with his mother, and the promiscuous female avenges the disappointments experienced with her father.

It is important to distinguish persistent promiscuity from occasional premarital or extramarital sexual experiences. According to the data of Kinsey and his collaborators (1948, 1953), 83 per cent of men reported premarital sexual experience and 50 per cent reported past or present extramarital sexual activity. Among women, the corresponding percentages were 50 and 27 per cent. The majority of the population is thus at some time legally guilty of a sexual offense, but only a minority displays the compulsive repetition characteristic of true promiscuity.

Deviations in the Mode of Sexual Behavior

Some of the deviations to be discussed in this section may be classified as at least partially genital, e.g., masturbation, exhibitionism or forcible rape, and some as "anatomical transgressions" in which a nongenital erogenous zone dominates the individual's sexual activity.

Masturbation. Sexual pleasure obtained by manual or mechanical stimulation of the genitals or other erogenous zones, e.g., the anus, is widely practiced by the higher animals and—among humans—by immature males who have not yet established adult heterosexual relationships or by adults of both sexes who have been deprived of accustomed heterosexual outlets. It may be accompanied by fantasies of a homosexual, heterosexual or other nature. Mutual masturbation may be practiced by males or females with members of the same or the opposite sex. The use of artificial genitals resembling those of the opposite sex has been reported in literature since the time of Aristophanes' *Lysistrata*.

During the Middle Ages the Church, following the strictures of the Old Testament, condemned all forms of sexual activity other than genital intercourse engaged in by husband and wife for the express purpose of conceiving children. Masturbation was regarded as evil, perverse and self-abusive. Even in the present century many well-educated persons, including physicians, thought masturbation led to insanity or other tragic consequences. In order to stop girls from masturbating, the clitoris was sometimes surgically removed. More recently it has

been realized that masturbation is a normal part of the process of sexual development. The Kinsey studies report that 93 per cent of males and 62 per cent of females admit to having masturbated. Masturbation is a normal outlet for sexual tensions for most persons and should properly be regarded as a sexual deviation only when it is practiced in public or typically preferred to heterosexual genitality or associated with intense feelings of anxiety and guilt.

Oro-genital and Ano-genital Activities. The technical terms for oro-genital activity are cunnilingus, the apposition of the mouth to the female genitals, and fellatio, the apposition of the mouth to the male genitals. Sodomy is the term for intercourse per anum. Any of these acts may occur heterosexually or homosexually. Fellatio was the preferred type of activity among homosexual offenders in Sing Sing prison. Sodomy is also a frequent practice between adult male homosexuals or it may occur between man and boy (pederasty). In most states all such acts are illegal whether they occur between partners of the same sex or opposite sex, and irrespective of whether or not both participants are consenting adults or in private surroundings, or even if they are married. From a psychological standpoint such legal definitions have little meaning. Mutually satisfying sexual activities between consenting adults of opposite sex in private as a prelude to more enjoyable intercourse can scarcely be seen as a sexual deviation by any scientific definition; even this statement may be too restrictive.

Voyeurism. Also termed *scoptophilia*, voyeurism consists of obtaining sexual gratification through observation of the genitals or sexual behavior of others. Increase in sexual excitement by visual stimulation is of course normal and nearly universal, particularly for the male. Society has long catered to the desire for visual stimulation through a variety of stage presentations, art forms, photographs and films, some pornographic and some not. The true voyeur is almost always a male whose behavior goes far beyond ordinary visual stimulation; his urge to look is stronger than his urge for sexual intercourse. He obtains a maximum of sexual excitement from clandestine observation of a female in a state of undress or in a sexual or excretory act. Under these circumstances, he experiences orgasm, either spontaneously or through masturbation.

The typical "peeping Tom" is a socially isolated, shy, schizoid individual who prowls after dark and looks through lighted windows.

Voyeurs fear women, but some find the danger of being caught exciting and do not respond sexually when observation is permitted, as in a burlesque show. For others, burlesque and pornographic pictures are satisfying. A minority are primarily interested in watching homosexual and other forms of deviant behavior. In the past it was not unusual to watch sadistic acts carried out on others, as described in the following account, dated 1792 and quoted by Hirschfeld (1944):

> There is a rich old banker in Broad Street who has arranged with the head mistresses of two girls' schools (one in Hackney, one in Stratford) to pay them a large weekly sum each for a most peculiar entertainment. At the time of his weekly visits at each school the children received their accumulated punishments. The old man stays in an adjacent room and watches through an aperture while the girls, one after the other, are brought in, bared behind, and chastised with the rod.

The dynamics of voyeurism are complex. Not only do voyeurs fear heterosexuality—contrary to popular superstition, they rarely attack women—but they seem to need constant reassurance that they are able to respond sexually. The excitement they experience in observing women convinces them that they are not asexual. In addition, many seem to identify with the women on whom they spy, so that a homosexual component is present. There is also an aggressive element in voyeurism which stems from its forbidden and stealthy character and from direct hostility toward the sexual object. Thus, a voyeur may get a special thrill out of social interaction with a woman whom he has previously spied on: he "knows a secret" about her and therefore feels a hostile type of superiority.

Exhibitionism. A rarity among females, exhibitionism may be defined as exposure in public of the male genital before a woman or child, with the exposure itself as the final sexual aim. Exhibitionism should be distinguished from exposure practiced for other purposes, for example, exposure as an aggressive act or a defensive counter-attack against women as practiced in some primitive tribes (Christoffel, 1956).

Exhibitionism is one of the most frequent of contemporary sexual deviations. In some jurisdictions it amounts to as much as one-third of all sexual offenses. Since exhibitionists are likely to be placed on probation, they constitute only a small fraction of imprisoned sexual offenders but a relatively high proportion of those receiving psychiatric treatment on an out-

patient basis. In an excellent study of exhibitionists treated at an outpatient clinic, Mohr et al. (1962) pointed out the importance of distinguishing between true exhibitionists and individuals who expose themselves prior to further sexual activities with a child (pedophilia). The investigators reported that the girls and women to whom exhibitionists expose themselves are almost always strangers. Among different individuals the act ranges from showing the penis, with no erection or conscious sexual feelings, to an intense sexual experience that includes masturbation and sometimes also obscene language and gestures. A frequent pattern consists of driving a car to a spot where one or more women may be found, e.g., a bus stop, exposure and masturbation without leaving the car, and then rapid flight from the scene. In many instances the female ignores what she sees or she laughs; this reaction may deflate and upset the exhibitionist, thus suggesting that the hostile shock value of his act may be an important element.

Exhibitionism is closely related to voyeurism, the only other deviation common among exhibitionists. In exhibitionism, as in voyeurism, there appears to be an identification with the sexual object.

The age distribution in Mohr's study of exhibitionists was bimodal, with one peak in adolescence and the other in the twenties. The adolescent patients were unmarried, but nearly all the young adults had married prior to the onset of exhibitionism. The major precipitants of exhibitionism in the latter group were an impending or recent marriage and the impending or recent birth of a child; unsatisfactory sexual relations or the threat of sexual deprivation attendant on the birth of a child are apparently important factors. Mohr's data are consistent with the impression of many investigators that the urge to exposure occurs when the individual is in conflict with a female—a domineering mother in adolescence and the wife or future wife in the twenties. It has been noted by investigators that the wife of the exhibitionist frequently is a mother substitute who dominates her self-effacing, unaggressive husband.

Many exhibitionists try to fight their tendencies but give way when tension mounts too high. Prior to an exposure, they may feel restless and apprehensive. They may experience headaches, palpitation and dizziness, and may perspire excessively. Following the act they are likely to be depressed and remorseful.

The following case history illustrates some of

the characteristics and background factors of a persistent exhibitionist.

A 24-year-old married man was hospitalized for evaluation after his third arrest for indecent exposure. He was the son of an alcoholic who had worked irregularly, spent all his money on drinking parties, and been inconsistent and, at times, cruel to his children. (There were three older sisters.) The patient's mother, on the other hand, was described as good, kind, long-suffering and easy to get along with. There was a great deal of open discord between the parents.

The patient's physical development was normal. He was a well behaved, overtly conforming boy who left school at 16 to be trained as an electrician. As a boy he had always been emotionally immature and shy, and avoided participation in athletic or social activities. He obtained little sexual information in childhood, but at 14 began to expose his genitals to girls in his age group and sometimes to masturbate in front of them. However, his behavior did not result in arrest until at age 20 he exposed himself in front of a mature woman. He was beaten up by her brother, arrested and fined. Nevertheless, he continued to exhibit himself frequently and at 23 was arrested again for exposure before an adolescent girl. This time he spent a month in jail.

Shortly afterward he met a pregnant woman who soon gave birth to an illegitimate child. The child was immediately adopted. The patient and the woman—clearly a mother-figure for him—were married. Their sexual relationship was at first satisfactory to him and his exhibitionism ceased. However, he soon began to manifest a pattern of behavior in which any trivial conflict with his wife caused him to feel childishly hurt and resentful and to refuse to have sexual relations with her even if she approached him. She soon became pregnant and he regressed to his former pattern of exhibiting himself; he picked up a woman in his car, began to masturbate, and once again was arrested. As is common with married exhibitionists, he had successfully concealed his deviant impulses from his wife, and his arrest and the subsequent revelations came as a complete surprise to her.

He was a quiet, mousy-appearing, self-effacing and tense young man. He was introverted and ridden by strong feelings of inadequacy. On a sentence completion test, two of his responses were, *"When I was a child* I always ran away or didn't fight back," and *"My greatest mistake was* running away from everything." The only trace of exhibitionism in his makeup was in his sexual behavior. His I.Q. was 118, he was not severely depressed, and there was no reality distortion, i.e., he was neither retarded nor psychotic.

The patient withheld from the hospital personnel as much information as he could about his sexual deviation and admitted to far fewer incidents than had actually occurred. (In general, exhibitionists withhold information about their sexual histories.) However, he reported that beginning at age 14, the age at which his exhibitionistic behavior had started, he had had

frequent migraine headaches associated with blurred vision, numbness on one side of the head, a buzzing in one ear and frequent nausea or vomiting. He felt that these attacks occurred when he was under emotional stress or tension; the same emotional factors apparently precipitated his exhibitionism. His regression when his wife became pregnant was a reaction to the frustration he anticipated because of her impending sexual unavailability. Furthermore, the child would be a rival for the attentions of his wife.

Diagnostically, the patient could be considered as a case of either neurotic anxiety reaction with sexual deviation, or psychophysiologic reaction (cardiovascular) with sexual deviation. Medication in the hospital relieved his headaches and psychotherapy resulted in considerable insight into the dynamics underlying his sexual behavior. It is not known, however, whether his exhibitionism recurred after discharge from the hospital.

6 **Transvestism.** Obtaining sexual gratification by wearing clothes appropriate to the opposite sex is called transvestism (literally, "cross-dressing"). It has been recorded among both men and women since antiquity, but, as in other deviations, males have attracted most of the attention of investigators. Hirschfeld (1944) studied a sample of male transvestites and concluded that 35 per cent were heterosexual, 35 per cent homosexual, 15 per cent bisexual and the remaining 15 per cent either restricted to autoerotic activities or completely asexual. The sexual orientation of female transvestites also appears to be very heterogeneous.

Transvestism in either sex has one of three major functions: (1) It may be a form of clothes fetishism—a deviation of object as well as mode—in an individual who is predominantly heterosexual or autoerotic. (2) In a homosexual or bisexual individual it may be a means of attracting other members of the same sex as well as expressing the homosexual's identification with the opposite sex (e.g., a male homosexual may identify so strongly with the female that he is happier when dressed as one). (3) In some homosexuals, transvestism is symbolic of *transsexualism,* that is, a conscious desire to change anatomically from one sex to the other. In recent years a number of homosexual, transvestite males have in fact been transformed surgically into anatomical approximations of females, and many others have requested such operations. Trans-sexualism, like transvestism, may have several functions. In a study of a group of male and female transvestite and trans-sexual patients, Randell (1959) concluded that most were either homosexual or both obsessive-compulsive and fetishistic.

Sometimes trans-sexualism also involves a paranoid, delusional reaction in which the individual denies anatomical reality; in other cases there are no psychotic features. In the following case of transvestism and trans-sexualism the patient was in good contact with reality.

A 31-year-old patient requested help from a physician specializing in endocrinology. The stated complaint was, "My sexes are all mixed up." The patient had had her first name legally changed to a common male nickname, dressed and acted like a man, and spoke in a low, hoarse voice. The medical history notes included the following contradictions:

"Patient raised as male but always has been aware of his 'female-like' sexual organs. He claims his 'mind and desires' are those of a male and always have been, which is the reason he was raised as a male, even though his sex organs are those of a female. His sexual development has been female. No penis. Urinates like a girl. . . . Breasts developed by age 15. No voice change. Some fine facial hair growth. Shaves twice a week but probably more because of desire than need. General physique is male-like—broad shoulders, husky, well-developed muscles in arms and legs. . . ."

Sexual confusion also appeared in a letter written by the patient's elder sister.

"In school she was one of the guys, playing basketball, baseball, football, and even boxing against the fellows—and always beating them. ——— has always been very strong and muscular . . . as far as ———'s ability on the farm—he could hold a candle to any and all. Any kind of mechanical work as far as tractors, cars, farm machinery, carpentering, etc.— even to 'pulling' calves, castrating small pigs, milking cows, butchering, etc.—are all part of his present and past. ——— has always had an unlimited amount of energy, never tiring from any amount of work or athletics. During corn picking season, he can work a week or two straight with only five or six hours sleep per night."

The patient reported that she had started to menstruate quite late, at the age of 16. Thereafter menstruation was reported to be of brief duration but periodic and regular. (Patients of this type frequently minimize menstruation and other feminine characteristics in self reports.) A medical examination showed that anatomically the patient was a normal female and a laboratory test revealed that the sex chromosomes were genetically female. In a urine sample, the 17-ketosteroids (hormones that are produced by the adrenal glands and gonads) were also those of a normal female.

On the MMPI the patient's responses indicated a masculinity of attitudes and interests extreme enough to be unique, but the scores on all other scales were within normal limits. In effect, she was psychologically a normal, even a very masculine, male. The patient wished to marry a woman four years younger than herself and had come to the physician to request a surgical operation to make her anatomically male.

Both she and her "fiancée" were very moralistic and inhibited. The patient was deeply in love with the fiancée and said she would like to put her on a pedestal. Neither of them smoked or drank and both were virgins, although they had unsuccessfully attempted to have sexual relations. Both were very introverted, both could be classified as neurotics with depressive tendencies, and neither manifested a psychotic denial of anatomic reality. They had been together for eight years; whenever they were separated during this period they both felt depressed and lost weight. The impetus for requesting surgery had come from the patient's fiancée. In an interview with a psychologist, she stated: "He [the patient] lost his mother last November and now he's afraid he's going to lose me. . . . He feels so alone."

The patient's family were in favor of the requested surgery. The patient herself wrote the following eloquent plea:

"I am banking everything on this operation. I know there is going to be a lot of pain and it isn't going to solve all of my problems, but it is the biggest step that I have to take toward solving them. This is not a spur of the moment decision. I have thought about it ever since I knew it could be done and I am 31 years old and I decided it was now or never. The whole family has got their hearts set on it. They think (and so do I) it is the best thing that could happen to me. My dad isn't going to be here forever and when the time comes I am going to have to go out into the world on my own and I always hire out as a man, so I want to be one. [The patient had worked as a hired hand all her life.] It's the only kind of life I know and it's the only kind I want to know. I know how men talk and act when they are in a bunch, and anything they would say and do wouldn't shock me in the least. I don't see how this could affect me spiritually. I am not religious and besides that I don't think God judges you by your body but by your soul. My morals have always been very high and this operation won't change me any, except I will be a lot happier and I will feel as though I am as good as anyone else. Doctor, I would rather die on that operating table as not to have this done."

In interview the patient stated that she had never worn a dress. She had always liked trucks and tractors and in school had taken manual training and found that she could successfully do anything mechanical. Her parents had accepted her psychosexual inversion and exploited her strength and endurance unmercifully. At one time, when still a child, she worked from 6 A.M. until 1 A.M. the following morning running a cornpicker; her mother had sent hot coffee out to the field where she worked. There was reason to believe that the fundamental basis of her problem was psychological. She had identified with a male role, had been rewarded for her mechanical talents, energy and strong physique, and had never been permitted to learn how to be a woman.

The patient's request for surgery had to be denied. Although surgery can convert a male to an anatomical approximation of a female by removal of the penis and testicles and construction of a functional vagina, it cannot successfully convert a female into a male (except for breast and uterine removal). The patient wanted removal of the uterus and breasts but she also made an impossible request for construction of an artificial, functional penis. She and her fiancée separated when the surgery was denied since they wished to remain together only if they could conform to social norms in a legal marriage. The patient responded to the frustration of her hopes with some depression. She had no interest in psychotherapeutic help and it is not known what happened to her subsequently.

Sadism. The attainment of sexual gratification through the infliction of bodily or mental pain on others by physical or verbal means is sadism. In a broader, nonsexual sense, sadism refers to any type of cruelty or extreme aggression. The term is derived from the Marquis de Sade (1740–1814) who practiced or fantasied a wide variety of perversions which he recorded in a novel entitled *Justine and Juliette, or The Curse of Virtue and the Blessing of Vice.*

Most societies assign a more aggressive role to the male than to the female. It is therefore not surprising that the male, in his sexual relationships, should sometimes obtain additional pleasure from aggressive behavior toward his partner. The practice of inflicting pain before or during intercourse is generally minimal in civilized societies, but some deviant individuals can attain a maximum of sexual pleasure only from the sight of blood or by the torture or even death of the sexual object. The greater the degree of sadism, the greater the probability that the individual is psychotic. Sex offenders in general are not sadists; only about 5 per cent of offenders harm their victims.

The following case history taken from Lindner (1955), who treated the patient psychoanalytically, illustrates the development of sadism leading to murder and violation of the corpse (necrophilia).*

If you had seen Charles on the street in your city you would not have known him for a vicious killer. In prison, he still has a freshness of face which belongs in a choir stall. When I last saw him, he was scarcely twenty-one. . . .

Before Charles came to prison I had read about him in the newspapers. The case had made headlines for

---

*Abstracted by permission from Lindner, R. 1955. Songs my mother taught me. *In* The Fifty-Minute Hour. New York, Holt, Rinehart and Winston, Inc. Reprinted 1956, Bantam Books, H-2304, p. 11.

many days: it was composed of elements that were "naturals" for arousing public interest—a boy, a pretty girl—"Not so pretty," says Charles—an empty apartment, an ice pick.

The girl was a stranger who had come to the door of Charles' apartment with samples of religious books and records and asked to see his mother. He waved her into the apartment, struck her on the head with a hammer and stabbed her sixty-nine times with an ice pick. Then he flung himself on her and raped her. Immediately afterwards, he went for a leisurely walk without locking the apartment door behind him, ate an ice cream cone, and then went to a police station and reported his crime in a nonchalant and emotionally flat manner.

When he was interviewed, it was suspected that he was a paranoid schizophrenic but no definite diagnosis was made. A pentothal interview was then conducted and during it he spoke of having heard a voice telling him to kill the girl. He subsequently claimed that he had told his mother about the voice but that she did not want him to report it and claim insanity. "She didn't want the publicity. She's a buyer in one of the big department stores and she was afraid she'd lose her job. She wanted everything kept quiet. She was afraid to have her name connected with it . . . you see, she has a different name than mine so nobody connected her with me. . . ."

Long before Charles was born the marriage between his parents was falling apart. They had not wanted each other nor the two children that followed. Under religious compulsion they maintained a semblance of harmony for over two years, but in the first month of their marriage both had known it could not last. . . . In Charles' third (his brother's second) year, a religious dispensation permitted the parents to separate, and the figure of their father disappeared from their lives. For a few months their mother tried to maintain the home, but since she herself was a harassed, conflicted, easily disturbed person, she found the task too great. On the advice of her confessor the children were placed in an orphanage. For fifteen years thereafter the two boys were to live in homes and institutions. . . .

Charles' life in one institution and home after another was miserable and shocking to learn about. He lived in constant fear and terror. He was brutalized beyond description. He was beaten unmercifully for the smallest infractions and made to do extravagant penances for expressing the ordinary playfulness of a small boy. . . . Before long Charles found himself regarding his person and his being with guilt; for under the warped codes and philosophies to which he was exposed he was forced to accept the idea that what was happening to him—his exile from normal life, his abandonment by his family—was somehow his own fault.

It was not long before Charles donned the only armor available to him. After a few years during which he had been the recipient of brutality, the target of assaults sexual and physical, the butt of sadisms that make a small boy's life a hell, he associated himself in spirit with his tormentors. The process of this identification began with a change in the fantasies he had so long employed for comfort when he nursed his wounds in the dormitory at night. In analysis, we learned that these first fantasies were heroic in stamp, epic with poetry and, though mean and pitiful from such a distance, panoplied with the glory that life lets us know only once. But they did not help against the harsh realities of his environments. The heroes of his mind could not hold out against the inquisitors in his real life, nor could their gleaming swords avail against the sticks and blows of his masters and fellows. Into his reveries, then, there crept a new note. Richard Coeur de Lion was replaced by Genghis Khan, the Dragon Slayers by Bluebeards, and instead of dreams of chivalry he came to cherish fantasies of revenge. As the character of his inner life changed, so did Charles. Growing meanwhile, and acquiring physical strength, he was soon able to express the vengeful hate in him. Toward those smaller and weaker he behaved as he could not toward those larger and stronger. He passed on his hurts: he became an afflictor, delighting in giving pain. Also, he learned shrewdness and cunning; and soon he was accomplished at diverting hurt from himself to someone else. In sexual activities, where he was once the target he became the arrow, and on the vainly protesting forms of others he discharged the venon of his frustration. By the age of ten he had become perverted in every way to the roots of his being—already his soul had been twisted into that of a murderer.

During these years, when Charles was undergoing the changes described, he saw his mother only infrequently. Her occasional visits on his birthday or a holiday were always hurried. They left him with a feeling of something incomplete, undone and unsaid. Always laden with gifts, she made a small, excited flurry in his colorless life. He said to me, "She was like a fairy princess when she came. She smelled so good." But at the same time that he looked forward to her visits and dreamed of her after she had gone, part of him hated her, too, for having placed him in the purgatory of his daily life. It was this that made of her visits the incomplete episodes they were. He wanted to ask her to take him with her when she left, but he feared to ask, knowing her reply in advance. So an emptiness would seize him when she went away. At such times he would cast about for victims on whom to vent himself, and the record I have of his life shows that every visit was followed by a display of aggression. . . .

On special occasions there were visits to his mother's home. Brief exposure to normal life, these were more confusing and destructive than solacing, for all they gave Charles was a taste of what he should have had, and they increased an appetite that, under the circumstances, could never be satisfied.

It later became clear that the visits to his mother's home were by no means exposures to normal life. For example, on one occasion at the age of nine he was removed from his mother's bed where he was sleeping by a strange man who then retired to the bedroom with his mother. Most of the time he was left alone in his mother's apartment while she went out. On one visit at age thirteen, he discovered a trunk containing old letters from which he learned that his father was not dead—as his mother had told him—but had remarried and was living in another city with a second family. At the same time he found his mother's wedding ring which he used for some time afterwards as a fetish to achieve sexual orgasm. Later, on a visit to a prostitute, he was impotent until she put on his mother's wedding ring. His attitude to his mother was a compound of hate and frustrated desire; in killing and raping the girl he symbolically destroyed and possessed his mother.

Closely allied to sadism is *forcible rape* or *sexual assault*. Glueck (1956) found that rapists were younger and more aggressive, outgoing and impulsive than any other group of sex offenders in Sing Sing. The assault itself frequently occurred when control was diminished by alcohol or a combination of sexual frustration and temptation. Many rapists are sociopathic and therefore have a low tolerance of frustration even when sober. In a number of assault cases, the female victim either deliberately or unconsciously tempts a sociopathic offender—who cannot resist this temptation—to commit the act of which she subsequently complains to the police. We shall return to the role of the victim at a later point.

Masochism. Sexual gratification obtained through suffering bodily or mental pain is called masochism, although the term is also applied in a wider sense to any type of acceptance of pain. The word "masochism" is derived from Leopold von Sacher-Masoch (1836–1895) who desired women to treat him as a slave. However, women more often than men exhibit masochistic behavior.

In the seventeeth and eighteenth centuries, a number of Englishwomen became addicted to flagellation, that is, whipping as a sexual excitant, perhaps as a continuation of treatment they had previously received at the hands of parents and teachers. Hirschfeld (1944) quotes a contemporary description of a homosexually oriented flagellation club whose members, mostly married women, met once a week to whip each other. Similar masochistic and sadistic practices were formerly widespread in monasteries, convents and boarding schools.

The masochistic behavior of heterosexually oriented males has frequently been attributed to a combination of pain and sexual stimulation experienced in childhood during punishment by sadistic females. Hirschfeld reports a case of masochism which began when a 13-year-old boy was a guest at the home of a schoolmate. The latter and his two elder sisters were in the care of a sadistic governess who beat the girls almost daily. The two boys took to observing the beating through a keyhole; in the evening they masturbated together.*

One evening they were surprised in the act [of masturbation] by the governess. She locked the door behind her and said: "You're now going to get a good hiding, and every evening for eight days, before bedtime, you're going to get the same." She fetched a stick, laid each of the boys across the arm of the sofa and raising his shirt—all that he was wearing—she laid on with the cane until his buttocks changed colour. Both boys submitted. "It burned my behind like fire, but at the same time it prickled so pleasantly, so delightfully. And it was the blows that did it, it had never been so nice when we masturbated, which we did again. And later I noticed that the governess's hands, during the now regular chastisements, frequently strayed between my legs and stayed there. So we were glad of the blows and when the happy days were over we longed for them."

As adults, male masochists may indulge their impulses in brothels that are equipped with a variety of ingenious machines for flagellation or torture. Not infrequently, male masochists have mutilated, castrated or even fatally injured themselves in attempting to experience suffering. Here, again, it should be noted that the more extreme the deviant behavior, the greater the probability that the individual is psychotic.

The term *sadomasochism* denotes the simultaneous existence in an individual of sadistic and masochistic tendencies. It is widely accepted that a masochist always harbors sadistic tendencies and vice versa: masochism may be a turning of sadism against oneself, or sadism may be a reaction-formation against masochism, or sadism and masochism may be bipolar manifestations of one drive. Occasionally a masochist will suddenly shift to sadistic behavior, or vice versa.

Deviations of the Sexual Object

In his pioneer work, *Three Contributions to the Theory of Sex,* Freud (1905) wrote:

The most striking distinction between the erotic life of antiquity and our own no doubt lies in the fact that

*Reprinted by permission from Hirschfeld, M. 1944. Sexual Anomalies and Perversions. Copyright, 1948 by Emerson Books, Inc., New York.

the ancients laid the stress upon the instinct itself, whereas we emphasize its object. The ancients glorified the instinct and were prepared on its account to honour even an inferior object; while we despise the instinctual activity in itself, and find excuses for it only in the merits of the object.

The contemporary emphasis on the object stems from the Judeo-Christian tradition and its condemnation of all sexuality that does not lead to procreation. Hence homosexuality, fetishism, pedophilia and bestiality are unacceptable. For somewhat different reasons, to be discussed later, incest is also unacceptable.

Homosexuality. It is widely accepted that all persons are in some degree bisexual, i.e., all persons have a greater or lesser tendency to homosexuality as well as heterosexuality. However, the homosexual tendency remains latent in the majority. In a large minority it results in occasional overt, homosexual behavior, and in a smaller minority—variously estimated at from 2 to 8 per cent of the population—homosexuality is persistent as well as overt. Our discussion will concentrate on overt rather than latent homosexuality.

One type of overt homosexuality, referred to as accidental or pseudohomosexuality, frequently occurs under circumstances in which the individual has no access to the opposite sex. Accidental homosexuality is found in military service, prisons and boarding schools. Its occurrence demonstrates the ability to substitute one sexual object for another and the role of frustration in precipitating such a substitution.

Homosexual activities have been observed in both the males and females of a variety of infrahuman mammals; the male animal who mounts another not infrequently reaches orgasm. Homosexual relationships between human males have at times been widely accepted and practiced in civilized cultures as well as in primitive tribes. Homosexual behavior in human females, also known as *lesbianism* or *sapphism,* has also been widely accepted at times; generally speaking, it is less likely to arouse social censure than male homosexuality. At present, there is considerable discrepancy in the attitudes toward male homosexuality in different localities. At the very same time that New York State reduced the category of a homosexual offense between two adult males from a felony to a misdemeanor, California increased the maximum imprisonment for the offense from 10 to 20 years.

The legal trend has been toward a more tolerant view of the private sexual behavior of consenting adults. One of the most influential documents in support of this trend with respect to homosexuality and prostitution was the Wolfenden Report (1963). This report was prepared by an interdisciplinary group of legal, social and medical experts who were appointed to consider the laws, practices and treatments relating to homosexuality and prostitution in England. Their report to Parliament in 1963 recommended, among other things, that "homosexual behavior between consenting adults in private be no longer a criminal offense."

Despite condemnatory social attitudes, the occurrence of mutual masturbation with members of the same sex is a very widespread phenomenon during adolescence. Males who reach puberty at an early age have a much higher percentage of homosexual activities than late maturers. Homosexuality may begin in adolescence after seduction by an older homosexual: the seduced adolescent develops homosexual habits before he has adequate opportunity to develop heterosexual habits. Kinsey et al. (1948, 1953) reported that 37 per cent of males and 13 per cent of females admitted having had some homosexual experience to the point of orgasm after the onset of adolescence. Eight per cent of all males in Kinsey's sample had engaged exclusively in homosexual activities for at least three years after age 16. Among single persons in the group aged 36 to 40 years, 40 per cent of males and 10 per cent of females reported current involvement in overt homosexual relationships. These figures were much higher than expected, but the investigators expressed confidence in their reliability: "Whether the histories were taken in one large city or another, whether they were taken in large cities, in small towns, or in rural areas, whether they came from one college or another, a church school or a state university, or some private institution, whether they came from one part of the country or from another, the incidence data on the homosexual have been more or less the same" (Kinsey et al., 1948). It is often asserted that homosexuality is currently on the increase. Whether this is indeed so or whether homosexual practices are less concealed today than formerly is uncertain.

A high proportion of older unmarried homosexuals is characterized by a true psychosexual inversion, that is, a psychosexual reversal of sexual role. Sexual inverts who are anatomically male tend to think and act as though they were female, and inverts who are anatomically female tend to think and act as though they were

male. Married homosexuals—many of whom are really bisexuals—are less likely to be inverts or are only partially inverted. In any case, inversion and overt homosexuality are by no means synonymous; many homosexuals do not assume the role of the opposite sex and many psychologically inverted persons do not engage in overt homosexual behavior but behave heterosexually, autoerotically or asexually. Inversion is closely related to childhood identification. The boy may identify with a mother whom he overidealizes; less often, he may be afraid of an aggressive mother and adopt the defense of identifying with the aggressor. In either case, cross-identification can result in inversion. Similarly, the girl may overidentify with an idealized or a feared father.

Inversion is closely related to the dimension of activity-passivity. The female who takes an active, aggressive role in thought, affect or overt behavior, either in a heterosexual or homosexual context, comes to what society defines as masculinity. (The reader will recall the case of trans-sexualism described earlier.) The male who takes a passive, submissive role with a heterosexual or homosexual partner comes close to femininity. The majority of overt homosexuals do not conform completely to either role but alternate between the two. The promiscuous homosexual who picks up members of the same sex in a public place does not know the role preference of a new acquaintance until they are alone. If both prefer an active role, one must be passive or they take turns.

Physical characteristics are of little use in identifying role preference. The male with a ruggedly masculine appearance may not only be a homosexual but may also prefer the passive role in anal or oral intercourse, and the effeminate appearing individual who happens to be a homosexual may prefer an active role. Nor are physical characteristics and related attributes very helpful in identifying homosexuals as such, regardless of role. Although some male homosexuals are effeminate, many engage in so-called "masculine" occupations and are truck drivers, soldiers, athletes and so forth. It has been estimated that about 85 per cent of homosexuals would go unrecognized on the basis of their ordinary, day-to-day behavior. The primary sex organs—the testes and penis in the male and the ovaries and uterus in the female—are anatomically no different in homosexuals than in heterosexuals. In a minority of cases, secondary sex characteristics are indicative of homosexuality: some male homosexuals have

PUPIL SIZE

wide hips and narrow shoulders and some female homosexuals have narrow hips, relatively undeveloped breasts and wide shoulders. Menstruation begins late in some female homosexuals. (Parenthetically, repugnance toward menstruation is very common in female homosexuals, as is repugnance toward the male genital; female homosexuals often state that the thought of sexual intercourse with a male is horrible enough to make them shudder.) Sometimes homosexuals are identifiable by clothing, gestures and vocabulary, but here, too, the majority are no different from heterosexuals. Male homosexuals may or may not dress freely and "artistically." Women homosexuals may appear to be completely feminine; even when they dress in mannish fashion and cut their hair short they are unrecognizable since social norms now permit heterosexual women to do the same.

Overt homosexuality may take the form of mutual masturbation, oro-genital activity or ano-genital activity (sodomy). The individual may have a preference for a single one of these activities or he may engage in all of them. Oral or anal sexual behavior may be active or passive. For example, the attitude of an active male homosexual toward a partner with whom he engages in anal activity may approximate that of a heterosexual toward a woman, with the anus substituting for the vagina.

Many homosexuals belong to groups that are amazingly well organized. A homosexual arriving in a strange city usually is told in advance where to go to meet other homosexuals or he may be given specific names and addresses. In large cities, homosexuals tend to have their own bars, beaches, shops, private vocabulary, and norms for acceptable and unacceptable behavior. The homosexual group is a source of psychological support as well as personal contacts. The motivation for such groups is understandable when it is recognized that the homosexual tends to have a chronic feeling of social alienation and a fear of detection and punishment.

A pervasive theme in the psychology of homosexuality is sexual disgust felt for the opposite sex. Homosexual males may get along with females socially but not sexually; homosexual females react in the same way to men. The differential response of homosexuals to males and females was clearly demonstrated in a study by Hess, Shlien and Seltzer (1965). Five homosexuals and five heterosexual males were shown pictures of male and female nudes, and

changes in pupil size were noted for the differing stimuli. Homosexuals showed greater changes in pupil size when viewing male nudes, while heterosexual males had greater pupil changes in response to female nude pictures (Fig. 15–1). Thus sex object preferences seem to have far-ranging consequences, including the influencing of physical responses not ordinarily thought of as being under clear voluntary control.

The majority of confirmed homosexuals have not been convicted of homosexuality in court nor have they sought psychiatric or psychological help. Those who seek help are more apt to do so because of neurotic anxiety or depression—intensified by social condemnation and fear of detection and disgrace—than because of any great desire to change a basic homosexual orientation. Some, however, keep fighting their homosexual propensities. The following case is that of an essentially neurotic homosexual who in typical fashion sought psychiatric assistance for neurotic symptoms.

The patient was the second of two boys, six years younger than his brother, born to middle aged parents of limited economic means. The father was an immigrant laborer described by the patient as a

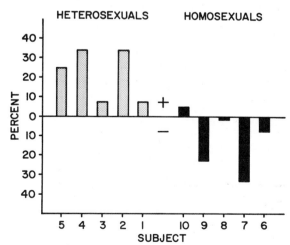

PUPIL SIZE CHANGE
PERCENTAGE DIFFERENCES
IN RESPONSE TO MALE & FEMALE PICTURES

Figure 15–1. *A positive score shows higher response to pictures of females; a negative score shows higher response to pictures of males. (From Hess, E., Seltzer, A., and Shlien, J., 1965. Pupil responses of hetero- and homosexual males to pictures of men and women. J. Ab. Psychol., 70:165–168. Copyright 1965 by the American Psychological Association, Inc.)*

surly, brutish man who would "as soon slap me as look at me." The patient was an unwanted child; the mother had wanted a girl or no further children. His birth was a difficult one and the mother nearly died. However, as a reaction-formation she soon became overprotective toward him. From the time he was born she had no further sexual relations with her husband and throughout childhood the patient slept with her while the displaced father shared a bed with the older brother. The mother unfailingly coddled and supported the patient and the two presented a united front against the father. The patient's family environment was a moralistic one. He grew up to respect his father, but, at the same time, felt hostile toward him and, as a result, the patient identified with his mother. His childhood thus fell into the classical Oedipal pattern typical of many neurotics and sexual deviates.

He was of average intelligence and made average progress in school but was somewhat withdrawn and inhibited and made few close friends with children of either sex. At the age of 14 he was seduced by an older man who lived in the same small town. His moralistic upbringing made it difficult for him to accept the relationship; he was shattered by an overwhelming sense of guilt but unable to talk about the incident with anyone. He became anxious and depressed, withdrew from school in the eighth grade, and remained at home where he could be close to his mother. Later he went to work at a variety of jobs, including those of janitor, desk clerk, gas station attendant, hairdresser and cosmetologist.

At 18 he fell in love with an older man and left home to be with him. However, it continued to be impossible for him to accept his sexual tendencies and within three months he returned home in a state of guilt and depression. For the next 20 years he was home most of the time. After his father died he continued to live with his aging mother and brother; the latter had a masculine identification but had also failed to marry. When troubled, the patient would sit on his brother's knee and weep. For a brief period he dated a girl and had sexual relations with her but he found them unsatisfactory and terminated the relationship. Living as he did in a small town, he could not associate regularly with a homosexual group. He suppressed most of his homosexual urges and usually felt acutely lonely. At intervals over the years he had close but guilt-ridden friendships with one or another homosexual individual. Sometimes he would flirt with a man up to what he described as "the danger point" but then would withdraw. His speech and overt behavior were extremely effeminate. At times he dyed his hair from dark to blond, used makeup and plucked his eyebrows. He had a strong interest in antiques and art. As an adult he converted from Protestantism to Catholicism and for a while considered entering a monastery to help keep his homosexuality in check.

At the age of 45 he was admitted to a psychiatric hospital following several episodes of amnesia in which he had awakened in strange hotels with no rec-

ollection of the antecedent events. Later reconstruction of these episodes during psychotherapy made it appear probable that they represented a defense against acknowledgment of unacceptable homosexual impulses toward a younger man of whom he was sincerely fond. He was afraid to approach this individual sexually and did not want to corrupt him as he had himself been corrupted, but he was also afraid of losing him. He denied any overt homosexual behavior over the past two years—it was not clear whether his denial was truthful—but in any event the conflict made him feel neurotically anxious and depressed. At one point his depression led him to take an overdose of sleeping pills. However, he responded rapidly to supportive psychotherapy, underwent a decrease of anxiety and depression, and returned home where he continued to have occasional homosexual relationships.

Fetishim. In this deviation, part of the body or an inanimate object (the fetish) habitually produces sexual excitement or gratification. The individual may overrespond to the buttocks, thighs, legs, feet, breasts or hair, or he may make fetishes of female underwear, stockings, shoes, furs or gloves.

Of course, many normal males attach special significance to various parts of the female body, especially in fantasy or heterosexual foreplay. Military censors have at times been inundated by female undergarments sent from home at the request of men in overseas service. However, these phenomena differ from the extreme forms of fetishism in which body parts or inanimate objects are the preferred or even the only objects of the individual's sexual behavior. True fetishists will kiss or fondle undergarments, snip off locks of women's hair, collect hundreds of photographs of women's feet, or respond to women's breasts but to no other part of the female anatomy. Both kleptomania (compulsive stealing) and pyromania (compulsive fire setting) occasionally serve a fetishistic function; the kleptomaniac steals objects that he has endowed with sexual significance, and the pyramoniac sets fires so that he will be aroused to orgasm by the blaze and the excitement of fire engines. Such cases are a minority, however, since kleptomania and pyromania do not usually involve conscious sexual motivation.

Pedophilia. Sexual activity of any type—masturbatory, oral, anal or genital—with a prepubertal child is called pedophilia. The offender is usually male. Pedophilia may be heterosexual or homosexual.

The heterosexual pedophiles in the Sing Sing study were found to be older on the average than other sex offenders. They had histories of poor marital adjustment and manifested considerable disturbance in reality perception, particularly under the influence of alcohol. Among heterosexual pedophiles treated in an outpatient clinic, Mohr et al. (1962) found a distinct trimodal age distribution, with peaks in adolescence, the thirties and the fifties. The adolescent patients were retarded psychosexually and socially. The patients in their thirties resembled many of the pedophiles in the Sing Sing sample: they tended to regression, severe marital and social maladjustment, and alcoholism. The oldest patients were characterized by loneliness and either actual impotence or concern about impotence. Elderly pedophiles sometimes manifest the generalized loss of behavioral control characteristic of senile psychotics.

In the following case the patient was poorly controlled, had both schizoid and sociopathic traits, and was given to promiscuous relations with both children and adults.

A man of average intelligence, married, the father of four children, was hospitalized for psychiatric evaluation on referral by his family physician. The patient described himself as lacking in sexual control. His sexual relationship with his wife had never been entirely satisfactory to either of them. Some years before hospitalization he had had a sexual relationship with a young sister of his wife. After the girl was killed in an accident he periodically engaged in sexual relationships with girls between the ages of 6 and 10 years. He also began to have extramarital affairs with adult females and two of them became pregnant; since they were both promiscuous it was not certain that he was the father. His wife became aware of his sexual activities and on a number of occasions threatened divorce unless he discontinued his infidelity and deviant behavior. He repeatedly promised to do so but each time failed to keep his word. Finally, she began divorce proceedings but he successfully persuaded her to postpone them and agreed, instead, to a legal separation. Shortly thereafter he came in for psychiatric evaluation. A psychiatrist who talked with him felt that he was far less interested in changing his behavior than in obtaining psychotherapy for the purpose of convincing his wife that since he was at least seeking help he should be permitted to return home.

The patient was the eldest of eight children with a gap of five years between him and the next child; quite naturally, he was relatively isolated from his siblings. The father was away from home much of the time and when he was home he and the mother quarreled a great deal. The mother was chronically tired and never wished to go anywhere; the father unjustly accused her of being a poor housekeeper.

From an early age the patient was given many responsibilities on his parents' farm and had neither the time nor the opportunity for social activities. His father was very strict and frequently beat him with a belt. Between the ages of 14 and 17 the patient left home twice but returned at his mother's request. He left school in the ninth grade, worked on the farm for three years, joined the Navy, returned briefly and then left home to work in a factory. His social isolation and fear of his father (possibly including unconscious castration fear) had furthered the development of both schizoid and sociopathic traits. On several occasions he had engaged in shoplifting.

The patient was ignorant of sex and afraid of it when he married at 21. Soon after marriage he discovered that his wife was "very cool" and unresponsive sexually. He felt that throughout their marriage she had pushed him away sexually and then had blamed him for seeking alternative outlets. He did not entertain the possibility that his infidelities and deviant behavior had intensified her frigidity by making her hostile to him. He was a poor husband and father who behaved as his own father had. Frequently he was away from home; when home, he withdrew socially from the family and was strict with his children, sometimes beating them as his father had done. He denied feeling sexually attracted toward his daughters (three of the four children were girls), but his wife expressed concern over this possibility. The psychiatrist felt that his impulse control was poor enough to make the wife's fear a realistic one.

While hospitalized, he was pleasant and cooperative in manner but in sociopathic fashion frequently ignored regulations that had been brought to his attention. When confronted with his behavior he either denied that he was breaking a rule or maintained that he had not known it existed. He spent a good deal of time with the adolescent female patients on the ward.

An intelligence test yielded an I.Q. of 88. On the MMPI there were marked elevations on the scales for schizophrenia and psychopathic deviation. The Thematic Apperception Test and the Rorschach indicated feelings of inadequacy and suspiciousness, poor masculine identification and a poor relationship with both men and women. He was anxious and conflicted; his perceptions of reality were inaccurate. The total picture on the TAT and Rorschach was suggestive of schizophrenia; a tendency to hostile acting out was also indicated.

In view of his schizoid characteristics, he was treated by a phenothiazine drug and on discharge was referred for outpatient psychotherapy. However, when it became apparent that his wife was determined to divorce him, he terminated both the medication and psychotherapy.

Hebephilia. Closely related to pedophilia is hebephilia, sexual activity by an adult with an adolescent up to the age of 16. (Hebe was the

Greek goddess of youth.) A sensitive story of heterosexual hebephilia may be found in Nabokov's novel *Lolita.* Glueck (1956) reported that men convicted of heterosexual hebephilia were aggressive, impulsive and also given to schizoid disturbances in judgment.

A common legal offense—*statutory rape*—overlaps the definition of heterosexual hebephilia. Statutory rape consists of sexual relations outside of marriage with a female under the legal "age of consent," usually defined as 18, even if the female participates voluntarily. It is often difficult to determine whether statutory rape is forcible or not.

Homosexual pedophilia or hebephilia involves any type of sexual activity between adult males and pre-adolescent or adolescent boys. Homosexual pedophilia consists of three deviations in one since the sexual object is inappropriate both anatomically and chronologically and the mode is also deviant. Anal intercourse with boys is known as *pederasty.* Among all the offenders in the Sing Sing study the homosexual pedophiles showed the greatest degree of psychiatric disturbance. A high proportion were overtly psychotic, with marked impairment of reasoning and judgment. The only individuals with whom they could form any sort of relationship were boys.

Zoophilia. Sexual relations with an animal is called zoophilia or bestiality. It is most common in rural areas where domesticated animals abound and where coitus between animals is frequently observed. Zoophilia is more common in adolescence than later. Kinsey et al. (1948) reported that 8 per cent of males had had at least one sexual experience to the point of orgasm with animals; for the subgroup of males who had been reared on farms, the percentage was 17. For all females, in whom zoophilia usually took the form of general body contact rather than coitus, the percentage reported by Kinsey was 3.6. However, *persistent* bestiality is much rarer than these percentages would indicate.

Incest. This is sexual activity between persons whose blood relationship is closer than is sanctioned by the culture. Some societies permit marriage between cousins, or between uncles and nieces or aunts and nephews, and some prohibit the marriage of persons of any degree of blood relationship, no matter how distant. In the course of history a few privileged groups have been exempted from incest taboos; e.g., in Egypt during the Ptolemaic period marriage between brother and sister in the royal family was not only permitted but was prescribed for generation after generation.

With such rare exceptions, one or another variation of the incest taboo is universally found. The most widely accepted explanation is that the taboo is designed to prevent a disruption of community and family life. A tribal group is strengthened both economically and militarily if its members marry outside of it. A family, whether primitive or civilized, is likely to be severely disrupted by the existence of intrafamilial sexual relationships other than that between husband and wife; such relationships breed open rivalries, threaten the structure of family authority and power, and endanger the emotional and economic security of the family members.

However, the near universality of the taboo does not mean that it is universally observed: a widespread taboo indicates that the urge toward the tabooed activity is also widespread. The Freudian theory of psychosexual development is built on the hypothesis that children universally experience incestuous urges which culminate in the Oedipal triangle. A violation of the incest taboo may take one of three forms: (1) Intrafamilial incest, including both Oedipal and non-Oedipal relationships—father-daughter, mother-son, brother-sister and so forth; (2) incest as a secondary aspect of an indiscriminate promiscuity that involves various sexual objects, both blood relatives and nonrelatives; and (3) incest as a secondary aspect of pedophilia, usually involving father and daughter.

Incest appears to be more common in lower socioeconomic groups. In part, it is a reflection of crowded family living. (Accurate statistics are difficult to obtain, as many cases go undetected.) Sometimes incest is substitutive, e.g., father-daughter incest occurs when the wife, the preferred sexual object, becomes unavailable. However, incest cannot be attributed solely to this or other precipitating factors. To quote from a study of father-daughter incest by Cormier et al. (1962), ". . . external reality such as the death or absence of the wife, disturbances in the marital relationship, the return of the father after a long absence, physical overcrowding, alcoholism, a relatively young father living close to an adolescent daughter, all these precipitating factors which are put forward are commonly found without leading to incest. In some predisposed fathers, however, they can reawaken concealed and suppressed incestuous temptation which is eventually acted out."

DAD & DAUGHTER ✳

In terms of the blood relationship involved, father-daughter incest is apparently the most common. Weinberg (1955) accumulated data on 203 cases; 159 involved father and daughter, 37 brother and sister, 5 both father-daughter and brother-sister, and only 2 involved mother and son. Weinberg's results are reasonably consistent with other data; in the Sing Sing study one-half the offenders who had committed incest were heterosexual hebephiles and most of them had had sexual relations with an adolescent daughter.

In a study of a group of girls involved in incest, Sloane and Karpinski (1942) found that more emotional damage appeared to be present when the incest occurred during adolescence rather than earlier. The adolescents generally became promiscuous and manifested various other maladaptive behaviors. A number of daughters who are involved in incest eventually rebel at the exclusive possessiveness of the father and seek their freedom. They either run away and form other emotional and sexual attachments or they reveal the fact of incest to the mother or the police. The following case history of father-daughter incest involved a pathologic relationship of the parents as well as the daughter's rebellion, the development of promiscuity, punishment of the father by disclosure, and punishment of other men onto whom the patient had displaced her hostility.

An attractive 15-year-old high-school girl of average I.Q. was admitted to a psychiatric hospital at her own request after she had charged five young men with getting her drunk and forcing her to have intercourse with them. Part of her statement ran as follows: "I started to menstruate when I was 11. At this time my father and I started to have intercourse about twice a week. I didn't know that it was wrong. My mother had never told me anything about sex. When I was 13 I went to baby sit one night. A fellow about 18 came and gave me something to drink. I knew it wasn't ginger ale but I didn't know what it was. I remember what happened but it is all hazy. The fellow had intercourse with me and it was about 4:30 A.M. by the time I got home. My mom had phoned the police and they were at my home when I got there. They tried to find out if I had had intercourse with this fellow. I wouldn't tell them but I told my mother that I and this fellow did what dad and I did. Mom didn't understand until I said, 'You know—what you and dad do.' Since this mom has been very jealous of my father and I and our relationship. About a week ago my father wanted me to have intercourse. When I refused he said he wanted me because my mother would only have intercourse with him about once a year."

She claimed that her mother had once told her that she could have intercourse with her father provided she first obtained the mother's permission. The father was sociopathic, had poor control of his impulses and was rejected by a neurotic wife who might well have made the statement attributed to her by the daughter. The latter felt unwanted at home where she was responsible for much of the housework, getting meals and looking after younger siblings. She resented the frequent arguments that took place between her mother and father and the close fashion in which they supervised her friendships. Her mother broke up several relationships with well-behaved boys by telling them in her presence that she was too young to go out. The daughter then rebelled; she went out by herself and picked up boys and men with whom she satisfied her increasingly strong sexual urges. However, she felt guilty over her promiscuous behavior and resented the behavior of her partners. Finally, she let herself be picked up by five men and spent a night with them. She then preferred charges against them and disclosed her relationship with her father.

In the hospital she felt guilty and somewhat depressed; she realized that she had been an inviting victim rather than a completely blameless one. However, she was able to benefit from psychotherapy and was soon placed in a residential school for girls with behavior problems in the hope that her emotional maturation would continue.

Deviations in the Social and Physical Context. The most important phenomenon in this category is prostitution. It is permitted in some countries and encouraged in some religions, but in our culture the male who regularly prefers prostitutes is psychologically deviant, even if his behavior is oriented to genital heterosexuality with adults. (The male who resorts to homosexual prostitutes or the prostitutes who will inflict punishment on him is obviously deviant in object, mode or both.) The prostitute herself may also be deviant; apart from economic and social factors in the causation of prostitution, there are personality factors, and many prostitutes are schizoid, sociopathic or mentally retarded. Many are also sexually frigid, at least with the great majority of their partners.

Pornography. Obscene literature, movies and the like have been frequently condemned as providing the stimuli for subsequent sexual aberrations. Concern over the effects of pornography was widespread enough in the 1960's that the U.S. Congress created a Commission on Obscenity and Pornography to study the casual relationship of such material to antisocial behavior and to recommend appropriate legal measures to deal with the problem. The report of the Commission was released in 1970 amidst much controversy. Nonetheless, the report stands as one of the few attempts to examine rationally the data with respect to any links between exposure to erotica and sexual deviations.

Not surprisingly it was found that opinions concerning the ill effects of pornography varied widely from group to group. Most professional workers, such as psychologists, psychiatrists and social workers, believed that sexual materials do not have harmful effects on either adults or adolescents. However, 58 per cent of the police chiefs surveyed believed that "obscene" books were a contributing factor to juvenile delinquency. 58%

It was found that most people are aroused by pornographic materials, particularly those depicting heterosexual intercourse. Both males and females are aroused by such exposure, although women are more reluctant to report such arousal and are more apt to report the physiological sensations associated with sexual arousal than directly report being sexually aroused. In general persons who are college-educated, religiously inactive and sexually experienced are more likely to report arousal than those who are less educated, religiously active and sexually inexperienced.

With respect to the effect on sexual delinquency, the evidence seems to point toward the conclusion that pornography has no impact upon moral character over and above that of a generally deviant background. The Commission cites data from Denmark which indicate that increased availability of explicit sexual

materials has been accompanied by a decrease in the incidence of sexual crimes. Other research has indicated: (1) that the decrease coincided with legal changes which permitted wider availability of explicit sexual materials; and (2) that the changes could not be attributed to concurrent changes in definitions of sex crimes or in public attitudes toward reporting such crimes or in police reporting procedures. Available evidence from other studies seems to suggest that sexual offenders had less adolescent experience with erotica than other adults, and also see less erotica as adults than do normals (see Figure 15–2). Goldstein et al. (1970) suggest that the sexual offenders' relative inexperience with erotic material as adolescents is a reflection of their generally deprived sexual environment. For example, the 20 convicted rapists in this study reported little nudity or discussion of sex in their original families. If caught with pornographic materials they were more apt to report having been punished by their parents than the control group. Many rapists had relied on their wives for much of their sexual information since it was not available in the home. As a group the rapists reported more extensive extramarital intercourse and a higher frequency of sexual relations than normal controls but less enjoyment of sex. After surveying this and other data the Commission on Obscenity and Pornography (1970) concluded:

In sum, empirical research designed to clarify the question has found no evidence to date that exposure

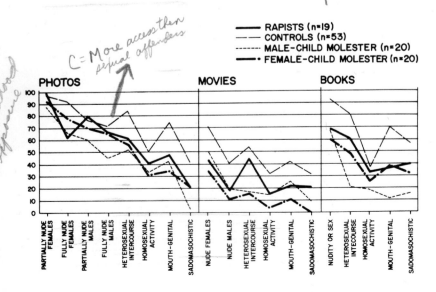

RAPISTS (n=19)
CONTROLS (n=53)
MALE-CHILD MOLESTER (n=20)
FEMALE-CHILD MOLESTER (n=20)

C = More access then sexual offenders

% of childhood exposure

PHOTOS   MOVIES   BOOKS

PARTIALLY NUDE FEMALES / FULLY NUDE FEMALES / PARTIALLY NUDE MALES / FULLY NUDE MALES / HETEROSEXUAL INTERCOURSE / HOMOSEXUAL ACTIVITY / MOUTH–GENITAL / SADOMASOCHISTIC / NUDE FEMALES / NUDE MALES / HETEROSEXUAL INTERCOURSE / HOMOSEXUAL ACTIVITY / MOUTH–GENITAL / SADOMASOCHISTC / NUDITY OR SEX / HETEROSEXUAL INTERCOURSE / HOMOSEXUAL ACTIVITY / MOUTH–GENITAL / SADOMASOCHISTIC

Figure 15–2. Percentages of rapists, child molesters, and control-group members who were exposed to pornography when they were teenagers. (Redrawn from Goldstein, M. J., Kant, H. S. Judd, L. L., Rice, C. J., and Green. R. Exposure to pornography and sexual behavior in deviant and normal groups. In *Technical Reports of the Commission on Obscenity and Pornography. Vol. 7, U. S. Government Printing Office, Washington, D.C., 1971.)*

to explicit sexual materials plays a significant role in the causation of delinquent or criminal behavior among youth or adults. The Commission cannot conclude that exposure to erotic materials is a factor in the causation of sex crime or sex delinquency.

THE ROLE OF THE VICTIM

Public opinion and the law have traditionally regarded a molested woman or child as the innocent victim of the male. However, it has been repeatedly observed that many victims deliberately invite or unconsciously provoke deviant behavior. Weinberg (1955) reported that while some victims of incest resisted it, others were compliant and cooperative. Hirschfeld (1944) pointed out that some children become remarkably astute in identifying male exhibitionists. One child may encourage the exhibitionist to expose himself while another fetches a policeman. Contrary to popular opinion, most sexual offenses against children are not committed by strangers but by persons known to the children. The child victim is usually attractive, charming and possessed of a strong need for attention. Many child victims have a history of behavior difficulties, particularly restlessness and rebellion against parents. In statutory rape, the victims tend to come from low income groups, disorganized neighborhoods and disorganized families, and to have strong needs for attention and affection.

An invitation to sexual assault by an adult female sometimes results from sadistically arousing the male with the deliberate intention of frustrating him, only to discover that he will not accept the frustration. In another pattern, a hysterical or otherwise neurotic female may quite unwittingly provoke a sexual response which she then attempts to reject. In either case, the subsequent hostility of the female victim may lead to legal charges and conviction.

ETIOLOGY AND DYNAMICS

Heredity

We have previously emphasized the fact that the psychopathology of deviates is very heterogeneous. A diversity of psychopathology is also found in the family histories of deviates. The parents and siblings of neurotic deviates have a high frequency of neurotic personality characteristics and symptoms; the families of

sociopathic deviates manifest a high frequency of antisocial behavior and alcoholism; the families of psychotic deviates have high rates of psychosis and suicide. As always, a high family frequency may reflect either heredity or maladaptive learning.

However, a number of investigators have speculated that sexual deviation itself, apart from personality and underlying psychological disturbance, may have a genetic component. Kallmann (1953) reported data for 95 pairs of adult male twins in each of which one member was predominantly or exclusively homosexual. Among 44 pairs diagnosed as monozygotic, Kallmann reported a concordance rate of 100 per cent for homosexual behavior in the co-twins. In contrast, among 51 pairs of dizygotic twins, only 40 per cent were reported to be concordant for overt homosexual behavior. However, due to the methodological weaknesses of twin studies, most investigators have not accepted Kallmann's conclusion that homosexuality has a hereditary basis.

Several large scale studies performed during the first half of the present century indicated a relative excess of brothers among the siblings of male homosexuals. On the basis of these studies it was first inferred that the excess of males was due to a genetic factor which produced anatomical maleness even when the chromosome pattern was female, thus implying that the homosexual is genetically neither fully male nor female. Direct inspection of chromosomes was not possible earlier in this century, but more recently it has become an available technique. Pritchard (1962) examined the chromosomes of a number of male homosexuals and found the normal male complement of one X and one Y chromosome in all his subjects. The earlier hypothesis that intersexuality between the male and the female is the basis of homosexuality must therefore be rejected.

Chromosomal analysis in recent years has also revealed the existence of a number of individuals who have neither the two X chromosomes of the normal female nor the single X and single Y chromosome of the normal male. A wide variety of chromosomal anomalies have been reported, two of the most frequent occurring in conditions known as Turner's syndrome and Klinefelter's syndrome. In Turner's syndrome there is only a single X chromosome; the individual is externally female but does not develop secondary sex characteristics, rarely menstruates and is sterile. Frequently there are malformations of the aorta (the main artery of the body) as well as deafness and mental deficiency. In Klinefelter's syndrome, on the other hand, there are generally three sex chromosomes, two X and one Y. Externally the individual is male although somewhat feminine in build, usually sterile and often mentally retarded. In both syndromes the individual may be asexual but is not homosexual or otherwise sexually deviant. The fact that these chromosomal variations produce bodily malformations and intellectual subnormality but not sexual deviations is strong evidence against the existence of chromosomal abnormalities in sexual deviates—homosexual or otherwise—who are physically and intellectually normal.

Other Biological Determinants

Coppen (1959) compared the body build of 31 male homosexuals, 22 male heterosexual neurotics and 53 male medical patients. Both neurotics and homosexuals deviated from the normal masculine physique, thus refuting the popular belief that peculiarities of physique are specifically related to sexual abnormality.

It has long been hypothesized in many quarters that deviant sexual behavior must be closely related to endocrine function. In the lower animals, sexual activity may be consistently decreased by castration. Administration of male hormones to male animals increases their sexual activity and results in generalization of the activity to include homosexual as well as heterosexual objects. In humans, however, the correlation between hormone levels and overt sexual behavior is very small. In females, the marked changes in endocrine activity during puberty and menopause are not necessarily accompanied by changes in sexual behavior. In males, the sharp increase in hormone level accompanying puberty is not necessarily accompanied by overt behavioral changes, and castration during adult life may have relatively slight effects on established patterns of sexual behavior. Sexual behavior may decrease in quantity after castration, but the kind of object that attracts the individual remains the same.

In a number of studies an excess of female hormone (estrogen) has been reported in the blood stream of male homosexuals, and an excess of male hormone (androgen) in the blood stream of female homosexuals. (The normal individual has both androgen and estrogen, but the male has more androgen and the female more estrogen.) However, some of the

homosexual subjects in these studies did not manifest a hormonal imbalance; in other studies no homosexual subjects had an imbalance; and in still others an imbalance was found in some heterosexual individuals. Furthermore, glandular treatment of homosexuality to redress an imbalance is not effective. It can be stated with confidence that *no consistent abnormalities of endocrine function have been observed in any group of sexual deviates.* Interestingly, the homosexual himself frequently believes in a constitutional explanation, endocrine or otherwise, "I was born that way and it's unfair to expect me to behave differently," is his claim. Other deviates also make this claim at times.

Following an extensive comparison of sexual behavior in many species of animals and in 190 human societies, Ford and Beach (1951) concluded that in the course of evolution the control of gonadal hormones over sexual behavior has become progressively relaxed with the result that human behavior is relatively independent of this source of control:

. . . the cerebral cortex has assumed a greater and greater degree of direction over all behavior, including that of a sexual nature. It appears that the growing importance of cerebral influences accounts for the progressive relaxation of hormonal control over sexual responses. At the same time, increasing dominance of the cortex in affecting sexual manifestations has resulted in greater lability and modifiability of erotic practices. Human sexual behavior is more variable and more easily affected by learning and social conditioning than is that of any other species, and this is precisely because in our own species this type of behavior depends heavily upon the most recently evolved parts of the brain.

Psychological Determinants

Deviant sexual behavior is too diverse to have a single psychological cause. A multitude of important contributing factors exist, among them: deprivation of opportunity to engage in normal sexual behavior; isolation in childhood; specific episodes in which deviation is learned in childhood or youth; castration anxiety, fixation on (or regression to) infantile sexuality, and fear of the opposite sex; defense against incestuous impulses; inappropriate sex-typing and identification; generalized inhibition and sexual ignorance; and fear of adult responsibility.

Deprivation of Normal Sexuality. Under conditions of deprivation, especially when there is prolonged segregation of the sexes, a

REGRESS - return to earlier
REPRESS - invol.
SUP - vol

certain amount of deviant behavior occurs. Mature adults often turn to increased masturbation as a sexual outlet when deprived of normal sex objects. Immature persons, when subjected to the added stress of deprivation of normal sexual outlets, may turn to deviant behavior. Hartman and Nicoloy (1966), for example, found that sexually deviant reactions were more frequent in expectant fathers. Apparently such fathers were more immature than others and the added stress of increased responsibility and sexual deprivation was enough to lead them to seek sexually deviant outlets. The individual who becomes involved may or may not abandon his deviation at a later time.

Isolation in Childhood. The child who is isolated from other children is handicapped in psychological development. Like the isolated monkeys in Harlow's study (1962) he may never acquire mature, heterosexual habits or he acquires them only with great difficulty. Among the possible deviations due to childhood isolation is a preference for pedophilia. Promiscuity may also occur if the individual overcompensates for his early isolation and insatiably attempts to obtain attention and feel needed.

Specific Episodes in Childhood or Youth. A sexual episode or a series of them may profoundly affect the later behavior of an impressionable individual. Homosexuality often begins when a child or adolescent "experiments" with someone of the same age or is seduced by an older homosexual. If a youngster's need for affection and protection is met by the seducer, the newly learned homosexual behavior is rewarded and is therefore more likely to become persistent.

Being beaten across the buttocks arouses both pain and sexual excitation in some children, and masochism may result. Fetishism is also likely to begin with specific learning episodes. Sexual excitement becomes conditioned to some object, especially if the individual masturbates when the object arouses him, and the object becomes a more and more powerful stimulant. Of course, this sequence of events can occur only if the individual's personality renders him vulnerable.

Castration Anxiety, Fixation, Regression, and Fear of the Opposite Sex. In his *Introductory Lectures on Psychoanalysis* (1920), Freud remarked, "If it is correct that the real obstacles to sexual satisfaction, or privation in regard to it, bring to the surface perverse tendencies in people who would otherwise have shown none,

we must conclude that something in these people is ready to embrace these perversions; or, if you prefer it, that the tendencies must have been present in them in a latent form."

The tendencies that survive are infantile and polymorphous perverse, that is, they include various objects and nongenital aims. Adult deviations are fixations on the infantile or regressions to it, i.e., failures in development. In the case of fixation there is no learning of mature sexuality at puberty; in the case of regression there is abandonment of learned, mature behavior. Freud distinguished between the pervert and the neurotic by the hypothesis that in the former the primary reaction to frustration is sexual fixation and regression, whereas the symptoms of the latter symbolize infantile sexuality but give the appearance of NEUROTIC being nonsexual.

In psychoanalytic theory, the ultimate cause of sexual fixation and regression is presumed to be castration anxiety (or penis envy in the female). To quote Fenichel (1945): "In perversions, adult sexuality is supplanted by infantile sexuality. Something must be repulsive in adult sexuality, and something especially attractive in infantile sexuality. While the latter factor is variable, the former is constant; it is always the castration complex that interferes with the capacity for enjoying full genital sexuality." The adult male's unconscious castration anxiety causes him to avoid women, for they remind him that he may be castrated. The female avoids males, for they remind her that she has already been castrated.

Fear of the opposite sex, often associated with hostility, is manifested in deviation after deviation. Masturbation and fetishism are means of avoiding other human beings, voyeurism is a timid method of putting distance between the individual and the sex object, homosexuality substitutes a familiar object—one's own sex—for the strange and fearful opposite sex, and pedophilia is a relationship with an immature and therefore less fearful object. A component of satyriasis and nymphomania is overcompensation for fear of the opposite sex. (The fear of the opposite sex felt by various types of deviates has led many theorists, including analysts, to hypothesize that all deviates have a basically homosexual orientation.)

Sexual deviations have also been hypothesized to be *direct* attempts to allay castration anxiety. For example, the masochist may invite a "symbolic castration through pain," as if to be reassured each time he is hurt that he is not *really* castrated. Pain may also be a price paid in advance to ward off castration. The sadist may symbolically castrate others before they can castrate him. The exhibitionist may repeatedly attempt to demonstrate that he has not been castrated. Psychoanalytic theory has in this manner derived a great many phenomena from castration fear; so many, in fact, that it can be questioned whether a single causal factor can possibly be so all-important. But whether it is invariably a cause of deviation or not, strong castration fear is undoubtedly present in many individual deviates. In the study by Hammer and Glueck (1955), sex offenders revealed feelings of genital inadequacy and anticipation of punishment which were apparently related to their castration fears. (However, their inadequacy feelings may have been in part based on reality, since many offenders are undersexed.) Furthermore, among the various subgroups in Hammer and Glueck's study, the intensity of castration fears was greatest for those individuals whose sexual objects were least like the mature female.

Defense Against Incestuous Impulses. In Freudian theory a major source of castration fear and penis envy is the child's unacceptable, incestuous urges toward the opposite-sex parent. Again, this factor is undoubtedly present in many deviates. A homosexual male often reacts to women as if each were a forbidden mother; consequently homosexual activity makes him feel less guilty than heterosexual activity. The masochist's suffering may in part represent an atonement stemming from a pervasive sexual guilt which had its beginnings in the parent-child relationship. Even pedophilia may be a defense against incest: the child-object is least like the forbidden parent.

Inappropriate Sex-typing and Failures in Identification. Sexual behavior in the narrow sense occurs within the context of a broader set of behaviors that are considered socially appropriate for men or women, respectively, and are learned through the process of *sex-typing* or sex role differentiation (McCandless, 1961). By sex-typing is meant the imitative or modeling activity in which the young boy in a particular culture practices behaviors characteristic of men and the girl practices behaviors characteristic of women. These include manner of speech, gestures, preferred play activities and many other behaviors other than the purely sexual.

Successful sex-typing depends on several factors. First, the consonance or dissonance of the individual's physical characteristics with the role to be adopted is important. The feminine-appearing boy, for example, has a harder time becoming appropriately masculine in his behavior than the masculine appearing boy.

Second, sex-typing depends on the psychological and social pressures to which the individual is subjected. Hampson (1963) and Money (1963) investigated the importance of these pressures by studying intensively the biological and psychological characteristics of a number of individuals who had one or another kind of hormonal or hermaphroditic (anatomically bisexual) disorder. Some of the subjects were females who, biologically, were excessively masculinized by an overproduction of male hormones; in others, the internal reproductive organs were female but the external genitals were sexually ambiguous; others had still other anatomical incongruities of sex. A sample of this sort is ideal for studying the relative importance of biological and psychological factors in determining psychosexual orientation, that is, the sex the individual attributes to himself and the masculinity or femininity of his interests, fantasies, mannerisms and goals. The investigators found that when there was a disparity between one or another biological variable and the role that the family had assigned to the individual and in which he had been reared, the resultant psychological orientation almost invariably conformed to the assigned sex role rather than to the biological variables. Psychosexual orientation was independent of the biological variables of masculinity or femininity of chromosome pattern, gonadal structure, male-female hormonal balance, nature of the internal reproductive organs (uterus, prostate and so forth) and external genital appearance. It was concluded that the human being is psychosexually neutral at birth and learns a masculine or feminine role in response to his life experiences.

A third and crucial factor in sex-typing is the presence or absence of an adequate male or female model, usually the father or mother, to serve as a basis for identification. In psychosexual inversion, the individual identifies with a parent or parent-substitute (an older brother or sister, for example) of the opposite sex. The earlier this identification is made and the more intense it is, the deeper the degree of inversion. A number of variables contribute to cross-sex identifications. Sears (1953) reported that preschool boys who chose a father role in a standardized play situation with a family of dolls had warm, permissive fathers. Boys taking the mother role had cold fathers and mothers who were warm but who disparaged the fathers and restricted the sons' mobility outside the home. Fouls and Smith (1956) found that siblings also furnished appropriate models. A boy with an older brother was more likely than an only child to choose feminine activities. Bronson (1959) found that boys 9 to 13 years old whose father-relationships were stressful showed surface patterns of behavior that either were *extremely* masculine—i.e., the boys rigidly and defensively copied their fathers—or else tended to be feminine. Regardless of surface masculinity or femininity, the boys with poor father-relationships rejected masculinity at a deeper level, as judged by TAT stories. In contrast, boys with rewarding fathers made satisfactory masculine identifications at all levels.

Bender and Paster (1941) reported that 90 per cent of a group of 23 actively homosexual children had same-sex parents who could not possibly serve as effective models for identification. They were physically absent from home, or grossly abusive, or domineering and over-solicitous yet basically weak. Consequently, the parent of the opposite sex was perceived as a source of reward and was emulated. Apperson and McAdoo (1968) collected data on perceptions of parents' behavior from a group of homosexuals who were functioning adequately in the community. Compared with controls the homosexuals saw their fathers as more critical, impatient and rejecting and less of a socializing agent. Thus the fathers were seen as poor models to emulate for identification purposes.

Kolb and Johnson (1955) emphasized the roles of parents in actively fostering psychosexual inversion and homosexual behavior. Mesnikoff et al. (1963) intensively studied the early parental attitudes and behavior of four pairs of male twins who, in adult life, were sexually discordant: one member of each pair was heterosexual and one homosexual. In each case the mother was the dominant parent and the father was openly and actively derogated or else he assumed a passive role. The twin who became homosexual was associated most closely with the mother, whereas the twin who became heterosexual was closer to the father.

Westwood (1960) studied the homes of 127 male homosexuals in England and concluded that a good identification could not be made in 75 per cent of them. In an extensive comparison of 106 homosexual males and 100 heterosexual

males undergoing psychoanalysis, Bieber et al. (1962) found marked differences in the parental relationships of the two groups. As shown in Table 15–1, the mothers of homosexuals were more demanding and more seductive (for example, they tended to dress and undress with the patient, kiss him sensually, fondle him and so forth). The mothers formed coalitions with the sons against the fathers; they did not encourage masculinity and interfered with heterosexual activities. In short, the mothers behaved as if they *wished* their sons to be homosexual, much as they might deny this. The fathers of the homosexual patients were distant, disliked and feared. A noteworthy aspect of the study is that the differences in parental relationships between the homosexual and heterosexual comparison groups were considerable even though the latter group also consisted of patients in treatment (mostly for neurosis and character disorder).

Deviants often form secondary identifications with sexual objects that mirror their primary identifications. For example, the heterosexual voyeur often identifies with the female he spies upon, thus betraying a basic inversion. A passive male homosexual may behave toward an active male as his mother did toward his father. An active male homosexual may choose young boys as a reflection of a narcissistic wish that

TABLE 15–1. Parental Relationships of 106 Homosexual and 100 Heterosexual Male Patients (All figures are percentages.)*

	Homo-sexuals	Hetero-sexuals
Mother		
Demanded that she be prime center of patient's attention	61	36
Was seductive toward patient	57	34
Spent a great deal of time with patient	56	27
Tried to ally with patient against husband	62	40
Was more intimate with patient than with other male siblings	56	29
Encouraged masculine activities	17	47
Interfered with patient's hetero-sexual activity during and after adolescence	58	35
Father		
Patient was father's favorite	7	28
Patient spent little time with father	87	60
Patient hated and feared father	57	31
Patient admired father	16	47

*Data from Bieber, I., et al. 1962. Homosexuality: A Psychoanalytic study. New York, Basic Books.

his mother might have chosen him, or he may choose passive males in imitation of a dominant mother and weak father.

Generalized Inhibition and Sexual Ignorance. Glueck (1956) found that the most markedly deviant offenders have been extremely modest in childhood. Throughout the developmental years their attitudes toward sexual behavior had been "continuously traumatic, prohibiting and inhibiting." They had been socially isolated and the most deviant had been the most shy and timid. The majority were ignorant as well as afraid and had misconceptions of normal sexual activity.

Fear of Adult Responsibility. A final factor is fear of involvement in the responsibilities of an adult relationship. Adult heterosexuality in our culture is likely to involve long-term commitments as a husband or wife, parent and provider. The unmarried deviate avoids these commitments and the married deviate periodically flees from them.

Sociocultural Factors

By and large, a culture that suppresses sexuality fosters deviations and a culture that is permissive tends to be relatively free of them. In the Trobriand Islands, for example, where almost no restrictions are placed on the sexual behavior of boys and girls, Malinowski (1927) found that sexual activity before and during adolescence was very frequent but almost entirely heterosexual.

Within western society there are class differences in sexual suppression. Lower-class children are punished more than middle-class children for behaving as the opposite sex is expected to behave; the apparently lesser frequency of homosexuality among adults in the lower than the middle class has been attributed to this difference in child rearing. Children in the middle and upper classes are taught a greater degree of control over their heterosexual and aggressive impulses than children in the lower class; the lesser frequency of heterosexual assault and incest in the middle and upper groups may be a consequence of this difference. In addition, a certain amount of promiscuity is accepted as normal by many members of the lower class, as long as the sexual act is genital, heterosexual and performed in a prescribed manner. By contrast, the more varied sexual behavior of the other classes—e.g., various types of heterosexual foreplay and variation in coital positions—is viewed as perverse in the lower class. Members of the lower class apparently have a greater fear of being considered perverse and sexually peculiar.

Sociocultural factors other than class affect sexual deviations. Observers have claimed that homosexuality is relatively frequent in Germany, both homosexuality and oral sexuality in France, and sadistic practices in England. The total number of convictions for sexual offenses is far greater for whites than nonwhites in the United States, but the incidence among some nonwhite groups—perhaps as a reflection of class membership—is higher than for whites. However, the importance of sociocultural factors in causation should not be overemphasized: deviations, like other evidences of psychological disturbance, are found within every national and racial group. The determination of who will and who will not be a deviate within a group depends on individual experiences and personality.

TREATMENT

The behavior of society toward the sexual offender, like its behavior toward other offenders, falls into three classes: (1) segregation and punitive retaliation; (2) a demand that the offender repair the damage he has done; and (3) therapy and rehabilitation. Of these, the traditional reaction to the sexual offender has been retaliation. When a major sexual crime is committed in a community, particularly the rape and murder of a young girl, there is usually a public outcry for indiscriminate imprisonment of all sexual deviates on the naïve assumption that they are all equally likely to commit a similar offense. It would appear that the persons who are most vociferous in making such demands tend to be those who have the greatest conflicts over the control of their own sexual impulses. It is true that society must sometimes defend itself by institutionalizing dangerous offenders, but the dangerous minority is vastly different from the harmless majority. It should also be realized that incarceration alone does not benefit the sexual offender; in fact, it is usually harmful psychologically. For some years past, there has been an increasing understanding of these facts and a tendency to evaluate the sexual offender objectively and treat him when possible.

Various somatic treatment measures have

been tried. Tranquilizers and anti-depressive drugs have been successfully used to provide relief from the anxiety and depression accompanying sexual deviation, but of course they do not change the structure of the individual's sexual motivation. ECT and even lobotomy have been employed for psychotic sexual deviates. Suppression of male sexual activity by the administration of female hormones results in diminution of sexual desire and activity, but there is no change in the direction of the residual sexual impulses. Castration—usually voluntary, but mandatory in some localities— also fails to change the individual's sexual aims although it diminishes the drive. Male hormones administered to homosexuals have failed to convert them to heterosexuality. In general, it appears that somatic treatment has not fared well with sexual deviations.

Psychotherapy is unlikely to change long-established preferences in sexual behavior, but it can help a patient whose deviation is of recent onset. Psychotherapy is also helpful when the deviant behavior occurs within a context of genital heterosexuality—for example, partial homosexuality in a basically heterosexual individual. In addition, psychotherapy can alleviate the anxiety and depression frequently associated with deviant sexual behavior. To quote from a letter Freud wrote to a woman who had appealed to him to help her homosexual son:

By asking me if I can help, you mean, I suppose, if I can abolish homosexuality and make normal heterosexuality take its place. The answer is, in a general way, we cannot promise to achieve it. In a certain number of cases we succeed in developing the blighted germs of heterosexual tendencies which are present in every homosexual, in the majority of cases it is no more possible. It is a question of the quality and the age of the individual. The result of treatment cannot be predicted.

What analysis can do for your son runs in a different line. If he is unhappy, neurotic, torn by conflicts, inhibited in his social life, analysis may bring him harmony, peace of mind, full efficiency whether he remains a homosexual or gets changed. . . .

A number of therapists believe that helping the confirmed homosexual to accept his homosexuality and to learn to be more comfortable with it is a legitimate therapeutic aim, provided the patient chooses adult sexual objects rather than boys or adolescents.

Psychoanalysis with sexual deviants is on the whole more difficult than with non-deviant neurotics because the deviant symptom is a pleasurable one and therefore becomes the basis for strong resistance to change. A complication of psychoanalysis and other types of psychotherapy is the sex of the therapist. Most neurotic patients can make therapeutic progress with either a male or female therapist, but many sexual deviates react totally differently as a function of the therapist's sex. A male homosexual may have great difficulty with a female therapist or with a male whose manner and appearance are not sufficiently masculine. A sexually sadistic male patient may find it impossible to be other than aggressive with a female therapist.

In addition to psychoanalysis, various types of psychotherapy have been used. A simple but often helpful procedure is to provide the misinformed deviate with adequate sexual information. The inhibited deviate can be helped to be less prudish. In some cases the patient can be shifted gradually from an undesirable to a desirable object. For example, the homosexual male can be encouraged to develop friendships with boyish looking females and then to move further and further in the direction of more feminine-appearing females. Hypnosis has also been tried, utilizing post-hypnotic suggestions that the patient will no longer wish to engage in deviant behavior and will prefer normal behavior, but in general the results have been unimpressive.

Reconditioning therapy has been employed with a number of deviations. For example, Lavin et al. (1961) successfully treated a male transvestite by administration of a nauseating drug which caused him to vomit while he viewed photographs of himself in female clothing. There were 66 reconditioning trials; 6 months later he still had no desire for female dress. In reconditioning sexual deviations, attempts may be made to substitute aversion for previous pleasure, in contrast to the substitution of pleasure for anxiety in the treatment of neuroses by reconditioning. Techniques of reconditioning have also been used to make fetishistic behavior aversive and to weaken homosexual and strengthen heterosexual tendencies. For example, Freund (1960) treated 47 male homosexuals by injecting a noxious drug while they viewed slides of males, and by administering testosterone (male sex hormone) before they viewed films of semi-nude and nude females. A follow-up several years later revealed either temporary or permanent weakening of homosexual tendencies in 40 per cent of the patients.

Desensitization has been used with exhibitionism, voyeurism and other deviations. An example is Wolpe's (1958) treatment of an anxiety-laden exhibitionist whose impulse to expose himself arose whenever he felt anxious or submitted to authority. Wolpe desensitized him by inducing relaxation responses and assertiveness rather than submissions while the patient visualized in imagination the authority and other situations that frustrated him. The result was a marked reduction of the patient's impulse to exhibit himself.

Group therapy has been used with some success. An illustrative example was reported by Cabeen and Coleman (1961). Of 120 hospitalized male homosexuals, pedophiles and ex-hibitionists, 69 of whom were diagnosed as psychopathic and 51 neurotic, 79 improved enough in analytically oriented group therapy to be returned to the community. Improvement was judged by changes in observed behavior in the hospital and changes in personality tests. The more group sessions a patient had, the greater was the degree of improvement. A follow-up six months to three years later showed that only three patients had been again apprehended and arrested.

Generally speaking, psychotherapy with sexual deviates is difficult, but it would appear that several of the methods just discussed have considerable promise.

what is chance prob?

16
ALCOHOLISM AND DRUG ADDICTION

O thou invisible spirit of wine! if thou hast no name to be known by, let us call thee devil! . . . O God! that men should put an enemy in their mouths to steal away their brains!

William Shakespeare, *Othello*

ALCOHOLISM AND DRUG ADDICTION

Man has used alcohol and other drugs for thousands of years. With time, excessive indulgence in them came to be considered as depraved or criminal behavior. In recent years, however, it has been recognized that alcoholism and drug addictions are psychiatric, psychological and social problems that entail a staggering cost to the individual and society, both emotionally and economically.

In its broadest sense, an addiction is any behavior that dominates the individual to a degree that excludes—in whole or part—alternative, normal forms of behavior. Excessive eating, drinking of water, reading, working, sexual activity, cigarette smoking or any other excess can be an addiction. In practice, however, the term is usually confined to alcohol and other drugs when they are used to the point of emotional and physiological dependence on them.

The concept of addiction implies an intense craving that the individual must gratify regardless of consequences. Psychoanalysts and psychiatrists generally stress the impulsive nature of the craving and view addictions as forms of character disorder marked by impulsiveness and by relative freedom from anxiety and psychotic misinterpretation of reality. It is true, as we shall see, that many

addicts are sociopathic, but some are neurotically anxious, some are psychotic and many are more compulsive than impulsive.

There are a number of similarities between alcoholism and other drug addictions and many alcoholics also use other drugs to excess. However, alcoholism is far more prevalent than addiction to other drugs and it has been studied more intensively. Alcoholism is discussed in detail in the first part of this chapter, followed by a briefer consideration of certain other forms of drug addiction. Five major problems will be explored:

1. What are the immediate physiological and behavioral effects of alcohol and other drugs?
2. What is the nature of addiction?
3. What are the long-term effects of prolonged addiction?
4. Why do people become addicts?
5. What treatment measures are available?

ALCOHOLISM

The Immediate Effects of Alcoholic Intake

An ancient Hebrew legend symbolically summarizes the nature of alcoholic intoxication.

One day, while Noah was plowing a field, the Devil approached and asked what he was doing. Noah replied, "I am planting a vineyard. When the fruit is ripe, the grapes are excellent to eat, either moist or dried, and when pressed the juices become wine which warms the body and the spirit." The Devil suggested that they become partners in the vineyard and Noah agreed. Thereupon the Devil killed a sheep, a lion, a monkey and a pig in such a manner that the blood of each animal flowed around the roots of the vines. The Devil's action was interpreted to mean that man is ordinarily like the sheep—mild and inoffensive; after he starts to drink, he feels like the lion—proud and confident of his strength; if he drinks deeper, he starts to chatter aimlessly and scampers about like the foolish monkey; and if he drinks still more, he falls to the ground and wallows in filth like the pig.

Contrary to popular belief, alcohol is not a stimulant but a sedative. Its immediate physiological effect is to depress the functioning of the higher brain centers. This results in (1) impairment of perceptual and intellectual functioning; (2) relief from anxiety, fear and sorrow; and (3) release from behavior normally inhibited by the cortex. (The superego has been defined as that part of the personality which is soluble in alcohol.) After a few drinks, most people experience a pleasant sense of unreality and a feeling of liberation from responsibility. The individual's speech may become rapid and slurred, and he may manifest either flight of ideas or a repetitive, obsessive concern with a single idea. His gestures and motor behavior are likely to become large and sweeping, although a big enough dose of alcohol will have a reverse effect and bring on a coma. The stimulation of thinking, speech and movement by a small dose is due to sedation of the cortical cells that ordinarily inhibit these aspects of behavior.

Incoordination, double vision, poor discrimination and judgment, and a dulling of the capacity to perceive discomfort—e.g., cold—are common effects of alcohol. If sufficiently intoxicated, the individual "blanks out" and subsequently is unable to remember what he said or did. Such blanks or "blackouts" are most frequent among chronic alcoholics but may also occur during an isolated episode of excessive drinking. (The individual is legally responsible for any antisocial acts committed while intoxicated, whether or not he remembers them, since the law holds that he placed himself in this position voluntarily and should have known the possible consequences.)

In sum, the effects of alcohol on the typical individual consist of a loss of efficiency but a temporary feeling of well-being. Samuel Johnson, in "The Life of Addison" (in *Lives of the English Poets*) wrote, "In the bottle, discontent seeks for comfort, cowardice for courage, and bashfulness for confidence." The following morning, however, retribution awaits most persons in the form of a hangover with varying degrees of intellectual impairment, physiological disturbances, a feeling of anxiety, and remorse.

A few individuals manifest an atypical reaction to alcohol that is known as *pathological intoxication* and is quite different from ordinary intoxication. Sometimes it follows a debauch and sometimes, in a particularly susceptible individual, a moderate dose. Emotional stress and convalescence from physical illness seem to contribute to susceptibility. The reaction consists of a state of acute confusion that lasts from several hours to a day. The individual may become hallucinated and disoriented. He is likely to fly into a blind rage and may commit assault or homicide, followed by complete amnesia. Apparently, alcohol merely precipitates pathological intoxication; the predisposing causes consist of the emotional and biological characteristics of the organism. Since pathological intoxication tends to recur, susceptible individuals should not drink even in moderation.

Blood Stream Concentration. A number of investigators have attempted to relate the concentration of alcohol in the blood to changes in behavior. Alcohol does not affect behavior until it passes from the gastrointestinal tract into the blood stream, primarily through the walls of the stomach and small intestine. As the level of blood alcohol rises, behavior is impaired faster and faster so that a small increase in blood alcohol results in a proportionately much larger increase in the degree of impairment. When the concentration is one-twentieth of 1 per cent, the average individual (there are many exceptions) feels euphoric and uninhibited. He loses the ability to be self-critical and may become boastful and aggressive. At one-tenth of 1 per cent, the average individual staggers, feels drowsy and behaves noisily. At two-tenths of 1 per cent, his emotions are out of control, he may feel nauseated and he cannot remember recent events. At three-tenths of 1 per cent, stupor is common. A higher concentration is likely to be fatal. These figures, however, are averages; psychological and physiological tolerance of alcohol varies widely from person to person. Chronic alcoholics, for example, generally acquire a tolerance that enables them to consume enormous quantities until liver damage or various nutritional deficiencies diminish the tolerance.

The concentration of alcohol in the blood is determined by a number of factors. (1) It increases as the amount swallowed in a given time increases. The rate of drinking is thus as important as the total amount drunk. (2) Concentration increases with the rate of absorption into the blood stream. The absorption process is much faster if the stomach is empty of food. (3) Concentration is lower for a large than a small person, since a given amount of alcohol results in a lesser concentration with increased weight. (4) Concentration is higher if the metabolic processes of the liver are slowed down by disease, because alcohol circulates in the blood until it is oxidized by the liver. (A number of chronic alcoholics suffer from cirrhosis of the liver and consequent metabolic defects.) Liver metabolism is also slower in small than large persons.

Personality Factors. In addition to blood stream concentration and physiological tolerance, personality factors also determine the effects of alcohol on the individual. The aphorism *in vino veritas* should not be interpreted to mean that an intoxicated individual will not lie, but that a man's true nature is revealed under the influence of alcohol. The eighteenth century novelist Henry Fielding described in *Tom Jones* the tendency of alcohol to intensify existing characteristics as follows: "It [drink] takes away the guard of reason, and consequently forces us to produce those symptoms which many, when sober, have art enough to conceal. It heightens and inflames our passions (generally indeed that passion which is uppermost in our mind) so that the angry temper, the amorous, the generous, the good-humoured, the avaricious, and all other dispositions of men, are in their cups heightened and exposed." Because it depresses inhibitory functions, alcohol may sometimes seem to produce behavior that is the reverse of the individual's "true" nature. The timorous person becomes aggressive; the considerate, selfish; and the shy, amorous. But these apparent changes merely indicate personality tendencies that are ordinarily inhibited. A statement by a character in the play *The Late Christopher Bean*—"A man's the same when he's drunk as when he's sober, only more so"—is basically true.

Temporary moods as well as long-term traits of personality influence the response to alcohol. The individual is likely to experience quite different effects if he drinks when depressed from those he experiences if he drinks when in a euphoric mood. Immediate events also make a difference: it has often been observed that an emotional shock may have a sobering effect on an intoxicated individual.

The Nature of Addiction to Alcohol

Tens of millions of persons in the United States use alcohol. The majority of these do not drink more than the mores of the community permit. A large minority, however, are excessive drinkers whose consumption of alcohol goes beyond community customs. A subgroup of excessive drinkers, in turn, may be classified as alcoholics. In 1949, a committee of the World Health Organization defined alcoholics as ". . . those excessive drinkers whose dependence upon alcohol has attained such a degree that it shows a noticeable mental disturbance or an interference with their bodily and mental health, their interpersonal relations, and their smooth social and economic functioning; or who show the prodromal [pre-syndrome] signs of such developments. They therefore require treatment." The number of alcoholics in the United States has been estimated as possibly 5,000,000, mostly male. The typical age is 35 to 50.

The committee investigated the development of alcoholism and concluded that excessive drinking begins with a stage of *irregular symptomatic excessive drinking* in which the individual drinks as a symptom of psychological, somatic or social pathology. In this stage he may behave pathologically when he is intoxicated but he recognizes the fact and can stop drinking when he wishes. He is not yet a chronic alcoholic. Many excessive drinkers never go beyond this state. Others, however, proceed to a state of *habitual symptomatic excessive drinking* which consists of either daily drinking, particularly in countries where wine or beer are customarily consumed, or intermittent bouts of heavy drinking, particularly in countries or social groups in which the consumption of hard liquor is common. (Some hard liquor drinkers drink every day and some do not.) The individual is now well on the way to losing control of his behavior. In the next and final stage he has lost all control and is unable to stop drinking once he starts. He may now be described as an *addictive drinker* or an *alcoholic addict.* Drinking has become a compulsion; he *must* drink regardless of consequences. Many addicts drink a quart or more of hard liquor every day, a consumption that seems unbelievable to the nonalcoholic.

E. M. Jellinek, an outstanding authority on alcoholism, analyzed the histories of more than 2000 male alcoholics and formulated a comprehensive account (1951) of the development of addiction which is, in the main, compatible with the formulation of the World Health Organization committee. (1) The *prealcoholic symptomatic phase* lasts from several months to two years and is characterized by occasional or constant drinking to obtain relief from excessive tension. Toward the end of this phase the individual begins to experience an increased tolerance for alcohol and needs a larger amount to reach the same stage of sedation.

(2) The beginning of the *prodromal phase* is characterized by the sudden onset of blackouts for some of the periods of drinking. During this phase dependency upon alcohol increases and is manifested in surreptitious rather than open drinking, preoccupation with alcohol, gulping down the first drink or two, guilt feelings about drinking, avoiding reference to alcohol in conversation, and a greater frequency of blackouts than in the previous stage.

(3) The *crucial phase of addiction* is initiated by a loss of behavioral control. Drinking becomes quite conspicuous and the drinker's parents, wife, friends or employer begin to reprove and warn him. He may respond with grandiosity and aggression, or with alibis designed to rationalize his drinking, or with persistent remorse and limited periods of total abstinence. He is likely to drop friends and lose jobs. As he becomes more and more dependent upon alcohol he manifests a loss of outside interests, concern over protecting his supply of liquor, and marked self-pity. He contemplates or carries through a flight to a new environment. He neglects his diet and is likely to be hospitalized for the first time. Metabolic changes and decrease in the sexual drive occur. If married, he responds to his loss of sexual drive by jealousy or even paranoid de-

lusions of infidelity. At about this time he begins to drink regularly in the morning in order to escape the increasingly intolerable burden of his misery, remorse, and deteriorating reality situation. (One of the authors was acquainted with an individual who began drinking every day on the stroke of 12 noon and continued until he passed out in the evening. "I never touch a drop in the morning," he proudly asserted.)

(4) The *chronic phase of alcohol addiction* is initiated by prolonged bouts of intoxication— "benders"—which often lead to marked ethical deterioration, impairment of thinking and, in about 10 per cent of chronic alcoholics, alcoholic psychoses (described in the next section). The alcoholic now tends to drink with anyone, regardless of social level or personal characteristics, who will accept him. He may drink anything that contains alcohol, even rubbing alcohol. At about this time a loss of tolerance for alcohol is likely to take the place of the previous increase in tolerance. The loss is usually related to a decreased ability of the liver to accomplish oxidation. Other symptoms of this stage listed by Jellinek are indefinable fears, tremors, psychomotor inhibitions, obsessive thinking and the development of vague religious desires. At this point the addict admits defeat but unless he receives therapy is likely to continue drinking.

The sequence just described is true for many alcoholics. Many others, however, skip some intermediate stages and pass very rapidly from total abstention to chronic addiction. Whether addiction is reached slowly or rapidly, it involves the use of alcohol as a drug, not as a beverage to be drunk like other beverages. To quote Bacon (1958), "He [the alcoholic] is no more a drinker than a kleptomaniac is a customer or a pyromaniac is a campfire girl. Alcoholics may consume alcohol. They do not drink." The essayist G. K. Chesterton once remarked that the alcoholic and the abstainer both make the same mistake: they regard wine as a drug and not as a drink. The powerful grip of alcohol is described in the following excerpt from *The Lost Weekend,** a novel about an alcoholic:

The windows are blue-white. Was it early morning or evening? He lay watching the panes between the curtains and wondered if they would whiten into day-

---

*Reprinted with the permission of Farrar, Straus & Giroux, Inc. from *The Lost Weekend* by Charles Jackson, Copyright Charles Jackson 1944.

light or thicken into dusk. He wondered what time it was, what day. The clock said 6:10 but that told him nothing.

He had awakened fully dressed on the couch in the living room. His feet burned. He reached down and unlaced his shoes and kicked them off. He rose to a sitting position and pulled off his coat and vest, untied his tie and loosened his collar. Automatically his hand groped beside the couch for the pint on the floor. His heart sank as he found it, and found it empty.

Had he been sleeping all night, or all night and all the next day? There was no way of telling till the light changed outside, for better or worse. If it were evening, thank Christ. He could go out and buy another, a dozen more. But if morning—He feared to find out; for if it were morning, dawn, he would be cut off till nine or after and so made to suffer the punishment he always promised himself to avoid. It would be like the dreaded Sunday, always (at these times) the day most abhorred of all the week; for on Sundays the bars did not open till two in the afternoon and the liquor stores did not open at all. Once again he had not been clever enough to provide a supply against this very thing; again he had lost all perspective and forgotten his inescapable desperation of the morning, so much more urgent and demanding than any need of the evening before. Last night it had been merely drink. It was medicine now.

He lifted the empty pint to his mouth. One warm drop crawled like slow syrup through the neck of the bottle. It lay on his tongue, useless, all but impossible to swallow. He thought of all the mornings (and as he thought of them he knew he was in for another cycle of harrowing mornings) when, at such times as these, he would drag himself into the kitchen and examine the line-up of empty quarts and pints on the floor under the sink, pick them up separately and hold them upside down over a small glass, one by one for minutes at a time, exacting a last sticky drop from one bottle, two drops from another, maybe nothing from a third, and so on through a long patient nerve-wracking process till he had collected enough, perhaps, to cover the bottom of the glass. It was like a rite—the slow drinking of it still more so: and it was never enough.

Though he hated this need of his, hated his dependency on the pick-up, so often impossible to get—hated it for what it did to him till he got it—all the same he had a profound and superior contempt for those who spurned liquor on the morning after, whose stomachs, shaken as they were by the dissipation of the night, turned and retched at the very thought of it. How often he had been dumbfounded—at first incredulous, then contemptuous—to hear someone say, after a night of drinking, "God, take it away. I don't want to smell it, I don't want to *see* it even, take it out of my sight!"—this at the very moment when he wanted and needed it most. How different that reaction was from his own, and how revealing. Clearly it was the difference between the alcoholic and the non-. He was angry to know this, but he knew it; he knew it far better than others; and he

kept the knowledge to himself. It would tell them too much about him, tell them he was the drinker who couldn't stop—an abhorrent thing, more shocking to the man who went in for the occasional heavy weekend spree than it ever was to the abstainer. The hair of the dog was no lighthearted joke with him as it was with the others; but he could kid about it with the rest, if need be, hiding his agonized impatience till such time as he was able to sneak a drink or, if offered one as a dare in the presence of others (dare!), quench his thirst with affected bravery amid the shudders of his hungover friends.

Thirst—there was a misnomer. He could honestly say he had never had a thirst for liquor or a craving for drink as such, no, not even in hangover. It wasn't because he was thirsty that he drank, and he didn't drink because he liked the taste (actually whisky was dreadful to the palate; he swallowed at once to get it down as quickly as possible): he drank for what it did to him. As for quenching his thirst, liquor did exactly the opposite. To quench is to slake or to satisfy, to give you enough. Liquor couldn't do that. One drink led inevitably to the next, more demanded more, they became progressively easier and easier, culminating in the desperate need, no longer easy, that shook him on days such as these. His need to breathe was not more urgent.

The Long-Range Effects of Addiction to Alcohol

Chronic alcoholism may culminate in severe disturbances of bodily and behavioral functions. The catalogue of disturbances includes damage to the endocrine glands, particularly the thyroid and ovary; cardiac decompensation (failure of heart functioning); hypertension; a tendency to capillary hemorrhages, often responsible for the redness and swelling of the face, especially the nose; shrinking and inflammation of the lining of the stomach; widespread tremors; autonomic disturbances; and cirrhosis of the liver, in which liver cells are replaced by fibrous tissue that contracts and strangles the blood circulation through the liver. In addition, the peripheral and central nervous systems may be disordered, and the central disorders may result in a number of neurological and psychotic syndromes. (Of all first admissions in 1968 to public hospitals for mental disease, 13.5 per cent were classified as alcohol addiction.) The major psychotic syndromes to be considered are:

1. Delirium tremens
2. Alcoholic hallucinosis
3. Wernicke's syndrome
4. Korsakoff's syndrome
5. Chronic alcoholic deterioration.

Some of these, e.g., delirium tremens, are short-lived and acute; others, e.g., chronic alcoholic deterioration, are long-lasting or irreversible. There is no sharp line between the acute and chronic consequences of chronic alcoholism, however, for the former often shade into the latter. An attack of delirium tremens or some other "acute" syndrome may mark the beginning of chronic deterioration.

Before outlining the nature of these syndromes, a word is in order regarding etiology. Alcohol is not necessarily the direct cause of "alcoholic" psychoses. Such psychoses are frequently due to *nutritional deficiencies* that tend to accompany chronic alcoholism, especially vitamin deficiencies, or to *sudden withdrawal of alcohol* from cells that have adapted to it over prolonged periods of times.

The evidence for this statement is considerable. First, it is known that independent of alcoholic intake, a deficiency of vitamin B_1 (thiamine) will cause cardiac decompensation, inflammation of peripheral nerves and acute or chronic brain syndromes; a deficiency of nicotinic acid (niacin, a member of the vitamin B_2 complex) will also cause acute or chronic brain syndromes; and deficiencies of vitamins C or K will cause a tendency to hemorrhage.

Second, most alcoholics suffer from nutritional deficiencies for a number of reasons. (a) Alcohol is expensive, and the typical alcoholic spends what money he has—he may have very little because he cannot hold a job—on alcohol rather than food. (b) Alcohol is itself high in calories—one pint of 100-proof whiskey contains approximately 1400 calories—so that it provides sufficient energy even without food. However, alcohol does *not* provide needed vitamins and minerals. (c) Alcoholics are prone to various infections and other bodily disorders that require an increased vitamin intake. The alcoholic needs more vitamins—but gets less—than the nonalcoholic.

Third, it is known that the abrupt withdrawal of a variety of sedative drugs (other than alcohol) after a lengthy period of usage may provoke an acute brain syndrome that resembles delirium tremens, sometimes accompanied by epileptic seizures (Kalinowski, 1958).

Delirium Tremens. About 5 per cent of alcoholics are susceptible to delirium tremens, the so-called "D.T.'s." Most often an attack is preceded by a period of heavy drinking, but it may occur as a consequence of sudden abstention from alcohol. Delirium tremens is a special case of delirium, an organic and behavior disturbance which may occur in nonalcoholics due to brain infection or the destruction of brain cells which sometimes result from a large number of diseases, metabolic disorders and so forth. (Delirium is one of two manifestations of acute brain disorder; the other is stupor or coma.)

Delirium tremens begins with a prodromal or warning phase in which the patient feels anxious and irritable and is oversensitive to external stimuli. This is followed by the phase of delirium tremens proper. The patient becomes confused, disoriented, excited and apprehensive. His consciousness is cloudy, his span of attention limited, and he is restless and unable to sleep. He becomes incoherent, loses motor coordination and displays a coarse tremor of the arms and legs ("the shakes"). He perspires profusely, has a rapid pulse, and experiences headache, loss of appetite, nausea and generalized weakness.

Most prominent of all the symptoms of delirium tremens, however, are the vivid illusions and hallucinations, mostly visual. The patient sees unpleasant or frightening creatures, such as snakes and cockroaches, climbing up and down the walls of his room or even crawling on his body. (Contrary to popular belief, alcoholics rarely hallucinate pink elephants.) The animals or insects change rapidly in color, form and size. Sometimes they are microscopic and sometimes large and so frightening that the patient may experience panic and harm himself in attempts to escape from them. Tactile hallucinations may also occur in which the terrified patient feels as well as sees creatures crawling on him.

Fortunately, delirious patients are suggestible and it is sometimes possible to talk them out of some of their symptoms for at least brief periods. However, delirium tremens is no light matter; it is fatal in 3 or 4 per cent of cases. The majority of patients recover in a few days to a week, particularly if vitamins and other nutritional substances are administered. Usually, the patient is so frightened that for some time he abstains from alcohol, but sooner or later he resumes drinking until the next attack.

The following passage from Mark Twain's *The Adventures of Huckleberry Finn* is a vivid and accurate description of tactile hallucinations and auditory illusions in delirium tremens. (The narrator is young Huck; the alcoholic is his father.)

I don't know how long I was asleep, but all of a sudden there was an awful scream and I was up. There was pap looking wild, and skipping around every which way and yelling about snakes. He said they was crawling up his legs; and then he would give a jump and scream, and say one had bit him on the cheek—but I couldn't see no snakes. He started and run round and round the cabin, hollering "Take him off! take him off; he's biting me on the neck!" I never see a man look so wild in the eyes. Pretty soon he was all fagged out, and fell down panting; then he rolled over and over wonderful fast, kicking things every which way, and striking and grabbing at the air with his hands, and screaming and saying there was devils a-hold of him. He wore out by and by, and laid still awhile, moaning. Then he laid stiller, and didn't make a sound. I could hear the owls and wolves away off in the woods, and it seemed terrible still. He was laying over by the corner. By and by he raised up part way and listened, with his head to one side. He says, very low: "Tramp—tramp—tramp; that's the dead; tramp—tramp—tramp; they're coming after me, but I won't go. Oh, they're here! don't touch me—don't! hands off—they're cold; let go. Oh, let a poor devil alone!" Then he went down on all fours and crawled off, begging them to let him alone, and he rolled himself up in his blanket and wallowed in under the old pine table, still a-begging; and then he went to crying. I would hear him through the blanket. . . .

Alcoholic Hallucinosis. This is a relatively rare syndrome to which some chronic alcoholics are subject. It has certain similarities to delirium tremens and certain differences from it; the patient with alcoholic hallucinosis is delirious but he has auditory rather than visual hallucinations and does not have tremors. The syndrome lasts up to several weeks, somewhat longer than delirium tremens. Essentially, alcoholic hallucinosis seems to be a release of latent paranoid or schizophrenic tendencies by alcohol. The patient hears voices which accuse him of sinfulness, particularly of a sexual type, and also threaten to punish and torture him. He misinterprets sounds: he hears a door closing as a pistol shot. He may become frightened and seek protection. In some instances patients suffering from alcoholic hallucinosis have committed suicide.

Wernicke's Syndrome. Named after the German neurologist Karl Wernicke (1848–1905), this syndrome is marked by ataxia (incoordination and inability to maintain balance in standing or walking), clouding of consciousness and paralysis of eye muscles. Wernicke's syndrome involves degeneration of the central nervous system, especially in the midbrain. It has an insidious onset, often following an attack of delirium, and may worsen with time until the

patient becomes stuporous. As with the other psychotic consequences of chronic alcoholism, Wernicke's syndrome occurs in nonalcoholics also as a result of vitamin deficiency but it has undergone a marked decrease in incidence since the early 1940's, apparently as a result of the enrichment of bread and flour with vitamins.

Korsakoff's Syndrome. This syndrome attacks about 1 per cent of chronic alcoholics, sometimes immediately following delirium tremens and sometimes not. It also occurs in nonalcoholics as a result of infections, ingestion of metallic poisons or anything that involves a vitamin B deficiency. The syndrome was named for the Russian neurologist and psychiatrist Sergei Korsakoff (1854–1900) who first described it.

Korsakoff's syndrome has three major manifestations: polyneuritis, amnesia and confabulation. Polyneuritis consists of an inflammation of a large number of peripheral nerves; in severe cases it is accompanied by diminished sensation, the wasting away of muscles and paralysis. Amnesia and confabulation are manifested in a loss of memory for recent events and the filling of the memory gaps by tales of imaginary events. Thompson (1959) cites the case of a patient with Korsakoff's psychosis "who was examined on a hot summer day in a psychiatric hospital. Her room opened on a courtyard into which refuse had been thrown by other patients, and the odor from it was quite obnoxious. When asked where she was, the patient said, 'You are a doctor, aren't you? You must be the ship's doctor.' When asked where she got aboard the ship she said, 'Yesterday in San Francisco. Yes,' she said, 'see, we are coming into New York harbor now.' The examiner asked her if she had enjoyed the trip and she replied, taking a deep breath of the stench-filled air from the courtyard, 'Oh, yes, isn't this sea breeze refreshing!'" As can be seen from this excerpt, the patient may be severely disoriented.

In many patients the symptoms can be arrested by administration of massive vitamin doses. Complete cures are rare, however, and a residue of permanent intellectual deterioration is common. The deterioration manifested in the following case is fairly typical:

A 65-year-old lawyer with a history of chronic alcoholism was admitted to a general hospital after three days of confused and irrational behavior. Eight years previously he had been hospitalized when the veins at the junction of the esophagus and stomach had ruptured due to cirrhosis of the liver. The patient's brother was also alcoholic and his wife was quite neurotic, partly a cause and partly a result of his drinking.

Two weeks before the second admission the patient's wife had instituted divorce proceedings. Frustrated and upset, he increased his already heavy alcoholic consumption and also began to take large doses of the hypnotic drug Nembutal. Four days before admission he suddenly stopped drinking; the following day he took several Nembutal capsules and that night he became violently excited and began to tear up the house and destroy furniture. (Basically, his excitement appeared to be precipitated by withdrawal from alcohol, complicated by the use of drugs.) The following morning he was aggressive and confused. His wife called an ambulance but he refused to get into it. By afternoon he was running around naked outdoors; he was overpowered and taken to a hospital where he was sedated, tranquilized and given intravenous fluids. However, he remained extremely confused and irrational. Moreover, he was found to have a large bruise on the back of the head, raising the possibility that his brain syndrome might have been caused, or at least complicated, by a head injury.

During the next few days he was incontinent, semicomatose and close to death. Tests for traumatic injury were negative and his confusion, therefore, was attributed to alcoholism.

As he began to recover, he displayed the clinical signs of Korsakoff's syndrome. His memory for recent events was extremely poor and he filled the gaps by confabulation. Polyneuritis was manifested in diminished sensation and muscular weakness. He was also disoriented for time and did not even know what year it was. Asked to subtract 7 from 100 successively—i.e., 93, 86, 79 and so on—his responses were "93, 89, 72. . . ." (The 100-minus-7 test is a standard, quick method of appraising intellectual impairment.) He maintained that nothing was the matter with him except that he must have been hit on the head, and he contradicted reality by denying both his alcoholism and marital discord. He had amnesia for his wife's divorce suit.

The patient was injected with large doses of vitamins, after which there was a marked and rapid improvement in intellectual functioning. However, one month after admission his I.Q. was only 107, clearly lower than it must have been when he had successfully practiced law. Vocabulary was relatively well preserved but there was considerable impairment in the nonverbal components of intelligence, a pattern typical of brain syndromes. Memory remained fairly poor and he showed evidence of concrete thinking and perseveration. Emotionally, however, he began to approach normality as his excitement dissipated. His wife dropped the divorce proceedings and he returned home after two months but was unable to resume his law practice.

Chronic Alcoholic Deterioration. After many years of excessive drinking—in some patients

30 years or more—a process of irreversible intellectual deterioration is likely to occur. The deterioration begins with judgment and the abstract capacities and then proceeds to the more primitive psychological functions such as simple attention and memory. Emotional deterioration also occurs and the individual manifests a loss of pride and a tendency to flatness of affect, irritability or impulsiveness.

Obviously dire social, occupational and familial consequences are inevitable with chronic alcoholic deterioration. The individual becomes ambitionless, egocentric and irresponsible and cannot hold a job. He tends to be touchy and critical of anyone who appears to disapprove of his drinking. At home he is likely to be surly and brutal. Almost invariably there is sexual difficulty, in most instances both contributing to the pattern of alcoholism and resulting from it. (Small amounts of alcohol lead to increased sexual interest and stimulation, due to removal of cortical inhibition, but larger quantities cause sexual incapacity.) A vicious circle sets in: the alcoholic's progressive incapacities lead him deeper and deeper into frustration and interpersonal alienation, and the latter lead him to drink more and more and therefore to further deterioration.

The Causes of Alcoholism

Heredity and Other Biological Factors. There is evidence that among the close relatives of alcoholics the frequencies of alcoholism, sociopathy and criminality are high. In a study of 645 Swedish alcoholics, Åmark (1951) found that approximately 25 per cent of their brothers and fathers were also alcoholic. Bleuler (1955) intensively studied the relatives of 50 American and 50 Swiss chronic alcoholics and found that for the two groups combined more than 28 per cent of the fathers, 5 per cent of the mothers, and 15 per cent of the brothers and 5 per cent of the sisters older than 40 were alcoholics. Neuroses and psychopathic personality were also unduly frequent. In contrast, schizophrenia, manic-depression, epilepsy and mental deficiency were no higher than expectancy, suggesting that certain specific tendencies to psychological disturbance are associated with alcoholism and others not.

Kaij (1957) studied the drinking habits of 26 monozygotic twin pairs and 56 dizygotic twin pairs of the same sex. The concordance rates for drinking were 65 per cent among the MZ twins and 39 per cent among the DZ twins, yielding an index of heritability for drinking behavior of 0.50. However, it should be noted that the variable here is drinking, not alcoholism. Mardones et al. (1953) found a positive correlation between the alcohol consumption of selectively bred parent rats and the amount consumed by their offspring, with body weight held constant. The results of this study are presented for the third through seventh generations in Table 16-1, modified from Mardones' original table. It is questionable, of course, whether these results can be applied to humans.

Several investigators have suggested that an important factor contributing to alcoholism is a congenital nutritional peculiarity. Williams (1957) postulated that some persons have unusually strong inborn requirements for certain food elements—vitamins, enzymes or minerals. If such a requirement is unsatisfied, the individual begins to crave alcohol as a substitute. (The craving is not the same as a liking for the taste of alcohol. Some alcoholics like the taste but some do not. The true addict will drink the most repellent concoctions provided they contain alcohol.)

In support of his theory, Williams gave adequately fed rats a choice of water or alcohol to drink. It was found that some animals drank the alcohol and some avoided it. A group of rats placed on a diet deficient in vitamins consumed more alcohol than a control group whose diet was supplemented by vitamins.

Williams' results are striking but it is dubious whether they support the theory that alcoholism is due to a combination of genetic and nutritional factors. First, the rats were limited to a choice of alcohol or water; other investigators have shown that given a third choice of a sugar solution or of fats in emulsion, vitamin-deprived rats will prefer either of these food elements to alcohol. Second, even if the theory were adequate to explain why rats drink, it would not necessarily be relevant to the origins of human alcoholism. Although various biochemical differences between alcoholic and nonalcoholic individuals have been found, leading to the speculation that alcoholics are congenitally different from other persons, it is possible and even likely that the biochemical differences are the result of excessive drinking rather than its cause. In order to demonstrate beyond question that a genetic basis exists for some bodily characteristic predisposing some persons to alcoholism, it would be necessary to make statistical comparisons of the characteristic among pre-alcoholics (to avoid the possibility that it has resulted from alcoholism), among various classes of their relatives and among nonalcoholic controls. To date, nothing of the sort has been done. The tendency of alcoholics to concentrate in families can be adequately explained, without assuming a genetic basis, by imitative learning, the sharing of similar experiences and the family transmission of neurotic or sociopathic characteristics. In a highly relevant study, Roe et al. (1945) found that children who have been separated from alcoholic parents and placed in foster homes are no more likely to become alcoholics in later years than children whose parents are not alcoholic.

A biological but not necessarily genetic variable that affects consumption of alcohol is sensitivity to it: many people are made ill by very small quantities. Since they lack a normal tolerance for alcohol, they cannot get drunk and cannot possibly develop into alcoholics.

It has also been speculated that endocrine factors may cause alcoholism. In Bleuler's study, a wide variety of endocrine malfunctions—particularly thyroid, pituitary and gonadal—

TABLE 16-1. Alcohol Intake of Offspring of Rats Selected with Respect to Alcohol Consumption*

| Parents' Consumption† | Percentage of Offspring Whose Alcohol Consumption Falls Within Indicated Range | | | |
	.00–.19	.20–.39	.40–.59	.60+
.00–.19	61.4	29.6	5.8	3.2
.20–.39	29.6	42.4	22.5	5.6
.40–.59	27.6	31.9	26.1	14.5
.60+	25.0	19.5	22.3	33.3

*Data from Mardones, R. J., Segovia, N. M., and Hederra, A. D. 1953. Heredity of experimental alcohol preference in rats. II. Coefficient of heredity. Quart. J. Stud. Alcohol, *14*:1–2.
†Consumption measured in cubic centimeters per day, per 100 grams of body weight.

were found in 28 per cent of both the American and Swiss samples. In some instances there appeared to be no causal relationship between the endocrine malfunction and the alcoholism; in others the malfunction seemed to result from the alcoholism; but in still others the endocrine defects appeared to lead to a personality disorder which in turn led to excessive drinking in order to obtain relief from anxiety and tension.

Psychological Determinants. The typical individual who drinks heavily does so to reduce anxiety. (A number of people avoid alcohol because, paradoxically, they find the feeling of relaxation and release from anxiety alarming and unpleasant.) Excessive drinking usually begins as a symptom of personality instability. It may also be a response to external stress; during World War II a number of relatively stable members of the Air Corps defended themselves against a consciousness of extreme danger by drinking to excess between missions.

In various psychoanalytic interpretations of drinking, the emphasis has been on its symptomatic and defensive nature, although each analyst has employed his own concepts. Freud (1912, 1917) interpreted drinking as a regression to the oral stage of psychosexuality in which the infant is dependent and free of responsibility. Adler (1941) emphasized the desire of the drinker to remove powerful feelings of inferiority as well as to escape responsibility. Rado (1933) noted that the euphoria produced by alcohol is a unique source of satisfaction in a life otherwise ridden with boredom, frustration and disappointment. Alcohol permits fulfillment in fantasy of the omnipotent and megalomaniac wish, persisting from infancy, to be the unchallenged master of a disorganized world.

A learning theory approach to the explanation of excessive drinking also emphasizes anxiety and frustration. As the drinker repetitively practices the sequence of anxiety, drinking, and immediate relief from anxiety, his drinking behavior becomes a stronger and stronger learned habit. In a series of experiments with cats, Masserman and Yum (1946) demonstrated the manner in which consumption of alcohol can be reinforced by relief from motivational conflict and anxiety. Cats were first trained to obtain food by operating a switch which opened a box in which the food was stored. They were then subjected to air blasts or electric shocks whenever they opened the box and they reacted with

"neurotic" fright, apprehension and avoidance of the switch. If given alcohol at this point, they once again operated the switch spontaneously for the food reward despite continued air blasts or shocks. More importantly, about half the cats learned to *prefer* milk containing alcohol to plain milk, and continued to do so as long as their experimentally induced "neuroses" persisted.

Using rats instead of cats, Conger (1951) replicated the work of Masserman and Yum and advanced it further. An approach-avoidance conflict was created by using food and electric shocks as the opposing reinforcements. Conger then demonstrated that, as with cats, alcohol reduced the conflict. Next, he performed an experiment in which one group of rats was taught to run to food and another to run away from pain. The strength of the tendency to approach food or avoid pain was measured by the subject's pull against a calibrated spring when temporarily restrained. Within the two groups, half the animals were given alcohol and half were not. It was found that alcohol produced a slight decrease in the pull of hungry animals toward food but a very marked decrease in the pull of frightened animals away from the area where they had been shocked in earlier trials. Alcohol thus acted not to heighten approach—in fact, it reduced it slightly—but to reduce fear and avoidance, just as it does in humans.

In contrast to these experimental designs, however, the human alcoholic in real life is not only rewarded by diminution of fear but also punished by negative consequences, from hangovers to illness, job loss, family difficulties and all the other woes previously discussed. He continues to drink because these negative consequences are *delayed,* whereas the rewards are immediate. It will be recalled as a basic principle of learning that the shorter the interval between a behavior and its reinforcing consequences, the more effective the consequences are. Furthermore, if an excessive drinker becomes apprehensive about later negative consequences, he has a simple method of reducing his apprehension: he takes another drink.

The explanation of excessive drinking in terms of a learned response to anxiety is highly relevant but incomplete, since only a minority of anxious persons acquire the habit. There must, therefore, be other factors, some of them psychological. In *Three Contributions to the Theory of Sex,* Freud hypothesized that repressed homosexuality led to alcoholism. (It will be recalled that paranoia was also attributed to repressed homosexuality.) Disappointment in a mother, wife or lover drives the latent homosexual to drink with other men in order to obtain the emotional satisfactions that he has failed to receive from women.

Abraham (1926) took a somewhat different yet related approach. Emphasizing the fact that prowess in drinking is widely regarded as the equivalent of sexual prowess, he interpreted alcohol as a substitute for sex and likened this substitution to perversions such as voyeurism and fetishism. Excessive drinking, according to Abraham, is due to fixation at the oral level. Orality, in turn, is hypothesized to be due to severe frustration by the mother. A homosexual element is also present, for the frustrated boy turns to the father and develops homosexual tendencies.

A number of critics of psychoanalytic formulations have felt that although orality and latent homosexuality plays a significant role in the problems of some alcoholics, these traits do not in themselves offer sufficient impetus for the development of alcoholism. Still other factors must be present. Among these, hostility is important. Menninger (1938) interpreted alcohol addiction as a form of self-destruction that is excited by a sense of guilt and a need for punishment which are ultimately due to aggressiveness. Other observers and theoreticians, including Fenichel (1945), have stressed the alcoholic's passivity and narcissism. The typical alcoholic is interested in receiving gratification, not in gratifying others. In addition, personality testing and interviews with alcoholics have repeatedly resulted in their being described as immature and deficient in the ability to endure frustration. Alcoholics are also deficient in self-esteem and many have a strong need to brag and boast in order to feel self-important.

Some marital interaction patterns seem to support alcoholism more than others. Ewing and Fox (1968), for example, describe an interaction pattern in which the alcoholic behaves in an immature, dependent fashion and such behavior is subtly supported by the spouse. The non-alcoholic partner in this marital style does most of the real decision making, takes on most of the family responsibilities, and fosters the helplessness and dependency of the alcoholic. The pattern is more similar to the relationship between a parent and child than to what one would expect between two mature adults. Often each partner is extremely dependent. The al-

coholic acts immaturely so that the spouse is forced to take care of him. The spouse, on the other hand, handles her own dependency needs through the defense of reaction formation and takes care of others as she wishes she could be taken care of. Often as alcoholic husbands improve, the wives have to be helped to express their caring needs elsewhere, such as in hospital volunteer work. Also the wives often appear to be more comfortable with a man who acts like a mischievous boy than with a mature male who makes more interpersonal demands than simply being cared for.

It should not be concluded that there is an invariable alcoholic personality. Some alcoholics are highly impulsive and tend to act out, some are guilt-ridden and some show much more hostility than others. Many are socially introverted and shy; others are extraverted in the pre-alcoholic years and only begin to withdraw later. Alcohol serves different purposes for different people.

A variety of poor home conditions in childhood may contribute to these varied personality characteristics. In Bleuler's study, 22 per cent of the American and 28 per cent of the Swiss alcoholics came from homes that had been broken by death or separation before the subjects were 10 years old. In a sample of Canadian alcoholics, Gregory (1959) found that by 10 years of age 23 per cent had permanently lost one or both parents and 7.1 had lost *both* parents. These figures were higher than for any other diagnostic category except sociopathic personality.

Undesirable parental attitudes have been related to alcoholism by many observers, e.g., Knight (1937). For example, the pre-alcoholic child may be overindulged by a permissive mother, fail to learn self-control and react to frustration with intense rage. His tendency toward rage may be further reinforced by an inconsistent father who unpredictably gratifies the child's needs at one time and denies them at another. The result is a personality pattern of dependence, intense desire for indulgence and deep feelings of rejection, inferiority and guilt. In adolescence, drinking may begin as a desperate expression of "manly" behavior in defiance of parental wishes. The father may attempt to forbid drinking even if he himself is alcoholic and irresponsible.

Alcoholism has also been linked to parental attitudes of direct rejection (e.g., Schilder, 1941). Ridicule, degradation, threats and corporal punishment may push the child deeper and deeper into the abyss of insecurity. He learns to fear interpersonal relationships and may retreat into alcohol as a substitute satisfaction.

Although, as just indicated, the early relationships and experiences of alcoholics are diverse, they are rarely favorable. In Bleuler's study, only 30 per cent of the alcoholics had had a favorable home environment in childhood. Neurosis and sociopathic personality are the two most frequent forms of pre-existing psychological disturbance in alcoholism. Neurotic alcoholics most often come from an over-controlling, demanding, anxiety-provoking family environment, and sociopathic alcoholics from homes marked by indifference, rejection and deprivation.

In the two cases of alcoholism described in the following paragraphs, many of the etiological factors just reviewed are present. By coincidence, there are a number of common factors in the two cases; some are widespread among alcoholics generally and some are relatively infrequent. Both patients were sociopaths; both became less sociopathic with time; both came from high-status but unsatisfactory family backgrounds, different though the backgrounds were in specific details; both used other drugs as well as alcohol; eventually both became suicidal. A number of personality factors were also common to both, particularly an inability to tolerate frustration, hostility, demandingness, and a tendency—at first latent, but eventually overt—to internalize hostility and become depressed.

At the time of his first admission to a state hospital at the age of 24, the patient, an unmarried and unemployed laborer, already had a long history of antisocial behavior, promiscuity and addiction to alcohol and other drugs. Beginning at age 14, he had been a frequent patient in a general hospital. There had been eight brief admissions to private sanatoria for alcoholics, a number of arrests for public intoxication and drunken driving, and two jail terms for assault.

The patient had been born into a wealthy and respected family in a small town. The patient's father, a successful and popular businessman, drank excessively and his death at the age of 57 was partly due to alcoholism. The mother also drank to excess. The parents exercised little control over the patient as a child, and he was cared for by nursemaids. His father taught him to pour drinks for guests of the family when he was very young and he reported that he began to drain the glasses at parties in his home before he was six; by the time he was 12 he drank almost a pint of liquor every weekend and by 17 was drinking up to three bottles every day. His father provided him with money to buy liquor and shielded him from punishment for drunken driving and other consequences of his drinking.

The patient was expelled from high school in his freshman year for striking a teacher. He then attended a private school until the eleventh grade when he changed the date on his birth certificate and joined the Army paratroops. After discharge, he was unemployed for six months; he drank heavily and needed repeated care at a sanatorium. When a job was obtained for him he quit within a month. On his third arrest for drunken driving he was jailed. His father bailed him out with the warning that no more money would be forthcoming. The patient left town and worked as a laborer—he had never acquired any useful skills—but returned home when his father died. During the next few years he was jailed for intoxication, for blackening his mother's eyes when he found a male friend visiting her, and for violating probation by getting drunk. He assaulted and badly hurt a prison guard in an escape attempt and was sentenced to two additional years in prison. When released, he began to use a variety of stimulant, sedative and narcotic drugs as well as alcohol.

The patient was extremely muscular, good looking, and above average in intelligence (I.Q. 115). Although any type of frustration led to extreme anger and impulsive violence, he was pleasant and friendly when not frustrated. Beginning at age 12 he had had a long series of heterosexual relationships; at 13 he had an affair with a women twice his age and during the next 10 years led a life of almost unbelievable promiscuity, never taking a girl out without having sexual relations with her and usually dropping her after one or two experiences.

On admission to the state hospital, he appeared surly, narcissistic, hostile and "tough." A report by a female staff member based on personality testing described him as manifesting "antisocial tendencies, inability to profit by experience, impulsive decisions, a lack of deep emotional responsiveness, and a rather shallow concern for other people and low frustration tolerance." She emphasized that his alcoholism was only a symptom of his deep psychopathic tendencies, but she undertook psychotherapy with him for the symptom. Ten months after admission, the patient was discharged; two weeks later he and his therapist —whom he had thoroughly succeeded in charming during the interviews—were married.

Although the patient was repeatedly admitted to various hospitals for alcoholism during the next 10 years, the marriage had a stabilizing effect and, contrary to expectations, he continued to live with his wife and the children she bore him. He provided adequately for them and changed residence only infrequently. His pattern of drinking and taking drugs also changed, becoming episodic rather than continuous. Like many sociopaths, he began to "burn out" as the years went by. His last recorded hospitalization followed an impulsive but nevertheless serious attempt while drugged to cut his throat with a razor blade; 42 stitches were required. The extent to which his sociopathy had diminished was indicated by his behavior in the hospital on this occasion: he was quite amiable, and intropunitively repentant.

* * *

A 28-year-old married woman of average intelligence with a lifelong history of egocentric and impulsive behavior was admitted to a state hospital after threatening to throw herself out of a moving car and superficially cutting one of her wrists. Personality testing in the hospital revealed a tendency to both sociopathy and hypomanic overactivity. For several years she had been increasingly dependent on alcohol and barbiturates (sedative drugs).

The patient was the only child of parents who had been in their forties when she was born. Her father, a university professor, was cold, distant and completely preoccupied with intellectual pursuits. When the patient started school, he criticized her academic performance and called her "beautiful but dumb." He was disturbed by her temper tantrums but unable to set firm and consistent limits for her. Sometimes he lectured her sternly and sometimes he let unacceptable behavior pass unnoticed. The mother died when the patient was a child and the father remarried; the stepmother was unable to get along with either the child or the father. The patient attended a series of private schools, each of which she left either because she disliked the school or because of behavior intolerable to the school authorities. Eventually she managed to graduate from high school.

The patient was a very charming, beautiful, narcissistic and demanding girl. After high school she worked as a model and led a very active social life; when she married at 21 she continued to work. Some years later she became dissatisfied with her husband, both sexually and because he did not advance in his career as rapidly as she wished. She had been considering a divorce for a year prior to hospitalization and had embarked on a number of extramarital sexual relationships. However, she found no lasting satisfaction in modeling, social life, promiscuity or anything else, and began to drink to excess and take large doses of barbiturates in the daytime as well as at night. Later she gave boredom and an effort to forget domestic and financial troubles as the reasons for her behavior. Asked about her temper tantrums, she said, "I always do that—if they do me some good, I have them." She was incapable of genuine affection and freely admitted that she used others only to gratify her immediate whims. The suicidal gestures which led to her hospital admission had been precipitated by anger with her husband.

On arrival in the hospital, she threatened suit for illegal detention, but in sociopathic fashion became composed and cooperative as soon as she found that her threats were ineffective. She accepted an invitation to participate in psychotherapy but used the interviews solely to inflate her ego and gratify her narcissism.

After three weeks she was discharged, but her addictions resulted in several additional hospitalizations during the following year. Then her pattern of life ended abruptly: while out with another man she suffered a severe facial injury in an automobile accident, thus losing one of her most prized possessions. Plastic surgery was performed and there was every reason to believe that in time there would be very little facial disfigurement. However, her fragile ego could not tolerate even a temporary loss of beauty and she became quite depressed, indulged in an orgy of self-pity and alcohol, and was readmitted to the hospital. Soon afterward she received a letter from her husband threatening to divorce her unless she controlled her behavior, and a week later, after managing to obtain a large quantity of sedatives in the hospital, she committed suicide by swallowing them all. Her suicide appeared to be a hostile act of retribution against her father and husband as well as a symptom of depression.

Sociocultural Factors. Clear-cut differences have been found in the frequency of alcoholism among males and females. The sex ratio varies from country to country, from as low as two alcoholic males to one female in England, to as high as 20 to 1 in some Scandinavian countries. In the United States the ratio is almost 6 to 1. The only reasonable explanation of these differences is a sociocultural one: there is a double standard which, although it varies considerably from country to country, objects to the female drinker more than to the male. As attitudes toward women change, the sex ratio for alcoholism changes; in recent years the proportion of female alcoholics in the United States has apparently increased. There is also reason to believe that alcohol addiction in women develops more rapidly than in men. When a woman begins to drink heavily she must overcome such strong cultural sanctions that she loses all inner restraints and progresses rapidly to chronic alcoholism.

Occupational differences are marked in drinking behavior. Bartenders, for example, have a high frequency of alcoholism although a great many bartenders are total abstainers.

Several studies have documented the high frequency of alcoholism in the United States among persons of Irish extraction and a low frequency among Italians, Chinese and Jews (although the frequency of neuroses and of addiction to other drugs is relatively high among Jews). The common factor in the use of alcohol among Italians, Chinese and Jews is that all three groups permit the use of alcohol but *regulate the occasions* on which it may be used —at mealtimes, in religious or holiday celebrations and so on.

The prevalence of alcoholism in various countries may be reliably estimated from the number of deaths caused by cirrhosis of the liver, since a fairly constant proportion of such deaths are attributable to alcoholism. Table 16–2 contains the estimates for a number of countries. The rate for the United States is comparatively high. The highest and lowest frequencies occur in France and Italy respectively; in France the estimated prevalence is more than 5 per cent of the adult population. The low rate of alcoholism in Italy corresponds to the low rate among persons of Italian ancestry in the United States. It is noteworthy that France and Italy are wine-producing and wine-drinking countries and are geographically close. There is widespread agreement that the important difference between them is that—according to a survey made in 1952—only 1 per cent of Italians consume alcoholic beverages apart from meals, whereas in France it is socially acceptable to drink wine at any time, both with meals and between them.

A variable that may affect alcoholism is the general level of anxiety in a culture. Horton (1943) analyzed 56 primitive societies and concluded that the greater the degree of subsistence anxiety, the higher the consumption of alcohol. Societies with strong anxiety over possible crop failure, drought, flood or interference by power-ful neighbors tended toward insobriety. Horton's conclusion is plausible but speculative, since the variable of overall subsistence anxiety is difficult to assess objectively. It is also doubtful whether his analysis is applicable to alcoholism in nonprimitive societies.

Bales (1946) analyzed cultural differences and formulated a theory in which three types of cultural and social influences on rates of alcoholism are specified. The first is the degree to which the culture arouses inner tensions and acute needs for adjustment in its members; the second consists of the cultural attitudes toward drinking for the relief of tensions; and the third is the variation across cultures in providing suitable satisfactions other than alcohol.

Cultural attitudes toward drinking—the second of Bales' three factors—are quite complex. Bales distinguished four attitudes: the *abstinent,* the *ritual,* the *convivial* and the *utilitarian.* Moslems, Mormons and some other groups prescribe complete abstinence from alcohol; the taboo is rarely violated since violation would be an act of strong aggression that the individual can commit only at the cost of experiencing strong counter-anxiety. A consistently ritual attitude toward drinking, generally associated with religious observances, as among orthodox Jews, leads to a perception of alcohol as sacred; the use of alcohol for getting drunk becomes indecent and anxiety-provoking. In the convivial attitude, drinking is social rather than religious. It accompanies economic transactions, informal social interactions or birthdays, individual achievements and other events that are celebrated in a nonreligious manner. Excessive drinking is common where a convivial attitude toward alcohol prevails. The utilitarian attitude regards alcohol as a means of promoting self-interest and individual, rather than social, satisfaction. This attitude is typical of alcoholics, particularly in cultures with inadequate substitute satisfactions. Apparently, then, two of the cultural attitudes described by Bales keep drinking in check and two do not.

A somewhat different analysis of cultural factors is that of Ullman (1958): "In any group in which the drinking customs, values, and sanctions . . . are well-established, known to and agreed upon by all, the rate of alcoholism will be low. . . . Lack of integration in the sphere of drinking activities and attitudes is directly related to higher rates of alcoholism." On this basis, a low frequency of alcoholism is eventually due to a *clarity* of cultural attitude, whether the attitude consists of abhorrence of

TABLE 16–2. Estimated Prevalence of Alcoholism in Various Countries

	Alcoholics per 100,000 Population (20 Years and Older)	Year	Source
France	5200	1954	Jellinek (1954)
United States	4360	1955	Keller & Efron (1957)
Chile	2960	1950	Popham (1956)
Sweden	2580	1946	WHO (1951)
Switzerland	2100	1953	Popham (1956)
Denmark	1950	1948	WHO (1951)
Canada	1890	1956	
Norway	1560	1947	WHO (1951)
Finland	1430	1947	WHO (1951)
Australia	1340	1947	WHO (1951)
England and Wales	1100	1948	WHO (1951)
Italy	700	1954	Jellinek (1954)

From Popham, R. E., and Schmidt, W. 1958. Statistics of Alcohol Use and Alcoholism in Canada, 1871–1956. University of Toronto Press, p. 120.

alcohol or ritual regulation of its use. When the cultural attitude is unintegrated and inconsistent with the rest of the culture, the individual feels ambivalent toward drinking; it is undesirable but permitted, and he may therefore drink excessively.

A hypothesis advanced by Jellinek and elaborated by Popham (1959) interrelates sociocultural and individual factors. The hypothesis asserts that in cultures or social groups with a low acceptance of drinking, the frequency of alcoholism is low, but among the few individuals who do become alcoholic in such groups, the frequency of severe psychological disturbance is high. In groups with a high acceptance of drinking there is a much higher frequency of alcoholism but a relatively low frequency of severe psychological disturbance among the alcoholics. The theory is plausible but lacks verification.

Treatment

Alcoholism may be treated by: disintoxication procedures to remove the effects of toxins; deterrents to halt the use of alcohol; and procedures that attempt to remove the causes of addiction.

Disintoxication. The typical method of disintoxication starts with a complete withdrawal of alcohol rather than a gradual tapering off. Tranquilizing drugs may be administered to help minimize any physical disorganization brought on by the sudden abstinence. Vitamins, glucose and nonalcoholic fluids are usually administered to compensate for the alcoholic's dietary deficiencies. He may also be given various stimulants, insulin or cortisone to improve his metabolism.

Deterrent or Suppressive Measures. These treatments are unlikely to be curative by themselves but they often insure a period of freedom from alcohol during which measures leading to more lasting remission may be applied. The deterrents frequently employed are compulsory institutionalization, all too often in jails rather than hospitals, conditioned reflex treatment, and drugs that react with alcohol to produce illness.

In conditioned reflex therapy the patient is repeatedly given a substance to produce nausea and vomiting while he sees, smells and tastes an alcoholic drink. A conditioned aversion to liquor is likely to result but it is often temporary, and repeated conditioning is necessary to insure a lasting aversion.

Certain drugs, such as disulfiram (Antabuse), alter the metabolism of alcohol in the liver. If the patient drinks any alcohol within as many as three or four days after taking the drug, a toxic product forms and makes him violently—even dangerously—ill. Blood pressure drops sharply, cardiac palpitations occur and the patient has a feeling of impending death. In the standard Antabuse treatment, these effects are first demonstrated to the patient and thereafter he takes a daily dose of Antabuse at home. Of course, by not taking the drug the patient can quickly overcome his drug-induced intolerance of alcohol.

Treatment of Causes. Somatic measures such as ECT or the administration of tranquilizing or anti-depressant drugs are often employed when the addiction is associated with a functional psychotic disorder—schizophrenia, manic-depression or others. Psychotherapy is usually fruitless with alcoholics who are basically sociopathic, but is feasible with those who are neurotic. The patient must stop drinking prior to psychotherapy, a prerequisite best accomplished by institutionalization or other deterrent measures. The usual goals of intensive therapy with an alcoholic are insight into himself and the strengthening of his ego so that he will no longer need to drink. He must understand that abstinence will have to be total and lifelong; there is no way of converting an alcoholic into a moderate drinker. Unless he learns that a life without alcohol can be more satisfying than a life completely submerged in it, he will continue to drink.

The effectiveness of psychotherapy with alcoholics is a matter of dispute. Some investigators have reported cure rates of more than 50 per cent, particularly for a combination of psychotherapy and conditioned reflex therapy, but other reports have been far less impressive. In a study by Gerard, Saenger and Wile (1962), a follow-up of 299 patients who had been treated by various psychotherapeutic procedures in alcoholism clinics revealed that only 18 per cent had remained abstinent for at least one year. Furthermore, most of the patients stopped drinking apparently because they were afraid of police arrest, liver disease, or death, rather than because of the therapy.

Much better results have often been reported for group therapeutic approaches to alcoholism. Alcoholics Anonymous (A.A.), an organization that was established in 1935 and has since grown to more than 100,000 members, employs a group approach with strong emphasis on inspirational and spiritual elements. The organization functions as a proselyting agency to bring in new members and old ones who have relapsed. Individual members often help considerably in interpreting the nature of an alcoholic's problem to his family and in enlisting family cooperation in treatment. The alcoholic who joins may come to feel that he is no longer isolated, misunderstood and mistrusted.

Alcoholics Anonymous encourages each individual member to recognize that he lacks the power to control his drinking and should turn to a power greater than himself. He is helped to make a frank autobiographical review of his drinking and from day to day is given emotional support for abstention. The specific character of A.A. meetings varies from chapter to chapter; in some, religion is emphasized, others resemble a social club with a good deal of fellowship, and still others come very close to a professional group therapy program.

Many alcoholics begin to attend meetings and then drop out. (Over half the patients discontinue within a month any type of voluntary treatment of alcoholism.) Among those who continue A.A. membership for a protracted period, over 50 per cent have been reported as ceasing to drink, either permanently or with occasional relapses. A number of therapists have urged alcoholics to attend A.A. meetings as an adjunct to various deterrent measures or individual psychotherapy.

DRUG ADDICTION

In seeking relief from pain or boredom, man has learned to use a variety of drugs with one of four effects on the organism—sedation, tranquilization, stimulation, or production of delirium.

A *sedative* drug slows the organism and diminishes its responsiveness. The major sedatives include hypnotics and narcotics. *Hypnotics* are drugs used mainly to produce sleep, *narcotics,* primarily to relieve pain, produce numbness and insensibility, and, eventually, stupor.

The action of *tranquilizers* is in many respects like that of sedatives. The tranquilizer most likely to result in addiction is meprobamate.

A *stimulant* drug acts on the brain and sympathetic nervous system to increase alertness and motor activity and to prevent fatigue and sleep. As a rule, stimulants also increase

neuromuscular irritability and the level of anxiety.

A *deliriant* drug produces an acute brain syndrome marked by confusion, illusions and hallucinations, and usually, also, temporarily increased psychomotor activity.

Table 16–3 lists the drugs within each of these four classes that most commonly lead to habituation or addiction. Each drug group is either derived from a specific source or its members have a common chemical structure. Opium and its various products, for example, all come from the opium poppy (called "the plant of joy" by the ancient Sumerians). The barbiturates are chemically similar to each other; the amphetamines also resemble each other chemically. It should be noted that the table lists cocaine as a stimulant, although federal drug authorities classify it as a narcotic because, like the true narcotics, its use easily leads to addiction.

In the United States the favorite drug of narcotic addicts is heroin, the narcotic with the greatest potency, and morphine is preferred next. Cocaine addiction is relatively rare. In recent years barbiturate addiction has become very frequent, and marijuana (Indian hemp) has been used more and more. In the United States the latter is usually smoked in cigarettes; in India it is chewed or mixed with liquid.

TABLE 16–3. Drugs Leading to Habituation or Addiction

SEDATIVE DRUGS

Narcotics (pain relievers that also impair consciousness)
Opium and its products
Morphine, heroin, codeine, etc.
Synthetic substitutes for morphine
Demerol, methadone, etc.

Hypnotics (sleep producers)
Barbiturates
Amytal, Nembutal, Seconal, etc.
Nonbarbiturates
Bromides, paraldehyde, chloral hydrate, etc.

TRANQUILIZING DRUGS

Meprobamate (Equanil, Miltown)

STIMULANT DRUGS *(response facilitators)*

Cocaine
Caffeine
Nicotine
Amphetamines
Benzedrine, Dexedrine, Methedrine, etc.

DELIRIANT DRUGS *(delirium producers)*

Marijuana (hashish; Indian hemp)
Mescaline (from peyote)
Psilocybin (from mushrooms)
Bufotenin

The immediate effects of these drugs depend partly on personality. In vulnerable individuals a single large dose of a strong stimulant, such as cocaine or an amphetamine, may release latent symptoms of psychosis which disappear when the effects of the drug wear off. The immediate effects also vary from drug to drug, over and above the basic effects of sedation, stimulation, delirium production and so forth. Opium makes the individual drowsy but at the same time gives him a mistaken sense of mental clarity. He experiences a feeling of relaxation and euphoria, a pleasant state of reverie, a decrease of sexual desire and a distortion of the sense of time and space—a state sometimes described as "a sense of infinity." When these effects wear off after several hours he craves the drug again. Cocaine often produces headache and restlessness which are soon followed by several hours of euphoria. Some individuals, however, experience frightening and unpleasant hallucinations, both visual and tactile, in response to cocaine. Marijuana typically creates a euphoric state in which time seems slowed and the individual's intellectual and motor activities are retarded. Contrary to widespread belief, however, there is no evidence that marijuana results in long-range damage to the organism.

Long-Range Effects of Drug Addiction

The prolonged use of narcotics such as morphine or heroin is accompanied by profound changes in bodily functions and personality. The entire body adapts to the presence of a narcotic and develops an increasing tolerance for it so that progressively larger doses are necessary to produce the same effects. Concurrently, the individual develops an increasing emotional and physiological dependence on these effects to the extent that he feels acutely miserable whenever his body does not contain a sufficient quantity of the drug. Prolonged use of narcotics also results in lack of appetite, constipation, loss of weight and disinterest in sexual and social relationships. A moral and ethical deterioration is common, although the superego development of many addicts is defective even prior to the onset of addiction.

The sudden discontinuation of narcotics after prolonged use results in a variety of *withdrawal symptoms* characterized by over-activity of various organ systems. During a narcotic addiction, the organism is profoundly sedated; sudden removal of this sedation is violently stimulating, disorganizing and dangerous. Withdrawal symptoms include restlessness, nervousness, agonizingly painful muscular cramps, uncontrollable flow of tears, excessive perspiration, shivering, nausea, vomiting, diarrhea and weight loss of as much as 5 to 15 pounds in 24 hours. The intensity of withdrawal symptoms reaches its peak 72 hours after the last dose and then diminishes during the remainder of the first week. By the second week the symptoms are gone except for some residual nervousness, insomnia and muscular weakness.

Like the narcotics, barbiturates and other hypnotics taken over a long period lead to increased tolerance and dependency; withdrawal symptoms follow abrupt discontinuation. The hypnotics act primarily on the brain and, unlike narcotics, have relatively less effect on the rest of the body, so that the outstanding signs of prolonged use are intellectual impairment and disturbance of the motor functions dependent on the cerebellum. The patient manifests a lack of coordination, ataxia, slurred speech, tremors, choreiform movements (resembling the involuntary movements of chorea), and nystagmus. These effects are cumulative, even for barbiturates that are ordinarily eliminated from the body within a few hours. Abrupt withdrawal of hypnotics may be even more dangerous than abrupt withdrawal of narcotics. The individual may manifest epileptic seizures or an acute brain syndrome that appears identical with delirium tremens and lasts for several days. If not treated promptly by substitute sedatives and anti-convulsant drugs, the seizures may result in death. (Seizures and delirium have also been observed following the abrupt discontinuation of meprobamate.) The following excerpt from a case record describes the behavior of a middle-aged woman who had been taking large doses of barbiturates for many years. On withdrawal

. . . the patient developed signs of an acute brain syndrome. She had a marked tremor and was unsteady on her feet. She hallucinated, thought she heard the voice of her husband telling her that he was coming to get her in a taxi and she cried out to him. Soon she began seeing people climbing trees and looking through the windows at her. She became violent and abusive to the staff. Even after receiving sedative medication she remained restless, muttering to herself incoherently. Her tremor increased, her face became flushed and she began to perspire excessively. At times she twitched convulsively. A little later she began picking up imaginary objects and muttering "thank you" as if someone were handing them to her.

Later she was observed reaching for an imaginary glass and drinking from it. She ate imaginary food and picked imaginary cigarettes out of the air; she heard nonexistent doorbells and an ambulance siren. Following several injections of a phenothiazine tranquilizer, her hallucinations ceased and she again became rational. . . .

Cocaine and other stimulants may also lead to increasing tolerance and dependency. Continuous overstimulation results in a loss of appetite and weight, increased anxiety and irritability, sleep deprivation and periodic episodes of delirium. Abrupt discontinuation of stimulant drugs is not followed by the withdrawal symptoms observed with sedative drugs but by profound fatigue and a tendency to depression.

Marijuana does not lead to increased tolerance and physiological dependence resulting in withdrawal symptoms when the drug is removed. Some individuals may become emotionally or psychologically dependent on the drug through using it to help them control anxiety or to escape anxiety-producing situations. When deprived of marijuana such persons may experience panic and intense anxiety but typically it is easier to give up marijuana than either cigarettes or alcohol. In fact some experts have presented impressive evidence for the proposition that alcohol constitutes a greater threat to society and to the individual user than does marijuana (Kaplan, 1970).

The Nature of Drug Addiction

Alcoholism and addiction to other drugs are very similar. A committee of the World Health Organization defined drug addiction as ". . . a state of periodic or chronic intoxication, detrimental to the individual and to society, produced by the repeated consumption of a drug (natural or synthetic)." The characteristics of drug addiction include an overpowering compulsion to obtain the drug by any available means; an increase in dosage with time; and a psychological, and sometimes physical, dependence on the effects of the drug.

The committee distinguished between drugs leading to true addiction and those that merely result in *habituation* (habit-forming drugs). The addictive drugs, notably morphine and substances resembling it, *always* produce compulsive craving, sooner in individuals whose psychological make-up leads them to seek escape in drugs, and later in other individuals, but ultimately in all. Withdrawal of drugs classified as addictive causes genuine disturbance. In contrast, the habit-forming but non-addictive drugs never produce compulsive craving, although the individual may find their effects desirable and may quickly acquire the habit of taking them. Their withdrawal need not cause significant disturbance. The best known of the drugs leading to habituation but not necessarily addiction are caffeine and nicotine. The addictive drugs are socially harmful; the merely habit-forming are not.

It should be added, however, that the line between addiction and mere habituation is not always a clear one. The authors have observed individuals who have used such large doses of coffee or caffeine tablets as to cause a marked accentuation of neurotic anxiety and depression, psychophysiologic disorders (hypertension and peptic ulcer), loss of appetite and weight, severe impairment of sleep and impulsive outbursts of hostile aggression. The use of nicotine may also be addictive in some cases. Knapp et al. (1963) have suggested that heavy cigarette smokers are true addicts who show mild but real bodily withdrawal effects when they stop smoking.

In the United States, in addition to a great many occasional drug users, estimates have been made of between 60,000 and 180,000 true narcotic addicts. (England, for reasons to be explored later, has been estimated to have only 400.) Among first admissions to mental hospitals, fewer than 1 per cent carry the diagnosis of psychosis associated with drugs; the majority of addicts are not psychotic enough to require hospitalization.

Addiction is most common in large cities. Far more males than females are addicted; most are unskilled workers, in part because early addiction interferes with school attendance and preparation for a skilled vocation. However, addiction is also frequent among physicians, nurses and pharmacists, obviously because they have easy access to drugs. Since World War II the use of drugs by adolescents appears to have increased rapidly.

Causation

There is no evidence that heredity affects drug addiction significantly. The important variables are the use of drugs in medical treatment and various psychological and sociocultural factors.

Many of the psychological factors in alcoholism also affect addiction to other drugs.

Medical Factors. Medical patients for whom drugs have been prescribed over a prolonged period of time—as in the case of morphine and synthetic narcotics that are administered for pain, hypnotics for insomnia, and various sedatives for relief from neurotic anxiety—often become addicted. Physicians, nurses and pharmacists who become addicts generally take hypnotic drugs but occasionally also narcotics.

Sociopathic Personality. Since sociopathic traits predispose the individual to methods of obtaining gratification that are illegal or do not conform with the prevailing cultural mores, many narcotic addicts are also sociopathic. In the following case of early and strong addiction to stimulants and narcotics, the individual's history and personality traits were markedly sociopathic.

A 21-year-old man was voluntarily admitted to a general hospital with a request for help in terminating his dependency on several drugs. He reported that he was employed as a musician and agreed to pay the hospital bills but never did. In retrospect, it appeared that he had sought hospitalization in order to escape from several difficulties in his reality situation: (1) his parents had threatened to have him committed to a state hospital; (2) his wife had threatened to divorce him; (3) a girl had recently given birth to an illegitimate child and alleged that he was the father; (4) he may have known that he was being investigated by narcotics authorities.

The patient was the eldest of four boys. His next younger brother was a delinquent and drug addict currently hospitalized. The parents had been extremely lenient with their sons and unable to provide limits for their behavior. The patient, nevertheless, described his father as "kind of strict" and made no reply when asked what he liked most about his father. The mother was friendly, warm, easy to get along with and religious. Interestingly, the patient was as fond of her as he was hostile to his father.

Although of at least average intelligence, the patient barely obtained a "D" average in high school. He had been expelled three times for playing hooky, selling contraceptives to other students and beating up a much smaller boy. He had also been arrested while in high school and placed on probation for driving without a license and selling stolen goods.

In early adolescence he began a series of sexual relations with a number of girls; while in the tenth grade, at the age of 17, he was forced into marriage with a girl he had made pregnant. He left school and worked as a busboy and truck driver. According to his own statement, he began to use drugs during this period for motives that can be described as clearly sociopathic: he was attracted toward the excitement of taking drugs and wanted to impress people by

doing something dangerous. He also began to go out with other women; his wife left him and he returned to his parents' home.

On admission to the hospital, he reported that until six months previously his daily drug intake had been 60 mg. of a stimulant (Dexedrine) and four ounces of cough syrup containing a narcotic (codeine). He had then increased his intake of Dexedrine to about 90 mg. daily and added 400 mg. of Nembutal and 400 of Seconal. (These are enormous dosages; one tablet of Dexedrine contains either 5 or 10 mg. and the usual Nembutal or Seconal capsule contains 100.) He took most of the drugs in the evening and was "high" all night, during part of which he played in a dance band. Later it was learned that he had also been taking morphine and the narcotic drug Demerol. He would steal either drugs or articles that he could sell for money with which he brought drugs.

Immediately after admission to a psychiatric ward, he became friendly with a male schizophrenic who was the only other drug addict on the ward, but for the most part he spent his time, as male sociopaths tend to do, socializing with young female patients. In appearance he was large, soft and unattractive. He was relatively quiet and composed on the ward and did not develop severe withdrawal symptoms, possibly due to the action of anti-convulsants and sedatives which were administered to him as substitutes for the drugs he had been taking. It is also possible that he had succeeded in bringing a supply of drugs into the hospital; addicts can be extremely tricky in hiding drugs about their persons. In any event, all therapeutic medication was withdrawn within a couple of weeks with apparent success.

Persona ity testing indicated a mild depression in a basically sociopathic individual. He was not motivated toward changing his antisocial personality characteristics and after a month was discharged. Not long afterward he was arrested for burglarizing a dentist's office and stealing gold, silver and drugs. He admitted the theft and also confessed to stealing drugs from two drug stores. He was placed on prolonged probation on condition that he seek admission to the federal hospital for drug addicts at Lexington, Kentucky.

Just as the typical sociopath has a delinquent and criminal record, so too, does the typical addict. Many are delinquents prior to the beginning of addiction. Once addicted, the expense of the drugs makes it necessary for them to steal. (There is reason to believe that in recent years drug "pushers" have been seeking bigger profits by cutting drugs with larger and larger proportions of neutral substances. This practice results in lessened potency; in consequence, the addict needs more money to buy larger doses in order to obtain the same effect.) Clausen (1957) quoted from a study of young drug users in Chicago that pointed to the complex interactions of addiction and delinquency:*

With few exceptions known drug users engage in delinquency in more or less systematic form. Contrary to the widely held view that the delinquency of the young addict is a consequence principally of addiction, it was found that delinquency both preceded and followed addiction to heroin. . . . Three observations may be made about the effects of addiction upon the delinquent behavior of the person: (1) The pressure of need for money to support his addiction impels the user to commit violations with greater frequency and with less caution than formerly. (2) Delinquents, after becoming addicted to heroin, do not engage in types of delinquency in which they are not already skilled. The post-addict delinquent, in other words, does not generally engage in more serious crimes than those he committed prior to his addiction. (3) Delinquents who as pre-addicts tended to engage in riotous behavior such as street fighting and gang attacks tend after addiction to abandon this kind of activity. Three elements are probably responsibile for the change: (a) the sedative effects of the opiate; (b) the desire to avoid attracting the attention of public and police; and (c) the tendency for adolescents to become quieter in their conduct as they approach maturity.

This description is quite different from the popular stereotype of the vicious addict who robs, assaults and kills uncontrollably.

Neurotic Personality. Neurotic anxiety may lead to drug addiction just as it may lead to alcoholism. Even cigarette smokers, as judged by several studies, have higher levels of anxiety and various neurotic characteristics than non-smokers. (Of course, smoking may cause tension just as readily as tension causes smoking.) Neurotic symptoms may be temporarily relieved by hypnotics, often with severe later consequences. The following case of barbiturate addiction in an extremely neurotic individual had a better outcome than many cases of drug addiction:

The patient was first treated for psychiatric difficulties as an 18-year-old college student. She had lost weight, was intensely anxious, fatigued, depressed and fearful, and could not continue in college. ECT treatments resulted in temporary improvement of mood, but it became evident that her depression and anxiety had been developing from early childhood. During the next decade she was repeatedly hospitalized and variously treated by ECT, tranquilizers,

*From Clausen, J. A. 1957. Social patterns, personality and adolescent drug use. *In* Leighton, A. H., Clausen, J. A., and Wilson, R. N. (Editors). Explorations in Social Psychiatry. New York, Basic Books.

sedatives, anti-depressant drugs, supportive psychotherapy and analytically oriented therapy. However, her depression and anxiety lifted for only brief intervals.

When she was 26, while working as an executive secretary, a medication containing several barbiturates was prescribed for the control of insomnia. She discovered that if she also used the medication during the day she felt much better. The physician who furnished the prescriptions failed to specify how many times they could be refilled by a pharmacist, and the patient obtained supplies at different drug stores, gradually increasing her tolerance and her dependency. Over a period of five years the drug enabled her to continue working and avoid hospitalization. At the age of 30 she became engaged to a man of different religion; her parents disapproved of the engagement and she felt ambivalent toward him. Her anxiety and depression increased and she became unable to work; she was hospitalized. In the hospital, withdrawal of the drug increased her anxiety still further.

The patient's parents were conscientious, overly conforming, insecure and relatively isolated socially. The parents had both been the children of ministers. The father could not express hostility outside his home but with his family he was an authoritarian tyrant. He frequently flew into violent rages yet did not permit any other member of the family to express anger or any strong emotion whatsoever. As a child the patient was shy and frightened. She hated her father more than any person she met then or subsequently. Automobile rides with him led to attacks of vomiting. However, demands for respect and obedience had their effect on her and she felt guilty for both her hostility and his anger. As an adult she defended him with the statement, "He had a hellish childhood. Children were to be seen and not heard. They had to sit quiet at table or be smacked in the face. He had to go to work and sell from door to door, and it nearly killed him because he's so shy." In retrospect, she also believed that her parents had wanted a boy and were disappointed when she was born. She had been unprepared for the onset of menstruation and thought she was ill when it occurred. She had had no sexual experience and relatively few dates prior to her engagement.

Apart from her neurosis, she had a number of personal strengths: she was intelligent, a good student and a fine pianist, well-built, pleasant in manner when not depressed, and able to socialize with other girls although not with boys. When free of depression she was attractive and had considerable sparkle and charm. She had been the first girl to be elected president of the senior class in her high school and, before dropping out of college, had been a candidate for president of her freshman class. The position she held as an executive secretary before being incapacitated by her neurotic symptoms was a responsible one.

In view of the failure of her chronic and severe neurotic symptoms to respond to all other available forms of treatment, a lobotomy was performed. However, in order to avoid damaging her intelligence and positive personality attributes, the amount of brain tissue cut was kept to a minimal level. At first she displayed considerable improvement of mood but soon became anxious and depressed again, resumed her dependency on drugs, and broke her engagement on the grounds that she could never be a satisfactory wife and mother. For a year she remained at home with her parents and took barbiturates. On the anniversary of her broken engagement she became so depressed that she attempted suicide by taking an overdose.

A second lobotomy was performed, only slightly extending the previous surgical cutting. This time there was marked and sustained improvement with no further recurrence of anxiety, depression or drug dependency. Her I.Q., as measured after two lobotomies, was 130. (Prior to the second operation it had been 117, obviously reflecting emotional interference with intellectual performance.) She was referred for vocational rehabilitation and found to have retained her skills as an exceptionally able stenographer. A year later she returned to work, moved into an apartment of her own and began to have a more adequate social life.

Psychoses. Pescor (1943) summarized the data on 1036 drug addicts treated at the federal hospital in Lexington, and found that 88.1 per cent were classified in categories equivalent to the current concept of sociopathic personality, 6.3 per cent were neurotic and the remaining 5.6 per cent mostly psychotics. The proportion of psychotics was thus quite small. However, the adult inmates at Lexington are a selected group who have previously spent time in correctional institutions. Among all addicts in the United States there are probably fewer sociopaths and more schizophrenics than in Pescor's sample. Overt or latent schizophrenia seems to be particularly frequent among adolescent addicts. Among 30 adolescents admitted to Lexington, Gerard and Kornetsky (1954) considered that no fewer than 14 showed evidence of overt or incipient schizophrenia. The social inadequacy, isolation and chaotic affective life of a schizoid adolescent may be the factors that lead him to take refuge in drugs.

Other Psychological Factors. Drug usage, like consumption of alcohol, is frequently a regressive defense against anxiety which becomes stronger with reinforcement. Both alcohol addicts and other drug addicts are often markedly oral, intolerant of frustration, narcissistic, hostile and low in self-esteem. Like alcoholics, drug addicts tend to come from unsatisfactory home backgrounds.

Chein et al. (1964) contrasted the family background of addicts and normal controls (see Table 16–4). The addicts tended to come more often from families characterized by emotional distance, poor father-son relationships, and instability. The authors concluded that family experiences play an important role in the etiology of addiction.

TABLE 16–4. Highly Contrasting Factors in Family Backgrounds of Drug Addicts and Controls

Item	Addicts (Percentage)	Control (Percentage)
1. Boy experienced an extremely week father-son relationship (30, 29)	80	45
2. For a significant part of early childhood, boy did not have a father figure in his life (29, 29)	48	17
3. Some father figure was cool or hostile to boy (23, 24)	52	13
4. Father had unrealistically low aspirations for the boy (late childhood and early adolescence) (16, 22)	44	0
5. Some father figure was an immoral model (early childhood) (26, 24)	23	0
6. Marked impulse orientation in father figure (23, 23)	26	0
7. Father had unstable work history during boy's early childhood	43	14
8. Father was unrealistically pessimistic or felt that life is a gamble (17, 19)	47	11
9. Lack of warmth or overtly discordant relations between parents (30, 29)	97	41
10. Mother figure was more important parent in boy's life during late childhood period (30, 29)	73	45
11. Some mother figure cool or hostile to boy (early childhood) (30, 28)	23	0
12. Some mother figure cool or hostile to boy (late childhood) (30, 29)	37	3
13. Boy experienced extremely weak mother-son relationship (30, 29)	40	7
14. Mother did not trust authority figures (29, 29)	38	10
15. Mother had unrealistically low aspirations for boy (late childhood and early adolescence) (29, 28)	31	0
16. Mother was unrealistically pessimistic or felt that life is a gamble (29, 29)	31	7
17. No clear pattern of parental roles in formation of disciplinary policy (adolescence) (30, 29)	23	0
18. Parental standards for boy were vague or inconsistent (early childhood) (29, 28)	55	4
19. Parental standards for boy were vague or inconsistent (adolescence) (30, 29)	63	3
20. Boy was overindulged, frustrated in his wishes, or both (30, 29)	70	10

All items differentiate addicts from controls at the .05 level of confidence. The total number of cases on which relevant information was available is indicated in parentheses for addicts and controls respectively. (From Chein, I., et al. 1964. The Road to H: Narcotics, Delinquency, and Social Policy. New York, Basic Books, Inc.)

One other possible determinant was incorporated into a theory of addiction by Rado (1958). Basing his speculations on the discovery by Olds (1955) of pleasure centers in the brain, Rado suggested that an addictive drug may acquire its hold by stimulation of these centers and induction of a self-perpetuating cycle of drug intake and reward. Rado's theory is plausible, but for the present it is not supported by direct evidence.

Sociocultural Factors.   Certain drugs are readily available in various societies and cultural groups. Opium, for instance, is widely used among some Asiatic people. In South America, cocaine is commonly obtained from chewing coca leaves. Among various segments of our own population, marijuana, barbiturates, heroin and stimulants are not too difficult to obtain, and have become "fashionable" to use.

Marijuana in particular has grown to be especially popular in this country in recent years. Whereas alcohol is the preferred drug among older segments of the population, marijuana is being used more and more by younger persons. In a 1967 survey of high school students in San Mateo County, California (Kaplan, 1970) 50 per cent of the male seniors and 38 per cent of the female senior students reported having used marijuana at least once in the preceding year. These figures represented a sharp increase over a similar survey taken a year earlier.

Surveys conducted in other parts of the country have shown somewhat lower incidence figures but a general increase is noted everywhere. The picture is the same with respect to college students. Blum and his associates (1969) report an overall incidence figure of 69 per cent in a large private California university in 1968 compared to only 21 per cent who reported having used marijuana in a similar study done at the same school in 1966. Most experts regard the figures from such surveys as underestimates because of students' natural reluctance to admit using a drug which is still associated with severe legal penalities.

The relatively high rates of narcotic addiction in the United States have often been attributed to punitive legislation and law enforcement rather than to the ready availability of drugs. (The United States has more stringent laws for the control of narcotics than any other nation.) In contrast, the low rates in England have been attributed to a benign system in which addicts secure a regular maintenance dosage of drugs from established clinics under medical supervision. However, the differences in frequency between the two countries may be due instead to the greater financial rewards for selling drugs in the United States, a more efficient criminal organization for distributing drugs, and less compelling cultural sanctions against addiction. Brill (1963) evaluated the situation in England and concluded that a low frequency of addiction preceded the adoption of current regulations, rather than vice versa. Whatever the cause, the fact is that the overall incidence of new drug addiction cases declined in England in 1969 while the incidence was still rapidly increasing in the United States.

Treatment

As in alcoholism, the treatment of addiction consists of: disintoxication; deterrent measures; and attempts to modify the personal factors responsible for addiction and its perpetuation.

Disintoxication of drug addicts may be achieved by the "cold turkey" procedure, i.e., sudden and complete removal of the drug. As we have seen, the withdrawal symptoms that ensue are distressing and even dangerous. Hence a more humanitarian procedure may be used consisting either of giving the patient progressively diminishing doses of his drug for several weeks, or substituting a less addictive drug until withdrawal from the latter can also be accomplished. Concomitantly, the patient may be given anti-convulsant agents, vitamins and glucose. A patient who has been tapered off is more likely to be motivated for later psychotherapy than a patient who is antagonized by the "cold turkey" method.

Compulsory institutionalization for a protracted period after the drug has been withdrawn is a common procedure. It is based on the assumption that isolation from society and enforced abstinence will act as deterrents to resumption of drug use after release from the institution. It is often argued, however, that compulsory institutionalization is self-defeating because it kills the motivation necessary for psychotherapy or other treatment measures. In general, voluntary cooperation is preferable to compulsion, but occasionally addicts who are confined under compulsion develop the motivation for active involvement in therapy.

For the psychotic addict, ECT or tranquilizing drugs may be helpful. For neurotic addicts, psychotherapy is possible but no easier to carry through successfully than with alcoholics. Estimates of cures using different methods are quite variable: for confirmed addicts treated only by institutionalization, cures have been reported for 1 to 15 per cent, depending on the particular sample; for patients willing to cooperate in psychotherapy, the estimates have run much higher. Addicted physicians have a particularly high rate of cure.

One of the problems in the treatment of drug addicts is the attitude of society toward them. Far too many persons, including a number of prosecuting attorneys, police and judges, would agree with the statement of a religious and otherwise compassionate individual: "The only way to deal with drug addicts is to get them in a state of grace and shoot them." In contrast, almost all psychologists and psychiatrists regard addicts as persons who are ill and in need of help. Addicts should be distinguished from the criminals who supply them with drugs and live off their misery.

More important than treatment is prevention. To be effective, a program of prevention must succeed in controlling the flow of addictive drugs and must educate the public to understand the causes and consequences of addiction.

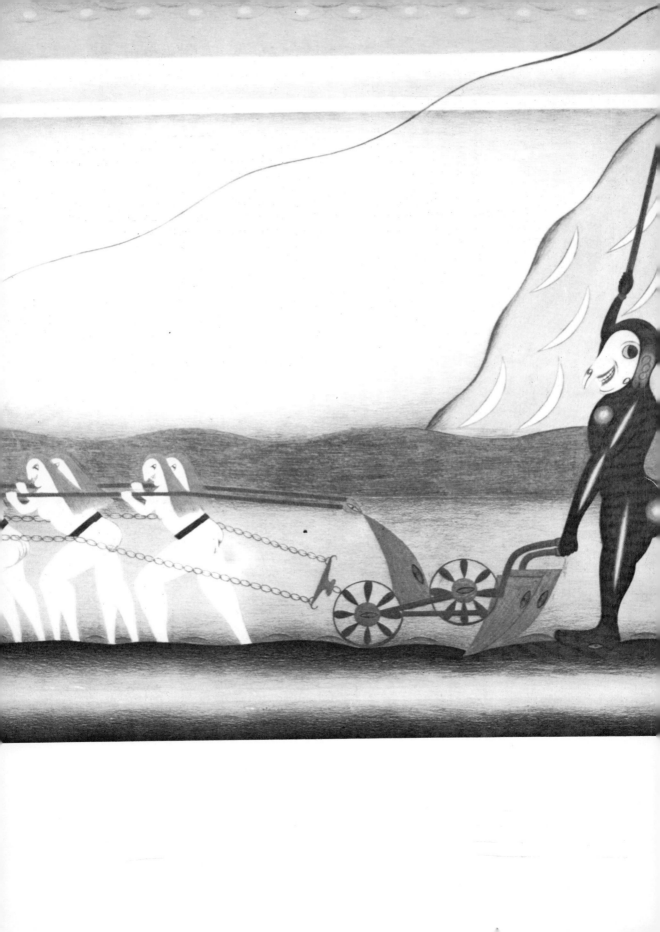

Body and mind, like man and wife, do not always
agree to die together.
Charles Caleb Colton (1780–1832)

17

BRAIN SYNDROMES

Organic brain syndromes are disturbances of behavior that are associated with pathological disturbances in the brain. Since the brain pathology is a necessary but not always sufficient cause of a brain syndrome—for example, a brain tumor does not always result in behavior disorganization—we shall be concerned, in this chapter, only with brain pathology that is associated with definite disturbances of behavior and that occurs later than early childhood. (Severe brain disturbance prior to or very soon after birth results chiefly in mental deficiency, which is discussed in the next chapter.)

Although brain syndromes, for the most part, fall within the compass of medicine rather than psychology, the psychologist is concerned with them for several reasons. First, an understanding of organic disorders puts functional disorders in a proper perspective. Second, the behavior of the brain-disordered patient is as much a response to the emotional and social effects of the brain changes he has suffered as to the brain changes themselves. Third, the symptoms of organic and functional psychoses overlap, and the psychologist, therefore, must be familiar with both, especially since various psychological tests are frequently used in the differential diagnosis of organic vs. functional disorders. Fourth, social and psychological factors are part of the etiology of brain disorders.

ACUTE VS. CHRONIC SYMPTOMS

An organic brain syndrome may be either acute or chronic. An acute brain syndrome is one in which there are reversible changes in brain functioning. The term chronic brain syndrome, on the other hand, is applied to those syndromes in which there are irreversible changes, often structural, in the brain and which are ordinarily manifested in a disruption of behavior that may be permanent. It is sometimes possible to determine whether a syndrome is acute or chronic by the nature of the symptoms. Certain symptoms are more frequently associated with an acute process while others are generally more characteristic of a chronic syndrome. However, there are many exceptions to these trends and considerable overlap exists between acute and chronic symptoms. For example, the same organic factor, such as a head wound or a toxic agent, may cause either an acute or a chronic reaction. Also, a residue of chronic effects may be observed after substantial recovery from what is usually an acute, completely reversible syndrome.

Table 17–1 lists the symptoms which tend to be associated with acute and chronic disorders. When a syndrome is acute in nature, the patient is often in a state of stupor and is lethargic, immobile and difficult to rouse. He talks little or not at all. If he responds to questions, his

325

Can both be organic or functional?

TABLE 17–1. Characteristics of Acute (Reversible) and Chronic (Irreversible) Brain Disorders

Acute Reversible Brain Disorders	Chronic Irreversible Brain Disorders
Usual clinical syndrome is delirium (sometimes stupor or coma).	Usual clinical syndrome is dementia.
Primary impairment of orientation, memory, all intellectual functions, judgment and affective response.	Primary impairment of orientation, memory, all intellectual functions, judgment and affective response.
Usually associated with disordered perception (especially visual illusions and hallucinations), consciousness (e.g., stupor) and psychomotor activity (excitement or immobility).	May be prominent secondary manifestations due to release or accentuation of latent personality characteristics— psychotic, neurotic, sociopathic, etc.
Due to temporary, reversible changes in brain cell function.	Due to permanent, irreversible damage to brain structure.
Frequently symptomatic of generalized toxic, infective or metabolic disorder, affecting other parts of the body.	May result from all the agents causing acute disorders; but also from localized intracranial lesion or degenerative process (sometimes hereditary).
Commonly encountered on medical and surgical wards of general hospitals.	Commonly encountered on neurological services of general hospitals or in mental hospitals.
Course brief, and may terminate in (1) death, (2) complete remission, (3) chronic brain disorders.	Course may be (1) prolonged or (2) progressive (with fatal termination).

answers indicate disturbances of orientation, memory and intellect. The maximal degree of stupor is *coma*, in which the patient is unconscious and cannot be roused. Most often, however, patients with acute brain syndromes become *delirious.* Whether stuporous, comatose or delirious, the patient looks physically ill. He is often in bed, is unkempt and haggard, and sweats profusely. His face appears expressionless or, if he is delirious, worried or fearful.

The major characteristics of deliria in acute brain syndromes are identical with those of delirium tremens, discussed in the preceding chapter, i.e., clouded consciousness, perceptual confusion, incoherence, tremors or psychomotor excitement and overactivity, disorientation, and visual illusions and hallucinations. Transient delusions sometimes accompany the hallucinations. Many delirious patients fluctuate rapidly between periods of confusion and brief intervals of lucidity. In severe delirium, the patient is unaware that he is suffering a primary impairment of intellect, memory, affective responses, and social and ethical judgments.

A patient's hallucinations in delirium are related to the emotional and social factors of his personality and may symbolize repressed impulses. Should there be auditory hallucinations, for example, women more than men are likely to hear the voices of babies and children. A delirious woman may hear herself accused of prostitution; a man is more likely to hear threats of physical injury or accusations of sexual deviations. In patients who experience repeated attacks of delirium, the hallucinations are likely to be similar from one attack to the next, even if several years elapse between attacks. The specific cause of the delirium does not matter: the symptoms are characteristic of the individual and not the cause. Occasionally a patient has an episode of delirium on one occasion and a schizophrenic breakdown on another, but the content of his hallucinations is likely to be repeated on each occasion.

Acute symptoms are often associated with biochemical brain changes, which may result from a tremendous variety of causes. Among them are diseases accompanied by high fever, such as malaria, pneumonia or typhoid fever; infections localized within the skull, such as meningitis or a brain abscess; excessive use of or withdrawal from alcohol, barbiturates or other drugs; carbon monoxide; toxic metals such as lead or manganese; head injury (trauma) that damages the brain or interferes with the blood supply; seizures in idiopathic epilepsy; brain tumors; circulatory failures or illnesses, such as pernicious anemia, that interfere with the supply of oxygen to the brain cells; vitamin deficiencies as in hypothyroidism; and the injection of excessive amounts of insulin.

Chronic syndrome patients typically manifest an intellectual deterioration. There are also several other types of symptoms which tend to be more frequently associated with a chronic, nonreversible process. A progressive loss of personal standards, control and inhibitions is common; for example, the previously meticulous dresser may become very sloppy, another person may lose his habits of cleanliness and table manners, and, in another, language may become rude and obscene. The observer receives the impression of a disintegrating superego. The chronic patient's manner of speech is certain to be disturbed in one of several ways. Most commonly, it becomes slurred and many

N.B.
ALL OD's have sec. symptoms

sounds are omitted or fused. A paretic patient, for example, cannot pronounce "Methodist Episcopal," a phrase widely used to test speech difficulties. A patient with cerebellar damage may speak in a scanning, sing-song manner and emphasize the wrong syllables. Some organic patients speak in a monotonous, expressionless voice and others in a series of explosive outbursts. As deterioration progresses, the stream of talk finally degenerates into gibberish.

In the affective realm, some organic patients are euphoric and some depressed, but most tend to be shallow and flat, giving the impression of dullness, listlessness and apathy. In a number of cases there is a marked lability; the patient responds to relatively innocuous external stimuli with irritability. Some patients also manifest so-called "catastrophic reaction," i.e., they become agitated and weep when faced with simple tasks or for no apparent reason whatsoever. Delusions and hallucinations are not particularly common in chronic brain syndromes, but when they do occur are consistent with other secondary symptoms. Should the patient have hallucinations, they are likely to be auditory rather than visual (in contrast with delirium). The depressed patient may have delusions of self-accusation; the euphoric patient, delusions of grandeur, and the paranoid patient, delusions of influence or persecution, often associated with auditory hallucinations. In the early stages of a chronic brain syndrome the patient may be aware that something is wrong. He may complain of poor memory and the inability to concentrate, and appear puzzled and bewildered by what is happening to him. In the later stages insight is completely absent.

Just as some brain syndromes are acute and others are chronic in nature, some syndromes are associated with psychotic symptoms and some are not. In some organic brain syndromes the patient's mental functioning is so impaired that he is unable to meet the ordinary demands of life. The impairment may result from a variety of factors. For example, hallucinations or delusions may distort perceptions; or alterations in mood may be so profound that the patient is unable to respond appropriately; or deficits in language and memory may be so extreme that the patient is unable mentally to grasp what is going on around him.

One of the most important facts to be remembered in organic brain syndromes is that all brain damage releases or accentuates secondary symptoms which may be any of the whole range of functional psychological disturbance: neurotic anxiety, affective disorders, schizophrenic or paranoid manifestations, sociopathic behavior, sexual deviations, addictions and so forth. An identical type and degree of brain damage in any two individuals may result in markedly different secondary symptoms depending on the personality traits of each individual prior to the damage. After six years of studying the effects of various cerebral lesions on the normal and experimentally neurotic behavior of 50 cats and 40 monkeys, Masserman and Fechtel (1956) observed, "The permanent effects of a cerebral lesion depend perhaps less on its site or even extent than on the personality of the patient, his significant pre-traumatic or preoperative experiences, and the physical and psychiatric care given him during the crucial period of rehabilitation." Indeed, it is the universal impression of clinicians that the more stable the premorbid personality of a patient with a brain syndrome, the better is his response to the disorder, i.e., the less likely he is to become highly anxious, irritable, depressed or paranoid, or act out antisocial impulses or have delusions or display other symptomatology.

2 guys could do opposit thing

GENERAL SYMPTOMS

Whereas functional disorders are classified primarily by symptoms, organic brain syndromes are classified according to cause or pathology. A large number of specific syndromes can be differentiated on the basis of precipitating causes or pathological processes. Precipitants may be traumas (injuries to the head), toxic chemicals, alcohol, fever, vitamin deficiencies, syphilis or other infections, and degeneration. Although from a medical point of view the biological causes of brain syndromes are very different from each other, from a psychological point of view the brain syndromes are relatively homogeneous. The delirium resulting from alcoholism resembles the delirium caused by malarial infection or ingestion of a toxic metallic substance. The dementia resulting from paresis resembles the dementia that is symptomatic of senility.

SYMPTOMS (ACUTE)

The patient with an acute brain syndrome often is in a temporary state of *stupor, coma* or *delirium* of which delirium is the most common. Another commonly noted symptom is pro-

①

gressive *dementia.* In both delirium and dementia several *primary symptoms of impairment,* temporary in the acute and irreversible in the chronic, may be evident. The most important are:

1. Impairment of orientation, especially for time but often also for place and person
2. Impairment of memory, notably for recent events and less so for events of the remote past, sometimes accompanied by confabulation
3. Impairment of all intellectual functions, including comprehension, learning ability, numerical ability and so forth; ideation tends to be impoverished, concrete and perseverative
4. Impairment of judgment, conscience and ability to plan
5. Impairment of affective responses, usually manifested in shallowness or lability.

As mentioned previously, a common manifestation of chronic brain syndromes is dementia. Dementia, the progressive deterioration of intellectual and other functions, may appear in the course of virtually any brain syndrome, regardless of the specific cause of the disorder. The severity of dementia varies from patient to patient. In mild cases the individual displays no obvious defects in casual conversation, but under careful observation or in testing reveals subtle signs of concrete thinking, memory difficulty, inability to concentrate, a paucity of new concepts and a tendency to repeat a restricted number of thoughts or phrases. On a test of abstract reasoning, the patient's score is poorer than on a vocabulary test. His thinking is rigid and he cannot easily shift from one point of view or method of classification to another. He has difficulty grouping or differentiating objects on a logical basis. The logic of simple classification appears to be lost to him; he may, for example, identify the picture of a somewhat ambiguous animal by saying. "It's an animal," or, "It's a dog," but not, "It's some kind of animal—maybe a dog."

In relatively severe cases of dementia, *overinclusion, interpenetration and fragmentation* are usually evident. The patient cannot discriminate relevant from irrelevant stimuli, perceptions or thoughts: e.g., if asked to name the members of his family he may begin to list them but then will shift overinclusively to persons outside the family. A thought or notion may interpenetrate a sequence of behavior and disrupt it, and a sequence of behavior may be fragmented into discontinuous segments. The net result of these processes is to make the patient's behavior seem quite irrational. It should

be added, however, that difficulty with abstractions, overinclusion, interpenetration and fragmentation are also found in delirium and often in schizophrenia, but in progressive dementia, they are particularly noticeable and not unique. In very advanced cases the patient is likely to regress to an infantile level. He lies in bed, incontinent, unable to speak or feed himself and completely indifferent to his appearance and surroundings. In many cases, such regression is soon followed by death.

In a detailed study of the effects of brain damage, Chapman and Wolff (1959) concluded that the greater the amount of tissue loss, the greater the impairment of the ability to integrate experience, reason abstractly, make judgments, plan and so forth. This finding supports the controversial hypothesis of *mass action,* that is, the hypothesis that large areas of the brain function as a whole to produce intelligent behavior. The contrasting hypothesis of *brain localization* asserts that each psychological function is dependent on a specific brain area and that damage to a specific area destroys its specific function. However, it is most likely that the brain is partly localized and partly not. Sensory processes, motor functions and language usage depend on relatively specific areas; vision, for example, is impossible without the occipital lobes of the cortex, and intellectual functioning stems from the frontal areas. It is also true, however, that if a particular lobe of the brain is damaged, the corresponding lobe on the other side may in time "learn" to substitute for the damaged area. Furthermore, there is some evidence that within a single large area of the brain one subpart is as important as another for the functions mediated by the large area: the subparts are *equipotential* for behavior.

Organic brain syndromes accounted for 25.9 per cent of all first admissions to public mental hospitals in 1968. Of that number 34 per cent were at least 75 years old. The figures for resident patients in public mental hospitals are almost identical: 25.8 per cent of all resident patients were diagnosed as organic brain syndromes and 31.8 per cent of this group were 75 years of age or older. In the last few decades the incidence of the organic brain syndromes which are associated with old age has increased rapidly. This increase is apparently due to the greatly decreased birth mortality, fewer deaths from childhood diseases and increased longevity; in addition, circulatory disorders themselves have increased in the general population.

PARIETOTEMPORAL—"language" (handwritten)

MULTIPLICITY OF CAUSES

While it is true that many brain syndromes are caused by specific agents or by injury of specific brain centers, the relationship between cause and effect is not always clear-cut. This fact can be seen most easily with respect to some of the language disorders such as aphasia. Aphasia is generally considered to result from damage to the parietotemporal area (the "language area") of the dominant cerebral hemisphere—the left hemisphere in right-handed persons, and vice versa. A number of investigators have distinguished various types of aphasia, each consisting of a different aspect of language defect. There are, for example, *motor aphasia,* an inability to express letters, words or sentences; *sensory aphasia,* an inability to understand the meaning of words or sentences; *alexia,* an inability to understand written language; *agraphia,* an inability to translate verbal sounds into corresponding written symbols; and, in addition, many other types corresponding to other language defects. Although it has been claimed that each type of aphasia results from injury to a very specific part of the parieto-temporal area, Schuell et al. (1964), in a recent exhaustive analysis, concluded that aphasia does not consist of a group of specific defects, but, rather, of a generalized language defect that may or may not be associated with an inability to hear words, a visual confusion that involves written language, or the evidences of other so-called types of aphasia. They wrote, "We consider aphasia primarily a language deficit upon which various perceptual and sensorimotor deficits concomitant with brain damage may or may not be superimposed."

The aphasic patient has a generalized impairment of vocabulary and ability to perceive and produce verbal messages. For example, if he is asked to name a designated piece of furniture, perhaps a table, he may be unable to say anything or, after a long pause, may say, "Chair, no—bed, no—eat—eat at the table—table—that's it, table" (Schuell et al.).

The damage to the parietotemporal area of the brain may result from the blocking of circulation, as by thrombosis (clotting, which often results from the narrowing of blood vessels and the slowing of blood circulation), tumors, infectious diseases or externally caused brain damage. The disorder was studied extensively after both World Wars I and II because of the large number of combatants who became aphasic. It can occur at any age but is most frequent in the later decades of life.

Unless other gross symptomatology is present, the aphasic patient is very much aware of his inability to understand or use language as he had formerly. As a result, he tends to become frustrated, anxious and depressed so that it is sometimes possible to mistake him for a psychotic. Frequently, however, aphasia is associated with primary symptoms of an organic brain syndrome, such as impairment of memory and orientation.

If the aphasia has been the aftermath of brain surgery, spontaneous recovery may take place. For most patients, however, recovery is a process of relearning. The treatment successfully employed by Schuell and her associates (1964) is directed to the central language process. It consists of auditory stimulation that progresses from the simple to the complex as the patient progresses from echo to discrimination. Specific language defects are treated within the context of the whole auditory-oral process. An integral part of the treatment is supportive psychotherapy.

SPECIFIC SYNDROMES

This section is devoted to a survey of some representative types of organic brain syndromes. Those syndromes resulting from alcohol will not be discussed here, as they were covered in the preceding chapter.

Senile and Presenile Dementia

Senile brain disease derives its name from the age group in which it is observed. Typically patients show some evidence of childish emotionality, self-centeredness, and difficulty in assimilating new experiences.

The brain of the senile patient shows considerable atrophy: there is a reduction in brain size, the cortical convolutions narrow, the fissures between them widen and functional cells are replaced by scar cells. It is possible that these pathological changes are caused by natural aging or they may be the cumulative effect of toxic processes. In a number of old people they are not accompanied by marked intellectual deterioration; in others there is an insidious onset of dementia along with irritability, insomnia and physical weakness, at any age after 60.

Of course, most old people show some decrease in alertness, breadth of interests, speed of performance on intellectual tasks and memory for recent events, but senile brain disease is an exaggeration of these "normal" symptoms. The patients exhibit a marked decrease in intellectual ability and a forgetfulness for recent events. Other symptoms are perseveration—as in telling the same story over and over—circumstantiality and rambling speech. In addition, a number of senile patients become very untidy and careless; others become incontinent, and still others lose control of their sexual impulses and, since they feel inadequate with other adults, may molest children. Another symptom is amnesia; the term *presbyophrenia* is sometimes used for a senile psychosis with severe amnesia but otherwise well-preserved personality and social behavior.

Secondary personality disturbances occur in approximately half the patients. Depending on individual premorbid personality traits, they may become neurotically anxious, depressed, delirious and confused. They may have acute neurotic reactions superimposed on the chronic impairment or paranoid reactions with delusions and hallucinations of a persecutory, erotic or grandiose nature. Approximately 15 to 25 per cent are paranoid.

The disorder ranges in severity from mild to severe. Deterioration is at a minimum in the mild cases, but superimposed on it may be psychotic, neurotic or behavioral reactions that may cause more disturbing symptomatology. Approximately 50 per cent of persons with the disorder follow a pattern of simple deterioration and a surprisingly large number of them can be helped by treatment. However, many are not brought into hospitals until they are in advanced stages of deterioration.

The course of the disorder proceeds through increasing physical and intellectual deterioration to a stage where the patient is bed-ridden, incontinent and incoherent. Fractures are frequent, perhaps because old bones are brittle or deficient in calcium. A large proportion of senile patients die within the first year of hospitalization but others survive for years.

The patient described below was a 73-year-old widow who was hospitalized five years after the onset of progressively deteriorating memory and other intellectual functions, confusion and loss of social habits:

The patient had been widowed at the age of 50 and thereafter lived with one or another of her five children. She had always been easygoing, happy and contented. Although she liked things to be neat and tidy, she was not exceptionally meticulous or compulsive. All her life she had been physically active and had had an excellent memory. The first indication of difficulty came in her late 60's when she lost some money that had been given to her. Soon thereafter she set out to visit one of her children but lost her way and needed police assistance. After this incident she was observed to lose her former interest in reading, writing letters and knitting. During most of the year preceding hospitalization she was unable to recognize her children and frequently her conversation was unintelligible. She ate without assistance but had to be dressed, undressed and taken to the toilet to avoid incontinence.

Consistent with her lifelong personality traits, her manner in the hospital was pleasant and cooperative. However, her comprehension and social behavior were grossly impaired. She walked down the corridor with her arm around a physician's waist and tickled his ribs. She misinterpreted everyday situations: when given her first bath in the hospital she said, "I don't want to get in the boat—the current is too swift." Her stream of talk rambled. The following is a verbatim sample: "While it is not so bad in the morning—that girl was over and she was saying that there was nothing better than the bottom one, and the cows and the calves were off and she was making out that . . . [unintelligible] . . . but I made out I never heard her. When they go out—you see—they don't bother taking the boxes. They just take everything with them." Her memory for both recent and remote events was close to zero. She was able to give her name correctly but when asked her age said, "I am 21 to 22 anyway, every minute." She could not give her birthday, the year of her birth, or any information about her previous life. Six months after admission she died of pneumonia, a frequent cause of death in senile patients. MOSTLY WOMEN

Presenile dementias are cortical brain syndromes whose clinical picture is similar to that of senile dementia but which appear in younger age groups. Two of the best known forms are Alzheimer's disease and Pick's disease.

A chronic, relatively rare syndrome with DIFFUSE progressive, widespread deterioration in the cerebrum, Alzheimer's disease (first described by the German neurologist Alois Alzheimer, 1864–1915) usually occurs between the ages of 40 and 60. It is often considered to be the equivalent of premature senile brain disease. The patient manifests a gradual intellectual deterioration, loss of memory, illogical reasoning, anxiety and depression, occasional hallucinations and labile affect with periodical episodes of forced laughter and tears. Serious speech disturbances are frequently evident as well as involuntary movements of the arms and legs, and convulsions. (A case of Alzheimer's disease was described in Chapter 1.) As neural degeneration progresses, the patient declines into a purely vegetative existence and wastes away. Death occurs within an average of four years of the initial onset. More women than men, in a ratio of approximately three to two, are subject to the disorder.

A pneumoencephalogram aids in the diagnosis of this as well as other degenerative diseases: the spinal fluid is removed and replaced by air which, on an x-ray, outlines the gross changes in the brain.

Pick's disease is a rare form of presenile dementia which was first described by a Czechoslovakian psychiatrist, Arnold Pick (1851–1924). Brain degeneration occurs in localized foci, mostly in the frontal areas. In Alzheimer's disease, on the other hand, degeneration is diffused throughout the brain. The age of onset is approximately the same as in Alzheimer's disease and the incidence among men is even lower. The disease is a slowly progressing dementia. The insidious intellectual impairment is characterized by distractability, easy fatigability, and the inability to deal with new problems and situations, although simple. Memory is little involved at first. During the course of the illness, interest and attention show marked fluctations. Depressive states are rare, but the patient's emotional reactions in general are reduced and blunted. As deterioration continues, restlessness, aimless activity and talkativeness sometimes develop. The talkativeness may be associated with various types of aphasia: speech may become a meaningless and hopeless jargon.

The duration of the illness averages five years. There is a gradual physical decline as well as the appearance of paralysis, contractures and epileptiform seizures.

Organic Brain Syndrome Associated with Intracranial Infections

Intracranial infections may be caused by epidemic encephalitis, syphilis or other conditions such as meningitis and brain abscess. For the present discussion we will use general paralysis as one example of such syndromes. General paralysis is caused by a syphilitic infection. Syphilis is caused by a spirochete, a microscopic organism that is usually transmitted by an infected individual during sexual intercourse. Since the discovery of

penicillin, the incidence of syphilis has decreased, but recently it has begun to rise again, particularly among adolescents.

Soon after the contraction of a syphilitic infection a hard pimple or open sore appears and is followed by a rash and, sometimes, headache, fever, and various other symptoms. If untreated, the disease becomes latent; the outward symptoms disappear but the spirochetes invade the heart, spinal cord, brain or other organs. Ten to 30 years later the latency stage ends and the individual may manifest very varied symptoms of this deadly disease. Neurosyphilis is the term for the form of the disease in which the nervous system is invaded by spirochetes; a subtype of neurosyphilis is paresis, also called general paresis of the insane, dementia paralytica and general paralysis. It is characterized by progressive dementia, which is caused by widespread destruction of the brain and its linings: the blood vessels are hindered from functioning properly, and scar cells (glia) multiply, narrowing the brain convolutions and widening the spaces (sulci) between them. The spaces become filled with fluid and the functional brain cells degenerate, particularly those

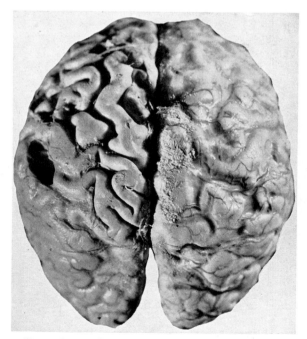

Figure 17–1. General paresis: widening of the sulci, extensive meningitis. (Courtesy of Dr. L. H. Cornwall. From Wechsler, I. 1963. Clinical Neurology. Philadelphia, W. B. Saunders Co.)

in the frontal areas. The paretic brain looks different to the naked eye. It has often been described as "moth-eaten."

The onset of paresis is typically insidious and occurs when the infected individuals are in their 40's and 50's. It is much more common in males than females, and in whites than Negroes, although the reason for the latter is not certain. Other mysteries of the disorder are why paresis develops only in less than 5 per cent of untreated syphilitics, and why it is more prevalent in certain racial groups and countries. One of the hypotheses advanced to account for the apparently selective susceptibility to the spirochete is that paresis is caused by a specific strain; another holds that spirochetes attack the individual's weakest organ which, in paresis, would be the nervous system and the brain; and still another holds that the spirochete is merely predisposing and the immediate precipitant is an injury to the brain.

Early symptoms of the disorder may be physical or psychological or a combination of both. The Wassermann and other laboratory tests for examination of blood and spinal fluid aid in diagnosis although they are not infallible: blood tests, for example, are sometimes negative in paresis. The patient may display any or all of the following symptoms: the pupil of the eye does not contract to light; there is a tremor of the tongue, lips, eye muscles and arms; in cases where the spinal cord as well as the brain is damaged, ataxia is present; and, frequently, reflexes such as the knee jerk are absent. The patient's speech is slurred, his writing shaky with many omissions and errors, and his abstract thinking, judgment, memory, orientation, and superego deteriorated. A loss of judgment may be reflected in very bizarre, "silly" behavior. Bruetsch (1959) cites a patient who took from its hinges the door of a waiting room in a public health center and then tore the linoleum from the floor. A second patient tried to buy an automobile in a five-and-ten-cent store; a third demanded that a bank cash a check for $25,000 although he had no account; and a fourth tried to plant a six-foot maple tree on a window sill. Some paretic patients become euphorically expansive and have grandiose, wish-fulfilling delusions of power, wealth or physical prowess. Some become depressed and hopeless, often with irrational, hypochondriacal delusions. Others show few secondary psychological symptoms, although occasionally they may have episodes of excitement. Secondary symptoms are dependent, in large part, on the

patient's occupation, education and previous pattern of adjustment.

If untreated, the paretic patient steadily deteriorates physically and intellectually; he becomes subject to convulsive seizures and paralyses, and dies within two or three years. Treatment—to be discussed in a later section—results in essentially complete recovery for approximately one-third or more of the patients, although often with some minor residual symptoms since destroyed brain cells cannot regenerate. In an additional large group the syphilitic process is arrested and dementia becomes no worse although it has already gone too far for the possibility of adequate functioning; for still other patients, treatment is ineffective and death ensues. In the following case the disease process was arrested, but permanent hospital care was unavoidable.

A 42-year-old man was admitted to a state hospital one year after he began to manifest a number of changes in his behavior. He used to lay things down and immediately forget where he had placed them. He became very dependent on his wife and seemed unable to do anything without her assistance. Although he continued to work until hospitalized, he often sat and brooded. He became irritable and assaultive when a member of the family asked him to do something and he struck out with whatever lay handy. He was hospitalized after he struck his wife in the face and swung a shotgun at his son. His wife reported that he had been a good husband and father until the onset of his illness.

On admission to the hospital it was noted that he had some memory loss and a slight impediment of speech so that paresis appeared to be a possibility. Physical examination revealed none of the typical neurological signs, however, and blood tests were negative. Laboratory tests of his spinal fluid indicated neurosyphilis. On psychological examination he showed confusion, disorientation for time, and marked impairment of memory for recent events. The patient heard people saying they were going to poison his food and drive him insane. Sometimes he thought his wife and son were in another part of the building waiting for him. His emotional reaction was labile and he was either jovial and euphoric, laughing for no apparent reason, or apprehensive, angry and aggressive.

The patient's illness occurred before penicillin was available and he received the standard treatment then in use. Over a period of several months he was given 50 fever treatments, during each of which his temperature was raised to 105 degrees for five hours, plus injections of bismuth and an arsenic compound. The disease process was arrested but still a great deal of brain damage had taken place and the patient continued to require hospital care. Fifteen years after admission he still showed marked impairment of memory and other intellectual functions. Most of the time he was apathetic or mildly euphoric and grandiose; in the latter mood he had delusions of wealth, freely wrote checks for several million dollars each and promised automobiles to everyone who made a request. At times he became acutely impulsive and violent; he repeatedly cut his hands and arms badly by thrusting them through windows. Following the introduction of the major tranquilizing drugs it became possible to control much of his excitement, but there was no essential change in his primary symptoms.

Organic Brain Syndromes Associated with Other Cerebral Conditions

Various cerebral conditions such as brain traumas, tumors, and "hardening of the arteries" can cause organic brain syndromes.

Cerebral Arteriosclerosis. Arteriosclerosis is not an ordinary concomitant of aging. Some elderly persons show no signs of the disorder even in their 70's. The disorder consists of the hardening and thickening of the walls of blood vessels, large arteries and small arterioles and capillaries, which reduce the supply of blood to the brain. In many respects the condition is similar to that found in general paresis. It typically occurs anytime from the 50's on with a median age close to 70, a few years before the onset of senile brain disease. The onset of symptoms may be gradual or sudden; in the latter instance they may follow a "stroke." In more than half the cases the first symptom is delirium.

When the onset is gradual, the clinical picture is very similar to that of senile brain disease. Personality changes are frequent: the patient is likely to become disinterested in his environment and to neglect his personal cleanliness and appearance; his ethical controls may disappear and he may become sexually deviant or paranoidally suspicious. Cerebral arteriosclerotic patients tend to have better insight than senile patients into the fact that they are ill and they often appear puzzled by their loss of memory and failures in comprehension.

When the onset is a sudden stroke, due to blockage of an artery, the initial symptoms include headache, dizziness, faintness, confusion and memory lapses. Occasionally, convulsions occur and in about half the stroke cases patients suffer temporary paralysis of one side of the body (hemiplegia). Usually the patient recovers from his first stroke with a remission of both physical and intellectual symptoms, but is

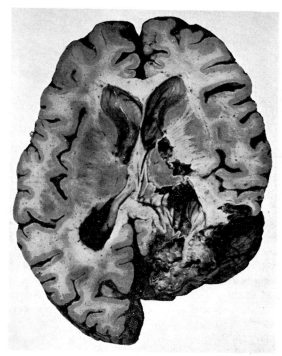

Figure 17–2. *Psychosis with cerebral arteriosclerosis. There is complete softening of the right occipital lobe. An area of infarction (tissue killed by obliteration of its blood supply) is also present in the right basal ganglia. (Reprinted by permission from Breutsch, W. L. 1952. Mental disorders arising from organic disease. In The Biology of Mental Health and Disease. New York, Hoeber-Harper.)*

likely to have repeated attacks of increasing severity, sometimes months or even years apart, as other blood vessels in the brain are blocked. The clinical pattern in such a case consists of long-term deterioration with superimposed episodes of acute, intense disturbance.

The duration of the disorder is difficult to determine. The average duration is considered to be about 3.5 years, yet, since the advent of antibiotics, some patients have lived for many years. The immediate cause of the patient's death tends to be pneumonia, cardiac failure or massive brain hemorrhage. Such complications of cerebral arteriosclerosis are responsible for about 6 per cent of all deaths in the general population.

Patients with cerebral arteriosclerosis differ from patients with senile brain disease in that among the first there is less profound physical and mental decay than in the second. Arteriosclerotic patients suffer fewer fractured bones; if they are confined to bed it is for reasons

SUDDEN
MORE TOGETHER

other than the disorder itself (except after a stroke or if hemiplegia is present); they tend to have emotional outbursts; and their blood pressures are elevated. In senile patients the memory defect is diffuse, but in arteriosclerotic patients the defect is often variable from one time to another. Both types of patients, however, tend to fabricate to make up for deficiencies.

Arteriosclerosis differs from Alzheimer's disease and Pick's disease in that the latter two always have a gradual onset; in arteriosclerosis a sudden onset is typical. In addition, Alzheimer's and Pick's diseases both occur earlier than most cases of arteriosclerosis. The intellectual impairment also differs: arteriosclerotic patients tend to show intermittent periods of improvement, the other two do not—they progress steadily to profound mental deterioration.

SUDDEN
EARLIER
IMPROVEMENT

Epilepsy. An epileptic is an individual who has recurrent episodes of altered consciousness accompanied by changes in the electrochemical activity of the brain. Convulsions may also occur as a result of high fever, intoxications, infections, tremors, uremia and a variety of other causes. With some exceptions, the brain changes are manifested in irregularities of the electroencephalogram (EEG). Some epileptics have involuntary movements or seizures during their episodes of altered consciousness and some do not. The disorder is equally common in males and females although the incidence is higher among children than adults, possibly because many children who are diagnosed as epileptic lose their symptoms with time. The age of onset varies from infancy to the middle decades of life, and later, but the median age is about 17. There is no difference between the intelligence of epileptics and that of the general population, although intelligence is affected if the seizures are unusually frequent and severe. If the seizures start early in life the patient has less chance of normal intellectual development than if the seizures start later. Persons with epilepsy, however, do not always manifest behavioral or intellectual evidence of a brain syndrome. At various times superstitition has endowed epileptics with magical or divine attributes. Some of the oustanding individuals of the past who were subject to seizures were Julius Caesar, Alfred the Great, Lord Byron, Algernon Charles Swinburne, Dostoevsky, Guy de Maupassant and Paganini.

= in
M+F
↑ in
Kids
50%, 17

An epileptic seizure is not a disease. It is an acute, usually repetitive symptom that arises out of a chronic predisposition, the cause of

ACUTE

which may be unknown, or, alternatively, out of many recognized brain disorders. It is widely believed that as a result of some unknown or focal irritation the neural tissue within the cerebral cortex is directly stimulated or irritated and whenever the tissue becomes overly sensitive to the irritation it triggers, in an unknown manner, an abnormal discharge of the neurones which, in turn, brings on the seizure. Some investigators have hypothesized that the irritation is metabolic in origin. In some cases of epilepsy no brain lesions are evident and the seizures are attributed to genetic, metabolic or other constitutional factors; such cases are referred to as *idiopathic*. When the organic cause of the seizures is known the case is labeled *symptomatic*. *ORGANIC*

a)
b)

Epilepsy is manifested in several different forms, and some patients suffer from more than one during their lifetimes. Each form has a typical EEG (see Figure 17–3), but in itself an abnormal EEG pattern is not necessarily an indication of the presence of epilepsy. Approximately 10 per cent of the population show some irregularity of brain wave patterns, yet only one-half of 1 per cent are subject to seizures. The most important types of epilepsy are described as follows.

1)

Petit Mal. This form of epilepsy is most common among children. The attack consists of a loss or diminution of consciousness, without convulsions, which lasts only a few seconds and is followed by the resumption of normal activity. The patient may not even be aware of the attack. He may just "freeze"—stop and stare—momentarily. He may maintain his posture during the attack or he may slip and fall. Small children who fall a great deal for no apparent reason are frequently found to be suffering from the disorder.

No CONV.

2)

Grand Mal. The most dramatic and, presumably, the most common form of epilepsy is grand mal. The patient falls to the ground unconscious, often with a cry, and then has a generalized convulsion that usually lasts less than a minute. Preceding the convulsion, in most cases, is a brief prodromal *aura* during which the patient experiences psychological, sensory or motor symptoms. The most common auras are illusions and hallucinations, mostly visual, but other individuals report auras made up of auditory hallucinations, unpleasant ideas, disturbances of memory, affective reactions, criminal thoughts, or impulses to walk, cry, sing, attack someone or exhibit the sex organs. Most epileptics experience the same aura before every seizure and sometimes experience the aura without a following convulsion.

The convulsion itself consists, in the beginning, of *tonic* rigidity of the entire body in which breathing ceases and the jaws are clenched, followed by *clonic* spasmodic contractions of various muscle groups. In the clonic phase the patient may foam at the mouth, bite his tongue, strike his head against the ground, and lose sphincter control. The contractions soon diminish in intensity and most patients sleep afterward for a few minutes or, occasionally, up to an hour. Patients temporarily manifest some symptoms of an acute brain syndrome after a convulsion (as in the case described earlier). Some patients are subject to grand mal seizures every few days or even oftener; others have one or two in an entire lifetime. Recent advances in drug therapy have made possible the prevention of convulsions in most cases. The following case* is an example of a post-convulsive trauma of an acute nature.

This man, aged 45, was brought by the police to the Emergency department of a general hospital. He had been found by the police in an empty garage beating his head against the wall and talking excitedly. His face was badly bruised and bleeding, evidently as a result of the self-injury.

It was difficult to examine him in the Emergency department because he was obviously reacting to hallucinations, shouting out that the Communists were going to kill him; that he had seen a skeleton hanging up on a neighbour's house; that he had seen a man sawing up another man. He was extremely terrified and so disturbed that admission to a mental hospital had to be arranged immediately.

Following admission to the mental hospital, he continued in a disturbed state, frequently knelt and prayed, cried, and clapped his hands together manneristically. He was impulsive and on one occasion smashed his fist through a window. Under heavy sedation it was possible to examine him physically. There were no signs of skull defects and although the possibility of a subdural haematoma [a swelling that contains effused blood and is situated beneath the dura, the outer-most covering of the brain] was kept in mind, all neurological findings were normal. The presenting clinical picture could be described as a delirium and yet in keeping with an acute manic or schizophrenic illness. The wife was interviewed both at the Emergency department and following the patient's admission to the mental hospital. She stated that the patient had been subject to seizures off and

on since childhood and that following a drinking bout, he had had a series of ten convulsions over a period of forty-eight hours preceding his discovery by the police. This information plus the statement by the wife that there had been no noticeable change in personality over the years raised the likelihood that this illness was of the nature of a post-epileptic furor or delirium.

For the next two to three days in hospital he continued to be disturbed. There were intervals of quiet but most of the time he appeared to be responding to visual and auditory hallucinations. He would mutter his prayers unceasingly. He said that he had visions of going up to Heaven and that a battle ensued between God and the Devil. On chlorpromazine his disturbed state subsided, the hallucinations disappeared, and he became pleasant, cooperative and clear in his thinking. It is interesting to note that the wife described a similar acute illness eighteen months previously following a series of seizures.

The delirious state persisted for four days on that occasion.

Although the patient was quite recovered from his disturbed state he was kept in hospital in order to obtain a more detailed history and to carry out further investigations. The points in his history of significance are as follows. When he was a small boy he is said to have fallen off a hayrick on his head. Whether this story of a head injury is of significance or not, he had seizures from that time on. The patient stated that preceding the fits he had a feeling of dizziness followed by an unpleasant odour and a vague feeling of abdominal discomfort. These prodromal symptoms were not always followed by a seizure. In the seizures, his wife had observed him to lose consciousness, froth at the mouth, pass through a tonic and clonic phase followed by apnoea [transient cessation of breathing] then stertorous breathing and confusion giving place to sleep; in other words a rather typical grand mal seizure. The fits had occurred three or four times a year but in recent years they had become more frequent. Detailed neurological examination and skull films were normal but the electroencephalogram revealed slow waves arising in the right temporal lobe. This finding was considered to be in keeping with an epileptic focus in this part of the brain.

Since the patient had never had adequate anticonvulsant therapy he was placed on an appropriate regimen of drugs. One year later he was well, working steadily and free of seizures.

(3) *Psychomotor Attacks.* This form of epilepsy is also known as an epileptic equivalent and may or may not involve loss of consciousness. Attacks manifest themselves as states of confusion, automatic behavior, feelings of unreality or any of a variety of mental disturbances. The patient may be docile, terrified or violently assaultive. He may have paranoid ideas and hal-

*Reprinted by permission from Dewan, J. G., and Spaulding, W. B. 1958. The Organic Psychoses, Toronto, The University of Toronto Press, pp. 99–100.

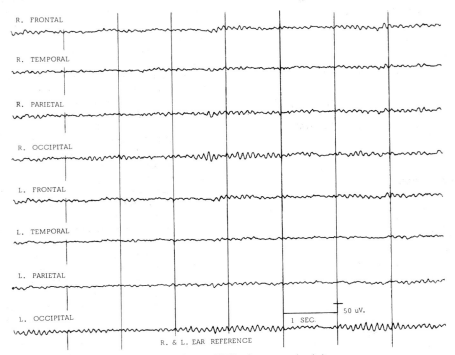

Figure 17–3, a. *EEG of a normal adult.*

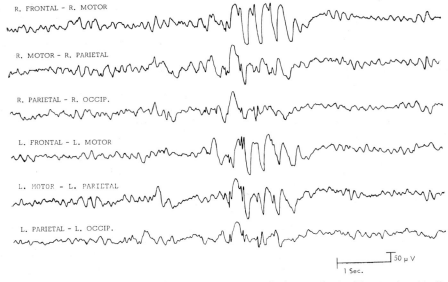

Figure 17–3, b. *One type of EEG found between attacks in a patient with grand mal epilepsy.*

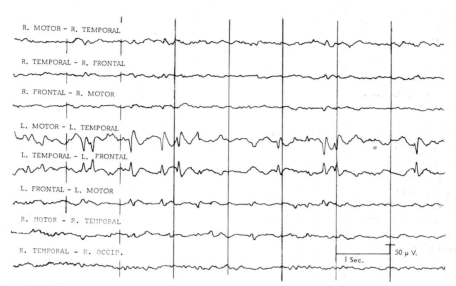

Figure 17–3, c. *EEG seen between attacks in a patient subject to psychomotor seizures of temporal lobe origin.*

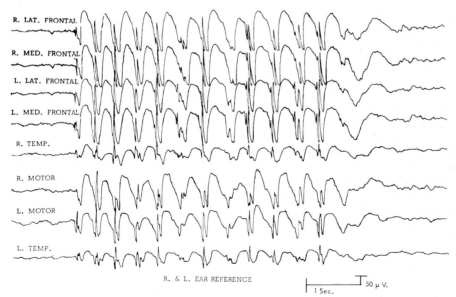

Figure 17–3, d. *EEG taken during a short, clinical, petit mal attack that began and ended abruptly. (From Noyes, A. P., and Kolb, L. C. 1963. Modern Clinical Psychiatry. 6th Ed. Philadelphia, W. B. Saunders Co.)*

lucinations, wander aimlessly about, or engage in bizarre behavior. The attacks may last from a few minutes to several days. They occur most frequently among adult males but the reason for this is not known.

Meier and French (1964) found that among psychomotor epileptics indications of personality disturbance, as measured on the MMPI, are more related to the presence of bilateral than unilateral EEG abnormalities. Subjects with bilateral EEG's scored higher on the scales indicative of schizo-adaptive and depressive behavior characteristics than subjects with unilateral EEG's. The analysis of MMPI elevations for the patients with bitemporal independent spike foci suggested a highly selective correlation between such EEG patterns and test indications for psychopathological patterns of behavior. The sample was comprised of 53 patients of whom 40 were later given temporal lobectomies—confirming the spike focus diagnosis—because of seizures that were poorly controlled by anti-convulsants.

Jacksonian Epilepsy. First described by the British neurologist John Hughlings Jackson (1834–1911), this form of epilepsy is a variant of grand mal. It consists of a motor seizure that begins in part of one side of the body, e.g., one side of the face or one arm or a finger, and then spreads to the entire side. It may or may not engage the other side also and end in a generalized convulsion. In the typical case of Jacksonian epilepsy, the patient has a structural lesion in the part of the brain that controls the movement of the area where the seizure begins.

Regardless of type of epilepsy, a number of patients with the disorder eventually develop personality disturbances of a neurotic nature that are apparently an emotional reaction to the seizures themselves. The extent of the disturbances are influenced by the patient's total life experiences as an individual. Overprotection by his family may prevent him from learning to adjust to his disorder. His ego development may be stunted because he has never developed, or loses, the sense of personal worth. He may be apprehensive because he fears the convulsions, being out of contact during the seizures, death, or the social stigma attached to the disorder. He may be anxious about having attacks in inappropriate settings or before disapproving people. Self-doubts and feelings of insecurity may arise over his unknown behavior during and after the seizures, for the future or for the achievement of different goals. He may become

evasive, lying to get jobs and hide his disorder, or defensive, aggressive or suspicious over imagined or real slights and taunts. His limited choices in education, vocation and marriage may lead to a sense of inadequacy, feelings of rejection or the desire to hide. To protect himself, he may become seclusive, egocentric or rigid and perseverative. The longer epilepsy persists, the more likely it is that the manifestations of personality disturbance will develop.

In a review of the evidence bearing on the personality of epileptics, Tizard (1962) concluded that most epileptics do not share a characteristic personality but that the incidence among them of one or another kind of personality disturbance is relatively high. Some patients, especially those who develop the disorder late, adjust to their difficulties without marked distortions of personality. True epileptic seizures are not hysterical in origin. In hysterical seizures the patient does not usually lose consciousness, or hurt himself when he falls, or bite his tongue or lose control of his sphincters. The majority of epilepsy patients do not have dementia. Epilepsy is far less likely to entail irreversible deterioration than a number of other chronic syndromes.

Psychotic reactions are rare in epilepsy and only about 1 per cent of first admissions to mental hospitals are diagnosed as having psychoses associated with epilepsy.

Intracranial Neoplasm. In the following case* of fatal brain tumor the patient manifested a psychotic reaction over and above the primary organic impairment. He was 41 years old and was hospitalized after his wife complained that he had been behaving peculiarly for about a year and had finally struck her. The patient's disorder must be classified as acute since successful removal of the tumor probably would have reversed his impairment and resulted in his return to a pre-illness level of functioning.

. . . On admission [the man] appeared confused, was unsteady and acted as if intoxicated. His memory for recent events was poor. He was untidy and would urinate on the floor. At times he complained of severe headaches, sudden in onset and of short duration. As these symptoms were strongly suggestive of organic disease of the brain, the attending physician was especially interested in learning of the onset of the mental illness with reference to previous per-

*Abstracted by permission from Dewan, J. G., and Spaulding, W. B. 1958. The Organic Psychoses. Toronto, The University of Toronto Press, pp. 110–112.

sonality and other symptoms indicative of cerebral disease. His wife stated that he had always been a well-adjusted, cheerful person who had many friends. He had worked as a florist's assistant for some years until fourteen months previously when he had a difference of opinion with his employer regarding overtime, the disagreement resulting in his discharge from the job. One wonders if this dispute with his employer, which was foreign to his usual behaviour, might not indeed have been the first sign of the developing mental illness. He was unable to obtain work quickly, appeared despondent and would sit by himself for long periods. His behaviour frequently would be facetious, he would laugh for no apparent reason and when questioned would make irrelevant remarks. Six months previous to admission, it was noticed by the patient's family that he had a squint and the patient complained of seeing double. His mental symptoms became more pronounced, he appeared sullen and preoccupied, sitting staring into space for long periods. In the four months previous to admission he often cried out, "my head, my head," and then would laugh. The last few weeks before coming into hospital the patient stated that he expected the Devil daily at 3 p.m. He thought people were outside the window. He complained of crawling feelings up the back of his head and misidentified relatives. It was only when he struck his wife that she finally consulted a physician and this led to his admission to hospital.

The significant findings were as follows: internal strabismus of the right eye; both pupils reacted to light but the right was sluggish; a questionable weakness of the right hand grip; a tendency to fall to the right side; marked papilloedema [optic neuritis due to intracranial pressure] bilaterally. . . .

The history and mental and physical findings were in keeping with a space-occupying lesion. At operation, a large meningioma [a benign tumor of one of the coverings of the brain] the size of an orange and weighing 105 grams was present. . . . The patient did not survive the operation.

Meningioma is the most favourable type of brain tumour to remove. An early careful examination might have indicated the organic lesion. In reviewing the case it would seem that there was a wealth of signs suggesting the likelihood of an underlying organic process involving the brain: striking personality changes a year prior to admission in a man of previous stable personality; six months before admission, strabismus and double vision; complaints of sudden, severe headaches of short duration; memory defect for recent events associated with a generally confused mental state with disorientation and deterioration of fine sensibilities and personal habits; and finally the neurological findings, particularly the advanced papilloedema.

Huntington's Chorea. This disease is a relatively rare, irreversible psychosis characterized by progressive chorea, impaired speech and intellect, and dominating emotional moods. It was first described by the American neurologist George Huntington (1862–1927) and has since been traced to inheritance of a single dominant gene (see Chapter 6). Post mortem studies of the brains of victims of the disease have revealed widespread cerebral atrophy and the presence of scar cells. The behavior and overt physical symptoms, generally not distinguishable until the patient is in his 30's, include progressive dementia, apathy, depression or irritability, sensory defects, choreiform

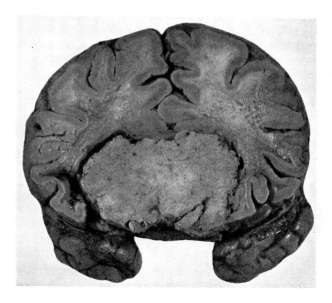

Figure 17–4. Psychosis with brain tumor (meningioma). Section through tumor mass in the frontal lobe area. (Reprinted by permission from Bruetsch, W. L., 1952. Mental disorders arising from organic disease. In The Biology of Mental Health and Disease. New York, Hoeber-Harper.)

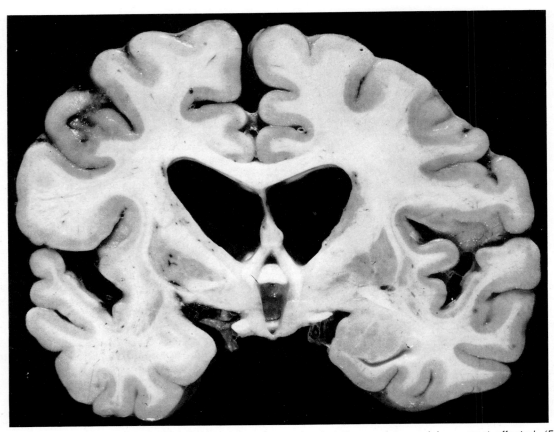

Figure 17-5. Huntington's chorea. There is diffuse atrophy, but the caudate nuclei are most affected. (From Robbins, S. L. 1962. A Textbook of Pathology. 2nd Ed. Philadelphia, W. B. Saunders Co.)

twitching of the arms or legs, ataxia and a bizarre gait, facial grimacing, smacking of the lips and tongue, and explosive speech. Delusions occur in a minority of patients and the more depressed may attempt suicide. Sometimes the physical symptoms appear without personality changes. Sometimes the psychological symptoms appear first and lead to a mistaken diagnosis of schizophrenia or other functional disorder. Hospitalization is inevitable with time, and death usually ensues within 20 years of the onset of symptoms.

In the following case the patient at first seemed to be suffering from a neurotic reaction to environmental stresses. The anxiety and depression she experienced throughout the course of her disorder, as well as the content of the delusions that eventually developed, appeared to be a reaction to her experiences prior to the overt disorder.

The patient's first psychiatric contact came at the age of 36. She was depressed over the deteriorating

relationship with her alcoholic and irresponsible husband. She also felt guilty because of their premarital sexual relations and had recently become sexually frigid. She appeared to improve with supportive psychotherapy but during the next four years had several further minor episodes of depression. She then divorced her husband and undertook to raise their three children with the financial assistance of welfare agencies.

Two years later she became increasingly anxious and depressed in a seemingly neurotic pattern. Further supportive psychotherapy and meprobamate medication resulted in symptom amelioration but soon she began to display involuntary movements of the arms and legs and forgetfulness; she also began to neglect her appearance and personal hygiene. The symptoms worsened with time and at the age of 46 she was referred to a neurologist who made the diagnosis of Huntington's chorea. Without any preparation, he informed her in a rather brutal manner that she had an incurable brain disease and that her children should be sterilized. Her reaction was a severe depression and, soon afterward, she was admitted to a state hospital.

With anti-depressive medication her mood improved and she was placed in a boarding home where she could receive simple nursing care. The uncontrollable movements in her limbs worsened and she developed increasing memory difficulty, particularly for recent events. Again she became severely depressed, lost appetite and weight, and attempted suicide by drinking a cleaning fluid. Readmitted to the state hospital, she was found to have gross delusions of self-accusation: she believed that she had killed her children and a number of other persons and that her deeds had been reported in the newspapers. She believed that her body was filled with deadly germs and she advised people not to touch her lest they be killed. Abstract intelligence, memory and orientation were markedly impaired and she became increasingly uncoordinated and weak until her death a few years later.

An investigation disclosed that her father had died of Huntington's chorea at the age of 54. The patient had four siblings, three brothers and a sister, of whom the sister was in another state hospital with a diagnosis of Huntington's chorea, and one brother was suffering from an undiagnosed "nervous disability." The patient's mother, who had been the dominant parent in the family even prior to the father's illness, had been strict, critical and physically abusive toward the children. In retrospect, it appeared that the patient's predisposition to anxiety and depression stemmed from her childhood relationship with her mother.

Organic Brain Syndromes Associated with Other Physical Conditions

A variety of brain syndromes are caused by general systemic disorders such as endocrine disorders, metabolic or nutritional disorders, systemic infections and drug or poison intoxication.

An acute brain syndrome caused by metabolic disturbance is illustrated in the following case of hypothyroidism. The patient's behavior was markedly psychotic, a reflection of her basic personality trends as well as of the disorder itself.

A 39-year-old woman was hospitalized after five years of emotional instability and outbursts of temper. During the previous two years marked changes had occurred in her appearance: her weight had increased, her face had become puffy, skin and hair had turned very dry and her voice had coarsened. She had become intolerant of cold, chronically fatigued, constipated and short of breath. Her ankles had begun to swell and she complained of headaches, nausea, vomiting and excessive menstruation. She slept 12 hours a day.

When hospitalized, the patient was disheveled and in an obvious state of anguish. Her speech was repeti-

tive and stereotyped and she blocked frequently. Her attention span was short and she could not concentrate well; her abstract thinking was impaired and her memory for recent events, poor. Her affective responses were very labile and fluctuated from a tearful, agitated depression to resentful hostility. Among the most striking of her symptoms, however, were the transient delusions of reference, influence and persecution, along with varied hallucinations. The latter ran the gamut of hearing, vision, smell and taste; relatives appeared to be talking to her and she told a nurse's aide, "I hear all these voices—all day I have—but you are the first voice I believe—yes, I do—I believe I can trust you. You are pure. I used to be like you—a nurse's aide helping people." She had had two illegitimate children before her current marriage to an alcoholic with whom she got along badly. The voices she heard talked about her, accused her of immorality, and threatened her. She felt that everyone was watching her. At one time she believed that all her relatives were dead.

Her MMPI was elevated on the paranoid and psychopathic deviate scales. An intelligence test yielded an I.Q. of 73 and a memory test yielded an even poorer score. On clinical examination it became obvious that she was suffering from a severe thyroid deficiency. Her basal metabolic rate was −32 per cent and other tests of thyroid functioning were consistent. Concomitantly, she suffered from anemia and impaired heart functioning which are common in advanced hypothyroidism. Treatment by thyroid extract was begun, and after two weeks marked physical and behavioral improvement was noted.

Six weeks after admission, the patient's measured I.Q. was 93, although her memory was borderline and she still manifested a defect in foresight and planning. On an MMPI retest the paranoid and psychopathic scales were normal. The delusions and hallucinations disappeared completely. Her anemia and cardiac functioning improved greatly and her weight went down. Soon afterward she was able to leave the hospital on a daily maintenance dose of thyroid extract.

CAUSATION OF THE BRAIN SYNDROMES

As indicated earlier, the classification of the brain syndromes is based, in part, on the particular pathological process involved (e.g., tumor, cerebral arteriosclerosis or senile and presenile degeneration) and, in part, on the precipitating cause (e.g., head injury, intoxication or infectious agent). Observation, however, leads to the conclusion that in a brain syndrome the precipitating cause is necessary but not sufficient. Only a minority of the individuals who are exposed to various precipitating causes develop the associated brain syndromes. Syphilis, for instance, affects the brain of only a small number of infected individuals and chronic alcoholism does not always result in delirium tremens, Korsakoff's syndrome, chronic deterioration or any of the other possible consequences. It is known, of course, that both animals and people differ in vulnerability to biological stress. Windle (1952) subjected guinea pigs to prolonged anoxia and found that after 100 to 150 hours of deprivation some of the animals underwent changes in brain structure, memory and ability to learn and some did not. Humans also differ in response to anoxia as well as to sleep deprivation and vitamin and hormonal deficiencies.

Among those individuals who do develop a brain syndrome, the correlation between degree of brain damage and degree of behavior disturbance is by no means a perfect one. Many individuals with minor brain damage evidence marked psychological disturbance; conversely, post mortem examinations have revealed severe brain damage in persons who had shown no evidence of dementia. Sometimes there is even a reversal of the correlation: a study of patients with acute head injuries revealed that after recovery from the acute phase, those patients who had experienced severe injuries had few residual complaints and those whose injuries had been minor had many (Ruesch and Bowman, 1946).

It appears, then, that a number of predisposing causes must necessarily influence the development and manifestations of organic brain syndromes. For convenience, these predisposing factors may be divided into three broad categories: (1) a general body susceptibility or lack of immunity to a specific agent (e.g., infection or intoxication); (2) the specific propensity of some persons but not others to react to pathological brain processes with symptoms of overt intellectual impairment; (3) the specific tendency of some individuals with brain syndromes to manifest various forms of functional psychological disturbance as a response to biological stress. In general, such predisposing factors depend on heredity and lifelong environmental influences.

Epilepsy is one of a number of organic syndromes in which heredity is an important factor. In a study of epileptic twins not specified as either idiopathic or symptomatic, Rosanoff (1934) found a concordance rate for monozygotic twins which was lower than the rates found in subsequent studies of MZ twins with idiopathic epilepsy but higher than the rates for MZ twins with symptomatic epilepsy. Studies of twins with idiopathic epilepsy have resulted in consistent findings of high concordance among MZ twins and a low concordance among dizygotic twins. In studies of twins with symptomatic epilepsy, a minimal concordance is found among both MZ and DZ twins (Conrad, 1935; Lennox and Jolly, 1954; see Table 17–2). These findings are consistent with the clinical observations that with sufficient provocation anyone can have an epileptic seizure; the seizure threshold varies from one person to another and in the same individual from time to time; and persons with idiopathic epilepsy have consistently low thresholds for precipitating stimuli. It also appears probable that the tendency to develop post-epileptic confusion following a series of seizures varies considerably from person to person.

In the disorders of old age an inherited tendency to longevity is a definite factor. In addition, cerebral arteriosclerosis and senile brain disease are found more frequently among the relatives of affected individuals than among the

TABLE 17–2. Estimated Concordance Rates in Monozygotic and Dizygotic Co-twins of Epileptic Twins

Type of Epilepsy and Investigator	Apparent Zygosity of Twins	Number of Pairs	Estimated Concordance Rate (Per Cent)	$H = \dfrac{CMZ - CDZ}{100 - CDZ}$
Unspecified	(MZ	23	70)	0.61
Rosanoff et al., 1934	(DZ	84	24)	
Idiopathic	(MZ	22	86)	0.85
Conrad, 1935	(DZ	97	4)	
Symptomatic	(MZ	8	13)	0.13
Conrad, 1935	(DZ	34	0)	
Without brain damage (idiopathic)	(MZ	51	88)	0.86
Lennox and Jolly, 1954	(DZ	47	13)	
With brain damage (symptomatic)	(MZ	26	35)	0.26
Lennox and Jolly, 1954	(DZ	49	12)	

EPIL + PICKS — DOM GENE

general population. According to Kallmann and Jarvik (1961), some investigators believe that a dominant gene is responsible for the specific biochemical deficiency that results both in cerebral arteriosclerosis and its particular localization. According to other investigators, arteriosclerosis may consist of at least two separate entities: (1) defective cholesterol metabolism or circulatory functions, and (2) a breakdown of the structure of elastic elements in the arteries accompanied by calcification. These investigators noted a familial concentration, in cases of arteriosclerosis, for allied pathological conditions, such as coronary artery disease, essential hypertension and cerebral arteriosclerosis, so that a simple dominant mode of inheritance might be considered. Kallmann and Jarvik (1961) concluded that although there is some evidence at present that a gene-specific metabolic error is the basic cause of arteriosclerosis, many important etiological aspects of the theory are still obscure. Since men appear to be more vulnerable to the disorder than women, Busse (1961) hypothesized that the difference is hormonal in nature and that estrogen and other female hormones play a protective role.

Earlier, Kallmann (1950) studied 33 pairs of MZ and 75 pairs of DZ twins of whom at least one member had developed a senile psychosis, and reported an age-corrected concordance rate of 43 per cent in the MZ group and only 7 per cent in the DZ group. Senility and Alzheimer's disease seem to be influenced by multiple minor genes. In Pick's disease, on the other hand, a simple dominant gene has been considered a likely determinant. The role of heredity in Huntington's chorea was discussed in an earlier chapter.

A number of studies have indicated the importance of psychological factors in organic syndromes. Rothschild (1956) observed that "Tissue damage, per se, does not produce a psychosis; it is rather, the person's capacity to compensate for the damage, as well as present social and situational stresses, which impair the individual's ability to withstand the cerebral damage."

Auerbach et al. (1960) investigated the post-traumatic syndrome in 50 subjects, aged 15 to 57, who had been hospitalized 24 hours or longer with head injuries. The interval between injury and investigation was 5 to 36 months with a mean of 12 months, although in 10 cases the mean interval was more than 18 months. The cause of the syndrome, they decided, was a

CAUSE = combination of physical and emotional factors. They were surprised to find no significant relationship between the severity of the injury and the severity of the syndrome; they offered as possible explanations that either their clinical impressions had been based on patients with residual neurological defects (many other patients with equally severe injuries had made good recoveries); or that the manner of rating the severity of the injury might have been faulty; or that many patients had relatively severe reactions to minor injuries. They found a definite relationship between the pre-traumatic personality disturbances of patients and their post-traumatic symptoms. Where personality disturbances existed, the head injuries were often enough to upset the patient's emotional balance and resulted in the prolongation of symptoms. Some patients showed neurotic reactions in addition to or in place of post-traumatic symptoms. Some patients with personality disturbances recovered promptly, however, and the investigators hypothesized it was because the injury had not been particularly stressful and did not involve the area of their conflicts, or that the patients had had no previous tendencies to somatize their anxiety. Injuries that were psychologically stressful seemed closely related to the severity of the post-traumatic symptoms. In cases in which financial compensation was involved, patients had worse symptoms. The implication drawn by the investigators was that emotional factors and the circumstances of an injury to the brain are relatively more important than the severity of the injury.

In many cases the existence of a functional disorder may be itself responsible for the individual's exposure to an agent that precipitates an organic syndrome. A schizophrenic, for example, may deprive himself of sleep and essential vitamins; a depressed patient who inhales carbon monoxide in an unsuccessful attempt to commit suicide may, instead, develop a brain syndrome; and a sociopath who seeks excitement is vulnerable to head injury as well as the disorders associated with alcohol and drug addictions. Dewan and Spaulding (1958) caution that "a long history of emotional upsets does not automatically rule out the need to consider a physical element in the present breakdown."

In epilepsy, psychological stress may increase the frequency and severity of seizures but by itself does not cause them. The stress is merely a precipitant for those organically predisposed individuals who have a low threshold to epileptic seizures. Caveness (1955) lists three psychological factors that he believes should be considered by clinical neurologists in the diagnosis and treatment of epilepsy: (a) emotional problems that precipitate seizures; (b) emotional problems that contribute to the pattern of seizures; and (c) emotional problems that develop as a reaction to seizures.

It has been hypothesized that in organically predisposed individuals, convulsions are a means of discharging psychic tensions that they are unable to discharge normally. Mayer-Gross et al. (1960) find that moods of depression or mounting irritability preceding an attack are not altered by a minor attack, but only by a major one. They relate this finding to the observation that in ECT a minor convulsion has no effect in the treatment of depression.

Alternatively, a seizure may be an unconscious attempt by a predisposed individual to escape from an unbearable situation. Petit mal attacks are most frequently triggered by frustrations or inactivity and boredom. Grand mal attacks also may be precipitated by frustrations but other precipitants may be depression, any strong emotion or an emotionally charged situation. Usually, however, psychological problems influence convulsions indirectly through physiologic states. For example, in individuals with a low threshold, seizures may be caused by hyperventilation that is brought on by severe anxiety states; by overactivity of the adrenal cortex that is brought on by severe stress situations; or by overactivity of the adrenal medulla that is brought on by great rage and hostility. Psychotherapists have found that in some patients the number of grand mal seizures can sometimes be reduced by alleviating psychological difficulties.

Psychological factors also contribute to the causation of the chronic brain disorders of old age. The distribution of the disorders is not random as would be expected if the causation were exclusively organic. Busse (1961) suggests that mental and physical stress may precipitate the abrupt appearance of the symptoms of cerebral arteriosclerosis. When individuals function at a marginal level the addition of unaccustomed stress may cause the organism to break down and the symptoms of the disorder to become apparent. Raskin and Ehrenberg (1956) studied 270 elderly patients of whom 93 were diagnosed as having mixed arteriosclerosis and senile changes. Examination of this group revealed that brain atrophy was not proportionate to the age of the patient or the diagnosed illness. The investigators stated, "The degree of brain atrophy was not always indicative of the patient's mental deterioration. Some patients with greatly atrophied brains showed better compensatory mechanisms than others with less pronounced atrophy." They concluded that psychological and social changes in an individual's life history which breed anxiety and insecurity, and lower his motivational level, account for the psychoses of old age better than anatomical changes. "It appears that senility is a pathological condition precipitated by many factors, not the least of which are emotional" (Raskin and Ehrenberg, 1956).

The disorders of aging may be a neurotic reaction to the sense of decreasing adequacy, security and prestige and of increasing difficulty in making adjustments. Goldfarb and Sheps (1954), working in a home for aged persons, noted:

Behavior disorders of aged persons often occur in a setting of chronic brain syndrome due to a process of doubtful pathogenesis called senile sclerosis. . . . In all of our cases we observed fear and rage arising in a context of increasing helplessness due to loss of physical, social and economic resources. This helplessness led to failure to relieve tensions, to achieve pleasurable gratifications, and to master the social and physical environment. These failures increased the maladaptation of the aged persons by adding psychological inhibition to the physiological inadequacy.

Among the most important factors that may contribute to the precipitation of a chronic brain disorder in an aging person is isolation. It may be separation from children and family, or separation from the world of productive activities and interactions with large groups of people, or a loss of perceptual stimuli as a result of fading vision and diminished hearing. As we have seen in other contexts, the isolated individual is more prone to psychological and physical ills; he is also more prone to be hospitalized for one of the disorders of old age. In England, an investigation into the costs of the National Health Service revealed that among mental hospital patients over the age of 65, single, widowed or divorced persons occupied over two-thirds of the beds. Although single persons made up only 12 per cent of the population aged 65 and over, they occupied 41.3 per cent of the mental hospital beds in that age group and constituted 53 per cent of all hospital admissions. The proportion of married persons over the age of 65 admitted to all hospitals did not reach a high level even after the age of 75 (Guilleband Report, 1956). Williams and Jaco (1957) found that a married person aged 60 is only one-third as likely to develop a disorder of old age as one whose spouse has died. Women tend to outlive their husbands by about five years which accounts for the larger numbers of women with organic brain syndromes of senility, although there is no higher frequency of these disorders among women than men.

Isolation breeds loneliness which Hazell (1960) considers one of the most serious hardships for the elderly:

The affliction is of a negative kind—just being left alone, of no interest to anyone, just waiting to die, or as if they never existed or their lives had any meaning. For those without relatives it is a hard thing to bear, and for those with relatives who never visit them it leads to cynical despair. Continued loneliness brings about, not only mental illness in the way of apathy, indifference, depression or even dementia, but also physical illness resulting from lack of reasonable exercise, inattention to diet with poor nutrition, and failure to obtain treatment for any accompanying illness. The physical ill-health worsens the mental state, and vice versa, so setting up a vicious circle of poor general health.

In another study, Williams and Jaco (1958) considered psychiatric disorders among the aged to result from the loss of personal identity. They analyzed the aged psychiatric patients admitted for the first time to various hospitals in Texas over a two-year period and found that among those over 65 years of age the highest incidence of disorders was among Anglo-Americans, next among Negroes and last among Spanish-Americans. The rate for males in each group was higher than that for females but the rate for Anglo-American females was higher than that for males in either of the two lower groups. The investigators hypothesized that the Spanish-Americans do not exclude the aged from the family unit but that the urbanized Americans do. They concluded:

Any ensuing psychiatric disorder may thus be the resultant of a sequence of unsuccessful attempts to cope with the effects of being old and may exhibit any one or a combination of three major components: (1) a withdrawal and insulation from a society in which they are experiencing a loss of personal identity, (2) a distortion of reality in an attempt to re-

gain or maintain identity, (3) a self-depreciation in response to their apparent lack of significance and worth.

An individual's response to an organic brain syndrome is, in part, determined by his intelligence. It is widely recognized that the lower the individual's level of intelligence before he develops a brain disorder, the more likely he will require long-term hospitalization.

There is also some indication that individuals of lower socioeconomic status are especially likely to develop organic brain syndromes. It has long been known that at the lower socioeconomic level the rates of mortality from many accidents and illnesses are higher throughout childhood and young adult life than at other socioeconomic levels. Hollingshead and Redlich (1958) also found high frequencies of senile and other organic psychoses in the lowest socioeconomic classes of a city. These greater occurrences may be a result of the higher frequency of exposure to the disorders than in other classes, or, if exposure is similar, of greater vulnerability, or of inadequate medical treatment. An individual exposed to the economic and emotional stresses of poverty may be more likely to develop hardening of the arteries; he may receive treatment too late, or be more likely to deteriorate intellectually than an upper-class individual with the same degree of arterial damage in the cerebrum.

Men and women tend to be exposed to different hazards and consequently have different rates for various syndromes. Men have higher rates for alcoholic psychoses, psychoses associated with industrial poisons, paresis and cerebral arteriosclerosis. Women have relatively higher frequencies for brain syndromes associated with hypothyroidism, senility and the diseases of degeneration.

There is considerable variation in the frequency of the illnesses and intoxications responsible for brain syndromes from one geographical area to another. The variation is apparently a function of the general level of nutrition, the development of industry and public health programs, and the nature of parasitic infestations, in the area. Brain syndromes associated with malnutrition, malaria and trypanosomiasis (sleeping sickness) are still prevalent in many under-developed countries of the world, whereas those associated with alcoholism and industrial poisons are more characteristic of countries that are technologically developed.

TREATMENT

In organic brain syndromes, as in other disorders discussed earlier, the prognosis for treatment is better the more acute the disorder is and the sooner after onset treatment starts. As a rule, therefore, the prognosis for the treatment of acute brain syndromes is generally good; for treatment of chronic brain syndromes, the prognosis is guarded because destroyed neurones in the central nervous system cannot be regenerated. Some amelioration of the patient's condition can be expected, nevertheless, because (1) early treatment often arrests the course of the disease, (2) vicarious brain functioning takes place to some extent and (3) psychological adjustment is often possible.

The treatment of organic brain syndromes is either specific or symptomatic and supportive. Specific therapy is directed toward eliminating the causal agent (as in a brain tumor or paresis), whereas symptomatic and supportive therapy is directed toward eradicating the symptoms (as in delirium, stupor or convulsions) and in making the patient more comfortable (as in Huntington's chorea or senile psychosis).

Treating the wide variety of diseases and intoxications that cause acute brain syndromes is more appropriate for discussion in textbooks of medicine and nursing than here. Wherever possible, specific treatments are used to eliminate infecting organisms or toxic materials, increase the blood supply to the brain, remove tumors, relieve the brain of pressure caused by blood clots or fractured skull, correct metabolic disorders and halt convulsions. General symptomatic and supportive treatments are used to minimize the symptoms of delirium, stupor, coma, confusion, agitation, fever, dehydration, malnutrition or distress. The accustomed practice is to treat patients with acute brain disorders in a stable environment, i.e., in quiet, cool rooms in which the lighting is constant and subdued and with a minimum of nursing attendants in order to avoid compounding the patient's confusion and, in cases of infectious disease, to facilitate isolation precautions. Patients must be restrained from injuring themselves or others and excessive agitation must be curbed. Tranquilizing drugs, particularly the phenothiazines which can be given intramuscularly or intravenously for quick effect, are widely used for this purpose. Supplementary vitamins (particularly members of the vitamin B complex) are frequently indicated; care must be taken that the patient's bodily functions are maintained at normal or near normal levels. If the patient displays symptoms of a functional disorder, he is treated as soon as possible; psychotherapy may be instituted on the basis of functional symptoms associated with an organic brain syndrome.

Patients with acute brain syndromes are usually able to return to their pre-illness levels of functioning. If an acute episode occurs in an apparently healthy individual (as in the case of the hypothyroid woman), he is able to return to his pre-illness activities; if an episode occurs in an individual with a chronic disorder, the patient can be no better after the acute episode than he was before. Any brain syndrome that does not respond to the available forms of treatment or leaves a residue of damage that disturbs the individual's behavior, is classified as chronic.

In the treatment of chronic brain syndromes it must be remembered that there is no one-to-one relationship between extent of brain pathology and symptomatology, that all individuals react uniquely to each disorder, and that not all individuals respond predictably to treatment. As in any disorder, the immediate treatment for a chronic brain syndrome is to alleviate whatever acute phase may exist, then eradicate, if possible, the cause of the disorder (as in paresis), and then try to eliminate the symptoms. On the whole, treatment tends to be symptomatic or supportive. Medication, except where indicated symptomatically, is kept at a minimum; sedatives increase the symptoms of intellectual impairment and depression. However, anti-depressives or tranquilizing drugs effectively minimize emotional disturbances in patients with functional or organic disorders. Chlorpromazine is widely used to control excitement and motor restlessness, agitation or depression, in such patients, and to prevent insomnia. It does not reduce the intellectual deterioration resulting from senility or arteriosclerosis. Where deterioration is not too advanced, electroshock treatments or psychotherapy may diminish secondary functional symptoms.

Sometimes a decision must be made whether the patient should be kept at home or removed to a hospital, a nursing home or a mental hospital. By and large, most patients are better off in familiar surroundings, for old people appear to die sooner in institutions than at home; but the decision must also consider the effects of such persons on other members of the household, the availability of proper care, the manifestations of the disorders, i.e., frequency of convulsions or extent of disintegration, and the activities of which the individuals are still capable. The major part of the management of patients with chronic brain syndromes consists of social, milieu, occupational and supportive therapy.

Delirium

Whatever the cause of the delirium, the symptomatic and supportive treatment is identical in purpose: to prevent or combat cardiac embarrassment and failure, maintain the patient's strength and control his restlessness. Aside from indicated specific medication, the most important therapy, perhaps, is procuring needed rest and sleep for the patient. Despite restlessness, physical restraints are rarely used; in the struggle against them the patient may become more restless, perspire more and become more delirious. Hypnotics are of limited use because they tend to increase confusion, and have a depressing effect on respiration and circulation; instead, tranquilizers, especially chlorpromazine, are usually administered.

Epilepsy

Medication, for most epileptics, is a way of life. Anti-convulsants are not a cure but a control; the medication suppresses or modifies the convulsions but it does not cure them. When the effective dosage of anti-convulsant has been determined for a patient he is impressed with the fact that the medication has become a part of his daily routine for an indefinite period. Anti-convulsants supplement the individual's metabolic balance as do ketogenic (high acid) diets. Because of the effectiveness of anti-convulsant drugs, the diets are seldom prescribed now.

The first medication used to reduce the frequency and severity of epileptic seizures was bromide, introduced approximately 100 years ago. Some 60 years later barbiturates began to be widely used. Unfortunately, both medications were highly depressive and often had deleterious effects on the personalities of the patients. The search for better anti-convulsants continued and was rewarded, about 30 years ago, with the discovery of Dilantin. Today, close to 20 anti-convulsants are available, of which the most widely used are Dilantin, Mysoline and Tridione. Not every one is specific for every form or combination of the disorder and not every

person reacts equally to every drug. Anti-convulsants are prescribed separately or in combination. The medication is administered under continuing medical supervision because patients sometimes suffer varying degrees of harmful side effects, although there is usually a wide margin between the dose necessary for control and one that will cause side effects. Most patients have good control and suffer no significant difficulties as a result of the medication. There is no standard dosage. The physician determines for each patient not only the amount of the drug to be taken but the hours of treatment as well. A sudden discontinuance of the medication will usually lead to frequent uncontrolled seizures, and patients are warned against the unfounded optimism from which the discontinuance stems. Patients must also refrain from alcohol and must exercise care in taking other drugs.

As a result of anti-convulsants, more than 80 per cent of all epileptics are able to live comparatively normal lives. In 50 per cent of all cases the attacks are brought under complete control and in the other 30 per cent the attacks are minimized. Of all persons with epileptic convulsions, approximately 15 to 20 per cent do not respond to the anti-convulsants and need to be cared for. A very small number recover spontaneously.

The use of ECT has been successful in some epileptics with functional psychopathology, particularly severe depression. The therapy has also been reported to be helpful in some cases in which convulsions or mental disturbances occur only at infrequent and regular intervals and are preceded by days of altered mood or physical disturbance. Patients with psychomotor epilepsy have sometimes been given ECT on the theory that their agitation and restlessness are caused by internal tensions that cannot be discharged normally.

Surgery is sometimes resorted to when all other means of control have failed. It cannot be used in cases of idiopathic epilepsy, of course, but in some cases of symptomatic epilepsy it has been specifically successful in abolishing seizures. Not all symptomatic cases are suitable for surgery, however. The epileptogenic lesion may be in an inoperable area of the brain or may consist of a scar that it is inadvisable to try to remove except as a very last desperate measure. The main indications for surgery are (1) failure of the medication to control the convulsions and (2) an EEG of a discharge that can be demonstrated to originate on one side of the brain. Thus, 1 to 2 per cent of persons with epileptic convulsions have been considered suitable for surgery. Different surgeons have reported results suggesting that in approximately 50 per cent of the suitable cases, seizures can be abolished and the patient's psychiatric state significantly improved; in an additional 25 per cent of the cases worthwhile improvement is reportedly obtained. Removal of one temporal lobe apparently leaves no easily discernible neurologic deficit or personality disturbance, although whether the latter is true over a long period of time is still in doubt.

Epilepsy is not necessarily a disabling disorder. Patients are encouraged to lead active lives and take part in social activities but to avoid mental and physical fatigue. As part of the therapeutic regime they are advised to regulate their lives for time and hours of sleep, rising, work and meals. Hunger or excessive fatigue often precipitates a convulsion.

In some individuals, convulsions are set off by particular conditions and can be circumvented. Children, for instance, may have seizures during periods of boredom and inactivity but not when they are occupied. Some adults report that they can prevent convulsions if during the aura they concentrate on an activity or the printed words on a page. Patients with Jacksonian epilepsy have forestalled general convulsions by squeezing the small area—for instance, the thumb or hand—of the beginning seizure.

Whatever manifestations of functional disorders an epileptic displays are usually a result of the stresses of his environment and his pre-illness personality, not of the disorder itself. Most individuals with seizures have tremendous psychological problems. Various forms of psychotherapy may be effective with such patients, unless, of course, the damage to brain and personality is too great. The later in life that an individual becomes subject to seizures, the more difficult it is for him to accept the disorder, and the more important the role of psychotherapy in helping him to adapt to it. All epileptics need acceptance and understanding from their families and friends, but more importantly, perhaps, need to accept and understand their own disorders.

Although the controlled epileptic is a good job prospect to whom employment is essential for the furtherance of social and emotional growth, relatively few employers are willing to hire him. There is no medical reason why he should not marry and, in most cases, have children, but the decision for the latter can only be made by prospective parents.

General Paralysis (PARESIS)

The most effective treatment for paresis today is penicillin, with or without artificial fever induced by malaria or other means. Until the discovery of the antibiotic, fever therapy was widely used. Approximately one-third of the patients so treated recovered; in another third the progress of the disease was arrested although not reversed; for the rest, treatment was ineffective and early death followed.

Penicillin was first used for the treatment of paresis in 1943. It was immediately successful although the proper strain of the drug and the dosage were not fully determined and available until after World War II. At present it is the preferred treatment in all forms of neurosyphilis. The recovery rate is over 80 per cent and approximately half the patients are able to return to some occupation. The balance require custodial care of one form or another. Use of the drug in the United States resulted in almost complete disappearance of new cases of general paresis within the decade following World War II. Prior to penicillin, paretic patients had been a major problem in mental institutions. In 1956, approximately 5000 veterans of World War I with syphilitic psychoses, and an additional 1000 with other crippling lesions of syphilis, were still being cared for in hospitals by the Veterans Administration.

Penicillin acts directly on the syphilitic organisms, while malaria and artificial fevers mobilize the body's defenses against the spirochetes, that is, the fever stimulates the reticuloendothelial system which combats foreign bodies. Penicillin is highly effective in large doses, is inexpensive and is practically without risks, and the course of treatment is short.

The prognosis for penicillin therapy is best among those patients who have an acute onset and positive symptoms—i.e., delirium and acute motor excitement, severe agitated depression or acute mania—and poorest in cases displaying symptoms of intellectual deterioration—i.e., simple dementia, and impairment of memory. When the results of the treatment are assessed, it is found that in some cases personality is little damaged and the patient is able to return to his normal activities; in others, some degree of personality defect is evident but, if dementia is not advanced and no psychotic symptoms are present, the patient may be able to work, although at a somewhat lower level than previously. Institutionalization is required when the patient is disabled or psychotic. Roughly 50 per cent fall into this category.

ECT has effectively reversed symptoms of depression, in some paretic patients. The therapy was also used formerly on agitated and delirious individuals, but, today, tranquilizing drugs are generally administered to reduce agitation, and paretic patients, as a result, tend to be quieter, less destructive and more manageable than in the past.

It is still most important to detect and treat syphilis in the primary stage. Unfortunately, in recent years, widespread complacency over the effectiveness of penicillin in treating venereal diseases has been associated with increasing numbers of new cases, and reinfections, particularly in the younger age groups.

Brain Syndromes of Old Age

Until fairly recently little or no attempt was made to treat elderly persons who carried diagnoses of organic brain syndromes. It was reasoned that the irreversibility of brain damage rendered futile any efforts to halt or reverse the progress of the disorders. About all that could be done, it was believed, was keep the patients as healthy as possible, make them comfortable, provide them with some kind of tranquil occupation and protect them from difficulties.

By contrast, it is now recognized that organic brain damage in itself may not cause a disorder of old age, and that the symptoms of organic damage displayed by many aged persons are, frequently, a wordless cry for help. This attitude is supported by the evidence of many general hospitals and nursing homes to which disturbed individuals are brought for diagnosis or treatment. A fairly large percentage of patients respond positively to nutritious diets, symptomatic medications and interested and reassuring care from the medical and nursing staff, improving sufficiently to return home. When aged persons, however, are sent directly to mental institutions, the rate of recovery is slower or nonexistent, and many of the patients die within the year. The difference between the two groups may be partly in the atmosphere of recovery that pervades a hospital and reinforces the aged person's desire to live, and the feeling of hopelessness that overcomes him in what appears to be irrevocable and hopeless confinement—although the group admitted to mental hospitals may also tend to have more severe and prolonged brain damage.

If the patient has an organic brain syndrome, his symptoms may be somewhat alleviated but the damage to his brain cannot be reversed. His level of functioning may fluctuate over a period of time as a result of many factors, including the disorder itself, and psychological and sociocultural forces. Those of his symptoms that are predominantly psychogenic in origin may respond to treatment, but his organic damage can neither be treated nor repaired. Because of stereotyping, however, it is possible that the diagnosis of organic brain syndrome is made in some patients with psychotic symptoms on the basis of age rather than symptoms. Mensh (1959) inferred from an investigation of psychiatric diagnoses that in aged and chronically hospitalized patients "there may be confusion of physical and psychologic diseases at administrative or medical levels or both." Roth (1955) distinguished an affective psychosis from senile or arteriosclerotic psychosis by age (senile psychosis was preponderant above the age of 75) and outcome of the disorder, six months and two years after hospitalization. Six months after admission, most of the patients with the affective psychoses were discharged, but most of the senile patients were dead and most of the arteriosclerotic patients were still hospitalized or dead. Two years later each disease manifested the same distinctive pattern, except for arteriosclerosis, in which the peak shifted to death. Some of the affective patients had returned in the meantime but the percentage of discharges had increased slightly.

In their first study, Williams and Jaco (1957) reviewed the literature on mental illness in old age and found that, according to statistical studies, 85 per cent of psychoses occurring after the age of 65 were categorized as either cerebral arteriosclerosis or senile dementia. In a survey of 1134 psychiatric patients over the age of 60 who were admitted to medical branch hospitals in Texas between 1950 and 1954, the investigators found that approximately one-half the total diagnoses were functional psychoses and only 20 per cent were cerebral arteriosclerosis or senile dementia; in public mental hospitals, on the other hand, diagnoses were closer to the national average with 78 per cent listed as cerebral arteriosclerosis or senile dementia and only 11 per cent as functional psychoses; and in teaching or private hospitals the diagnoses were 37 per cent cerebral arteriosclerosis or senile dementia and 51 per cent functional psychoses. From their analysis (Williams and Jaco, 1958) of the patients admitted to the different institutions, the authors concluded that the figures "could hardly be interpreted to mean a differential rate in development of cerebral arteriosclerosis." While it may well be that more stereotyped diagnoses are made in public than in private institutions, it is also true that the latter tend to exclude the most chronic and impoverished patients.

The basis for present day treatment of persons with disorders of old age is that in addition to medication they need adequate nutrition, a stimulating environment in which they can feel accepted and useful, and some form of psychotherapy. Wolff (1959), after noting that most psychoses starting after the age of 60 are considered the result of arteriosclerotic changes and are diagnosed as chronic brain syndromes with senile brain disease or cerebral arteriosclerosis, started an active treatment program in a California hospital in 1952 for elderly female patients and found that the mental condition of a patient was improved if the patient's physical condition improved. He treated every physical condition, instituted measures to build up each patient's general strength and discovered that many acutely disturbed patients were helped if moved to new surroundings. In psychotherapy the patients' egos were built up through the process of transference. Freeman (1959) found that patients in a custodial ward of geriatric patients were considerably helped by an inter-disciplinary team that engaged in individual and group therapy, electroshock therapy, tranquilizing drugs and physical medicine, as well as occupational, recreational and musical rehabilitation therapies. During the experimental period, 15 patients were discharged as compared to 6 during the control period. Wolf et al. (1959) also reported a combined research and treatment program, in a Veterans Administration Hospital for mentally ill, that was beneficial to extreme chronic and regressed mentally ill patients, and similar results were reported by Sklar and O'Neill (1961).

Patients with the syndrome of cerebral arteriosclerosis respond to carefully regulated patterns of life and some kind of employment to prevent irritability, overt manifestations of hostility and depression with possible suicide. Bonner (1959) advocated physical rehabilitation, beginning within 24 to 48 hours after the cerebrovascular accident, to counteract the lethargy and pessimism usually displayed in treating patients with strokes.

ECT has been reported to benefit patients with marked agitation, paranoid and depressive states, but tends to accentuate primary symptoms of intellectual impairment. Gallinek (1948) administered ECT's to 36 patients over 60, the eldest 84, who were diagnosed as psychotic with cerebral arteriosclerosis or senile psychosis. The majority of the 36 received less than 10 shock treatments each and most of the patients were reported to show good, lasting results. The 84-year-old, a woman, had shown evidence of generalized arteriosclerosis, yet she apparently made a complete recovery but died seven months later of a blood stream infection. In each patient, behavior was reported improved, temporarily in some and permanently in many.

Reviewing the senile cases treated with ECT at Boston State Hospital, Ehrenberg and Gullingsrud (1955) reported results similar to Gallinek's. Their subjects were 112 patients ranging in age from 65 to 83. After ECT, 88 were discharged from the hospital and 55 per cent of them remained out for more than one year. Although some of the discharged patients had two or more readmissions after the therapy, they responded well to additional treatment each time. Wolff (1957) treated almost 700 chronic mental patients, some with organic disorders, with maintenance doses of ECT and noted no cardiovascular or other serious complications. In the ward containing the most disturbed patients he reported that the atmosphere changed so that attendants were able to spend time discussing the patients' problems with them instead of preventing fights and destructiveness. In the total sample, a considerable number of patients were able to remain out on convalescent leave for over 18 months while receiving their maintenance doses on an outpatient basis. Previously, such patients had been returned to the hospital every three or four months because of relapses. When the doses of ECT were discontinued, disturbing elements again appeared in the patients' behaviors. In recent years, however, the administration of ECT to patients such as these has been largely superseded by the widespread use of tranquilizing and anti-depressive drugs.

Since the disordered behavior manifested by the patient with an organic syndrome cannot be attributed solely to the structural damage of his disorder, it is important to know his prepsychotic psychological makeup and the stresses and conflicts that precipitated the onset of his behavior. For many years it was widely believed that the irreversibility of organic brain damage and the rigidity and inflexibility of the aged made them ineligible for psychotherapy. Yet individual, group and attitude therapies with hospitalized patients have proved to be feasible and beneficial. Psychotherapy for the geriatric patient is discussed in the next section.

GERIATRICS

Growing old has become a problem in the countries of western Europe and the United States because more people are living longer. In 1900, the proportion of persons over 65 years of age in the population of the United States was 1 in 25; in 1960 the proportion was close to 1 in 12. During the half century noted, the total population of the country doubled, but the number of persons aged 65 or over almost quadrupled. In 1960, the population aged 65 and over in the United States was 15,800,000; by 1980, the number should approximate 24,500,000, a further increase of 55 per cent.

Growing old has always been regarded as the least favorable period in life. Historically, the attitudes to old age have correlated with attitudes toward the mentally ill and women. In cultures where the mentally ill were considered to be touched with a bit of magic or divinity, the old were respected and cared for. In our own history the aging process has been considered a dreadful experience, and during periods of witch-burning the old have been almost natural victims (Rosen, 1961). The essentially negative attitude of our culture toward the aging process is reflected in the failure of early personality theorists to structure comprehensive systems that covered the span of life from birth to death. Their theories embraced life only to maturity. It has been just during the last two decades that psychology has become concerned with aging as a subject for investigation.

The aged have long been considered a burden emotionally, economically and socially. In urban centers the family has lost its cohesiveness and the generations have been separated by social mobility, exaggerated social strivings, changes in fads and fashions, and diminished communications. According to the findings of Williams and Jaco (1957), a 60-year-old person who lives on a farm or in a town of under 2500 inhabitants is only one-third as likely to develop a disorder of old age as an inhabitant of an urban area. The difference may be, in large part, attributable to employment or lack of it. Ours is a culture in which work is not only an occupation but also a source of status and social interaction. The man who works is part of society; without work he is an alienated individual. The urban industrial worker reaches the age of 65 to face compulsory retirement, inactivity, loss of status as the family breadwinner, loss of self-esteem, loss of social interactions and a diminished income. Many retirements are involuntary; approximately one-third the unemployed aged would be willing and are able to work (World Health Organization, 1959). The rural and small town laborer, on the other hand, is usually permitted to continue working as long as he can and to match his activities to his diminished vigor. Whitehorn (1956) considers the stress of congenial employment to be beneficial and necessary to the aging individual:

Job retirement, with illness or without, separates one from a sustaining context of activities and meaningful personal relationships. The narrowed circle of contacts, although kind and benevolent, may demand so little response as to leave one feeling unwanted and futile. Individual ingenuity may not be sufficient to devise or discover tasks and problems which sustain one's sense of dignity and worth, particularly when the vague need is not understood as a tension state, for which more idleness and futility are prescribed.

For the aging individual with poor familial and social relationships, retirement from work may be disastrous. He tends to become withdrawn and increasingly frustrated in his attempts to gain pleasure from his environment. He may develop psychotic symptoms that are exaggerations of his lifelong emotional patterns: complaints may become hallucinations, and paranoid trends may become delusions of persecution (Sheps, 1959).

Isolation may be intensified by physical infirmities. As the individual grows older and his eyesight or hearing fail he may be cut off from the rest of the world physically as well as socially. If there is no one to take an interest in him, he may, out of sheer inertia, make no effort to secure proper spectacles or a hearing aid. Unable to hear or see efficiently he loses interest in his surroundings and the world and, instead, centers his interests upon his body, resulting in hypochondriasis, or in his memories of the past, resulting in loss of contact with reality. Hypochondriasis is more prevalent among the aged than in any other group. The restrictions and discomforts of illness may be used both as a punishment and partial atonement for the guilt that results from hostile, vengeful feelings against people who are close. The aged individual shifts his anxiety from a specific psychic area to the less threatening concern with bodily functions (Busse, 1961).

For many old people the fear of illness is greater than the fear of death. Few persons reach an advanced age without having experienced some incapacitating illness or surgery that has left a residue of fear. The isolated individual becomes aware of his physical debilitation and may begin to brood over real or imagined impaired bodily functions and real or imagined aches and pains. This fear of illness is greater for the individual who lives alone, for then he worries about helplessness or lack of care.

Another frequent complaint among geriatric patients is insomnia, which becomes a source of great anxiety. Chronic insomnia may be traceable to unsolved emotional conflicts that involve feelings of guilt and hostility with fears of retaliation. Nocturnal restlessness sometimes accompanies the symptom. The individual is unable to remain sleepless in bed so he gets up and wanders about the house, opening and shutting doors, searching cupboards, or may even go out into the streets. The symptom is usually found in persons with decreased vision and hearing who also show signs of mental deterioration. When old persons wander away from home aimlessly it is sometimes an attempt to reduce inward tensions. They apparently miss the feeling of having a significant role in their environments and wander to make their lives interesting and exciting or to be missed and valued more in the home environment. If they cannot find relief from their tensions they may manifest irritability and hostility.

There appears to be a special relationship between suicide and old age. Statistically, the peak for suicides appears in late middle or old age. Aging persons take their own lives because of social or psychological factors, such as an awareness of physical and mental decline, loneliness, forced idleness, inability to adapt to changes in life and incurable disease. Suicide is also related to depression and a history of hardships. It is higher in urban than agricultural areas, lower in Catholic than Protestant countries, higher among unmarried than married individuals, increased during unemployment and depression, decreased during war, and higher in the early part of the summer.

Obviously, the healthier psychologically the individual has been throughout his life, the more readily will he be able to adapt to the stresses of aging. The prevention of a senile psychosis depends in large part on the individual's ability to adjust to life before senescence as well as on his ability to adjust to the deprivations and strains of old age. It has been said that anyone who wants to be a healthy old man must start by being a healthy young boy.

The vicissitudes of aging tend to accentuate existing and latent psychological tendencies. The dependent individual may become wholly so and revert to infantilism; the compulsive individual may try to find in overt obsessions a means of holding onto the world he once knew; the paranoiac may try to deny his inadequacies in self-aggrandizing delusions; and the schizoid may withdraw from his unpleasant reality completely.

Until fairly recently, psychotherapy for the aged person was considered with pessimism and reluctance. For example, Freud (1904) believed that psychoanalysis was valueless for persons beyond middle age, for they no longer had the mental or emotional capacity for change upon which treatment depends. This purported lack of resilience is in strange contrast to the fact that men in their fifties, sixties and over are the political, economic and social leaders of our society.

A greal deal of interest is now being taken in the psychotherapeutic needs of aged persons. The actual practice of such therapy is less frequent than with younger patients, but, according to Rechtshaffen (1959) "considering population trends, the prevalence of maladjustment in the aged, and current attempts to change cultural attitudes toward the elderly, it would not be surprising if, before long, psychotherapy might be as widely applied to old people as it is today to children."

Psychotherapists may have shied away from working with aged persons because of their unconscious fears of intimacy and identification with them and because of a fear of the connotations of aging: physical decline, loss of intellectual or emotional powers, sterility and eventual death. These fears, according to Rosenthal (1959), are a reflection of our cultural attitudes. Similarly, LeShan and LeShan (1961) noted that most therapists also avoid working with patients in terminal illnesses, apparently because of the fears evoked in them.

Alexander (1944) discussed two broad types of pschotherapeutic treatment for the aged: insight therapy and supportive therapy. If the patient's ego was too weak for the first, he advocated the latter. In supportive therapy the patient's need for assistance is answered by actual guidance; his inferiority feelings are met with reassurance, his anxiety is relieved by the protective role of the therapist and his guilt is relieved by the permissive attitudes of the therapist. Rechtshaffen (1959) reported that aged patients were observed to profit most from supportive therapy and that the greatest benefits of geriatric psychotherapy were in-fluencing the patients' goals rather than in at-tempting to squeeze happiness for them out of their currently rejecting environments. Craw-shaw and Peterson (1961) reported a successful course of supportive psychotherapy with a 71-year-old male who had many physical problems, some confusion and an old psychoneurosis of the anxiety type.

Rosenthal (1959) treated 30 neurotic patients from the age of 58 on. The length and depth of treatment was the same as for younger patients although the pace was slower. He reported that he rarely felt it necessary to restrict therapy to shortened, simplified or merely supportive tech-niques. He found that to the extent that the patients sensed, consciously or unconsciously, the inadequacies of their lives, the better they became motivated for change. The most signif-icant impediment to change, however, was the image of themselves that was projected upon them by society and their immediate environ-ments. The elderly neurotic is a ''hopeless case'' largely because he is so perceived by others. ''If psychologic treatment of the aged could be popularized and brought into the public eye, these people might find it worth while to seek such treatment for their depressive moods and their general feelings of inadequacy'' (Rosen-thal, 1959). Busse (1961) believes that treatment for the aged person should be directed toward restoring him to a level of functioning at which he can take advantage of the substitute sources of gratification that are available to him.

Successful psychiatric treatment has been re-ported in a home for the aged where the majority of residents were 80 to 90 years of age and the youngest referral for treatment was 63. The referred patients were argumentative, re-bellious, demanding, complaining, relatively im-mobilized, actively or passively sabotaging, querulous, openly depressed, potentially or actually suicidal, assaultive, abusive or threaten-ing. According to Goldfarb (1957) ''. . . as the amount of psychiatric aid available increased, as psychiatric techniques of treatment improved, as the home's staff acquired more psychiatric understanding, the transfer of cases to mental hospitals dropped sharply, and patients who would formerly have been considered intolerable, unmanageable, or risky were well handled with-out locked doors or barred windows and with relatively little augmentation of nursing and medical care.'' The psychotherapy did not re-quire lengthy or regularly scheduled sessions: ''a great deal can be accomplished toward re-

lieving mental suffering, improving social be-havior, and relieving symptoms of emotional overaction by means of short, infrequent inter-views or even by means of seemingly catch-as-catch-can sessions here or there on the ward or in the corridor.'' Earlier, successful treatments had been reported (Goldfarb and Sheps, 1954) in sessions of five to 15 minutes ''as widely spaced as the status and progress of the pa-tient permits.'' Each of the interviews, however, was structured so that the patient left ''with a sense of triumph, of victory derived from having won an ally or from having dominated the therapist.'' The patients pressed parental powers on the therapist. ''The role of powerful parent which the aged sick in their helplessness thrust upon the therapist gives opportunity to foster the illusion, a perceptual distortion of the patient, that the therapist is indeed such a figure. . . . By utilizing the role that the security-seeking aged force on him, guilt, fear, rage and depression can be meliorated or their social manifestations altered. The patient's sense of helplessness is then decreased'' (Goldfarb and Sheps, 1954).

The recognized importance of psychological factors in the precipitation of disorders of old age has emphasized the need to prepare people for the aging process and help them make the transition to old age. Most persons lose their physical and mental powers so slowly that they are not even aware that deterioration has taken place or that their powers of adaptation have been lowered. A concomitant change in oc-cupation or compulsory retirement may result in severe damage to self-esteem and bring on symptoms of emotional distress, especially de-pression. As a compensation, these individuals need sympathy and understanding for their plight as well as restoration of a feeling of im-portance; they must be convinced that they are loved and wanted and that their lives are still as important to other individuals as to themselves.

Public sentiment, at the present time, is be-coming more and more supportive of the aged. The old have become ''senior citizens'' and their retirement from active affairs, the ''golden age''; welfare and private funds have been used to organize social and occupational groups of ''senior citizens'' and in some cities, special rates are in effect for them at theaters and other places of public entertainment. In some sections of the country adult education courses are especially designed to aid aging persons make the transition to lowered activity levels.

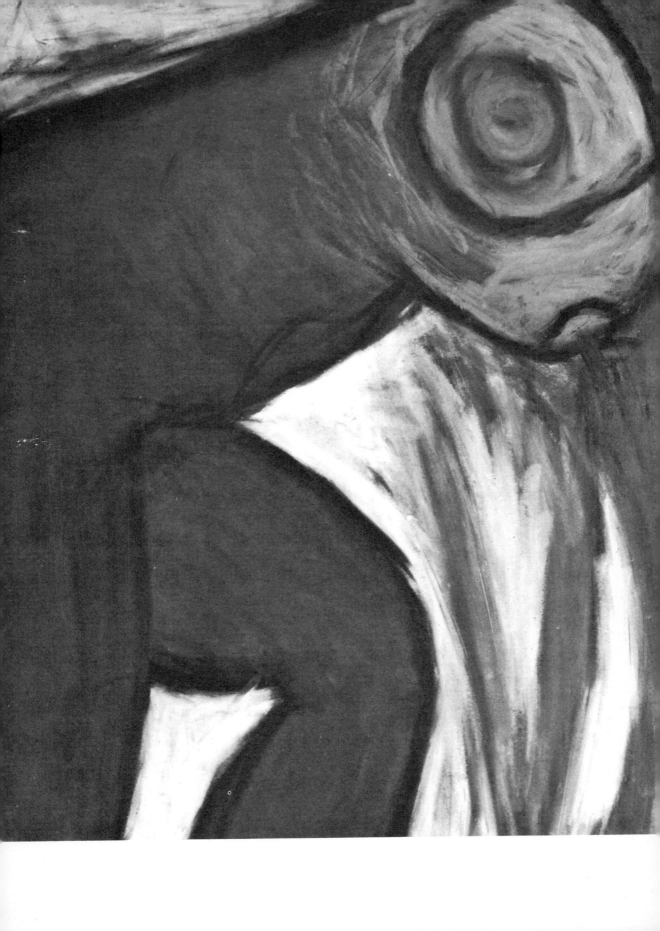

There are three kinds of brains; one understands of itself, another can be taught to understand, and the third can neither understand of itself nor be taught to understand.

Niccolo Machiavelli (1469–1527)

18

MENTAL SUBNORMALITY

DEFINITION AND DESCRIPTION

Mental subnormality has been recognized as a serious social and scientific problem since the early nineteenth century. Before then, mentally subnormal persons had been considered fools or degenerates and, sometimes, mentally ill. During the Renaissance, however, some societies in western Europe began to recognize differences between life-long intellectual subnormality and mental illness. Legislation was passed in England in the fourteenth century for the management of the "born fool" (fatuus naturalis) and his estate, which distinguished him from the insane. Several hundred years elapsed, nevertheless, before mental deficiency began to be investigated objectively and humane treatment was accorded its victims.

The scientific study of mental subnormality began in the early 1800's with Jean Marie Gaspard Itard (1774–1838). He attempted to educate and socialize a boy thought to have lived in isolation in a forest. Itard's attempts were largely unsuccessful but the published accounts of his work stimulated an interest in the mentally retarded. His work was continued by his now well-known student Edouard Séguin (1812–1880), who was interested in describing and evaluating the retarded as well as educating them. Since Séguin, two trends can be identified in the study of the mentally defi-

cient: one toward more complete and accurate diagnosis, characterized by the development of intelligence tests, techniques of describing social competence, genetic studies, investigations of various functions (such as perception and thinking), and a wide variety of medical approaches that analyze physiological and neurological characteristics; the second toward more adequate care, both in institutions and the community, and the development of more efficient and useful educational techniques.

Attempts have been made to define various levels of intellectual and social functioning among the mentally subnormal and apply meaningful descriptive and diagnostic labels to them. A great deal of confusion has arisen, however, because many different terms have been introduced and used interchangeably or in association with etiological factors that have often been hypothesized rather than established. The most common terms now in use are "mental deficiency," "mental retardation," "feeblemindedness" and "mental subnormality," in the United States; "mental deficiency" and "amentia" (absence of mind, literally), in England; and "oligophrenia" (small mind, literally), in Europe. In this chapter the terms in common usage in the United States are used interchangeably and no etiological significance should be attached to them.

Many students have attempted to distinguish

between those conditions in which organic brain damage is present and those in which etiological factors are not known or are presumed to be inherited. The term "exogenous" has been applied to the former and "endogenous" to the latter. This distinction has stimulated a great deal of interesting research (to be discussed later), but the results are controversial. So far no clear-cut criteria for separating the two groups according to etiology or test performance have emerged. The problem is further complicated by the fact that in most cases of mental subnormality the etiology remains unknown. For this reason the trend in the last decade has been toward defining mental subnormality in operational terms, i.e., in terms of intellectual and social performance rather than according to hypothesized etiological factors. In those cases in which the etiology has been definitely established, of course, specific diagnoses can be made.

Thus, the Group for the Advancement of Psychiatry (1959) used the term "mental retardation" to refer to a chronic condition present from birth or early childhood which is characterized by both impaired intellectual functioning as measured by standardized tests, and impaired adaptation to the daily demands of the individual's social environment. In its annual meeting of 1960, the American Association on Mental Deficiency adopted the following definition: "Mental Retardation refers to subaverage general intellectual functioning which originates during the development period and is associated with impairment in adaptive behavior."

The development of intelligence tests during the first part of the present century led to definitions of varying degrees of mental subnormality in terms of intelligence quotient and mental-age performance. The best and most widely accepted intelligence tests are individually administered. They are the Stanford-Binet intelligence scale, recently revised, and any of the several forms of the Wechsler Intelligence Scales. On both tests the assumption is made that intelligence at each age level is distributed in a normal or Gaussian curve. The mean I.Q. score is arbitrarily placed at 100, therefore, and one-half the population is assumed to have scores above 100 and one-half below. An I.Q. score indicates by how much an individual ranks above or below the average of his age group. Despite the many criticisms that can be made of intelligence tests, the scores derived from them are sufficiently valid to warrant their use both for research and practical purposes. I.Q.

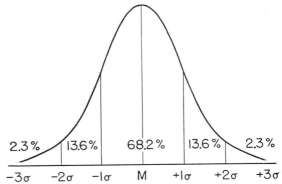

Figure 18–1. *Normal probability curve with theoretical distribution of I.Q.'s. (Adapted from Hebb, D. O. 1958. Textbook of Psychology. Philadelphia, W. B. Saunders Co.)*

scores are the most objective, efficient and easily communicated measure of intelligent behavior.

Persons who rank on intelligence tests in the lowest 2 to 3 per cent of the population are labeled mentally subnormal (see Fig. 18–1). The cut-off point is usually somewhere between an I.Q. score of 65 and 70. Thus, at present, there are between five and six million mentally subnormal individuals in the United States. On the basis of performance on intelligence tests it is customary to subdivide further the category of mental subnormality according to degree of severity.

Table 18–1 lists the categories currently used along with their corresponding intelligence quotient range.

The practical implications for education, for development and for socialization of four levels of retardation formerly in use were delineated some years ago by Sloan and Birch (1955) and are reproduced in Table 18–2.

In this chapter, for purposes of discussion and exposition, we will use three broad groupings of mental retardation: severe (I.Q.'s under 20), moderate (I.Q.'s of 20 to 49) and mild

TABLE 18–1.   Degrees of Mental
Retardation

Level	Descriptive Term	I.Q. Range
I	Profound	Under 20
II	Severe	20–35
III	Moderate	36–51
IV	Mild	52–67
V	Borderline	68–85

TABLE 18–2. Adaptive Behavior Classification*

	Pre-School Age 0–5 Maturation and Development	School-Age 6–21 Training and Education	Adult 21 Social and Vocational Adequacy
Level I	Gross retardation; minimal capacity for functioning in sensori-motor areas; needs nursing care.	Some motor development present; cannot profit from training in self-help; needs total care.	Some motor and speech development; totally incapable of self-maintenance; needs complete care and supervision.
Level II	Poor motor development; speech is minimal; generally unable to profit from training in self-help; little or no communication skills.	Can talk or learn to communicate; can be trained in elemental health habits; cannot learn functional academic skills; profits from systematic habit training. ("Trainable")	Can contribute partially to self-support under complete supervision; can develop self-protection skills to a minimal useful level in controlled environment.
Level III	Can talk or learn to communicate; poor social awareness; fair motor development; may profit from self-help; can be managed with moderate supervision.	Can learn functional academic skills to approximately 4th grade level by late teens if given special education. ("Educable")	Capable of self-maintenance in unskilled or semi-skilled occupations; needs supervision and guidance when under mild social or economic stress.
Level IV	Can develop social and communication skills; minimal retardation in sensori-motor areas; rarely distinguished from normal until later age.	Can learn academic skills to approximately 6th grade level by late teens. Cannot learn general high school subjects. Needs special education, particularly at secondary school age levels. ("Educable")	Capable of social and vocational adequacy with proper education and training. Frequently needs supervision and guidance under serious social or economic stress.

*Reprinted by permission from Sloan, W., and Birch, J. W. 1955. A rationale for degrees of retardation. American Journal of Mental Deficiency 60, 258–264.

(I.Q.'s in the 50 to 69 range). Because intelligence is normally distributed, it follows that the number of persons at each level of subnormality must decrease as the degree of severity increases.

Severe Subnormality. Historically, the legal-medical term for this group is *"idiot."* It includes persons with I.Q. scores below 20 who never attain a mental age greater than that of the average two-year-old child. They number approximately 0.1 per cent of the total population and 3.5 per cent of all retarded persons. It is estimated that in the United States only 25 per cent of this group are institutionalized, yet they account for 30 per cent of the institutionalized mentally deficient population.

Severely subnormal persons are grossly retarded in development from birth or infancy onward. Their capacity to develop resistance or immunity to infection may also be limited, which results in frequent or severe infections and increased mortality rates. They tend to be small in stature and often have facial or bodily deformities or both. They may have physical characteristics associated with a specific form of defect (e.g., the facies of mongolism, cretinism, gargoylism or hypertelorism; or the size and shape of the head indicative of microcephaly, hydrocephaly or acrocephaly). They are grossly delayed in dentition, walking, ability to feed and dress themselves, and in bladder and bowel control; many of them never master these skills and functions. Marked disturbances of gait and involuntary movements are frequently present. In the most grossly subnormal, speech is limited to a few unintelligible sounds; those with I.Q.'s close to 20 are sometimes able to say a few simple words or phrases. Many of them display relatively little interest in their surroundings, but those who are less severely incapacitated may be fairly active and attentive to their environments. They look dirty and untidy unless they receive a great deal of nursing care. They are unable to protect themselves against common dangers and throughout their lives are totally dependent on others for physical care, nourishment and protection.

In the following case the patient's severe subnormality is associated with organic brain damage. It is possible, of course, that her mental deficiency, apparently genetic in origin, was less severe earlier, but that it was exacerbated by the onset of epileptic seizures. It was noted in the previous chapter that the early onset of epilepsy frequently leads to the deterioration of intelligence.

The patient, unmarried, was first admitted to a state institution at the age of 27 with a history of mental subnormality since birth, epileptic seizures since the age of five and purported increasingly difficult behavior during the preceding year.

She was the seventh of eleven children of whom four

had failed to progress beyond grade seven in school. Her father had completed only four school grades and her mother six; nevertheless, the patient was the only member of the family to be institutionalized for any reason.

The parents reported that the patient started walking by the age of about two years and talking by three. They only became aware of retardation in her development after she fell at the age of five and struck her head hard. From then on she was subject to epileptic seizures which were largely controlled by anti-convulsant medication. The patient never attended school and remained at home with her parents. She was unable to help with household duties and required constant care and attention; she was unable to dress or wash herself. The family regarded her as dull, but quiet and good natured. She spent much of her time sitting and rocking in a chair and talking to herself; at times she laughed, cried or became angry. The patient's behavior had not changed during the year preceding her admission to the hospital, but the mother's health had deteriorated so that she was less able or willing to look after the patient.

In the hospital she was found to have some signs of brain damage. She lacked coordination, was unable to walk without assistance and had involuntary movements of the arms. She gave her age as five and when asked where she lived replied, "Mommy lives on the corner." She was able to count to eight but was unable to recognize any letters of the alphabet. The Stanford-Binet test of intelligence showed considerable intra-test variability, but her overall performance was at about the level of the average one-year-old child. She made a satisfactory adjustment to long-term institutional care.

Moderate Subnormality. This category, traditionally labeled "imbecile," includes persons with I.Q. scores ranging from 20 to 49; they have mental ages equivalent to average three- to seven-year-old children. They make up 0.3 per cent of the total population and approximately 11 per cent of the total category of mental subnormality; only 15 per cent of them are institutionalized, but they make up 50 per cent of the total mentally subnormal institutionalized population. Signs of delayed development occur very early in life but sometimes they are not recognized by unsuspecting, unperceptive parents until the child is a year or more old. An expert observer, however, is usually able to identify the symptoms of retarded development in the first weeks or months of life. The child is severely retarded in all areas of development; he does not begin to talk or walk until two or three years after the usual age. Imbeciles are somewhat smaller in size than average, usually ungainly and poorly coordinated, and frequently have some physical abnormality or deformity.

Those with I.Q.'s in the upper limits of the range often learn to talk—their vocabularies are very limited—but none manages to acquire the basic skills of reading and writing. Attendance in a conventional school is far beyond their abilities as is any work that requires initiative, originality, abstract thinking, memory or consistent attention.

Like idiots, imbeciles are dependent upon others throughout their lives. They are regarded as "trainable" in that they can master certain simple, routine tasks, such as doing laundry or sweeping, can learn to care for themselves and help look after less adequate individuals, can guard themselves against common physical dangers and participate in simple games; nevertheless, they require constant supervision. They cannot support themselves or take any position outside a highly sheltered environment.

Mild Subnormality. This category, traditionally called "moron," includes persons with I.Q. scores ranging from 50 to 69 and mental ages equivalent to average 8- to 12-year-old children. They make up somewhat less than 3 per cent of the total population, approximately 85 per cent of the total category of mental subnormality and 20 per cent of the total subnormal institutionalized population, although in the United States only about 1 per cent of them are institutionalized.

In contrast with the other two groups, the mildly subnormal do not usually show physical abnormalities or deformities. Statistically, they tend to be somewhat smaller than average. Their appearance, behavior and conversation are closer to the norms expected for their particular ages and sex but are comparable to those of persons of limited socioeconomic status. They may converse spontaneously and answer simple questions relevantly and appropriately, but their general information, comprehension and interest patterns are childlike. Their capacity for abstract thinking is limited and their concepts tend toward the concrete (as in the patient with organic intellectual impairment or schizophrenia). If they are not psychologically disturbed, they show no more evidence of magical, paralogical thinking than the average child.

Their general development is slower than average all through infancy and childhood. They learn to walk, talk, feed and toilet themselves eight or nine months later than the average. They continue to engage in solitary play after their age group has acquired the techniques of sharing and play participation. At the age of six they are ready only for play at the nursery-school level and they are eight and one-half before they are able to learn to read and write. Although a mildly subnormal person shows signs of delayed development very early in life, the extent and severity of his retardation sometimes is not apparent until he is in school. He is soon identified as a slow learner who cannot keep up with the others or master elementary academic subjects at the appropriate age, and frequently he is required to repeat early grades. It is not uncommon for him to have speech difficulties (most often involving articulation and voice) that add to his problems. He is incapable of achieving beyond the sixth grade level and remains in school two or three grades below that of his chronological age group and then may drop out as soon as it is legally permissible. At the lower end of the range (where I.Q. scores are close to 50), failure is so obvious and so severe that institutionalization is frequently recommended.

The mildly subnormal individual is regarded as "educable" in that he is able to participate in elementary school activities (although at a more advanced age than other children), learn to read and write at a rudimentary level and acquire minimal vocational skills by which he can support himself at the unskilled or semi-skilled level. If accepted for military service, he is sometimes discharged prematurely.

Among the more severely subnormal groups, the individuals do not mature sexually and remain infertile; among the mildly subnormal, sexual development and fertility are usually within normal limits. At the same time, the mildly subnormal are generally immature, have poor control over their impulses, lack good judgment and fail to anticipate the consequences of their actions. As a result, their sexual behavior may lead to a variety of difficulties. The males are often unable to find satisfactory or permanent sexual partners and, since they are easily frustrated and have poor control, may become involved in deviant sexual behavior with animals, or attempt assault on girls and women, or engage in window peeping and indiscreet masturbation. The women experience less difficulty. There is little or no pressure on them to demonstrate economic independence. They often make fairly satisfactory marriages, are able to perform routine household tasks and care for children in a borderline manner. In some cases, however, they produce illegitimate children or become victims of sexual aggression. Because their deviant behavior is so visible, society tends to institutionalize them more often than the mildly retarded male.

TABLE 18–3. Comparison of Mental Subnormals by Intelligence, Percentages of Total and Subnormal Populations and Institutionalization

I.Q. Scores	0–19	20–49	50–69
Mental development (in years)	2	3 to 7	8 to 12
Per cent of total population	0.1	0.3	3.0
Per cent of subnormal population*	3.5	11.0	85.0
Per cent institutionalized	25.0	15.0	1.0
Per cent of institutionalized mentally subnormal population	30.0	50.0	20.0

*Does not equal 100 because of rounding of figures.

Table 18–3 summarizes the differences among the three classifications of mental subnormals according to intelligence, percentages of the total and subnormal populations and institutionalization.

Among the more severely subnormal are a number of distinguishable syndromes. *Mongolian idiots* are so-called because individuals with the disorder have facial characteristics similar to members of the Mongolian race. Most of them are not idiots but imbeciles with I.Q.'s between 20 and 50. They tend to be small in stature with small, round heads and dysplastic features; their eyes are slanting and almond shaped and their noses short and flat (the Mongolian features). In addition, they have

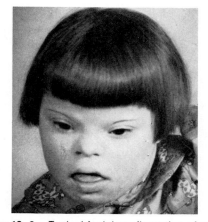

Figure 18–2. *Typical facial configuration of mongolism in a 7-year-old girl. (From Nelson, W. E. [Editor]. 1964. Textbook of Pediatrics, 8th Ed. Philadelphia, W. B. Saunders Co.)*

marked clefts between their first and second toes, unusual patterns of creases on the palms of their hands, and many other physical characteristics that are evident upon examination. Approximately 1 in every 500 births is a mongoloid; they account for between 10 and 25 per cent of all mentally defective infants and about 10 per cent of institutionalized subnormals (Benda, 1960). The typical mongoloid patient, such as the one described in the following case, is born to an older mother.

The patient was 35 years old when she was admitted to a state institution for the first time. Her lifelong mental deficiency and associated behavior pattern had not changed, but economic difficulties in the family had necessitated her institutionalization. Her elder sister cared for four children and an aged father, in addition to the patient, and had been forced to go to work to support the family after her husband became ill.

The patient was the third and youngest child in the family. Her father had been about 47 and her mother about 40 years old when she was born. The birth apparently had been a normal full-term delivery. Her development, however, was retarded from birth; she began to walk when she was nearly five and talked at the age of 9 or 10 but had difficulties with articulation. At the age of 10 or so she was enrolled in school, but, unable to make any progress, was sent home after a few weeks. She was never able to help with any work and was wholly dependent upon the family. Her mother died when she was 27 and she and her father moved in with the sister. The patient was able to dress and feed herself and her toilet habits were satisfactory.

She liked to play with a doll, guitar and skipping rope, and to scribble on paper. She also watched television and listened to the radio. She was mongoloid in appearance, good natured, cheerful and cooperative. There was no history of antisocial behavior. On arrival in the hospital she talked little and frequently laughed for no apparent reason. She answered questions to the best of her ability, but many of her replies were unintelligible. She gave her name correctly but said she was three years old. She could not tell where she lived.

She said that she went to school and could read but was unable to name letters of the alphabet or numbers. Formal intelligence testing by means of the Stanford-Binet showed her to have an I.Q. of 26 and the mental development of an average three and one-half to four-year-old child. She was in the lower part of the imbecile range. Her adjustment to institutional routine was uneventful.

Another disorder occurs in some individuals as a result of brain injury and is sometimes called *cerebral palsy.* Its frequency is about the same as that of mongolism. The syndrome embraces a wide variety of motor disorders (incoordination, paralyses, tremors and so forth)

and, sometimes, defective intelligence; these symptoms result from brain injuries that occur before or during the birth process or early in life. Not all cerebral palsy patients are mentally subnormal; many have normal or even superior intelligence; others range from the lowest levels of intelligence on up, depending on the severity of the injury to the brain. Because of the often severe motor and speech handicaps, the psychometric evaluation of children with cerebral palsy is extremely difficult. No doubt many errors are made in classifying their intelligence since the effects of their physical and communication handicaps cannot be properly assessed.

Other syndromes of mental deficiency are rare and are found in less than 1 per cent of the institutionalized population. *Microcephaly* is a type of subnormality associated with failure of the cranium to attain normal size. The microcephalic has an unusually small head (rarely exceeding a circumference of 17 inches) that is characteristically of a "sugar-loaf" shape. Such patients fall into the severely and moderately subnormal categories.

Hydrocephaly develops from the accumulation of an unusually large amount of cerebrospinal fluid within the cranium, resulting in damage to the brain and enlargement of the skull. In some cases the circumference of the head has exceeded 30 inches. The degree of intellectual impairment varies, depending on the size of the

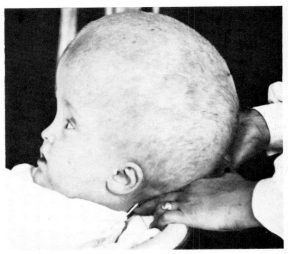

Figure 18–3. *Congenital hydrocephalus. (Courtesy of Prof. Otto Marburg. From Wechsler, I. S. 1963. Clinical Neurology. 9th Ed. Philadelphia, W. B. Saunders Co.)*

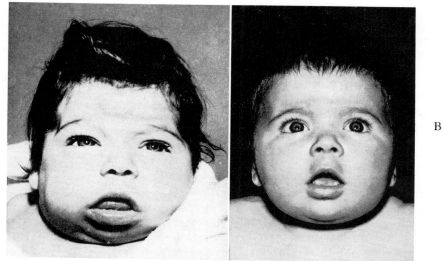

Figure 18–4. *A, Congenitally hypothyroid infant at six months of age. B, Four months later, after treatment with thyroid medication. (From Nelson, W. E. [Editor]. 1964. Textbook of Pediatrics. 8th Ed. Philadelphia, W. B. Saunders Co.)*

head and the extent of neural damage. In some cases hydrocephalics become severely subnormal and require complete care.

Cretinism results from a failure of the thyroid gland to function properly. When the thyroid deficiency is present at an early age, sometimes before birth, and is not treated, the patient manifests characteristic symptoms: a small, thick-set body, coarse and thick skin, short and stubby extremities, large head with abundant hair of a wiry consistency, and thick eyelids that give a sleepy appearance. The cretin has a protruding abdomen and does not mature sexually. Depending on the severity of the thyroid deficiency and the age at which treatment is begun, cretins range in intelligence from the severely subnormal through the moderately subnormal categories.

Another very rare syndrome is *phenylketonuria* (PKU), an inability to metabolize phenylalanine (amino acid) that is caused by a hereditary metabolic disorder. It is identified by the presence of phenylpyruvic acid in the urine. The mental subnormality is severe and is usually accompanied by motor symptoms; it has a frequency of about 1 in 5000.

Still another rare hereditary metabolic disorder is *amaurotic idiocy*. This is, in fact, not one but a group of disorders that appear at different ages in childhood and differ, to some extent, in symptoms and degree of intellectual impairment. Among the major symptoms are visual difficulties, often blindness, seizures and

neurologic manifestations. The disorder differs from the usual mental deficiency in that the patients appear normal until the onset of symptoms. Its incidence is never more than 1 in 1000. *Infantile amaurotic idiocy,* also known as Tay-Sachs disease, is frequent among but not exclusive to Jewish infants of eastern European extraction. The disorder appears at about six months of age and death occurs between the age of two and three. If the onset appears later in infancy, the patient may survive for a longer period. *Juvenile amaurotic idiocy* occurs at five or six years of age and the patient may survive for 10 to 13 years. In *adolescent amaurotic idiocy* the disorder begins to manifest itself between 14 and 16 years of age. Intellectual functions and vision may deteriorate at a slower rate than in the earlier forms, but the loss of motor functions may be more severe.

Other rare symptoms are listed under Causation.

Functional Psychopathology

Many persons who are diagnosed and even institutionalized as mentally subnormal are, or at one time were, potentially capable of more adequate intellectual performance; presumably they function on a lower level because of adverse psychological and sociocultural factors. Sometimes these patients can be identified by test responses above their general intellectual, verbal and social level of functioning, or by unexpected responses to educational or therapeutic programs. In other instances, the patient's history indicates, for instance, early deprivation or lack of stimulation; it is hypothesized that the effects of these early experiences prevent normal intellectual development. Such abnormals have been labeled, in the past, *pseudo-retarded* or *pseudo-feebleminded* because no organic basis for their handicap could be found: with the operational definitions of mental subnormality the labels fell into disuse. Because psychological and sociocultural factors may play a prominent role in the determination of their mental subnormality, these patients are the subjects of a great deal of interest and study at the present time. Much has already been written about the children who have many of the characteristics of severe subnormality (lack of responsiveness, inability to speak and retardation in many areas of development), but who may be seriously psychologically disturbed rather than lacking in innate ability. These cases, however, are more appropriately classified as abnormal personalities and will be discussed in the following chapter.

For a number of years, observers of mentally subnormal children have noted that many of them appear to be highly anxious. The anxiety is expressed in, for instance, the inability to attend to assigned tasks, nervous mannerisms, high incidence of habits such as nail-biting and bed-wetting, and unusually strong needs for reassurance. A number of investigators (Carrier et al., 1962; Feldhausen and Klausmeier, 1962; and Cochran and Cleland, 1963) have found that low I.Q. children are more anxious than normal or high I.Q. children, as measured by the orally administered Children's Manifest Anxiety Scale (CMAS) which is a revision of the Taylor Manifest Anxiety Scale for Children (Castaneda et al., 1956). It has also been observed that moderately and mildly retarded persons have poor self concepts, feelings of inadequacy and little self-confidence (to be discussed later).

The following description is of a *mild subnormal (moron) with a neurotic depressive reaction* who evidences feelings of inadequacy and lack of confidence. The precipitating causes and symptoms do not differ essentially from those found among persons of normal intelligence, nor does the patient's response to treatment differ. In the answers to the sentence completion test, however, she manifests a deep feeling of inadequacy which may be a result of an unverbalized awareness that subnormal intelligence is the source of most of her life problems. Her depression, however, is more likely a function of her personality, as influenced by her mother, than of her mental retardation.

A 39-year-old unmarried woman was admitted to the state hospital after a year of increasing depression. A few months earlier she had taken a few sleeping pills in a possible suicide attempt but suffered no ill effects. She was eating and sleeping poorly, weeping quite frequently, fearful of becoming a burden and convinced that life was not worth living. The apparent cause of her depression was her inability to obtain anything other than temporary employment.

The patient was the second of five children; the only brother had died of meningitis in infancy so that the patient was raised as one of four girls. Her parents were still living together at the time of her admission to the hospital. The father, a shoe repairman for many years, was currently employed as a night watchman. He was described as quiet and stubborn but always lenient with the children. The mother, on the other hand, had a "nervous temperament" and was a chronic nagger, always demanding, criticizing and trying to control everyone.

The patient was slower in learning to walk and talk than her older sister and before many years it was recognized that her development was behind that of her siblings. She obtained poor grades in school, hated studying and was quickly surpassed by the sister three years younger. The patient finally left school at about the age of 14 with the equivalent of a sixth grade education. She remained at home for a year or two and then worked at a number of different jobs as a domestic but stayed home a great deal between jobs. At about 19 she left home to obtain employment on her own. Between 21 and 25 she was a novice in a convent. The order was rigidly cloistered and the patient said she left because it was too much of a strain; she lost 40 pounds and became "nervous" during her last year. After leaving the convent, she went to stay in a nursing home for a few days but remained for several months to help the owner who was kind to her. During the next 14 years she went in and out of a variety of jobs in factories and domestic service but had difficulty holding each one, evidently because of her limited ability. She was conscientious and religious and denied having had any form of sexual experience.

On arrival in the hospital she said, "I was getting along fine until five days ago when the doctor took me off night medicine and I haven't slept period. It's not the way I live but the way I feel. I can't see anything to live for in life." She admitted that at times the future had looked hopeless and she had contemplated suicide, but that she felt this was wrong. When asked about the overdose of sleeping pills, she replied, "I didn't really mean to do away with myself. I just meant to sleep on." There was no evidence of illusions, hallucinations or delusions. She was correctly oriented and showed no gross impairment of memory.

Her intellectual function was estimated in the upper limit of the mentally subnormal range, and she obtained an I.Q. of 69. The following are some of her responses to a sentence completion test:

1. *I always wanted* to be a nun.
2. *If I were ever in charge* I would not try to be a boss.
3. *Most of my friends* don't know that I am afraid of life.
4. *My greatest mistake* was not being educated.
5. *My greatest weakness* is not having confidence in myself.

She was also discouraged over her failure to marry and raise a family. She said, "I soon won't be able to have any children. I'm too old now. My hair's growing gray. I've been teased about being 'just an old maid' and it hurts."

Her depression rapidly improved following a short course of ECT and she left the hospital three months later to work in a nearby convent. Within three months her depression returned and she was readmitted to the hospital. On this occasion she remained only three weeks and again returned to the convent. For some time afterward she continued to receive a small dose of tranquilizing medication to relieve her symptoms of anxiety and irritability, but she made a satisfactory adjustment and there was no recurrence of acute symptoms during the next five years.

It is generally agreed that all symptoms of psychological disturbance are found in retarded persons and some symptoms are found at all levels of subnormality. The incidence of mental illness is thought to be much higher in the subnormal than general population. Penrose (1938) surveyed the psychological disorders among a population of institutionalized defectives and reported that exclusive of epilepsy, approximately 16 per cent of the patients evidenced some sort of neurotic or psychotic pattern. His results are comparatively conservative, for similar studies (Neuer, 1947, and Angus, 1948) report higher percentages of psychological disturbances among subnormal patients.

These data are supported by surveys conducted among the hospitalized mentally ill. Pollock (1945) studied the first admissions to state hospitals for the mentally ill in New York and found that over a three-year period the annual admission rate for persons diagnosed as subnormal was several times as high as for persons within the range of normal intelligence. The most frequent diagnosis was "psychosis with mental deficiency" for 40 per cent of the new patients and "dementia praecox" for 18 per cent. The investigator concluded that the general rate of incidence of mental illness was higher among the subnormal population than the general population and that the rate of mental illness declined as the degree of intelligence rose.

It is difficult to interpret and generalize from such studies for at least two reasons. First, mentally subnormal persons do not reside in any one type of setting. While some of them are in institutions for the retarded or the mentally ill, the majority (especially those at the upper levels of subnormality) remain in the community. Any institutional survey, therefore, necessarily omits this large segment of the mildy subnormal population and is overweighted with the severely and moderately subnormal. It is true that such surveys do provide information about the institutionalized population, but the findings cannot be generalized to the total subnormal population. Second, an even greater difficulty in interpretation occurs because diagnostic procedures and criteria vary greatly from setting to setting and, in most instances, are not adequately described in the report of the survey results. The studies just cited are among the best available, yet none reports diagnostic criteria and Pollock does not give his method of determining the existence of subnormality.

Only a few studies are concerned with the psychological adjustment of noninstitutionalized defectives. One such study (Weaver, 1946) was based on a sample of 8000 persons in the United States Army with I.Q.'s below 75. Of the sample, 62 per cent of the females and 56 per cent of the males were able to make satisfactory adjustments to military life. The remainder showed some symptoms of psychological disorder—psychotic, neurotic, psychosomatic or sociopathic in nature. The median I.Q. of the successful group was 72 as compared with 68 for the unsuccessful. Weaver concluded, however, that personality factors far outweighed the importance of intellectual level in the individual's adjustment to military service.

Some of the symptoms of *schizophrenia* and *mental deficiency* are very similar. A number of subnormal patients manifest the same disturbances of affect, unresponsiveness, limited speech or mutism and silliness, for example, that is observed in schizophrenics. (Most patients with mental deficiency, however, will not develop schizophrenia or other psychotic symptoms.) When schizophrenia and mental deficiency occur in the same person it often cannot be determined which symptoms arise from the intellectual limitations and which stem from the psychological disorder. The diagnostic problem is further complicated by the fact that many schizophrenics cannot utilize their intellectual capacities efficiently and consistently; they continue to deteriorate as the illness progresses, or deteriorate and level off. Not infrequently, schizophrenics obtain test scores that place them in the subnormal range. In some studies, for example, Böök (1953), Larsson and Sjögren (1954), results apparently indicate an increased frequency of mental deficiency among patients developing schizophrenia (and possibly vice versa) which has led to speculation of a possible genetic connection between the two syndromes.

Some investigators (e.g., Tredgold and Soddy, 1963) believe that it is sometimes impossible to distinguish between schizophrenia and mental subnormality and that both conditions may be clinical manifestations of the same organic abnormality. Others hold that schizophrenia and mental deficiency should be differentiated and considered as two separate conditions. Penrose (1964), for example, states that theoretically a person at any level of intellectual capacity can experience any degree of psychological disturbance. A majority of psychologists and psychiatrists today agree with the latter opinion, yet, it must be emphasized, the evidence is by no means clear.

The following case is typical of many which are seen. It appears that the patient had brain damage as a result of anoxia at birth, but no neurologic signs were obvious. Her parents did not notice any retardation in her early development, and, although school was difficult for her, she progressed from grade to grade until early adolescence. It is possible that her symptoms of mental subnormality were actually early evidences of schizophrenic deterioration.

The patient was born after prolonged labor that terminated in a difficult instrumental delivery under deep anesthesia. It is probable that during this period the blood supply to her brain contained too little oxygen. At the time of birth her face was badly marked by the instruments, unlike her two younger siblings, and some degree of mild facial deformity remained. Her parents did not notice any retardation in her early development. She was a little slower than the younger siblings in starting to walk and talk, and her speech was more difficult to understand, but there was no evidence of obvious damage to her nervous system. She entered school at the age of six, and, although she had some difficulties, particularly in arithmetic, was advanced from grade to grade each year until she reached seventh grade. She repeated the grade but made little progress beyond that of the preceding year. As no special instruction was available for retarded children, her parents were advised to keep her at home. Her brother and sister both went on to complete high school as the parents had.

The patient remained at home and never went out to work. She helped her mother very little and complained of nervousness and an inability to concentrate. Her parents did not consider her behavior abnormal until one day, when she was 19, she went out and failed to return home. She was found standing in a lane and did not seem to know why she was there. During the next three years she became increasingly seclusive, stopped going to church, and remained in the house most of the time.

When she was 21 her parents thought there was an improvement in her condition because she started to become more talkative, but her conversation soon became quite disconnected and unintelligible. In addition, she started to destroy her clothing, throw dishes and furniture about the house, scream and shout without apparent reason, and move about constantly. Suddenly, her condition changed to one of stupor and withdrawal and she remained in bed for several weeks. When she again became acutely excited and disturbed she was admitted to the state hospital for the first time. She was 22.

When asked how old she was, she replied, "I must be 99. It's my great grandmother. I knew one in the first battalion." When asked her age again, she replied, "Somewhere in the millions. At the barracks. That's all I know since I died on the first of May." When asked the year, she said, "Leap year. I don't know. Over 99 millions. It's the boy and girl question. I think my sister is doing this. They went all through the barracks. I went to Europe."

She was given convulsive therapy (induced by injections of Metrazol) which controlled her episode of catatonic excitement. Because of additional episodes of both stupor and excitement, she remained in the hospital for over two years before she stabilized and was able to return home to live with her parents. During the next 13 years she was at home without any recurrence of acute symptomatology. She had no outside interests or friends. Then, again, she became uncommunicative, inactive, spent all her time in bed, stopped eating and lost weight; she was readmitted to the hospital at the age of 39.

ECT had become available, in the meantime, and she was given a short course of treatment to which she responded promptly. When she was rational and had been off treatment for several weeks, a full scale I.Q. of 55 was obtained and it was estimated that her intellectual function had never been higher than the moron level. She subsequently went home with her parents but promptly had another attack of acute excitement which was readily controlled by chlorpromazine. Long-term medication, however, did not control her tendency to recurrent catatonic episodes, particularly the states of stupor. After repeated visits at home she was readmitted to the hospital for long-term custodial care with periodic symptomatic treatment for her acute episodes.

Criminal Tendencies

Early writers in the field of mental subnormality were impressed by the high incidence of crime, immorality and poor living conditions among the mentally subnormal and their families. Most experts in the first decades of the 1900's believed that many persons in the moron category were potential criminals and needed only the proper conditions and opportunity to develop their antisocial tendencies. Goddard (1912), in his classic work on the Kallikaks (a large family with an extremely high incidence of mental subnormality), asserted, "The best material out of which to make criminals, and perhaps the material from which they are most frequently made, is feeblemindedness." He cited a number of studies that indicated that high percentages of young people in detention homes and reformatories were mentally retarded. Wallin (1956), reviewing the studies of criminality among mental subnormals, including studies made and reported prior to 1930, noted that the estimates of percentages of mental defectives in prisons or courts ranged from 22 to 90 per cent. The high estimates were, in part, a result of surveys in which the diagnosis of mental subnormality had been erroneously based on faulty intelligence data secured from unstandardized tests that were neither valid nor reliable and, also, from varying interpretations of test results. It is very possible, of course, that more mental subnormals were imprisoned then than now.

A violent reaction occurred to the claims for a high incidence of crime among the mentally subnormal. Studies began to appear that indicated that the incidence of mental subnormality among prison and court populations was about the same as for the general population. One of the best and most comprehensive investigations was conducted by Tulchin (1939) among more than 10,000 inmates of correctional institutions in Illinois. The results of intelligence tests for this group closely approximated those for the Illinois army draft during World War I; the percentages of inferior, average and superior men were highly similar in the two populations. It is interesting that some relation was found between level of intelligence test scores and type of crime. The highest median intelligence test scores were obtained by the men committed for fraud; the lowest scores were obtained by those committed for sex crimes.

In New York City, Bromberg and Thompson (1937) studied approximately 10,000 prisoners who were referred to the psychiatric clinic of the Court of General Sessions. The sample comprised all prisoners indicted for and found guilty of felonies. A psychiatrist examined those considered to be mentally deficient and administered two or more psychological tests to them. Subnormals were defined as those persons with I.Q.'s below 66, and only 2.4 per cent of the cases were so classified.

Glueck and Glueck (1934) studied 1000 juvenile delinquents and reported that only 13.1 per cent of them were mentally retarded. Kvaraceus (1945) estimated that 12 per cent of the delinquents in his study were mentally subnormal. These and many other studies (for instance, Healy and Bronner, 1926; Zeleny, 1931) that belittled the importance of intelligence in crime caused Wallin (1956) to assert that probably as a reaction against the early exaggerations, the pendulum had now swung too far in the opposite direction and the intelligence factor in criminality was being neglected.

Recent follow-up studies in the area indicate that the moderately subnormal are seldom involved in antisocial behavior (because they are usually under supervision) but that a somewhat higher delinquency and criminal rate occurs among the mildly retarded than would be expected from their general prevalence in the population. Thus, Wattenberg (1954), comparing the records of 99 pre-adolescent "repeaters" with those of 235 boys who had had only one police contact, found that repeating was highly associated with low intellectual ability, poor school work, membership in gangs and a reputation for trouble. Baller (1936) and Charles (1953) followed up the same group of "opportunity room" students in Nebraska; the first study was made when the subjects were 22 years old, the second when they were 42. The investigators found that the number of court records for the subjects were several times higher than for a "normal" group; by the time of the second study 60 per cent of the males had police records although most of the citations were for minor violations.

Peterson and Smith (1960) compared 45 mildly subnormal adults who had once been in public-school special classes, with 45 normal controls, matching the groups according to socioeconomic status. Among the retarded adults, 62 per cent had committed illegal offenses and of a more serious nature as compared to 31 per cent for the normal group.

Most follow-up studies of educable mentally retarded persons indicate a higher delinquency

TABLE 18–4. Estimated Concordance Rates in Monozygotic and Dizygotic Co-twins of Institutionalized Mental Defective Twins

Investigator	Apparent Zygosity of Twins	Number of Pairs	Estimated Concordance Rate (Per Cent)	$H = \dfrac{CMZ - CDZ}{100 - CDZ}$
Rosanoff et al. (1937)	MZ	126	91	0.81
	DZ	240	53	
Juda (1939)	MZ	71	97	0.93
	DZ	149	56	

and criminal rate among them than would be expected from their prevalence in the general population. Smith (1962), reviewing the studies in this area, pointed out that the problem of delinquency among the subnormal population is complicated by school failures, early school drop-outs, difficulty in finding and retaining employment, low socioeconomic status and other variables. Limited intellectual capacity in itself does not necessarily imply nonconforming behavior, but because the mentally deficient individual also lacks insight and normal comprehension, his inability to conform to our increasingly complex society is penalized. School or probation office psychologists often discover predelinquent or youthful offenders with limited intelligence and recommend their commitment to institutions for the mentally subnormal instead of imprisonment. Apparently, however, some youthful subnormals thrive under the security of institutional care so that they are considered reformed and are returned to the complex world with which they are unable to cope and then commit additional or more serious crimes.

CAUSATION, DEVELOPMENT AND DYNAMICS

In the beginning a child's potential intelligence is determined by the interaction of many biological factors that are hereditary and environmental in nature. After birth, biological forces continue to operate, of course, but in conjunction with psychological and sociocultural factors. Together they determine the manner in which the individual develops, how efficiently he utilizes his intellectual resources and how adequately he adjusts socially.

Heredity appears to be the prime factor in the determination of intelligence. It was indicated in Chapter 6 that, in general, intelligence meets the three criteria considered to be indicative of polygenic inheritance, i.e., (1) continuous quantitative variation; (2) appropriate sequence of correlations between different classes of relatives; (3) positive results from foster child and twin studies. There are also studies of mentally deficient twins that affirm the importance of heredity. Rosanoff et al. (1937) and Juda (1939), investigating mental deficiency in the co-twins of institutionalized mentally deficient twins, found much higher concordance rates for monozygotic than dizygotic pairs (see Table 18–4).

Other biological factors, however, are also known to be the cause of some mental deficiency. Severe and moderate mental subnormality is usually the result of central nervous system damage that occurs during prenatal maturation, at birth or early in infancy. Sometimes it is possible to obtain a history of the significant injury, but the probable causation can be assigned in only about 20 per cent of the cases; in the remaining 80 per cent, severe retardation is only known to have been present from birth or infancy onward.

Among persons who are mildly subnormal, the majority of the mental deficient population, central nervous system damage is difficult or impossible to determine. Generally, the brains of the mildly subnormal are a little smaller in size and weigh slightly less than the normal. The convolutions tend to be wider and simpler. However, the gross abnormalities that are found in the brains of the more severely retarded are absent. Microscopic examinations do not show the paucity and imperfection of neurones that are found in the severely subnormal. According to Tredgold and Soddy (1963), the brains of many high grade feebleminded persons would be classified as normal, although it is possible that present techniques are not good enough to discover abnormal characteristics that, in fact, may be present. On the other hand, it is also possible that mental subnormality is not in all cases the result of brain abnormalities.

The mildly subnormal have often been described as having a "familial" type of mental deficiency, i.e., they tend to come from families in which parents, siblings and other relatives are also of low intelligence. Thus it has often been assumed that a genetic factor is responsible for their subnormality. In recent years, however, there has been an increasing interest in the role of sociocultural factors in the determination of mild subnormality (Sarason, 1953). As knowledge increases in this field the category will unquestionably be subdivided into several types according to the different etiologies that may be discovered.

Strauss (1939), Strauss and Lehtinen (1947) and Strauss and Kephart (1955) were pioneers in the attempts to differentiate exogenous (brain-damaged) from endogenous (non–brain-damaged) mental subnormals by their intellectual and perceptual functioning, and to design educational programs based on the special handicaps of each group. The terms exogenous and endogenous were used in a restricted sense, i.e., excluding all cases in which gross neurologic symptoms, such as those found in specific clinical syndromes, were present. The exogenous cases were identified through a history of prenatal or postnatal accidents, premature or difficult births, or infectious diseases in early life. The endogenous cases were identified by intellectual defects without evidence of neurologic damage and were cases that are sometimes called familial or common garden variety defectives. The subjects were equated for mental age.

The findings of Strauss and his associates suggested that the exogenous retardates manifested disorders of perception and concept formation that were not so apparent in the endogenous group; the exogenous performed better on verbal than on nonverbal tasks, on the whole, while the reverse performance was usual among the endogenous; and the behavior of the exogenous was more often rated as uncontrolled, erratic and uninhibited. The testing procedure was similar to that of Goldstein (1939) who worked with brain-injured adults and noted the same trends as Strauss and his associates. The Strauss series of studies, however, has been criticized for a number of reasons, and attempts to replicate the results have been generally unsuccessful (Gallagher, 1957).

A recent study by Hetherington and Banta (1962) suggests that although the results of such experimentation were controversial, it may be useful, nevertheless, to probe distinctions between exogenous and endogenous subnormals; when they compared normals and the two types of retardates on intentional and incidental learning, they found no difference between normals and endogenous subjects on either acquisition or retention for intentional or incidental learning, but the exogenous group did significantly poorer on incidental learning than either of the other groups. There was no difference for intentional learning.

A number of difficulties are inherent in such research, not the least of which is the separation of exogenous from endogenous cases. Brain injuries are not homogeneous in terms of extent and site of lesion, and it must be expected that the differences will be reflected in the various kinds of behavior or symptoms found in the individuals. The neurologic criteria of minimal brain injury are by no means perfect; unquestionably some cases classified as endogenous actually have unobservable brain injuries. In addition, if there are hereditary factors in the etiology of the endogenous cases, then it may be presumed that the subject has a genetically transmitted defect in the structure or functioning of his central nervous system. As Spitz (1963) has pointed out, such a subnormal child is no less brain damaged than the subnormal whose neural mechanisms are insulted by trauma or disease, although the damage is different. By the same reasoning a child who is retarded as a result of disease early in life is differently damaged from a child who suffered a birth injury, and to group them together for research purposes seems questionable. At any rate, because of these numerous and complex diagnostic problems, the psychologist who attempts to differentiate and compare exogenous and endogenous mental subnormals is in the position of comparing test results with a criterion of unknown validity.

Heredity

Reed and Reed (1965) have reported on the incidence of mental retardation in 289 families of which at least one member was institutionalized between 1911 and 1918 for mental deficiency (i.e., with I.Q.'s of 69 or below). The existence of early, detailed records made possible the recording of family pedigrees from grandparents, parents and siblings through children and grandchildren, and showed a total of 82,217 individuals spread over three to five generations. The investigators concluded that "retardation and some of its concomitant social consequences are not distributed at random through the population." Mental deficiency is clustered in families and perpetuated by assortive matings resulting in a concentration of bad genes and bad environment. Many retarded persons, 9 per cent of the sample population, took retarded marriage partners.

The 289 probands were classified according to the etiology of their subnormality; 84 were listed as primarily genetic, 55 as probably genetic, 27 as environmental (including biological) and 123 as unknown (isolated cases). For each classification the percentage of retardates among relatives of the probands was estimated according to degree of relationship, i.e., first degree, comprising parents, siblings and children; second degree, grandparents, aunts, uncles, half-siblings, nieces and nephews and grandchildren; and third degree, half-aunts and -uncles, half-nieces and -nephews, great-nephews and -nieces and first cousins. The findings are shown in Table 18–5. (In 37 of the 289 families the proband was the only known retardate.) The table shows a clear-cut and sharp drop in percentages of retarded relatives as the degree of relationship becomes more distant, evidence that is consonant with a polygenic theory of inheritance (a drop of 50 per cent with each decrease of one degree of relationship).

The one-family pedigree method, exemplified by Goddard's (1912) study of the Kallikaks, did not resolve the nature-nurture issue. The study is of historical significance as a fascinating portrayal of a mentally subnormal family and as a source of material on the high incidence of

TABLE 18–5. Percentages of Retardation Among Relatives of Retarded Probands According to Classification of Etiology and Degree of Relationship

| Etiology | Degree of Relationship | | |
	1st	2nd	3rd[*]
Primary genetic	33.6	9.2	3.7
Probably genetic	50.7	16.8	5.3
Environmental	21.4	2.0	1.1[†]
Unknown	15.6	2.6	2.1
All	28.0	7.1	3.1

[*]Many too young to test.
[†]Lower than expected percentage in general population.
Adapted from Reed, E. W., and Reed, S. C. 1965. Mental Retardation: A Family Study. Philadelphia, W. B. Saunders Co.

TABLE 18–6. Percentages of Siblings of Mental Defectives, According to Level of Intelligence[*]

| Grade of Subject | Grade of Siblings | | | | |
	Normal (or Superior)	Dull	Feeble-minded	Imbecile	Idiot
Dull	77.4	16.2	4.9	1.0	0.5
Feeble-minded	76.8	11.9	8.3	2.5	0.6
Imbecile	83.5	7.6	4.6	3.5	0.7
Idiot	81.0	9.9	4.2	1.7	3.2

[*]Data from Penrose (1938) condensed by Roberts. Reprinted by permission from Roberts, J. A. F. 1950. The genetics of oligophrenia. In Congrès International de Psychiatrie, Paris, VI, Psychiatrie Sociale, Génétique et Eugénique. Paris, Hermann, pp. 55–117.

retardation in such a family. The Reed study is important in that it is predictive rather than explanatory: it establishes empirical risk figures that can be used to determine the probability of mental deficiency among different degrees of relatives given a subnormal parent or sibling. This is similar to the work of Kallmann (1953) on the psychoses.

A number of investigators have tried to differentiate the weight of heredity in severe subnormality as opposed to mild subnormality. Wildenskov (1934), dividing his mentally deficient subjects into mild and severe groups, found that in the mild group subnormality existed in 51 per cent of the siblings, but in the severe group, in only 26 per cent. Penrose (1938), in an extensive study of 1280 mental defectives, reported on the intelligence of his subjects' siblings according to the subjects' levels of retardation. His results were summarized by Roberts (1950) and are shown in Table 18–6. The dull and mildly subnormal subjects had a high proportion of dull and subnormal siblings, whereas the subjects classified as imbeciles and idiots had relatively lower proportions of siblings with severe degrees of subnormality.

Following an investigation of 562 siblings of feebleminded (mildly subnormal) and imbecile (moderately subnormal) patients falling within an I.Q. range of 30 to 68, Roberts (1952) presented his results graphically (see Fig. 18–5) to show that the siblings of the feebleminded are lower than average in intelligence and include a high proportion of mildly subnormal persons. The siblings of the imbeciles, on the other hand, more closely approach the normal distribution of intelligence but have proportionately more members in the severely

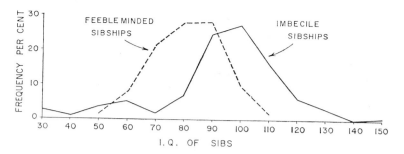

Figure 18–5. Frequency distributions of the I.Q.'s of 562 sibs of feeble-minded and imbeciles of the I.Q. range 30 to 68. (Reprinted by permission from Roberts, J. A. F., 1952. The genetics of mental deficiency. Eugenics Review, 44:71–83.)

subnormal range than in the superior. Usually, the I.Q. range of imbeciles is considered to be 20 to 49; if moderate subnormals with I.Q.'s between 20 and 39 had been included, the conclusions would probably not have been changed perceptibly, for it is generally agreed that the more severe the subnormality, the less important is the factor of heredity.

Similarly, it has been found that the parents of mildly subnormal patients are lower in average intelligence and more likely to be mildly subnormal themselves than the parents of the severely subnormal. Penrose (1964) estimated the mean I.Q.'s of the parents and siblings of his large series of mentally defective patients and found that when the parents are considered to be normal in intelligence, the siblings are also normal and a wide separation exists between the intelligence of the patients and their relatives; when the parents are subnormal in intelligence, the gap is narrower but the patients are closer in intelligence to their parents than to their siblings. In summary, severely subnormal patients have parents and siblings who are frequently within the normal range of intelligence. The parents and siblings of the mildly subnormal, on the other hand, are more like the patients in range of intelligence.

A number of surveys of the occupations and socioeconomic level of parents of mental subnormals consistently show that the high grade cases tend to come from low socioeconomic levels but low grade cases have parents who represent a wide random sampling of the general population socioeconomically (Paterson and Rundquist, 1933; Bradway, 1935; Halperin, 1945; Roberts, 1952). Anastasi (1958) has also pointed out that large-scale surveys reveal that the distribution of intelligence test scores closely approximates the normal curve when the mildly retarded are included with normal and superior people; however, the distribution deviates significantly from normal when the moderately and severely retarded are added

to the group. The number of persons with I.Q.'s below 45 is much greater than would be expected by chance. This is, of course, because of the high incidence of biological insults to the brain, and suggests that organic brain damage is the pre-eminent factor in the severely subnormal group, but that in the mild group heredity factors are more important.

Simple mendelian inheritance, nevertheless, is responsible for the development of a number of the rare syndromes that are associated with mental subnormality. The degree of retardation accompanying these rare syndromes is usually severe enough so that affected persons seldom reproduce and thus do not transmit their defective genes. The analysis of family data, however, has indicated that certain forms of severe mental subnormality are attributable to the presence of a single dominant gene arising by new mutation. Examples of these disorders include epiloia (tuberous sclerosis), ocular hypertelorism (greater than normal width between the eyes), and other syndromes associated with lesions of the skin, blood vessels and bones.

Mental subnormality that is attributed to a single pair of recessive genes is found in individuals with parents who are apparently normal but carry the condition, and in 25 per cent of the siblings. This form of inheritance has been found in certain patients with microcephaly (which, however, may also be caused by infections and other environmental processes), amaurotic familial idiocy, phenylketonuria (PKU), gargoylism (a disorder of carbohydrate metabolism associated with facial and other deformities), and other forms of metabolic disturbances.

These rare syndromes constitute a minority of all cases of severe subnormality which, itself, occurs much less frequently than the milder degrees of subnormality. By contrast, the genetic factor in the causation of mild mental subnormality appears to be approximately the same in degree (one-half to two-thirds the overall variance) and in nature (polygenic transmission) as it is in the overall determination of intelligence in the general population.

Knowledge of the importance of genetic factors in the causation of mental subnormality has been increased, over the past decade, by advances in cytogenetic techniques that have led to the discovery of several chromosome anomalies. Normally, females and males have 22 pairs of autosomes each, but the female has two X chromosomes while the male has one X and one Y chromosome. Among the chromosome anomalies that have been identified, for instance, are Turner's syndrome (in which the patient is externally female but lacks gonads) that is caused, as a rule, by the presence of only one X chromosome; and Klinefelter's syndrome (underdeveloped testes) in which most patients have two X as well as one Y chromosome. A variety of other anomalies have been found of which the most common appears to be the presence of three X chromosomes. Maclean et al. (1962) found that in a large sample of both male and female mental defectives the presence of the extra X chromosome was several times as frequent as in a large sample of the general population. The presence of the extra sex chromosome, however, is still quite rare among mental defectives and is usually accompanied by mild rather than severe subnormality.

Mongolism stems from a different anomaly. Since the identification of the syndrome approximately a hundred years ago, little has been known, until recently, of its etiology. At the beginning of this century it was observed that mongoloids tended to be the offspring of elderly mothers; more recently Penrose (1964) reported that the frequency of mongolian offspring was over 100 times as great for mothers past the age of 45 as for mothers under the age of 20. The possibility of a genetic basis was suggested by the very high rate of concordance in monozygotic twins and the very low rate in dizygotic twins, and by the observation that the mongolian mothers who reproduced gave birth to about 50 per cent normal and 50 per cent mongolian children. This was frequently interpreted as evidence of transmission by a single dominant gene.

Using cytogenetic techniques, Lejeune et al. (1959) established the transmission of a whole extra chromosome as the primary cause of mongolism. The extra chromosome is present in many mongoloids but not in all. It is not a sex chromosome, but a small autosome. In mongolism the first discovery of an autosomal aberration in man was made. When it was found that mongoloids did not possess the extra chromosome, the belief arose that in certain cases of mongolism the syndrome occurs as a result of the translocation, or exchange, of segments, between nonhomologous chromosomes. On the basis of cytogenic studies of six families, each containing more than one mongoloid, Shaw (1962) concluded that familial mongolism stems from many different causes and that in every family with more than one mongoloid careful investigation is warranted.

Other Biological Determinants

Just as mild and severe mental subnormalities tend to be associated with differences in genetic transmission and chromosome anomalies, so are they also associated with differences in environmental determinants. The mildly subnormal tend to grow up in families that are limited in intelligence and socioeconomic status, and to experience difficulties in social adjustment as a result of emotional and social deprivation. The severely subnormal, in contrast, tend to have learning and adaptation difficulties because of any of a tremendous variety of biological insults that may lead to a chronic brain syndrome. Such brain damage may occur during intra-uterine life or the birth process, or during early postnatal life, and may be the result of infections, intoxications, physical injury, uncontrolled seizures or deficiencies of oxygen, essential vitamins, or hormone imbalances.

Four main types of maternal and fetal *infection* have been regarded as important causes of mental subnormality: the spirochete causing congenital syphilis, the virus causing rubella (German measles), the protozoon causing toxoplasmosis (as parasitic infection) and virus infections that cause cytomegalic inclusion disease (which affects cells in the blood). Brain infections occurring shortly after birth may also cause life-long mental subnormality.

Congenital syphilis may result in stillbirth, prematurity, bodily deformity or brain damage. It was formerly the main intra-uterine infection recognized as a cause of mental subnormality. Rubella is generally a mild infection except during the first three months of intra-uterine life. Approximately 10 to 20 per cent of the living infants born after maternal rubella have anomalies that most often affect the eyes or heart, but in some cases involve the brain and result in mental subnormality.

The protozoon responsible for toxoplasmosis has a worldwide distribution among a variety of animals. Infection probably occurs from swallowing contaminated water or by transmission prenatally, from the mother. It may result in a variety of brain lesions that lead to hydrocephaly, microcephaly, or epilepsy, associated with mental retardation. The virus infections responsible for cytomegalic inclusion disease also may result in a variety of brain lesions with associated mental subnormality.

Among the *toxic agents* responsible for mental subnormality, Jervis (1959) included large doses of x-ray therapy to the abdominal region of the pregnant mother, severe jaundice caused by incompatibility between the blood of the mother and child, lead poisoning, usually acquired by ingesting paint or other substances after birth. In the case of hemolytic jaundice, the brain damage is to the basal ganglia (kernicterus) and apparently results from the presence in the infant's blood of large amounts of bilirubin, a breakdown product of hemoglobin. The best known form of this serological incompatibility is that of the Rhesus (Rh) blood group factor. Mental subnormality can be prevented if recognition of the disorder is prompt and the affected infant's blood is exchanged for normal blood of the same group.

Cerebral palsy commonly implies the influence of two major conditions: mechanical trauma and brain damage due to anoxia. The effects of the two agencies are extremely difficult to assess. During the first half of the present century a number of ingenious experiments were performed on animals which clearly demonstrated that the birth process obeys the physical laws of hydrodynamics and that brain lesions could be produced by subjecting the head of the animal to a lower pressure than that of the rest of the body. In accordance with these findings, Schwartz (1957) reproduced all cranial and cerebral changes occurring in normal and pathological births by placing a suction cup on the heads of newborn animals. Dekaban (1962) intensively studied 15 brains of human infants with acute hemorrhagic lesions that were related to the birth process and advanced the opinion that a combination of various adverse factors is usually responsible for the occurrence of cerebral palsy. A particularly difficult and hasty delivery, however, may lead to obvious mechanical injury and is the major or sole cause of severe intra-cranial hemorrhage.

In his experiments on the production of *anoxia* in adult guinea pigs, Windle (1952) demonstrated that changes in brain structure were associated with impairment of memory and learning. In a subsequent series of experiments on monkeys, Windle et al. (1962) demonstrated that structural changes in the central nervous system, neurologic abnormalities including epileptic seizures and behavior deviations followed asphyxia at birth.

Premature birth sometimes results from various complications of pregnancy, i.e., toxemia or bleeding, or a variety of other conditions that may impair the mother's health. Regardless of its cause, however, premature birth exposes the child to an increased risk of brain damage from mechanical trauma and anoxia. In a longitudinal study of 500 single-born premature infants and 492 full-term control infants, Knobloch et al. (1956) found that the frequency of neuropsychiatric abnormality increased as the birth weight of the infant decreased. Among those infants with a birth weight of less than 1501 gm. (approximately 3 lb. and 3 oz.) neurologic or intellectual defects were present in 50.9 per cent, and some infants also had a major visual handicap.

Postmature birth also appears to result in an increased risk of anoxia for the child, during both the later weeks of pregnancy and the birth process. Turnbull and Baird (1957) in a study of the oxygen content of venous and arterial blood from the umbilical cords of 100 first deliveries that followed clinically normal pregnancies found that the average oxygen saturation of the blood decreased as maternal age and length of gestation increased, and was sometimes dangerously low, especially in women giving birth to their first child after the age of 40 and after the forty-first week of pregnancy. There is a relatively high rate of death among post-mature infants born to older mothers pregnant for the first time, and it appears probable that there is also a relatively higher frequency of neurological abnormality and intellectual subnormality.

Vitamin deficiencies in experimental animals have been demonstrated to result in infertility; if the animals did become pregnant the offspring had high rates of death and deformity. Almost all the congenital defects that occur in man have been faithfully reproduced in experiment animals maintained on a diet deficient in vitamin A.

Studies of the effects of maternal diet during human pregnancy were reviewed by Toverud et al. (1950). In some, dietary supplements (mainly vitamins A, D and B, phosphorous, calcium and iron) were administered to the women and resulted in a significant reduction of still-birth and neonatal mortality rates. Harrell et al. (1955) conducted an extensive diet study involving 2400 pregnant women living in Kentucky and Virginia. In order to secure four equivalent samples, the four types of dietary supplements were administered in serial order to women as they registered in the cooperating clinics. The supplements were (1) ascorbic acid, (2) thiamine, riboflavin, niacine and iron, (3) inert material, (4) thiamine. Neither the participants nor the person who later tested their offspring knew which supplements had been administered. In the Norfolk, Virginia, area, 518 offspring were tested at the age of three with the following results: children of mothers who had received supplement (2) obtained the highest average I.Q., 103.4; children of mothers who had received supplement (4) obtained 101.9; supplement (1), 100.9, and the nonsupplemented group, (3), 98.4. A year later 370 of these children were again tested and again a significantly larger mean I.Q. was obtained for the children of the women who received supplements as compared with the children of the women who were given only inert material. The authors concluded that in the Norfolk study the supplementing of pregnant and lactating mothers' diets significantly increased the average intelligence quotient of their children, at the ages of three and four, above the average I.Q. obtained by offspring of mothers whose diets were not supplemented. Statistically significant differences were not obtained in the Kentucky portion of the study, probably because of the better general diets of this group. The results of many other studies of maternal diet, conducted in the past decade, are often not clear-cut, because of inadequacies in the experimental design. A general trend, however, strongly suggests that women with good dietary habits, both before and during pregnancy, tend to have healthier babies than those with one kind or another of diet deficiency.

Deficiency or excess of certain *hormones* has been shown to produce developmental defects in experimental animals. In women, certain endocrine disorders are known to result in infertility or fetal death. Uncontrolled diabetes in the mother may lead to fetal death or postmaturity with its accompanying hazards. Several endocrine disorders in the infant may also result in mental subnormality; the most frequent, by far, is hypothyroidism. In adults this leads to myxedema, described in the preceding chapter, and in children the comparable disorder is known as cretinism.

Psychological Determinants, Development and Dynamics

The primary needs of the severely subnormal child are physiological, that is, to be fed and kept comfortable. In addition, there may be a primitive contact need, for he usually demonstrates greater contentment if he is handled or held, for example, or rocked or caressed. These needs are no different from those of the normal infant, but the normal infant's needs change with maturation; in the severely subnormal child the needs remain basic throughout his life.

The needs of mentally deficient children tend to become more varied and complex as the extent of the subnormality decreases. The mildly subnormal child has virtually all the needs found in persons with normal intelligence: needs for acceptance, approval, achievement, love, sex and nurturance, for example. Like the normal child, he goes through all the stages of emotional growth except that he remains longer in each stage because of the immaturity that is a result of the slower development of his nervous system.

The mildly subnormal child experiences greater difficulty in giving up present gratification and modes of adjustments for more complex levels of interaction. His perceptions and motor responses remain vague and diffuse longer than those of a normal child; his skills develop slowly and much practice is often necessary to reinforce them. He remains dependent on his parents long after normal children have begun to take care of their own physical needs, or venture out into the neighborhood or exhibit other independent behavior. He develops control over his impulses slowly, and often his tolerance of frustration seems hardly to increase at all. Weaning and toilet training are necessarily delayed (because of biological immaturity and his inability to understand his mother's requests) and may be accomplished in an atmosphere of such pressure and anxiety that he has frequent lapses and is vulnerable to regression for the rest of his life. As he approaches school age or is enrolled in the early grades, his limitations become more apparent and the differences between him and other children are more pronounced. In a school with normal children he may be regarded as odd and called "dumb," or "stupid," by his schoolmates. The gap widens between him and his peers as he reaches puberty: he is not able to converse at their level, is not accepted into their interest groups and is left behind as the others go on to high school. Younger siblings have begun to "catch up" with or even surpass him. He is expected to make vocational plans, yet has not mastered the rudiments of social adjustment at the grade-school level.

Because of his dependency and limitations, he is even more the victim of parental and community attitudes than the normal child. He reacts to his retardation as it is interpreted and communicated to him. He often develops a poor self-concept and thinks of himself as being a "bad" person because there is a discrepancy between his level of aspiration and capacity for achievement and because he experiences repeated failure and few successes and rewards. He feels guilty about his failures and tends to anticipate rejection.

Beier, Gorlow and Stacey (1951) studied the fantasy life of subnormal children as revealed in TAT stories and found that the themes of the retarded group were less aggressive than those of the normals. Their stories more often contained themes of self-accusation, rejection and problems of socialization. They were more concerned with family relationships and their own perceived "badness." The bad self concept, as noted in Chapter 12, is often seen among schizophrenics. There is reason to believe that this poor self image of the retarded child is fertile ground for increased withdrawal.

The child's retarded development evokes several patterns of response from parents. Kanner (1953) found that the parents of mentally deficient children characteristically react by *acknowledgment, disguise* or *denial* of the child's condition. The first response, of course, is the mature one. The parent accepts the reality of the child's retardation and recognizes his limitations. He approves of the needs of his retarded child, as well as those of his normal children, and tries to fulfill them. He does not make excessive use of repression, reaction-formation, projection or denial.

In the second response, the parent tries to hide from himself the existence of his child's limitations. He searches for some circumstance or cause to which he can attribute the deficiency. He may deny the extent of the impairment and sometimes perceives the child as lazy, uncooperative or hostile. Such a parent often engages in a continuous search for a doctor, treatment, regime or miracle that will restore his child to normal; he ignores the recommendations he dislikes. This reaction contradicts the best interests of the subnormal child. It puts him under pressure to perform at a level that is impossible for him to attain and he becomes frustrated and anxious. As a result, he is unable to make a comfortable adjustment and becomes increasingly incapable of using the limited resources he has. In some cases he appears to become more retarded and to develop new symptoms of maladjustment. Quite often, because of the unwarranted optimism for his eventual improvement or recovery, he may be denied the special training from which he could profit. The following case illustrates an attitude of denial in the mother of a moderately subnormal child.

A mother brought her seven-year-old daughter to a psychologist for a second psychometric examination within the year. The child had previously been seen by another psychologist who specialized in the evaluation of mental subnormality, but the parents were unable to accept his test findings, interpretations, prognosis or recommendations. The patient, about six years old then, had done about as well on the Merrill-Palmer scale (an intelligence test that requires very few verbal answers) as the average two- to three-year-old child. It was predicted that in adulthood her level of mental maturity would be comparable to that of the average child of five to seven and one-half years old. She was considered to be trainable in that she was capable of acquiring some basic habits of self-care and learning to do some useful work in a protected situation under supervision, but it was not expected that she would be able to compete with normal children or adults. The child had been examined a number of times by a neurologist also. The mother requested the new psychological evaluation as a slight change had been made in the child's thyroid dosage and she felt that considerable improvement had resulted. Essentially the same results were obtained in the second evaluation.

The child had suffered prolonged anoxia at birth. Although the mother's pregnancy had seemed normal, the labor and delivery had been very difficult and the child did not breathe for 12 to 15 minutes after birth. She was in an incubator for more than a month with additional periods of not breathing. During the first year of life she had many fevers as high as 105° and 106° as well as a number of convulsions. At the age of four months a severe thyroid deficiency was detected and from then on she was given thyroid medication.

The girl manifested symptoms of a chronic brain disorder: she had a gait disturbance, poor motor coordination and strabismus, and was retarded in all areas of development. She learned to walk at the age of four. Her speech was limited; she could say her name and three or four other words that were understandable to the family alone. She kept a musical toy with her at all times and frequently pointed at it to indicate that she wished to have it wound. Although she was able to feed herself, she could not dress or undress. She played with two- and three-year-olds and usually got along well with them.

In the past few months some changes in her adjustment had become apparent. When she was separated from her musical toy she cried and was inconsolable until it was found; although she had been toilet trained at about four and a half, lapses had become frequent; when playing with other children, especially older ones, she became very irritable and cried or struck out at them; she would lie on the floor screaming and kicking if anyone took something from her; she awakened many times during the night whining and crying. Although the mother appeared to be concerned about the changes, she did not recognize them as symptoms of psychological disturbance, nor was she able to relate them to any events.

The girl had two older sisters and a three-year-old brother who had already advanced beyond her in many areas. The father had a traveling job and was seldom at home. The mother and sisters were very protective toward the girl but also seemed to push her. They instituted a kind of educational regime in which, for instance, they spent hours teaching her to color within the lines of a picture. As the patient finally mastered the skill it seemed to the mother to be an indication that the girl was able to learn, that the extent of her handicap had been exaggerated and that she was capable of attending school. The mother mentioned the child's coloring proficiency many times during the interview and insisted that the child be permitted to demonstrate it.

The mother had not followed any of the earlier recommendations and was angry with their validation. She refused to believe that the child had not improved. She seemed, also, to be unable to recognize any relation between her increased demands (including the enforced educational regime) on the child and the child's symptoms of psychological disturbance. She reported that she and her husband were going to take the child to a clinic in Canada for further evaluation; they hoped to find some treatment there so that the child could be enrolled in a regular school the next year.

In the third response described by Kanner, the parent is unable to accept the reality of the child's subnormality and flatly denies it. He expects the child to meet the standards of normal children. He may become rigid and a persistent disciplinarian, punish the child for failures and fail to perceive his successes, which may result in severe emotional problems. The following case is an illustration:

A 35-year-old man was admitted to the psychiatric service of a private hospital because he had become physically abusive toward his mother and had threatened to take her life. He was below average in intelligence, used language poorly with a limited vocabulary and had an infantile manner. He was friendly, talked about his "Mommy" and "Daddy" and liked to play with cap guns. He had a mild physical handicap that was the result of a birth injury.

In an interview with a psychiatric social worker, his parents said that they were wealthy people and had been able to give him everything he wanted as he grew up, but now they felt they had erred by preventing him from developing ambition. Their son was very helpful around the house, they emphasized, but he was so close to them he had never wanted to leave home to get a job. They implied that he was employable. He was "spoiled," they said, but they had liked having him around before his temper outbursts made his behavior so unpredictable.

Although the parents withheld the information, it was discovered that the patient had been examined by a number of doctors and psychologists. His I.Q. on a variety of tests administered at different ages was consistently between 60 and 70. He had attended a public school for a time and had been placed, against the parents' wishes, in a special class for the retarded. His teachers, however, felt that he functioned at a level below that to be expected from his test performance, and institutionalization was recommended. The parents became angry, withdrew him from school and kept him at home with them.

In late adolescence he was apprehended for making sexual advances to young children and was brought to court. Again, institutionalization was recommended, but the parents promised to keep him out of trouble and he was placed on probation. Apparently they kept close watch on him and virtually allowed him no freedom. He complained of being kept in his room and not being allowed to go out alone. It is likely that his anger toward his mother developed out of his frustration and that he struck out at her because he lacked good impulse control.

He said, in the hospital, that he felt very guilty and would never hit his mother again. He had been a "bad boy," he said, and he did not know how he had gotten to be so bad.

The mildly retarded experiences anxiety and learns to develop defense mechanisms to deal with it. Hutt and Gibby (1958) have pointed out that while it is possible for such a child to use all the defense mechanisms, actually he tends to rely on the more primitive mechanisms out of an inability to use those that depend on a maturer level of ego development. They feel that the retarded child shows a preference for such defenses as denial, regression, introjection, undoing and repression, and uses projection, reaction-formation, isolation and sublimation to a lesser extent. Stephens (1953) has studied the defense reactions of the mentally subnormal and believes that the primary defense utilized is *denial*; this is the manner in which the mentally deficient try to protect themselves from the knowledge of their inadequacies. Employing this defense may lead to difficulties, however, for then the individual does not accept the reality of his limitations and sets impossible goals for himself. It may be that the person who is able to use denial successfully maintains some self-esteem and does not develop the fragile personality organization of the individual who perceives the reality of his limitations and develops the bad self concept to accompany it.

Sociocultural Determinants

Group differences in average intelligence are indisputably associated with sociocultural factors (the entire range of intelligence, however, appears in each group). Members of the upper socioeconomic classes have a higher average intelligence than the middle classes who, in turn, are higher in average intelligence than members of the lower socioeconomic classes. Persons in high prestige occupations have higher average I.Q.'s than those in low prestige jobs. Children from urban areas test somewhat higher on the average than children from rural areas; whites obtain average I.Q. scores higher than Negroes and people living in the northern United States score higher than people living in the South. The groups with lower average intelligence appear to have lower incomes, less adequate living conditions and limited opportunity for interactions with persons outside their own groups. Their schools tend to be characterized by fewer and less well trained teachers, poorer physical plants and facilities, fewer and older books and crowded classrooms.

Although the feebleminded tend to inherit their intellectual capacities, it must also be remembered that children grow up in environments created by their parents: the parents determine social status, opportunity for education, intellectual stimulation and goals, as well as genes. Low socioeconomic class membership does not cause mental subnormality but it provides the environment for the perpetuation of subnormality. Selective mating operates so that people tend to marry spouses highly similar to themselves and to produce children like themselves. Genetic factors are important in the initial determination of intelligence, but the persistence of inherited potential and the extent to which a person is able to utilize and develop this potential may be dependent upon sociocultural and psychological forces. Reed and Reed (1965) have summarized the interaction of forces as follows: "the result of each gene and each environmental factor is as-

TABLE 18–7. Rejection Rates per Thousand Registrants, by Region and Race (United States Armed Services, World War II)

Region	Total	White	Negro
Total U.S.	40	25	152
New England	17	16	65
Middle Atlantic	15	11	67
Southeast	97	52	202
Southwest	60	54	107
Central	14	12	61
Northwest	14	13	40
Far West	10	9	50

Adapted from Ginzberg, E., and Bray, D. W. 1953. The Uneducated. New York, Columbia University Press.

sumed to be so small that individual identification is impossible. The picture is the same as that for the polygenic traits of height or size in men and the laboratory animals." An individual with the potential to function at the lower end of the range of average intelligence may actually function in a mildly subnormal manner or lower because of chronic anxiety or a poverty of stimulation and experience.

For many years it was recognized that mental subnormality constituted a major social problem in the United States, but the astonishing proportions of the problem did not become apparent until World War II. Man-power was desperately needed for the armed services, yet hundreds of thousands of men were found to be unqualified because of mental deficiency. Ginzberg and Bray (1953) analyzed the records of the men rejected because of mental deficiency and those of the illiterate or semi-illiterate men who were inducted. According to statistical estimates (based on the normal probability curve), the expectations are that about 2 per cent of the population will fail to meet a minimum performance standard because of mental subnormality. From the beginning of selective service until World War II ended, however, more than 700,000 men, or about 4 per cent of the total number examined, were rejected for mental deficiency. The average was not stable for the entire country; in some states nearly 14 per cent were rejected as opposed to only 0.5 per cent in others. Table 18–7 lists the rates of rejections per thousand registrants by region and race. The rejection rates varied according to region and race depending upon the concentration of minority groups (Negroes in the Southeast and Southwest and Indians and Mexicans in the Southwest) and the availability of educational and cultural facilities. The rejection rates for Negroes in the Northwest and Far West, for example, were considerably below the rates for Negroes in the rest of the country and for whites in the Southeast and Southwest. (Included with whites in the Southwest were Indians and Mexicans.) The rejection rates for whites in the Southeast and Southwest were more than twice the national average.

The majority of men rejected for mental deficiency appear to have come from specific regions in which segments of the population live in economically marginal circumstances and where educational facilities are minimal and school attendance is not rigorously enforced. It is quite likely that a sizable number of individuals in the United States do not belong in the category of mental deficiency, in terms of inherited intellectual capacity, but are so classified because they have never learned to function efficiently. If so many persons with lower class membership function so poorly in the United States, millions of persons in the poverty-stricken areas of the rest of the world must also be functioning at mentally subnormal levels, a vast reservoir of wasted human resources.

The influence of environment on intellectual development is also mirrored in the relatively isolated group. Gordon (1923) investigated the intelligence test performance and educational achievement of a group of English canal-boat children who spent most of their lives on boats with their parents (many of whom were illiterate) and siblings. Special schools had been set up for the children, which they could attend while the boats were tied up for loading or discharging, but it was estimated that they attended only for about 5 per cent of the regular school year. The mean Stanford-Binet I.Q. for the 76 canal-boat children studied was 69.6, at the upper end of the mental subnormality range. Analysis of the data, however, revealed that the I.Q. in the group declined sharply with age: the four- to six-year-olds obtained an average I.Q. of 90 while the oldest group, composed of 12- to 22-year-olds, obtained an average of 60. Even in children within the same family, the drop in I.Q. was consistent.

The same trends were observed in gypsy children living in England (Gordon, 1923). Their average I.Q. was somewhat higher (74.5) and did not drop so markedly, perhaps because they attended school more frequently (34.9 per cent of the year) than the canal-boat children, and generally had more interaction with the outside groups.

Studies of isolated groups living in mountain areas in the southeastern sections of the United States have tended to corroborate these findings (Asher, 1935; Edwards and Jones, 1938; Wheeler, 1932 and 1942; Chapanis and Williams, 1945). Mean I.Q.'s were markedly below average and scores tended to decline with age. Age decrements have also been reported for other underprivileged, isolated groups, such as children admitted to an orphanage after varying periods in their own underprivileged homes (Skeels and Fillmore, 1937) and children in a high delinquency area in a large city (Lichtenstein and Brown, 1938).

There is reason to believe that the I.Q.'s of children in a particular community can improve noticeably when conspicuous improvements are made in environmental conditions, educational facilities and community opportunities. Wheeler (1942) administered group intelligence tests in 1940 to more than 3000 children in 40 rural schools of the East Tennessee mountains. Children from the same areas and largely the same families had been previously tested in 1930. The results of the two programs were compared and it was found that the median I.Q. score had risen from 82 in 1930 to 93 in 1940. Over the decade the social, economic and educational conditions of the communities had been greatly improved.

The weight of sociocultural factors is also substantiated in studies of monozygotic twins reared apart. The data of Newman, Freeman and Holzinger (1937) (see Chapter 6) and similar studies were analyzed by Woodworth (1941), who directed his attention to the differences in the environments of the twins reared apart. In a number of cases the I.Q. differences in a pair of twins were much greater than the average differences between all pairs. To determine whether the environmental differences were greater for twins with more disparate I.Q.'s than for those with less, five judges were asked to rate the social and educational qualities of the environment for each person, and to estimate on a 10-point scale the amount of difference for each pair. According to the results, educational differences were directly related to differences in I.Q.'s: the I.Q. score of the better educated twin was six points higher on the average than his co-twin (a statistically significant difference). In six pairs of twins with a difference in school of four years or more, the average I.Q. difference was thirteen points in favor of the better educated twin. The largest difference was 24 I.Q. points between a twin raised in a backwoods area who had only two years of regular schooling and his co-twin reared in a good farming community who went to college. This study proved that educational factors can produce I.Q. differences in persons with the same heredity. It indicated further that the large rather than the small environmental differences are important. In addition, Tyler (1956) noted that the 24-point disparity in I.Q. found in the one case was still much smaller than the disparity encountered between groups with different socioeconomic and educational backgrounds in the population as a whole.

A number of studies of foster children (Freeman, Holzinger and Mitchell, 1928; Burks, 1928; Leahy, 1935) agree that the I.Q.'s of adopted children are somewhat higher than those of children brought up in homes at the educational level of the adopted children's origins. Again, marked educational differences were associated with moderate I.Q. differences.

It is apparent that when children are relatively isolated in their own low socioeconomic class groups and receive little stimulation, whether in interactions with other individuals of different classes or in educational opportunities, their I.Q.'s, on the average, decline with age to such an extent that many of them are classified as mentally subnormal adults. When the sociocultural climate of such a group improves, however, the average I.Q. increases.

TREATMENT

A few syndromes of severe mental subnormality respond to specific treatment if the symptoms are recognized early enough. Patients so treated may be enabled to function intellectually at levels above the range of severe subnormality and, in some cases, within the range of normality.

If phenylketonuria (PKU) is diagnosed within the first month of an infant's life, the treatment, a diet relatively free of phenylalanine (found in most protein foods), will usually prevent the child's becoming mentally subnormal. The initial diagnosis is very simple and has become routine in many hospitals. Phenylpyruvic acid is detected in an infant's urine if his diaper turns a characteristic green when a diluted solution of ferric chloride is added.

Prompt penicillin therapy prevents many of the unpleasant effects of congenital syphilis. As a result of the routine blood testing and treatment of pregnant women found to have syphilis, mental subnormality and other manifestations in their children have become less frequent during the past generation.

Cretinism, if recognized at birth or in its early manifestations, can be ameliorated by the institution of thyroid therapy. The dosage prescribed is usually as high as the patient can tolerate, that is, until mild toxic symptoms appear (rapid pulse, diarrhea, loss of weight and irritability). If the treatment is begun early, severe subnormality can be prevented. The effect of the medication on physical growth is quite marked; in some severe cases, structural anomalies often disappear completely. The patient's intelligence also improves, although it seldom rises to the level of normality.

The administration of anti-convulsant medication may minimize intellectual deterioration in patients subject to epileptic seizures. If, however, the seizures are present at a very early age, the patient may be severely subnormal as a result of brain injury incurred before or during birth.

A number of surgical procedures have been devised in attempts to arrest the development of various forms of hydrocephaly. They are directed to the reduction of the normal production of cerebrospinal fluid or to the channeling of the fluid past the obstructions that have resulted from congenital malformations or postnatal infections. The early techniques of surgical intervention carried a very high mortality rate, but subsequent refinements reduced it to about 15 per cent. Recently, the initial success of various operative procedures has been in the neighborhood of 60 to 65 per cent, but the frequency of severe complications—particularly those caused by obstructions or infections in artificial drainage tubes and valves—following the postoperative period is quite high. Surgical intervention, however, may successfully reduce the mortality rate from hydrocephaly and prevent the development of severe mental subnormality.

When mental subnormalities are associated with disturbed behavior, the administration of tranquilizing drugs, especially the phenothiazines, may result in considerable benefits to the patient. The abatement of the behavior disturbances may permit the patient to function at a higher intellectual and social level.

Many investigators have experimented with nonspecific forms of medical treatment—for example, vitamins, hormones and brain stimulants—but the attempts have been unsuccessful. There is no known treatment to raise the level of intellectual functioning for the majority of mentally subnormal individuals. For them, and for some of those who are on remedial medical regimes but are still intellectually handicapped, decisions must often be made regarding their education, care and management.

In both the severely and moderately subnormal groups, impairment is so extreme that the necessity for care and supervision is obvious. While the child is still very young the family usually decides whether to care for him at home or place him in an institution. Intelligence tests are administered to determine the baseline of his intellectual functioning and to evaluate the efficacy of treatment (such as thyroid therapy). At the level of mild mental subnormality the intelligence test is also used as part of the basis for recommending appropriate training and education. Most urban schools have adequate psychological testing services so that children with learning disabilities are evaluated routinely. If limited intelligence appears to be the source of a child's problem, recommendations are made for special classes, a special educational program, or, in some instances, institutionalization. Social criteria as well as the level of intellectual functioning determine whether the child should be institutionalized or kept at home and educated in special classes. Rural schools are less likely to have appropriate diagnostic services or special classes for children with limited intelligence. In agricultural areas, however, mentally deficient individuals who are not too severely subnormal may find suitable employment and acceptance by the community so that, in a sense, they are better off than their urban counterparts.

In order to make decisions for the management of the retarded persons, trained workers usually interview members of the family and gather information on the subnormal child's psychological adjustment, his relationships with his parents, siblings and community, and his skills, abilities and aptitudes. In addition to such interviews and the usual intelligence tests, the Vineland Social Maturity Scale provides much useful information. It measures the individual's "social age" from 0 to 25 years and provides a method for evaluating his everyday behavior (dressing, feeding, playing, working and so forth) in terms of age norms. In addition, consideration must be given to the child's family and community environment. For example, if he is to remain at home it is important to determine the family's motivation for keeping him with them and their ability to provide necessary care and supervision. Community resources for education, recreation and supervision, and community attitudes toward retarded persons, must also be evaluated before reasonable decisions regarding placement or institutionalization can

be made. Mental subnormality should never be diagnosed by intelligence tests alone. Physical and neurologic examinations, personality and social adjustment evaluations, interviews with members of the family, observation of the person in his environment, and assessment of family and community resources and attitudes, are all essential in the diagnostic process. Although these procedures are important at all levels of mental subnormality, they are crucial for persons at the upper end of the subnormality range. At this level some mildly retarded persons can remain in the community because of adequate adjustments, their ability to work steadily at a job and the willingness of the family and community to provide some support and guidance. Institutionalization may be necessary for other subnormal children with similar intellectual resources if they have personality problems, poor emotional control, unsympathetic families and community environments or are unable to support themselves economically.

Only a relatively small percentage of the mildly subnormal are institutionalized; most remain in the community. A number of follow-up studies reveal that most mildly subnormal persons who receive training in special classes in the public school system remain in the community and make reasonably adequate adjustments. Baller (1936) was able to locate 95 per cent of a group of children with I.Q.'s under 70 who had been in special public-school training classes in Nebraska. They were over 21 years of age when he studied them in comparison with a "high-normal" group who had I.Q.'s ranging from 100 to 120. (This and the following study were quoted earlier.) They were studied again by Charles (1953) when their average age was 42 (he located 73 per cent of the original group). Both studies revealed that 7 per cent or less of the subjects had been institutionalized and that 83 per cent of them were at least partially self-supporting; as the economic situation had improved, fewer of them remained on relief. Not all held jobs at the lower, unskilled levels; some worked at jobs that covered quite a range of skills and salaries. During the later study, 80 per cent of the subjects were married with an average of two children (both statistics are below the national average). The children, for the most part, were doing successful work in school. It is interesting to note that the death rate for this group was high; at the time of the second study 25 of the 151 who had been located were dead, many by accident or violence. Highly similar results were reported by

Muench (1944), Kennedy (1948) and McIntosh (1949). O'Connor (1953) found a similar pattern in England.

Perhaps, in part, as a result of the successes revealed in studies such as the preceding ones and, in part, a growing realization by educators that more than 50 per cent of the jobs in our society do not require schooling beyond the elementary level, there is today an increased emphasis on integrating retardates into the community. Accordingly, DiMichael (1956) formulated a comprehensive program to facilitate the integration. He urged that each community institute a program of (1) diagnostic-treatment clinics with professional counseling for the family; (2) home-visiting counselors to help parents in training the retarded infant or child; (3) nursery classes; (4) special education, with improved vocational training and (5) improved social training for the "trainable retarded"; (6) training centers and sheltered workshops; (7) community centers to fill in gaps left by other services; (8) integration of the retarded in society, including selective placement in regular employment; (9) residence centers within communities for the retarded; and (10) an adequate program of research and training. There is reason to believe that considerable progress is being made in a number of these proposed programs.

During the past two decades the possibility of doing psychotherapy with the mentally subnormal has been gaining many enthusiastic supporters. Cowen (1955) reviewed reports of successful outcomes claimed by therapists who represented a variety of theoretical approaches and worked in many different kinds of settings. However, there are many problems in evaluating these results. Test data are absent, objective descriptive accounts of patients before and after therapy are not given, and control groups are rarely used.

Healy's and Bronner's (1926) finding that psychotherapy failed in 66 per cent of children with I.Q.;s between 70 to 79, but in only 10 per cent of children with I.Q.'s above 110, has been dismissed by Gunzberg (1958) and others as indicating only that the "usual" type of psychotherapy is unsuitable for mental defectives, not that mental defectives are unsuitable for psychotherapy. In general, therapists have moved away from nondirective and uncovering types of therapy because it is difficult for retarded individuals with limited verbal facility to describe fantasies, feelings and reactions. (Sarason, 1953, however, believes that too little attention has been paid to using a psycho-analytic, uncovering approach, and that it is premature to say it is unsuccessful as a method of treatment for the mentally subnormal.) Current emphasis is on directive counseling, providing meaningful rewards for behavior changes, and environmental manipulation. Gunzberg (1958) feels that although individual and group therapy can initiate and lay the foundations for readjustment, environmental therapy in the institution or the community is necessary to complete the adjustment.

PREVENTION

It is often argued that our knowledge of the causation of the various forms of abnormal behavior is too incomplete to justify preventive action; nevertheless such action has been proposed and even initiated by many men. Among the more controversial of the measures so initiated have been control of hereditary factors and removal of the individual from society.

Neel and Schull (1954) pointed out that for the majority of man's time on earth he must have been engaged in a constant struggle with his environment (including other men) and that he survived by a process of natural selection. Rigorous natural selection, however, has been offset by dysgenic (opposite of eugenic) influences, such as warfare between armies that exclude the physically and intellectually handicapped; preservation of the handicapped by humanitarian attitudes and medical advances; differential fertility, which has become relatively higher among those of low intelligence and socioeconomic status; and increased mutation, which may result from any increase in ionizing radiation.

The main dysgenic influences known to have operated during the past century may simply be summarized as differential mortality and differential fertility—in both instances favoring certain physically handicapped, intellectually subnormal, emotionally inadequate or socially incompetent groups of individuals. In recent years, the majority of persons who are interested in this problem have predicted a decline in the physical vigor and intelligence of the population, although the prediction has not been substantiated by studies hitherto undertaken. Higgins et al. (1962) reported on the first large sample, 1016 families (of which at least one member was hospitalized for mental retardation between 1912 and 1915), in which I.Q. data were known for parents, their offspring and unmarried or nonreproducing siblings, and stated:

The inclusion of these siblings allowed us to resolve the old paradox presented by the failure of the general intelligence level to decline in accord with the large negative correlation (−.30) between intelligence and the number of children in the family.

The explanation of the paradox is that when the single or non-reproductive siblings of the parents are included the negative correlation disappears. The higher reproductive rate of those in the lower I.Q. groups who are parents is offset by the larger proportion of their siblings who never marry or who fail to reproduce when married. Thus, the I.Q. level of the whole population should remain relatively static from one generation to the next, or at least not drop rapidly.

In addition, natural selection appears to operate in favor of persons with relatively high intelligence and socioeconomic status in that mortality rates, particularly marked during infancy, are higher for persons with lower intelligence and socioeconomic status.

Competent geneticists have tended to emphasize our ignorance of the precise significance of heredity, and the theoretical consequences of negative selection (the breeding to eliminate a trait), in mental subnormality and common psychiatric disorders. They have concluded that sterilization of the mentally defective is difficult to justify on genetic grounds. Yet it is on these grounds that a number of states and countries have based their adoption of laws that permit sterilization or abortion. Kemp (1957) reported that in Denmark in recent years just over two-thirds of the individuals submitting to sterilization on a voluntary basis were mental defectives, of whom about two thirds were female.

It cannot be overlooked that some parents are unable to provide normal, wholesome environments for their children, aside from a healthy inheritance. A number of scientists have concluded that the environmental argument in favor of various forms of family planning is stronger than the genetic. Regardless of which is the more important, the empirical fact remains that in certain families and social groups parents have a higher proportion of children with mental subnormality or other forms of psychiatric disorder.

Part of the legal justification for compulsory sterilization of subnormal individuals is contained in the following excerpt from a Supreme Court decision by Justice Oliver Wendell Holmes (1927):

We have seen more than once that the public welfare may call upon its best citizens for their lives. It would be strange if it could not call upon those who already sap the strength of the State for those lesser sacrifices, often not felt to be such by those concerned, in order to prevent our being swamped with incompetence. It is better for all the world, if instead of waiting to execute degenerate offspring for crime or to let them starve for their imbecility, society can prevent those who are manifestly unfit from continuing their kind. The principle that sustains compulsory vaccination is broad enough to cover cutting the fallopian tubes.

Kanner (1957), on the other hand, has made the following case for voluntary family limitation rather than compulsory sterilization:

More harm comes to children from parental instability than from low I.Q.'s of their parents. Sterilization laws, desirable though they are, can—and should—reach only a small group of people who combine feeblemindedness with the inability to rear children properly. This inability is not restricted to those of lower intelligence. It is found among highly educated, sophisticated people as well; among them are persons who have sense enough to know their emotional shortcomings and their lack of readiness for parenthood.

Up to this point we have been concerned with the problems of preventing the transmission of the hereditary determinants of mental subnormality. However, mental subnormality can also be prevented in some cases by using our knowledge of its environmental determinants. Among the most important are the provision of an adequate diet for all women of child-bearing age; the control of infectious diseases by isolation, antibiotic treatment and immunization programs; the prevention of exposure to poisonous chemicals; and the provision of a high quality of obstetric and pediatric care for the pregnant woman and newborn child. Such care can prevent premature and postmature births, excessive use of anesthetics, mechanical trauma and anoxia during birth.

Rubella may be reduced in frequency among pregnant women by guarding them from exposure or, if they have been exposed, by the administration of gamma globulin for temporary passive immunity. No woman of child-bearing age should receive large doses of abdominal x-rays unless it has been established that she is not pregnant, or unless her condition is so serious as to override this consideration.

The many infections and intoxications that may occur during infancy and cause mental subnormality are best prevented by a suitable program of immunizations for the child and a high quality of pediatric care which includes both expert diagnosis and appropriate treatment. Pediatricians and other persons who work with children are more sensitive to the possible effects of emotional deprivation on intellectual, psychological and social development, particularly among institutionalized children. This growing awareness has resulted in early and permanent adoptive placement, programs of "mothering" for institutionalized children, and a growing use of foster homes for children of inadequate parents.

Pasamanick and Knobloch (1961) reviewed an extensive series of epidemiologic studies on the complications of pregnancy and the birth process. They concluded that the evidence was sufficient to indicate the existence of a continuum of reproductive insult that is, at least, partly socioeconomically determined and that results in a continuum of reproductive casualties ranging from death through varying degrees of neuropsychiatric disability. This evidence is strong enough, apparently, to warrant the institution of preventive measures during the prenatal period and even, preferably, before conception. The authors stated:

These programs should be geared to the elimination and modification of such results of poverty and deprivation as malnutrition, infection and other forms of stress, prenatally in the mother and postnatally in the child. In addition, it seems apparent to us that psychosocial deprivation and faulty stimulation in childhood require fully as much attention, if not more, in preventive programs.

Freedman (1962) reported on the results of a long-range anterospective study of 445 premature infants and 50 full-term infants in Brooklyn, New York. Earlier studies of prematurity had concentrated on social factors in the children's environment because the high rate of premature births in the low socioeconomic classes, and the poor development of the infants, had sometimes been attributed to their environments. Freedman, however, found that the most significant difference between the mothers of full-term infants and the mothers of prematures, living in the same underprivileged area and subjected to similar stresses and deprivations, was the amount of prenatal care the mother received; this finding, he concluded, called for an energetic and well-directed program to provide adequate medical supervision during pregnancy for all women.

When prenatal care is available without cost through a community welfare program, it is interesting to speculate on the psychological and intellectual characteristics that separate the women who participate in the program from those who do not. It is possible that the women who participate are brighter, better adjusted, and concerned with their own health and the health of their offspring. Those who do not participate may be intellectually subnormal, discouraged, disorganized, and consciously or unconsciously rejecting motherhood. These factors may also be associated with the maternal anxiety level before and during birth and to the health and subsequent well-being of the offspring.

Unfortunately, the largest group of mildly subnormal children tend to live with parents who are unable to provide either the highest quality of prenatal and postnatal care, or favorable emotional relationships and examples, or stimulating educational opportunities. The combination of these factors makes the prevention of mild degrees of subnormality more difficult than the prevention of severe forms.

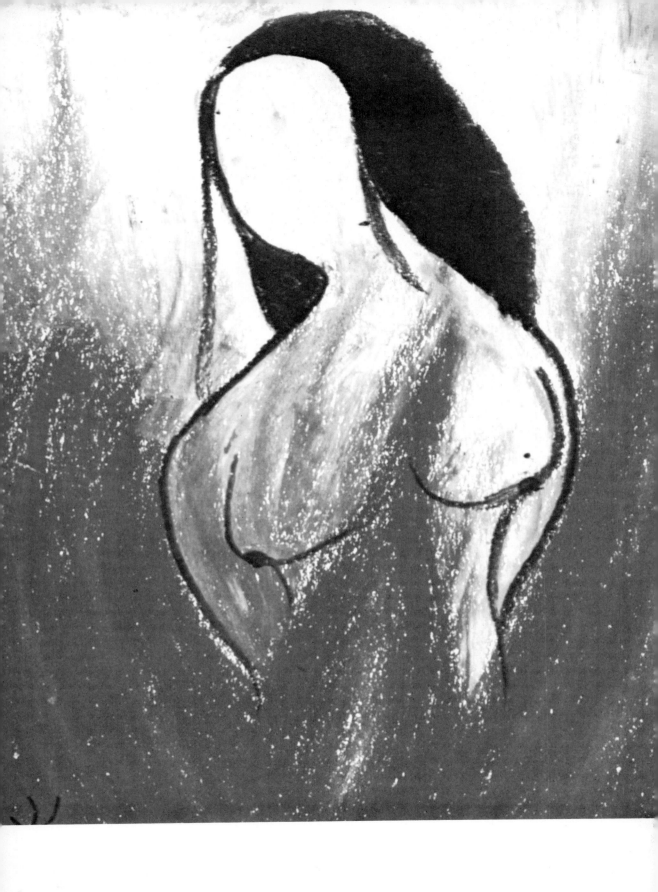

A little sorrowful deserted thing,
Begot of love, and yet no love begetting.

Thomas Hood, *Midsummer Fairies*

DISORDERS OF CHILDHOOD

Although mental subnormality in children was recognized as a problem some 200 years ago, other disorders of childhood were ignored until the beginning of the twentieth century. Psychiatric descriptions and classifications of mental illness, first compiled in the nineteenth century, noted the behavior problems of children, if at all, only as they could be fitted into the diagnoses devised for adults. Neither Kraepelin nor Bleuler even mentioned children's disorders. A few texts were published on the psychological disturbances of children, but, for the most part, were limited to superimposing adult categories upon the disorders of children. Kanner (1959) pointed out that the nosological preoccupation of the times was associated with a nihilistic attitude toward treatment and a widespread belief in the universality of biological causation. The disorders of childhood tended to be regarded fatalistically as the irreversible results of heredity, degeneracy, excessive masturbation, overwork, or religious preoccupation.

In the beginning of this century, developments in a number of different areas led to the delineation and establishment of child psychiatry and child psychology as fields in their own right. Freud and his associates, in Europe, began to emphasize the influences of early life experiences on later maladjustment. Adolph Meyer, in the United States, also noted the importance of the past in the problems of his adult patients. There was growing recognition that mental illness was the end product of a developmental history in which one could trace the pattern of an individual's reaction to his particular life situation. The biographical history became an important part of every psychiatric examination.

As a result of the resurgence of interest in the original theories of two early educators, Johann Heinrich Pestalozzi (1746–1827) and Philipp Emanuel von Fellenberg (1771–1884) — who had emphasized the individual needs of school children, particularly those with physical, intellectual or psychological handicaps — a group of educators in Germany, Austria and Switzerland founded a remedial education program to study and treat the learning and behavior problems of children. At the same time, in France, Alfred Binet (1857–1911) pioneered the development of psychological measurement — psychometry — which led to the scientific study of individual differences.

Children began to receive legal recognition. Prior to the 1890's a child who broke the law was treated like an adult offender. At the turn of the century, however, the clamor of aroused humanitarians in Australia and the United States resulted in the establishment of a number of juvenile courts. Presiding judges became interested in the motivations of the children brought before them, especially since a large proportion came from homes in which conflict, rejection, severe punishment and deprivation appeared to be prevalent. Psychologists and psychiatrists were called upon to make special studies of these children. Because of these requests, they were stimulated to develop the professional exploration and evaluation of children with psychological disturbances.

With the growing recognition that mental illness was a social problem, the mental hygiene movement began to emphasize the prevention of mental illness, and, consequently, fostered an interest in the childhood origins of adult disorders. In 1921, the Boston Habit Clinic was founded, and over the next few years was followed by the establishment of a number of "demonstration child guidance clinics" in other cities across the country. These clinics were originally financed by the Commonwealth Fund (a private foundation organized in 1918 to promote health and encourage better and more comprehensive health care), and were intended to "demonstrate" their usefulness to the community so that eventually they would be supported by local funds. Each clinic was staffed with a "team" consisting of a psychiatrist, psychologist and social worker. The psychiatrist usually functioned as the administrative head and medical director of the clinic and was in charge of much of the psychotherapeutic work with children; the psychologist was in charge of diagnostic services and research; and the social worker dealt most directly with parents and the community. (The idea of the professional team still exists although there is increasingly greater overlap in the roles and functions assumed by each team member.) Interactions between parents, between parents and child, and between school and community and child, were found to have material implications for the diagnosis and treatment of the young patients and, consequently, became important areas for study and research.

The first publications by Gesell (1925) marked the beginning of his monumental work on the psychological and physical development of children. A decade later, the first modern book on child psychiatry was published by Kanner. Thus, child psychology and child psychiatry were established as special fields, a culmination of all the early influences that ranged from psychoanalysis to education to psychometry to law to the mental hygiene movement and the establishment of special clinics.

Initially, childhood had been viewed solely as part of an adult's past, that is, as the precursor of adult maladjustment. (Freud formulated all his theory of infantile sexuality without ever having seen a child as a patient.) As a result, the mental hygiene movement set its goal of prevention by directing its attention to the future, that is, to altering or eliminating the beginnings of maladjustment in children in order to prevent future disorders in them as adults. But beginning in the 1930's, emphasis was placed on the present: children as children became the objects of research, diagnosis and treatment in both child psychiatry and child psychology.

CLASSIFICATION AND INCIDENCE

It is possible to recognize in children manifestations of the various syndromes that are found in adults (one of the reasons why children's disorders were not separated from adults' in the beginning). Children may show typical symptoms of neurosis, psychophysiologic disorders, depression, schizophrenia, delinquency, addiction, acute or chronic brain syndrome or various forms of mental subnormality. In the young child, however, symptoms are difficult to evaluate. The younger he is, the less likely are his symptoms to be persistently characteristic of one specific syndrome. Moreover, he frequently manifests abnormal behavior that is not characteristic of any syndrome but may lead to the development of any of a number of syndromes. Thus, for instance, enuresis (involuntary urination after the age of three) may be either a relatively isolated symptom or a manifestation of disturbance preceding the development of symptoms of neurosis, psychosis or delinquency.

As a result, the disorders of childhood have not been uniformly classified. Some psychiatrists and psychologists adhere to the adult classification system, with some alterations, and make diagnoses of depression, various neurotic reactions, schizophrenic reactions and so forth. Additional categories, such as "school phobia" and "reading problems," are often listed separately because of the frequency with which they appear and because they do not clearly fit into the other diagnostic categories. Other psychiatrists and psychologists consider that the adult categories overgeneralize and do not properly describe the problems of children. As a result, they have abandoned all formal diagnoses and, instead, describe in a brief paragraph the child's symptoms, the characteristics of his adjustment and his interactions with members of his family, school and community. Still others use summary sentences, such as, "Rebellious, antisocial behavior in a pre-adolescent boy in reaction to a hostile alcoholic father," or "Extreme withdrawal in a preschool child developed in a setting of parental rejection."

Some clinics and hospitals have developed a list of common symptoms that are seen in the children who are referred to them, and these symptoms are used as classifications. Thus, if a child is brought in with a presenting complaint of psychosomatic symptoms, sleep disturbance, eating difficulties, or school failure, he is classified according to his most disturbing symptom rather than by a syndrome. In one clinic, the five most frequent complaints were inability to achieve in school, poor peer relationships, nervousness, sleep disturbances and fearfulness (Marks, 1961).

The diagnostic manual of the American Psychiatric Association has a somewhat traditional approach to the diagnosis of the disorders of childhood, but places a great emphasis on the transient nature of many of the symptoms. A distinction is drawn between acute, transient reactions to an overwhelming environmental stress and behavior disorders. The term behavior disorders in this context is reserved for those childhood or adolescent disorders which are more stable and enduring than the transient, situational reactions but less fixed than the symptoms found in the neuroses and psychoses. This intermediate level of stability in the diagnostic schema for children calls attention to the fact that there is a greater fluidity of behavior in young people. Typical behaviors which are placed in the behavior disorder category are hyperactivity, withdrawal and chronic over-anxiousness.

Because of lack of uniformity in classifying children's disorders and dissatisfaction with current procedures, a total revision may be achieved in the future. Kanner (1957) believes that children's disorders may be classified on the basis of parental attitudes and their effects on the children. It is well known, for example, that children who experience parental rejection, expressed in overt hostility and neglect, often show not only physical disorders (malnutrition, broken bones, scars and so forth) but severe psychological disturbance as well. They are frequently withdrawn, show shallow affect and often are considered to be psychotic. Parental

overprotection is frequently associated with overdependence and immaturity in the child.

One possible schema is a coordination of developmental theory and diagnosis. According to a number of theories, particular conflicts occur at certain phases of development. In Freudian theory, for instance, the child experiences conflict between conformity and nonconformity at the anal stage which may be a determinant in the formation and development of his personality. For the schema, a means would have to be devised of identifying, recording and perhaps even "measuring" such conflicts in the child as well as his reactions to them, and then, if the occasion arises, diagnosing his disturbance in terms of his early developmental conflicts.

The incidence of behavior disturbances among children is almost impossible to assess. Difficulties in identifying cases, differences in diagnoses and differences in diagnostic criteria combine to obscure the numbers of disturbed children in the population. In addition, a cultural relativity confuses the issue. What is considered insignificant in one culture is regarded with alarm in another. In our society, the recognition of abnormalities and the decision to seek psychiatric or psychological evaluation are related to the socioeconomic status, sex and age of the child. Most psychiatric clinics for children see two or three times as many boys as girls, perhaps because more boys than girls display aggressive or delinquent behavior. (Interestingly enough, more women than men seek psychiatric help.) Similarly, the age of the child determines to a great extent the kinds of behavior problems with which parents will be concerned. Resentment and frustration may lead to breath-holding spells in infancy, for instance, but between the ages of three and 10 they lead to temper tantrums, and to sullenness and arguments during adolescence. Most parents regard as a problem only those behaviors that pose threats to them, and, as a result, the quietly disturbed tend to be ignored or tacitly encouraged.

O'Connor and Franks (1960) have estimated that approximately one in three English children needs attention or care. This estimate is based on the probability that 10 per cent of all children display some educational subnormality, 1 to 2 per cent are delinquents, 1 per cent suffer some severe maladjustments and 5 to 20 per cent manifest milder disturbances. The authors are quick to admit that the difficulties inherent in the problems of identifying disturbed children, defining disturbances, and diagnosing them, make their own figures far from certain.

Accurate incidence figures are not available for the United States either. A number of surveys of child guidance clinic populations indicate that in many communities the clients come more from the middle and upper socio-economic classes; low-cost clinics designed to serve the general public do not draw equal proportions from the lower classes (Maas et al., 1955; Roach et al., 1958; Marks, 1961). In communities where this imbalance exists, clinic statistics, of course, cannot provide much information on the incidence or nature of childhood disorders in the groups not proportionately represented. As a result, our knowledge of the problems of lower class children is severely limited.

There is no "typical" disturbed child. Because of the wide variety of symptoms manifested, a typical, or composite, picture of such children cannot be drawn. But since certain kinds of symptoms are more frequent and certain socioeconomic groups are more heavily represented, a description of a usual or "average" child who is most often referred to a child guidance clinic can be hypothesized. Marks (1961) constructed such a description in his study of 42 cases that represented 90 per cent of consecutive referrals accepted for treatment (excluding cases of mental deficiency and cerebral impairment) in a child guidance clinic in Minnesota over a period of above five months. He described the "average" child patient as:

. . . a Caucasian, 10-year-old boy in the fourth grade. His intelligence was average but he was referred to the clinic by the school because of academic deficiency. He was described by his parents as nervous and fearful, and was reported to have sleep disturbances and poor peer relationships. The average child was a Protestant and came from a home that had not been disrupted by death, separation, or divorce. His mother and father were 37 and 41 years of age, respectively. Both parents had received a tenth grade education. The child's father was employed in a skilled clerical or business (Class III) occupation.

DESCRIPTION

Some of the habit and behavior problems in children that arouse concern in the adults responsible for their care are enuresis, encopresis (involuntary defecation that is not attributable to physical illness), constipation, psychogenic vomiting, eating problems, breath-holding, head rolling, head banging, nose picking, ear pulling, thumb sucking, temper tantrums, irritability, involuntary spasmodic movements or tics, speech and language difficulties, overactivity, destructiveness, demanding of attention, overdependence, physical timidity, moodiness, specific fears, restless sleep and disturbing dreams. These symptoms are sometimes within the normal range of problems displayed at various stages of development, but with the addition of stress may become extreme and more persistent. The sources of the stress vary, of course, but characteristically are caused by difficulties in familial relationships.

Macfarlane et al. (1954) summarized the incidence of problems of over 100 normal children as reported by mothers in a 35-item open-question interview. Some of the problems were reported so frequently at certain ages that they appeared to be normal to the development of children in our culture. The incidence of some problems increased with age, others decreased, while others occurred with high frequency at more than one age. Nail biting increased with age; in girls, the peak, 40 per cent, was reached at age 11 and then the incidence decreased and leveled off; in boys, at the time of the last interview at age 14, 33 per cent were still nail biters. The problem of controlling elimination decreased with age. At 21 months bed-wetting was reported by three-fourths the mothers, daytime wetting by about one-half and soiling by one-fourth. The percentages decreased markedly with age. At about three to three and one-half, speech difficulties, temper outbursts and specific fears were most commonly reported. At about the age of five, overactivity and destructiveness (observed in far more boys than girls) reached their peaks and then declined. Some problems had two periods of high frequency: during the preschool age and in late pubescence. Examples were restless sleep and disturbing dreams, physical timidity, irritability and the demanding of attention.

For most children, the problems appeared at certain periods and then disappeared or became minimal. The greatest persistence was found in characteristics such as moodiness, somberness, overdependence and irritability. When oversensitivity was reported at about the age of five, the problem persisted as a characteristic of the child in about one-half the cases.

Parents react differently to the occurrence of these problems. Some respond casually, apparently assuming that they are part of the child's normal development and will be resolved and disappear naturally; others may also regard the problems as usual but make an active effort to help the child cope with the specific problem. For example, they reassure the child about his fears, minimize his frustration during the periods in which he is controlling anger with difficulty, and reward him for whatever progress he does make. Others become alarmed at the manifestation of problems because they consider them unusual and the child abnormal. Such parents may, for example, be overanxious about completing toilet training, or upset over any show of hostility, or unduly worried when the child eats very little. Many cases come to the attention of the pediatrician, child psychiatrist or child guidance clinic from this last group. Frequently the parents' complaints reveal a great deal about their attitudes toward the child and their own levels of anxiety or tolerance of inconvenience and frustration. Kanner (1957) remarked that:

The high annoyance threshold of many fond and fondly resourceful parents keep away from clinics and out of reach of statistics a multitude of early breath-holders, nail biters, nose pickers, and casual masturbators, who, largely because of this kind of parental attitude, develop into reasonably happy and well-adjusted adults. But, in clinic statistics, these same symptoms, figuring among "the traits" found in the histories of "problem children," are apt to be given too prominent a place, far out of proportion of their role as everyday problems or near-problems of the everyday child.

Still other parents either do not notice or are indifferent to the problems of their children. They seek psychiatric evaluation only at the instigation of teachers, physicians, law enforcement officers or other authoritative figures.

Adjustment Reactions

When the child is brought to a psychiatrist, psychologist or clinic for evaluation and treatment, the overt symptoms instigating the visit are never regarded as the entire problem or focus of disturbance. The presenting symptom, Kanner (1957) pointed out, fulfills several interdependent functions: it is an admission ticket to the physician's curiosity, a signal that something is wrong within the child, a safety valve to keep the child's inner resources intact, a partially effective means of solving his inner problems and a nuisance to the adults in his environment. The complaint, of course, often reflects the problems of the complaining adults. School teachers, for instance, have traditionally been more concerned about behavior that is noisy, disruptive and annoying, than the quiet

symptoms of severe emotional disturbances that do not upset classroom routine.

Some of the diagnostic categories for the disorders of children are given in the following sections and are illustrated with typical case histories.

Adjustment Reactions of Infancy. This classification includes transient reactions of a psychogenic origin in infants without organic disease. Such reactions are usually the outgrowth of the infant's reaction with significant persons in his environment, or a response to a lack of such persons. Undue apathy or excitability, and feeding and sleeping difficulties are common manifestations of such psychological disturbances in babies. In the middle and upper socioeconomic classes, most of these problems come to the attention of the family doctor or pediatrician rather than to the child psychiatrist or child psychologist. In lower socioeconomic groups, these problems are often untreated. The results of failure to deal with the adjustment reactions of infancy are not clearly known. Sometimes the problems decrease as maturation proceeds, but in many other cases the problems increase.

Adjustment Reactions of Childhood. This classification includes transient symptomatic reactions of children to some immediate situation or internal emotional conflict. The predominant symptoms may be repetitive activities, such as nail biting, thumb sucking, enuresis, masturbation or tantrums. Many "normal" children, of course, have these problems also, but in the child who requires professional help the problem is annoyingly persistent, becomes more severe, and frequently is associated with a high level of anxiety. In many cases, the symptom becomes a focal point of battle between the child and his parents. When parents fail in their efforts to deal with the problem, they may become irritated and hostile toward the child because of the persistence of the symptom.

The following case illustrates disturbances that largely disappeared as a result of a therapeutic regime and adoptive placement. It is an example of a transitory disturbance of children. It should be noted that many agencies would have placed this child in an adoptive home shortly after her birth despite the fact that no background information was available for her.

The six-year-old girl was referred to a residential child guidance clinic by the county welfare board primarily because enuresis, nail biting and a lisp made her a poor adoption possibility. She had been abandoned shortly after birth and nothing was known of her parents or her prenatal history. Immediate adoption had not been considered possible because of the unavailability of the information, and she had been placed in numerous foster homes until her admission to the clinic.

On examination, the girl was attractive but somewhat underweight, and scored an I.Q. of 114 on the Stanford-Binet, Form L. Initially, her nail biting was excessive. She seemed unaware that she was doing it until it was called to her attention and then she would burst into tears. Apparently an issue had been made of the habit by her different foster parents. She cried easily and frequently at the slightest reprimand, criticism or frustration, and was enuretic nearly every night.

She was enrolled in the first grade of the public school and was well liked by the other children but could become close to only one child at a time. Her school behavior and adjustment were considered satisfactory although she insisted that she did nothing well. She became extremely dependent upon and affectionate toward the teacher, demanding her help in putting on her coat and boots and going to the bathroom. She kissed the teacher hello and good-bye each day and frequently asked to sit on her lap. She looked for praise and reassurance in everything she did. Limits set by the teacher were interpreted as disapproval.

This same kind of dependency existed in her relationships with all adults who had any responsibility for her. The social worker from the county welfare board visited her monthly and the child anticipated each visit, and the possible treats or new clothes, for days in advance. Prior to each visit, she would tell children that she was going to leave the residence clinic and live with the social worker and her husband, and at the end of each visit would cry bitterly.

Her adjustment to the residence clinic was fairly satisfactory. She was much younger than the other girls in residence at the time and it was necessary for her to share a bedroom with a 12-year-old girl who manifested schizophrenic symptoms, and a 13-year-old who showed pre-delinquent behavior. Although, sometimes, she was the focus of her roommates' aggressions, they did not seem to resent sharing the room with her and were generally solicitous. Because she was the youngest, other children were quite accepting of any extra attentions she received from the staff.

The directors in residence placed few limits on her demands for attention and affection. She was an appealing child and most people responded favorably to her. Within a year she regarded the residence as her permanent home and said she planned to stay there forever. She chose one director as her mother and her psychiatrist as her father. During this period, it was noted, she became happier and more relaxed. She bit her nails only when she was overtired or upset. Her lisp disappeared after a course of speech therapy in school. In the interviews with the psychiatrist, she

talked more about friends and school activities and less about her desire for real parents. She became less demanding of physical closeness to him and showed interest in toys and play activities. The enuresis, however, decreased only slightly during this period.

When the child had been in residence for about 16 months, the county welfare board, which knew of the improvement of her habit disturbance and general adjustment, informed the clinic that they had prospective parents—a childless couple approaching middle age. During the next six weeks the couple made three visits to the clinic and took her out each time for part of the day. She was told of the possible adoption after the second visit and immediately all her former symptoms reappeared. She insisted that the couple did not want her and that if they did take her they would send her away shortly. At the same time, she seemed to want more than anything else for the adoption to take place, and began to refer to the couple as "Mommy" and "Daddy."

Because of the severe recurrence of nail biting, enuresis, and increased crying spells, there was a period in which it seemed that perhaps the adoptive placement should be delayed. Since the adoptive parents as well as the child were so eager, however, they were finally permitted to take her. At the time of the legal adoption, a year later, the parents and county welfare board reported that she was happy and no unusual problems had appeared. There was only occasional bed-wetting and a complete absence of other symptoms. School adjustment, both social and academic, was reported to be good. The girl continued to be dependent and affectionate in behavior; she liked to sit on her parents' laps and hold their hands, for instance, and seemed to want to spend little time away from them.

Unsocialized Aggressive Reaction. Some reactions are manifested by disturbances in the child's social conduct or behavior, such as truancy, stealing, destructiveness, cruelty, sexual offenses or the use of alcohol. The disturbed behavior may occur in the home, at school, in the community, or wherever the patient has a need to act out his problems. The following case illustrates a disturbance that disappeared during the patient's placement, for several years, in a residential treatment program. The boy undoubtedly had angry feelings and impulses toward his parents but was never able to vent these feelings toward them and apparently displaced his hostile impulses to children and adults who were emotionally unimportant to him. It is interesting that, although his antisocial behavior disappeared, he did not seem able to develop psychological closeness to other persons.

The patient, a 10-year-old boy, was referred to the residential child guidance clinic because of a severe behavior disorder. By the fourth grade he had attended three different public schools because teachers were unable to and refused to cope with his cruel behavior to other children and his destruction of school property.

He was an only child and had been born when his parents were in their early forties. The father was an executive in a national firm and traveled extensively. The mother, a very beautiful woman, had grown up on a large southern estate, primarily under the care of a governess, and had been a model before her marriage. Both parents were unusually conscious of social class: they were careful to mingle with and entertain the "right people," and were concerned about exposing their son to the proper social milieu. The mother refused to send him to a private boarding school, the father's plan, because she said she wanted him at home with her.

When the patient came into residence he was extremely polite to the staff, quite formal in speech and for the first few days tended to ignore the other children. He was a handsome boy and tall for his age. Physical and psychological examination indicated that he was in good health and had an I.Q. of 142 on the Stanford-Binet, Form L. Within a few days his destructive behavior became evident. He was abusive to the other children, particularly smaller boys, and to the nonprofessional staff, and was destructive with toys and furniture. At times he hit, kicked and pulled the hair of the other youngsters without apparent provocation. Once he tore the telephone and wires completely from the wall because the line was busy when he wanted to make a call. Again, he threw a pitcher of hot syrup across the table because the cook did not serve his pancakes first. When he discovered, one day, that the cleaning woman had put away some of his belongings in his room, he literally kicked her and her bucket of water down the stairway. When questioned about these behaviors by the professional staff, he stood at attention, said he was sorry, and guessed he had lost his temper. At no time did he become abusive in language or behavior toward the professional staff, except to kick and hit when someone physically tried to stop him in the middle of a tantrum. He showed respect for directions, such as returning from a movie at a designated time, and accepted, without question, the small weekly allowance that was given to all children his age. While in residence he and the other children attended public school. Academically, he did exceedingly well. He did his homework each night, sometimes did work for extra credit, played in the school band and maintained an excellent grade point average. There were several incidents of acting-out behavior that were brought to the attention of the residence staff, but none was as serious as the behavior reported previously to referral.

Initially, the patient was seen by the psychiatrist four times a week, and, after the first year, three times weekly. He, himself, kept the sessions on a rather quiet, interview-type level. He occasionally be-

came interested in a toy or game but engaged very little in play activity unless directed to do so. He was not inhibited in expressing himself but did not become aggressive toward the psychiatrist or the play materials. For example, when given the dolls and the doll house, he constructed a family with no apparent relationship problems in terms of aggressive feelings or behavior toward one another.

He was aware that he had been very much wanted by his parents. He felt, however, that primarily they wanted a son to carry on the prominent family name and the father's successful business. He had a certain emotional closeness to both his father and mother and wanted very much to please them; he was usually able to do so with his perfect manners and his gallantry in the presence of their friends. He had dreams, however, of a professional career that was different from his father's and this both pleased and upset him at the same time.

Although he had spent much time with his mother, he had been taken care of, for the most part, by other women whom he referred to as governesses or maids. From the time he was four, none of the women had stayed with him for more than a few months because they could not accept his abusive behavior. He spoke of them in a matter-of-fact manner, expressing neither particular closeness nor distaste for any of them.

His mother tended to infantilize him by the manner in which she dressed him, spoke to him, and protected him from his immediate surroundings; at the same time, nevertheless, she expected adult behavior from him. He had been with her much of the time but could scarcely remember having been alone with her. She entertained at parties constantly and lavishly, and always had her little boy on hand to amaze the guests with his gallantry. He helped women with their wraps, opened doors for them, gave up his chair and participated in their conversations.

The child did not seem particularly to resent his parents' expectations of him. More of a problem was the fact that their expectations and his gallant behavior seemed to permeate the parent-child relationships at all times. He did not have an acceptable outlet for negative or hostile feelings. His relationship with his father was of more concern to him than that with his mother. The father spent little actual time with the family, because of his extensive traveling, but each time he came home he brought expensive gifts for his son. He rarely, however, took the time to talk with him, even to tell of the places he had visited. Neither parent felt that the child was disturbed or had serious problems. They felt that his acting-out behavior was a response to mistreatment, and the proof of this view was his conforming behavior whenever he was with them.

Social contacts with other children his age were mostly confined to school and school hours and most of them were unsuccessful and unrewarding. He could not remember ever having had a best friend for more than a day or two at a stretch. He spent much of his time on school work and other reading, but his interests were not limited to them. He took music lessons for a while and showed a real appreciation for music. He was an excellent skater and bowler and was learning to ski. He followed team sports closely, both on a local and national level. His interests were primarily in activities he could do by himself and he shied away from participating in team sports.

He was in residence for almost four years. During this period he showed gradual improvement in relationships with children and a greater respect for the rights and feelings of others. His adjustment to the children in school improved more rapidly than to the children in the clinic, probably because he knew of the latters' imperfections and was intolerant of them. The parents cooperated by keeping scheduled appointments, and, although any change in them seemed quite superficial, the fact that they took the time to come and displayed an interest, together with the child's increased awareness of their personalities and motivations, apparently combined to improve the parent-child relationships and bring them closer.

Follow-up information revealed that the boy continued to be a bright and conscientious student after leaving the clinic, and was successfully completing his final year in law school. No known behavior problems or problems in his relationships were indicated. He had no plans for marriage but dated occasionally. There was some indication that he continued his "psychological distance" from others and that he was greatly involved in academic work and professional plans.

Adjustment Reactions of Adolescence. This category includes those transient reactions of the adolescent that reflect his emancipatory strivings and the vacillations of his impulses and emotional tendencies. Superficially, the pattern of behavior may resemble any of the personality or neurotic disorders. Transient adolescent reactions of this nature are often differentiated with great difficulty from deep-seated personality disorders or neuroses. The diagnosis is used initially in the hope that the disturbance will prove to be transient, but if difficulties persist, the diagnosis is revised.

In the following case the girl's behavior suggested a developing sociopathic personality. Treatment and placement in a congenial foster home, however, appear to have curbed the tendencies. Her initial difficulties may have been caused by rejecting, hostile parents, inability to establish satisfactory relationships with surrogate parental figures, and the fact that her early adult models were disorganized and, in the case of her father, sociopathic.

The patient was first referred to a psychiatrist at the age of 13 shortly after having been placed in a new foster home. She complained of numerous vague and varying pains, inability to hear or see clearly, great variability of mood, and momentary dizzy spells or "black-outs." One night when she was coming home from a meeting she apparently became confused and urinated on the street. The foster mother also reported temper tantrums. During one tantrum, she attacked a foster sister and for two hours afterward muttered to herself and banged on the walls and furniture. It was suspected that at least some of her symptoms might be attributable to a form of epilepsy, but the results of several electroencephalograms made this doubtful, and medication failed to control her outbursts of violent behavior. In any event, it gradually became apparent that her disturbed behavior was related to the interpersonal relationships within her current foster home. Two other foster children, girls, had been in the home since infancy, and, although the patient seemed to get along quite well with the younger one, she displayed intense rivalry and hostility toward the older girl who was just six months younger than she. The inevitable rivalry was unquestionably accentuated by the foster parents, who tended to favor this child. The patient had frequent fights with her and sometimes remained disturbed for as much as two hours afterward. Subsequently she claimed to have no clear recollection of these incidents. After several months she ran away and was placed in another foster home with an 11-year-old-boy who was a far worse behavior problem than she. Her outbursts of intense anger and violence continued, but the foster mother felt that there was always some provocation. Nevertheless, it was considered necessary to admit her to a psychiatric hospital for evaluation.

The patient had a sister three years older than herself and a brother one year younger. Her mother had apparently completed grade eight by the time she left school at age 16. One year later she married a man with a sociopathic personality. He had been unemployed at the time of the marriage and during the four years they were together he was unemployed and on relief most of the time. When his wife told him of each pregnancy, he became furious and afterward consistently rejected the children. He joined the army when war broke out but became a deserter. After the war he held a variety of brief jobs and lived temporarily with a number of different women.

Although the patient's mother consciously attempted to supply her with affection, her actions were rejecting. She breast-fed the patient during the few days she was in the hospital and then bottle-fed her. When the brother was born, the patient was sent to live with a maternal aunt for four years. She returned to the mother for two years between the ages of six and eight. The father returned from overseas then, and requested that she and her sister live with him. The arrangement lasted only about two months, for he beat the girls frequently and was finally sent to jail for sexually molesting the patient. The two girls returned to their mother, now living with a common-law husband, but two years later she became pregnant again and the three children were made wards of a child-protection agency.

The mother reported that at the age of one year the patient had developed a sore on her nose and picked at it constantly so that it remained raw for several months. In early childhood she had cried at night a great deal. After she started school she frequently pretended to be ill and was permitted to stay at home until the mother tired of the practice. She was advanced to another grade each year, however, and at 14 was attending the eighth grade. She had been subject to temper tantrums from a very early age, the mother said, and would scream, yell, kick and bite if she was not allowed to have her own way. The mother had tried spankings, but since they only made matters worse, she resorted to shutting the door on the patient and letting her cry. The patient was very disobedient, had to be reminded several times to do chores, and was always able to wind people around her finger.

Between the ages of 10 and 14 the patient had been placed in a total of nine different foster homes. Her foster parents and social worker considered her tense, highly excitable, unstable and unpredictable in her moods. In her first contacts with adults, her manner was very ingratiating, but subsequently she would quickly develop violent hostility toward them. She never received any formal sexual information, although her father had molested her when she was eight, and subsequently she was known to have made a number of sexual explorations with various boys. She also claimed that in two of the foster homes the men had approached her sexually and it was suspected that she had acted in a seductive manner and then rejected the approaches.

In the hospital there was no evidence of psychotic reality distortion or of severe depression. Her full scale I.Q. was 94. It was possible to establish an effective therapeutic relationship with her which led her to reappraise the idealized picture she had of her mother. The patient's attitude swung from one of idealization of her mother to marked hostility which subsided gradually as therapy progressed. During her months in the hospital there were no episodes of violent, uncontrollable behavior, and her frustration-tolerance and emotional maturity gradually increased. She was placed in a foster home with a fairly young couple who had several children younger than she and was able to establish more satisfying relationships than with any of her previous foster parents. No further difficulties were reported during the next few years.

Neuroses in Childhood

The major neurotic syndromes found in adults, such as conversion reactions, phobic reactions and compulsive reactions, are sometimes seen also in children and adolescents and, conse-

quently, may be the forerunners of adult neuroses. Like the neurotic adult, the neurotic child has a central problem with anxiety, and the symptoms he manifests are indicative of his attempts to handle it.

The neurotic child is inhibited in one or more of his activities, i.e., in his schoolwork, play or participation in activities. He is frequently shy and self-conscious and feels inadequate and inferior to others. It is difficult for him to assert himself or to make his feelings and wishes known. He tries, instead, to conform to the expectations of others and his efforts are often unusually conscientious. He is usually very well behaved. Evaluations of his family often reveal that one or both parents are demanding, strict and impose very high standards of behavior on him. Such a child often feels ashamed and guilty; he seems to be more comfortable when he is doing things for others, such as giving gifts, and is uneasy when he is the recipient of gifts and favors. In general, he is inhibited in his expression of feeling, especially if any hostility is involved. He does not have outlets for his anger. His fantasies, however, are often hostile and even sadistic. He may be preoccupied with sexual thoughts, but his fantasies often are disturbing to him and add to his feelings of guilt.

The neurotic behavior of the patient described in the following paragraphs reflects personality changes rather than a temporary emotional upset. The symptoms had been developing over a period of years. The mother's emphasis on physical symptoms and her unwillingness to allow the boy to become more independent, plus the poor identification model provided by the father, seem to have been important etiological factors. The child was not returned to his parents after treatment in the hospital, for his new reaction and behavior patterns were not strong enough for additional exposure to his mother's neuroticism and his father's hostility and lack of sensitivity.

The patient entered the child psychiatry ward of a general hospital at the age of 12 with a three- or four-month history of chest and stomach pains and headaches that had kept him from attending school. Physical examinations and laboratory investigations were essentially negative, and it was recognized that the boy's bodily complaints were emotional in origin and a means of avoiding school. He had many other fears, however, apart from school. His mother reported that he frequently cried out of sheer fright and the boy confessed that he was afraid of crowds, big open spaces, auditoriums, little places and being alone, particularly at night. He said he had difficulty sleeping and woke up three or four times every night when he would see "millions of dots of light moving real fast" in front of his eyes.

He was the second of three boys. The elder, 18 years old, had completed high school and was in military service. The other brother was less than 18 months younger than he and over the years considerable rivalry had grown up between them for the attention and approval of the parents. With each pregnancy the mother had apparently hoped for the birth of a girl, but was a conscientious woman and gave no behavioral evidence of rejecting any of the boys. On the contrary, she was an anxious, oversolicitous and overprotective woman (often considered manifestative of reaction-formation against hostile and rejecting impulses). She was subject to migraine headaches and, since the birth of her youngest son, high blood pressure; over the years she had had a number of other somatic complaints also. She was not only excessively concerned about her own health, but also about the health of her children; she kept them home from school for trivial reasons, rewarding and reinforcing their dependency on her and their tendencies to use bodily complaints as an escape from unpleasant situations. Psychological testing results were consistent with a diagnosis of conversion reaction.

The father appeared less obviously neurotic than the mother. He was a salesman and spent many evenings away from home. He gave the impression of being conscientious and apparently had never been unfaithful to his wife, but he was undemonstrative toward her and the boys. The mother stated that he never praised the children "for fear that they would get a big head." According to the patient, he was afraid of his father because the latter had a bad temper. The overall picture obtained was of a frustrated and hostile man who was generally critical and frequently punitive. His attitude toward the boy's sickness was that he should be pushed and he would get over it.

There was no evidence of retardation in the boy's early development. He was toilet trained by 18 months but continued to wet his bed on occasion until he was nine years old. From an early age on he had been afraid of the dark and continued to have a light in his room until he was admitted to the hospital. He was overcontrolled and overconforming. He was eager to please the teacher when he started school, and was regarded as a well behaved, hard working child, very attentive to detail.

When the boy was four years old he had an illness that was diagnosed as rheumatic fever (which frequently attacks the heart) and was hospitalized for two or three weeks. He received penicillin for the following 18 months and since there was no evidence that his heart was involved, the physician did not restrict his activities. The mother reported that he became less active and sociable, nevertheless, and it appears likely that this behavior was related to her excessive concern over his health. She treated him as a delicate child, thereafter, and kept him home for minor ailments on an average of two weeks a year, while he was in elementary school.

In spite of extreme anxiety during the psychological testing, he obtained a full scale I.Q. of 118 and gave no evidence of psychotic ideation or behavior. On projective tests he perceived his environment as extremely frightening and potentially destructive; he was ambivalent and indecisive, and gave evidence of conflict over sexual identification; he perceived father-figures as rejecting and frightening and his feelings toward mother-figures involved both dependency and hostility. It was suggested that there were two reasons for these feelings about his mother: (1) she was dominating and overprotective and he resented her control, and (2) she was seductive and erotically stimulating, leading him to fear his father as a hostile, destructive rival.

In the hospital the boy attempted at first to obtain rewards by means of somatic complaints, but these were investigated and then ignored. Social participation was reinforced, and he learned that he could express his feelings verbally without retaliation. His anxiety soon diminished greatly and he participated actively in physical as well as social activities. Unfortunately, the parents displayed no evidence of change in attitudes or behavior, and after five months of hospitalization the boy was transferred to a residential treatment center for long-term therapy and education.

Many child guidance clinics and private psychotherapists are concerned with the comparatively high frequency of a disorder that has been termed, for want of a better, "school phobia." Because this disorder has many characteristics of a phobic reaction, it is classified under neurotic reactions of childhood. The condition is manifested as an extreme anxiety over going to school and resembles an acute panic state. Its onset appears to be sudden. Without any warning, the child, after apparently having made a good adjustment, refuses to attend school. The refusal usually follows an illness or vacation that has kept him at home for some period. If he is urged or forced to return to the classroom, either the physical symptoms of his illness reappear or he develops new ones, often vomiting or dizziness. If he is brought to school by force, he may refuse to do any work or participate in any activity. Because of the child's adamant attitude toward school, attempts to handle the problem directly are notoriously unsuccessful. Lippman (1962) recounts the case of a frail boy who defied his father's order to return to school and locked himself in his room. In desperation, the father called a policeman who agreed to carry the child to his classroom. Although the boy was terrified of the police, he kicked and fought so hard that the officer decided force was a mistake and that the boy probably would not remain in school even if he was brought there.

Years of experience in exploring and treating this syndrome have indicated that while some reality factors may exist in the child's distaste for school (such as, for example, an overly strict or poorly prepared teacher, poor achievement, or unrealistic demands on the child), the actual source of his anxiety is often related to his fears of leaving home and being separated from a parent, usually the mother. The fear is displaced from the parental relationship to the school. In some cases that were diagnosed and treated, the child was afraid to leave his mother for fear she would be beaten by his alcoholic father, or he did not wish to leave her alone with a younger child, perhaps a newborn infant, who, he feared, would get all her affection. Such a child often becomes extremely dependent on the mother and attempts to restrict her activities as much as he can. The anxiety may also become so generalized that it is attached not only to the school but often, as well, to church, peer group activities or anything that may take him from his mother. Johnson et al. (1941) found that the school phobia in a child is often associated with a complementary neurosis in the mother. Any physical complaints in the child are emphasized and even encouraged by the mother in her attempts (unconscious) to keep him home. This aspect of the problem has been elaborated by Goldberg (1953), Suttenfield (1954) and Estes et al. (1956).

In the following case of a school phobia there were a number of characteristics highly typical of this disorder, such as an abrupt refusal to attend school, the use of physical symptoms as an excuse and a pathological relationship with a parent. The refusal to attend school had little if anything to do with the school itself, but arose out of the child's relationship with a parent, in this case, her father. He, in a well-meaning manner, allowed, and even subtly encouraged, his daughter to take the role she attempted to create for herself in relation to him. He really did not see what she was doing or the nature of the relationship that resulted. The problem was approached therapeutically by giving attention to the primary source of the child's disturbance—the parent-child relationship—and not attacking the school problem directly. After certain environmental and psychological changes had occurred, it was expected that the girl would return to school, and, in due course, she did.

The patient, a 10-year-old girl, was brought to a child guidance clinic because of her refusal to attend school. About five months earlier, her mother had died following a lingering illness and hospitalization. Although the child had completed the remaining six weeks of third grade without apparent problems, she refused to attend school after the summer vacation. She went to her fourth grade room the first morning with some reluctance but came home at noon and would not return. Sometimes she used physical symptoms as an excuse and at other times was slow to get ready. When urged to go she became very anxious, cried, refused to move from her chair and said she hated school. She remained home with only a neighbor to come in occasionally, and her father made arrangements at work for an extended noon hour to have lunch with her. The one other child in the family was a boy of 18.

Physical examination revealed an attractive but obese youngster who was otherwise in good health. She scored an I.Q. of 109 on the Stanford-Binet, Form L. Her school adjustment had been considered good, although she was unusually conscientious and perhaps an over-achiever. Her relations with other children were thought to be rather superficial; she was sweet to everyone, was accepted by others, but had no close friends and rarely brought other children home. Although her weight, a problem since she had been four years old, caused her some minimal concern, her father always assured her that good behavior was more important and that her behavior was just like her mother's.

The fatner stated that the patient had always been a conforming, rather quiet child, especially with people outside the family. Her reaction to her mother's illness and death had been amazingly adult-like, he considered, despite what he termed a close mother-daughter relationship. What many girls shared with friends, she had shared with her mother and had always shown an interest in helping with household chores, such as cooking and cleaning.

Following her mother's death, however, the patient did little but sit around the house and look at books and magazines. Her interest in toys was minimal and she took no initiative in helping with household tasks, even those she had performed during her mother's hospitalization. She became dependent upon her father for everything, and he, out of sympathy and concern, complied by doing all the chores and, in addition, planning joint excursions. She particularly enjoyed expeditions to buy clothes for her and to attend movies. At no time did the father question her changed mood and behavior except to suggest that she return to school. He also urged his son not to tease her for laziness.

She talked and laughed at home as much as usual and showed no signs of depression other than inactivity. About two weeks before the beginning of school she decided to give up her own room and sleep with her father. He thought the move inadvisable, but, again, complied when she rebelled against his objections. He reassured himself that the move wqs only temporary.

The girl was assigned to a female therapist and for many weeks related only superficially. She was very

TABLE 19–1. Ten Differential School Phobia Symptoms

Type 1	Type 2
1. The present illness is the first episode.	1. Second, third or fourth episode.
2. Monday onset, following an illness the previous Thursday or Friday.	2. Monday onset following minor illness not a prevalent antecedent.
3. An acute onset.	3. Incipient onset.
4. Lower grades most prevalent.	4. Upper grades most prevalent.
5. Expressed concern about death.	5. Death theme not present.
6. Mother's physical health in question: actually ill or child thinks so.	6. Health of mother not an issue.
7. Good communication between parents.	7. Poor communication between parents.
8. Mother and father well-adjusted in most areas.	8. Mother shows neurotic behavior; father, a character disorder.
9. Father competitive with mother in household management.	9. Father shows little interest in household or children.
10. Parents achieve understanding of dynamics easily.	10. Parents very difficult to work with.

(From Kennedy, W. A., 1965. School phobia: Rapid treatment of fifty cases. J. Ab. Psychol. 70:285–289.

polite, answered questions, accepted and followed all suggestions for activities, and displayed little initiative. As time went on, however, she became less inhibited and volunteered information about her family and feelings more freely. On one occasion, when cleaning up after painting, she commented that she used to pick up her things and help her mother but that now she did nothing because the amount of work to be done discouraged her. Since she tended to be a perfectionist, she chose to do nothing rather than attempt to do things she felt she could not do well. She had tried to take over her mother's role but felt guilty because she had failed at keeping house. As therapy progressed, it became evident that she tried to make up for this failure by doing other things her mother had done, such as sleeping with her father, accompanying him on activities that he enjoyed and staying at home while he was at work.

The disturbance in the child and in the parent-child relationship turned out to be less severe than had initially appeared. The father was able to see how he had permitted the problem to develop and continue, and was able to take some immediate steps to change the situation.

He hired a woman to help with the household chores and made arrangements for a neighbor, who appeared to be interested in the girl, to shop for clothes with her and help fix her hair. These acts not only relieved him of unwelcomed responsibilities but helped change the nature of the relationship that had developed between him and the girl after the mother's death. He joined a bowling league that met one night a week and encouraged the girl to bring friends to the house. When she became concerned about her weight problem and was able to follow the doctor's prescribed diet, he was able to give her much more encouragement than in the past.

About eight weeks after the beginning of therapy, the child returned to school and, at the father's suggestion, willingly gave up sleeping with him. She also began to take a little more responsibility at home, but never regained her earlier interest. The family itself decided to share cooking responsibilities, although the father actually did most of it.

The girl completed the fourth grade satisfactorily. Both she and her father remained in treatment for about 14 months and she developed an increasingly good relationship with the therapist. She confided in the therapist more and more and looked to her for guidance. The therapist, apparently, served as a mother substitute. The father needed support during this period for his new firmness with his daughter.

Follow-up evaluation two years after the case was closed revealed that the improved family relations were maintained: the child was active in school and attended freely; the brother was married to a young woman who took a great interest in the girl; and the changes made in the father's life pattern during treatment had become fairly permanent.

Kennedy (1965) has noted that there seem to be two types of school phobias. Type 1 is more sudden in onset and occurs in a relatively stable family environment. The general picture is that of a neurotic crisis precipitated by the child's anxiety. Type 2 school phobias (see Table 19–1) have a gradual onset of non-school attendance which becomes chronic and the family picture is unstable. Over a period of eight years in a child outpatient clinic Kennedy found only six cases which met seven of the ten criteria for Type 2 phobias. All had families in which one or both parents were seriously disturbed. Over the same period, 50 cases which met the criteria for a Type 1 diagnosis were seen. Kennedy describes a rapid, three day treatment program based on learning theory concepts, which led to a complete remission of school phobia symptoms in all 50 cases. Follow-up study indicated no evidence of recurrence or substitution of symptoms.

Psychoses in Childhood

Although affective psychoses are very rare before the age of 15, psychotic depressions and suicide are not unknown in early adolescence and childhood. Successful suicide is about three times as common in boys as in girls. Among white boys aged 5 to 14 years, in the United States, the annual rate of suicide has been reported as approximately four per million. Only about one in 40 of these is a boy under 10 years of age. The incidence rate is higher than this, however, since some child suicides are reported as accidents. Severe grief and depression may also be observed in very young children, particularly after prolonged or permanent separation from loved parents. Such a depression may result in self-imposed starvation or in death by some means not easily attributable to suicide.

The similarity between certain psychoses in children and schizophrenia in adults was recognized at the beginning of the present century. Between 1905 and 1908 De Sanctis reported a number of cases among children which he termed dementia praecocissima. Despert (1954) found the first reference in the American literature to childhood schizophrenia in 1933. One of the earliest definitions of child schizophrenia was formulated in 1937 at the first international congress concerned with child psychiatry. It read, ". . . a disease process in which the loss of affective contact with reality is coincident with or determined by the appearance of autistic thinking and accompanied by specific phenomena of regression and dissociation" (Despert, 1954).

This broad definition has been generally accepted. Because no clear syndrome is implicit in it, the definition has been variously elaborated by a number of different investigators, such as Bradley and Bowen (1941), Bender (1947), Despert (1952) and Kanner (1957). The following characteristics are the most often noted: defects in emotional rapport and inability to relate to other people; dullness of thought and feeling; blocking, retardation or inhibition of speech, sometimes with complete mutism; alterations in activity level—in some cases retardation to the point of complete immobility and in others extreme restlessness and excitement (perseveration and stereotypy are sometimes observed); and withdrawal of interest from the environment.

Bender (1947) found a number of physical and organic characteristics in a group of schizophrenic children. They include: disturbances in negative functioning (sympathetic nervous system); marked growth discrepancies; abnormal

EEG records in many cases; motor awkwardness; and retention of certain primitive reflex patterns.

Goldfarb (1961) also noted organic symptoms in many children who are diagnosed schizophrenic. He worked out some diagnostic criteria for dividing the category of childhood schizophrenia into two groups, and suggested separating them accordingly. In one, symptoms of organic brain damage appear to be present and in the other no such symptoms are apparent.

In general, it is agreed that schizophrenia in children varies in initial manifestations and in age of onset. In some cases the onset is sudden and there is a rapid change in the child's appearance (a waxy complexion has often been observed) and personality; in others, the onset is insidious, and the child displays a gradual withdrawal and refusal to eat, communicate and participate in activities. Frequently he does not look at people but gazes into space. He may show special interest in one object or toy and examines it for long periods or perhaps takes it apart and puts it together again in repetitive fashion. Some of these children do not tolerate any separation from the mother but others seem unaware that their parents exist. The active schizophrenic child is often aggressive, uncontrolled, and destructive; he may engage in a great deal of rhythmic activity, body swaying or rocking, chair rocking and bed rolling. Sexual preoccupation and constant masturbation are commonly observed symptoms.

Certain forms of childhood psychosis that closely resemble schizophrenia but have certain special characteristics have been described by Kanner (1944). He applied the term *early infantile autism* to a group of children in whom withdrawal tendencies were noted during the first year of life. Many cases of this type have since been described. The most common characteristic of such children is failure to relate to other people and situations in a usual manner starting in the early months of life. While they may relate skillfully and even affectionately to objects, they withdraw from any interpersonal stimulation or relationship. They have an obsessive desire for the preservation of sameness and do not tolerate change. They usually appear intelligent, are often attractive and are pensive in manner. About one-third are mute and the remainder use unintelligible language. Eisenberg and Kanner (1956) differentiated between autistic children who acquire language before the age of five and those who do not; about one-half the first group make some degree of scholastic adjustment, but in the second group only 1 in 20 subsequently acquires language and makes at least a mediocre adjustment in a protected school setting. They also tried to investigate the siblings of autistic children and reported that of 131 known siblings of 100 autistic children, three were regarded as probably autistic (on the basis of information supplied) and seven others were regarded as emotionally disturbed. In general, a high incidence of psychological problems was not found among the siblings.

In the same study (Eisenberg and Kanner, 1956), the family data on 120 cases of early infantile autism were reviewed. Of 200 patients, only 6 were diagnosed as having clinical psychiatric disorders. This finding contrasted sharply with the high incidence of psychiatric problems reported by Bender (1947) in families of older childhood schizophrenics and in families of adult schizophrenics reported by various authors. The parents of the autistic children also tended to be well educated; 87 of the fathers and 70 of the mothers had been to college. A control group of parents (parents of private patients selected solely on the basis of being next in call numbers after each of the first 50 cases of early infantile autism) had considerably lower levels of educational achievement and professional status.

Earlier, Kanner (1944) described the parents of 55 autistic children. They were dignified, polite and undemonstrative; they tended to be formal in all interpersonal relationships, including marriage, and indicated no major animosities. Divorce was rare among them. The mothers were not warm hearted and the fathers, although outwardly friendly, did not engage in childish play with their children, but taught, admonished and observed the children "objectively." Many of the parents were described as perfectionistic. The children were not rejected in the usual sense but were exposed from early infancy on to parental coldness, obsessiveness and a type of mechanical attention to material needs only.

Cases evaluated and reported later (Eisenberg and Kanner, 1956; and Kanner, 1957) revealed the same characteristics in family background and environment. Consequently, the authors concluded that emotional factors in the homes of autistic children are influential in, but not sufficient to account for, the genesis of the disturbance. Assuming that autistic children were somehow different at birth, they hypothesized that autism was a result of the interaction between hereditary and environmental factors. The supposition of an innate difference in the autistic child means relatively little, however, unless the nature and meaning of the difference can be specified.

Few disagreements with Kanner's descriptions of autistic children and their parents have been voiced. Kestenberg (1954) reported one case history of an autistic child and observed, in her introductory statements, that she found a variety of psychiatric problems in the parents of autistic children, especially depression, schizophrenia, neurosis and psychosomatic disturbances, and that she had not noted either a uniform type of parent or parental reaction to the child.

Early infantile autism is so similar to childhood schizophrenia in its manifestations that sometimes the two disorders cannot be differentiated except on the basis of historical data. By definition, fixation and not regression is involved in cases of infantile autism: the child never has a period of "normal" development and never manifests the responses of normal children to parents. In childhood schizophrenia, on the other hand, the child regresses from a relatively more complex, better integrated level of behavior to an earlier, more primitive one.

In the past, many schizophrenic and autistic children have been considered and treated as mentally subnormal. In the preceding chapter these children were referred to as the "pseudo-retarded." Some are placed in institutions for the feebleminded at any early age and others are kept at home without the benefits of treatment or special education. Such diagnostic errors undoubtedly still occur but are becoming less frequent as the syndrome becomes better known to more physicians and social workers, as well as psychiatrists and psychologists. For purposes of illustration, a case history of childhood schizophrenia and one of lifelong autism are presented in the following paragraphs. In the first case, the absence of peer relationships is notable. As is true of so many childhood schizophrenics, the boy had symptoms suggesting the possibility of neurologic involvement, i.e., the peculiar gait and an extreme language handicap which appeared early in life; he was also highly distractable. While the mother appeared to be fairly normal, little is actually known of her relationship with the child. It may be significant that she was unable to be more articulate about their relationship.

The boy was referred to a speech pathologist when he was nine years old because of problems in language comprehension. His mother reported that he had started using short phrases by the age of two and one-half years, but by four seemed to have difficulty in comprehension and in expressing himself; he did not ask questions or talk as much as would be expected for this age level. He was also hyperactive and distractable so that he could not attend school; for the past few years he had been tutored at home. His development in other areas also indicated abnormalities. He had started walking alone at the age of 17 months but walked on his toes until he was six or seven years old. He had had no contact with children his own age and had never learned to relate to them.

He was extremely distractable during the interview and avoided looking at the examiner's face. His attention span was brief but his performance improved on academic tasks, such as reading and arithmetic. He showed a marked impairment of language comprehension. His responses to short concrete questions and single-step oral directions in a closely structured stitution were inconsistent. Frequently, his responses revealed echolalia or perseveration. He was unable to attend and recall short stories ten sentences in length, but the repetition of digits and words was intact. He read second grade material fairly fluently but with poor comprehension. His sentences reflected intact formulation, vocabulary and articulation, but there was little attempt to initiate conversation, and his verbalizations were largely self-directed and inappropriate in content. He was able to work simple arithmetical combinations and to print and spell words at approximately the second-grade level. It was concluded that his peripheral speech mechanism was normal in structure and function but that he was emotionally disturbed. He was admitted, therefore, to the child psychiatry ward of a general hospital.

He was an only child, born out of wedlock, and lived alone with his mother, who worked as a waitress. During his first six months she remained at home to care for him but then returned to work. During the next three years she left him in the care of a baby sitter in the same apartment building and during the following three years, with her childless sister. For the two years preceding hospitalization he had been left with another middle-aged baby sitter. He was reported to have related fairly well to each of these women but never had the opportunity of learning to socialize with other children of his own age. For a year prior to hospitalization he had become increasingly anxious and tearful when it was time for his mother to go to work. An interview with the mother revealed no obvious psychopathology except in the area of interaction with the boy.

In the hospital, after he was separated from his mother, he whimpered like a puppy and for several days was obsessed with the idea of going home immediately. He avoided all contact and communication with other children but spoke briefly with the adult staff members who approached him. He was fearful of

new situations: the first time he was invited to attend occupational therapy he indicated distress, and the first time he was approached by a psychologist he ran away. The next day, however, the psychologist took his hand and the boy accompanied him without resistance.

He was distractable and his responses to questions were quite variable. Sometimes he responded appropriately, sometimes not at all, sometimes with echolalia, and sometimes with irrelevant and autistic replies. He cooperated sufficiently with testing so that he obtained an I.Q. of 66 on the Wechsler Intelligence Scale for Children but there was marked inter- and intra-test variability, and his performance on different subtests varied from average to a defective level. There was no clear-cut evidence of organic intellectual impairment. Projective tests indicated marked ambivalence; people were feared, but he needed their protection; the home was a source of refuge but was also restrictive and confining; he was overdependent on his mother, but his feelings toward her combined love and hostility.

After he became accustomed to the surroundings, he was much less fearful and participated in all available activities. He was still quite incapable of interacting with other children, however, and remained preoccupied with his own goals which led to parallel play situations. On one occasion he drew pictures of himself and his mother which were almost identical, including the fact that both figures were in skirts. Neither individual psychotherapy nor social and milieu therapy effected much appreciable change in his social isolation, and after two months of hospitalization it was recommended that he be transferred to a long-term treatment center for children. His mother was unable to accept this recommendation and took him home to live with her in the same situation as before.

The following case depicts an autistic child whose early behavior was indicative of mental retardation. (In the preceding chapter a discussion of the similarity between the symptoms of subnormality and schizophrenia in children was presented.)

The girl was first admitted to a child psychiatry ward of a general hospital at the age of nine years. Her history was one of lifelong developmental retardation and deviant behavior that, hitherto, had been attributed to mental subnormality. The parents reported that during the first year of life she had been quiet, passive, and unresponsive to the parents and older sister. She did not sit up by herself until the age of nine months and only started to crawl when she was 15 months old. She was able to stand alone at 18 months but did not walk by herself until she was 30 months old. At this time she was tested psychologically and obtained a Cattell Infant Intelligence Scale I.Q. of 58.

When she was three years old the only words she spoke were "Mommie" and "Daddy," but at the age of five she suddenly began speaking whole sentences. A Stanford-Binet test administered at the time showed her I.Q. to be 77. On this basis, she was still considered to be mentally subnormal and was placed in special classes in the public school system for several years. At the age of eight she obtained a Stanford-Binet I.Q. of 85 and her teachers became increasingly concerned about her complete preoccupation with self-directed activity and with her inability to participate in any group activities. When she was nine she was able to do the work in the basic first level reader and workbook, despite inattentiveness during reading instruction. Her workbook exercises were sometimes completed accurately and sometimes the page was decorated with scrolls, curves, pictures or drawings of bugs. She appeared happiest when looking through books on or pictures of science, birds, animals or insects. She had a remarkable memory for details which was demonstrated in a most unusual ability to cut out freehand any bird or animal in a matter of minutes.

When she was admitted to the hospital, her two outstanding characteristics were self-isolation and an extreme need for sameness. Other deviant behavior that was observed or reported included: not talking aloud anywhere except in her home setting; refusing to exit through a door unless someone else opened it, and refusing to enter through a door unless she herself opened it; refusing baths because of a fear of water; fear of television, which had kept her parents from buying a set until recently; standing in one place and insisting that she was unable to move; negativism, that resulted in her doing the opposite of what was requested; responding to any physical contact with people by touching or hitting them; complete egocentricity or narcissism, with disregard for the feelings or wishes of others; interpreting any accidental hurt or discipline as a withdrawal of love; compulsive behavior, such as touching things or jumping off the last step when descending stairs; obsessional preoccupation with the letter K (with which she replaced her middle name) and the number 8; restricted interest patterns involving animals, birds, flowers, masculinity, femininity and pregnancy; enuresis, habitual at night and occasional during the day.

The patient was the second of four children; she had an older sister and two younger brothers. Her parents maintained that the pregnancy was planned and she was wanted, but it appeared that they might have preferred having had a boy and that the patient experienced some rejection following the birth of the older son. Psychological testing of the parents showed defensiveness but no gross personality disorder, and the only abnormal behavior identified in interviews with them was their excessive compliance with the patient's demands and their inability to set limits or reward her for more normal behavior.

In the hospital her deviant behavior was discouraged by ignoring it, whenever possible; every slight manifestation of social participation was reinforced and rewarded with increased attention and other means. For example, she was given second helpings of food at mealtimes only when she asked for them out loud; within three months she was talking out loud most of the time. Gradually, she learned that human relationships could be satisfying but could not always be obtained on her own terms.

About four months after admission she obtained a Stanford-Binet I.Q. of 95, and a few weeks later obtained a full scale I.Q. of 116 on the Wechsler Intelligence Scale for Children (verbal score 104 and performance scale 127). She was now ready to participate far more fully in school classes held in the hospital, and worked at a grade three level. After a little more than eight months in the hospital she was discharged to her parents but continued to attend a special class in public school for the remainder of the academic year. She and her mother also continued to see a child psychiatrist at approximately monthly intervals. During the next two years both academic performance and social participation improved. She remained at a disadvantage in her relations with other children, however, as they were inclined to tease her and ridicule her behavior. Continuing difficulties were anticipated for her during adolescence and adult life.

Delinquency and Addiction

The various forms of persistent delinquency, sexual deviation and addictions were discussed in detail in Chapters 14, 15 and 16. Sexual deviation and addictions are frequently associated with neurosis or psychosis, but also with sociopathic personality characteristics. The manner in which these disorders develop is found in the adjustment patterns of childhood and adolescence. A determining factor in the kind of addiction a child may develop is availability. Children and adolescents have become addicted to such practices as glue sniffing, gasoline sniffing, drinking cough syrups containing codeine and using benzedrine inhalers. These addictions often do not have the permanency of addictions noted in later adolescence or adulthood—they may be unverbalized demands for attention which cease if the child's needs can be met satisfactorily—but they often progress to other forms of persistent psychological disturbance. The following case is fairly typical, except perhaps for the happy ending. It is interesting to note that the mother expected her son to be imprisoned, and it is possible that this expectation was of etiological significance in his behavior. It is also possible that some of his delinquent behavior had some relation to her partially unconscious antisocial impulses.

A 13-year-old boy was admitted to the child psychiatry ward of a general hospital with a history of intoxication caused by the inhalation of gasoline fumes. For the preceding two or three years he had intoxicated himself at least once a week by taking deep breaths of the fumes from gasoline cans or automobile gas tanks. He would become dizzy and feel as though he were "tingling all over" and "drifting in space"; he would usually hear an "eerie" sound, which he could only describe as a humming, which often increased in intensity for five to ten minutes after he started breathing fresh air again. When gasoline fumes were not available, he inhaled carbon monoxide from the exhaust pipes of cars. At times he had continued inhaling beyond his usual end point and had "keeled over" in brief periods of unconsciousness or stupor.

His mother was at first hostile and uncooperative, but subsequently gave the impression of physical attractiveness and seductiveness toward both the boy and male members of the hospital staff. It was learned that her father had died when she was a small girl. When she was about 17 she had given birth to an illegitimate child and two years later married the boy's father. The patient was the only boy and grew up with his half-sister who was three years older than he, and a full sister, three years younger. The half-sister was partly responsible for his care and discipline, and he was very hostile toward her.

The father came from a home broken by his father's desertion, and appears to have had a sociopathic personality disorder. He had been discharged from the army for psychiatric reasons and had had a number of extramarital affairs. He was divorced by the patient's mother when the boy was only five years old. The mother then started working full time as a secretary. She was involved in a relationship with a man, when the boy was first seen, whom she later married. The boy was her favorite child although she was resigned to the expectation that he would spend his life in prison and apparently conveyed this attitude to him. She was quite seductive toward him, and he greatly resented the intrusion of the man who was to become his stepfather.

The boy's mother considered his early development to be somewhat slower than that of his two sisters. He had walked by the age of 14 months, had bowel control by the age of two years and bladder control slightly after that. He had continued to wet his bed at night, on occasion, until his admission to the hospital. He had not been weaned from bottle feeding until the age of 14 months and did not talk until he was about three years old. His behavior had not become a problem to his mother, however, until he was about seven, when he repeatedly set fires in the house and slashed furniture with a razor blade, but the behavior gradually diminished without professional help. He was disinterested in school work and had had to repeat both grades one and five.

At the age of 12 he became involved in a number of delinquent activities and appeared in juvenile court charged with seven offenses of theft from parked automobiles, and breaking and entering private homes and stealing property, although of little value. He was

placed on probation and enrolled in a therapy program for delinquent boys in which he was required to spend weekends at a nearby ranch. He was polite and well behaved there, and apparently did not engage in further delinquent activities. He continued to underachieve at school and frequently lied to the teachers. In two group tests of intelligence administered at school his I.Q. was recorded at just under 90. It was felt that he completely disregarded the effects of his behavior on himself or on other people, and although he responded to correction he never showed any real feeling of guilt. He definitely responded to group pressure from his peers, nevertheless.

About six months prior to referral to the hospital the boy suffered an accidental head injury that was followed by a brief period of unconsciousness. Neurologic examination and an electroencephalogram were negative, but his performance on psychological tests was considered suggestive of organic intellectual impairment. His full scale I.Q. was 97 (verbal 108, performance 86) but he had some difficulty with the Bender-Gestalt test of reproducing designs. If the difficulty was a result of organic brain damage, it was considered that the damage might have been caused by either his prolonged inhalation of gasoline or the more recent head injury. Following his admission to the hospital, however, another electroencephalogram was negative and psychological testing did not provide conclusive evidence of organic intellectual impairment.

Projective tests suggested that his main problems concerned his self concept, difficulties in sex-role identification, unsatisfactory attitudes toward his mother and authority, and a combination of aggression with some depression. He perceived himself as a bad boy, and felt that others regarded him as such and that he must live up to this image. He regarded his head injury and other unpleasant experiences as having been deserved and as partial atonement for his guilt. He expected to be punished and felt that adults were captious beings who could not be trusted. At times he was able to express open hatred of his father for abandoning him and he demonstrated sexual confusion in his relationship with his mother. Most of the stories told in the Thematic Apperception Test involved unhappy endings.

On admission to the hospital, the patient was markedly hyperactive and at times attempted to grab at the breasts of the nurses as he did at his mother's. He was, at first, sullen and resentful of limits and discipline but gradually established relationships of trust with his psychiatrist and other staff members. At first he appeared isolated from his peer group and to relate better to children much younger than himself, but there was evidence of gradual improvement in his peer relationships during the six weeks that he was in the hospital. In view of his mother's ambivalent combination of erotic dependency on and hostile rejection of him, placement in a foster home was considered, but his mother did not accept this recommendation and insisted on taking him home with her.

Weekly interviews were continued with both of them,

and nine months later his mother remarried. Although the boy's stepfather was never involved in therapy, it appeared that he was very understanding of the boy's problems. He provided both a satisfactory model for identification and an accepting authority figure who could set consistent, firm limits on the boy's behavior. The mother's seductive behavior toward the boy diminished as she established a more mature erotic relationship with her husband. Therapy was terminated six months after the mother's remarriage and apparently there were no recurrences of delinquency or gasoline inhaling.

Organic Brain Syndromes in Childhood

The incidence of organic brain syndromes, it will be recalled, reaches a peak in childhood as it does in old age. These syndromes may be caused by the same infections, intoxications, convulsions, trauma, cerebrovascular accidents and intracranial tumors as organic brain disorders in adults, but especially by the high fevers and convulsions that may result from childhood infections. As in adults, severe damage to the brains of children may lead to chronic, irreversible syndromes, but, in young children, the latter syndromes usually result in lifelong mental subnormality of some degree. The younger the child when the damage occurs, the more likely he is to remain intellectually retarded and the more severe the retardation is likely to be. Congenital anomalies of the brain, for instance, usually result in some degree of mental subnormality that may or may not be associated with physical handicaps, such as paralyses, contractures, blindness or deafness. Brain lesions occurring after birth may result in partial or complete arrest of intellectual development, loss of functions already possessed, or behavior disturbances.

Damage to a child's central nervous system may be temporary or permanent. It may eventuate in spontaneous or therapeutic restoration of the disordered functions, although seldom at the level of the prepsychotic personality, to stabilization of the condition, or to progressive deterioration with or without periods of remission. The behavior of a child with brain damage is the result not only of intellectual changes or deficits, but also of emotional and social consequences of the interaction among biological, environmental and psychological forces. Children with physical handicaps resulting from congenital abnormalities may also manifest behavior disturbances as a reaction to their handicaps, rather than to the brain damage that caused the handicap.

The average child is exposed, during the course of normal development, to a number of acute infections that may result in typical manifestations of acute reversible brain syndromes, including delirium, mild drowsiness, stupor and coma. Apparently the nervous system of some children is more vulnerable than that of others to high fevers and various disturbances in metabolism, although acute brain syndromes resulting from childhood infections are less frequent now than formerly. The decrease in incidence has been a consequence of the combination of successful preventive measures, such as immunization against some infections, and the availability of antibiotic therapy that is effective against some others. Convulsions frequently are precipitated by high fevers or any condition in which the brain cell functions are altered. Lennox (1953) has estimated that about 2 per cent of children have one or more convulsions associated with fever within the first five years of life.

A form of intoxication that causes brain syndromes in children more often than is realized is lead poisoning. It is frequently a result of *pica*, an abnormal craving for unnatural articles of food, such as sand, hair, paint, plaster and various materials that may contain lead, a disorder more common among mentally subnormal or deprived children. Young children may ingest toxic quantities of lead from toys, furniture and the smoke from the burning of leaded objects.

Brain tumors are rarer in children than in adults, occurring only about one-fifth as often. They are sometimes difficult to diagnose, for the consequent behavior disturbances may depend more on the personality of the patient than on the size or location of the tumor.

Syndromes which are chronic in nature typically result in a deterioration of comprehension, memory, judgment and capacity for verbal communication. If speech was acquired before the illness, it may be partially or wholly abolished; if the illness takes place before speech is acquired, the child may remain mute, learn to speak late or learn to speak only rudimentarily. The child's intellectual processes are impaired and he may develop epilepsy. Among other common results are extreme restlessness, confusional states and the inability to use experience and recognize and avoid danger. Many children manifest antisocial trends. Some chronic syndromes are described in the following paragraphs.

Postencephalitic Syndrome. As the name indicates, the disorder is a result of encephalitis (inflammation of the brain) which may be of the epidemic variety or the aftermath of many children's infections. It includes a wide variety of neurologic, personality and behavior disorders. Damage is more pronounced in younger than in older children. The organic damage appears to destroy areas of the brain that regulate inhibitions that have been set up by training, so the child may become extremely restless, impulsive, intractable, unmanageable, antisocial, brutal, destructive and dangerous. Drug therapy is successful in reducing some of the excitement, but in severe cases institutionalization is necessary.

Juvenile Paresis. This brain disease is caused by congenital syphilis. As a result of the routine serological testing of mothers, however, it has become rare in the United States. Although syphilis among adults is more frequent in males than in females, in children the distribution is almost equal between boys and girls. It is still not known why some children with congenital syphilis develop paresis and others do not. The clinical symptoms are very similar to those of adults, and penicillin is the preferred treatment.

Epilepsy. In over half of all persons with epilepsy the onset occurs in childhood. The incidence among school-age children has been estimated as approximately 7 per 1000. Although the disorder has been noted to begin at almost any time in a child's life, three periods have been especially marked: during the first two years of life, at the beginning of school attendance, and at the start of puberty.

Children appear to have fewer attacks of grand mal than of other types of epilepsy. The seizures themselves are identical in nature with those of adults except that auras are less common among children. They may, however, display prodromal symptoms for hours or even days before a seizure. Usual symptoms include irritability, dullness, headache or digestive disturbances. Some children may have but one or two grand mal seizures in a lifetime, but in others the attacks may be so frequent and severe that the child becomes severely subnormal mentally and requires permanent hospitalization.

Prodromal symptoms do not precede petit mal seizures. Pyknolepsy is a variant of epilepsy resembling petit mal, except that the attacks are brief and mild; they occur frequently (from several up to 100 or more a day); they do not interfere with mental development; and they disappear spontaneously after three or four years and, at the latest, by puberty. Psychomotor attacks are uncommon in children.

Most epileptic children have normal intelligence. Lennox (1949) studied 1640 epileptics in clinics and private practice and found that 67 per cent were normal in intelligence, 23 per cent were slightly subnormal and only 10 per cent displayed severe intellectual deterioration.

Behavior problems and personality disturbances occur in about half of all epileptic children. The traits displayed, however, appear to be as much a result of the child's premorbid personality, or the reaction to his disorder, or the attitudes displayed by the adults around him, as of the disorder itself.

Minimal Brain Dysfunction

A term which is increasingly used in the diagnosis of children is minimal brain dysfunction. This diagnosis refers to children who have some central nervous system deficits which affect their behavior and their ability to learn in several different ways (U. S. Public Health Service, 1966). Such children may be of normal or high intellectual level and yet have school learning difficulties. Typically the difficulties arise from impairments in perception, conceptualization, language and memory, either singularly or in various combinations. Since such deviations may be slight they are difficult to detect except on very careful examination. Behavioral descriptions may include hyperactivity, distractibility, short attention span, impulsivity and aggressiveness. Typically, minimal brain dysfunctioning does not leave the child so impaired that his difficulty is readily apparent. Consequently he is often believed to have other problems. For example, a hyperactive boy of above average intelligence who is easily distracted, disinterested in school, prone to temper tantrums and reads poorly may be misdiagnosed as having an emotional problem resulting from a lack of consistent, firm controls. In fact, he may have minimal brain damage resulting in perceptual deficits which make learning to read overly difficult if he is taught in the same manner as children without such problems. This in itself can lead to frustration and aggressiveness when the child is unable to measure up to his own expectations as well as those of his parents and teacher. A child with perceptual problems may be able to learn to read by learning to use other perceptual cues, such as wooden letters he can feel as well as see in learning the alphabet. By using both the sense of touch and vision some bright children with perceptual problems can learn quite readily. Likewise, a child is likely to be seen as spoiled, rebellious and a bully because of his low frustration tolerance and aggressiveness when such behaviors may be the result of a central nervous system deficit. The symptoms shown in minimal brain dysfunction are also found in organic brain syndromes but are less extreme and more difficult to detect.

Reading Problems

The most common reason for referring a child to a guidance clinic, in the United States, is some school difficulty. Most often, the difficulty is academic failure, which, in a high proportion of cases, is accompanied by a reading problem that may or may not be the cause of the failure. In some instances, the child does not learn to read at all; more commonly, he acquires some minimal reading facility, but at a level markedly below most of the children in his grade. His reading deficiency becomes more and more of a problem as he progresses through the grades because so much learning in the majority of school subjects is based on the ability to read and comprehend what is read.

Reading problems are very prevalent in the school-age population, and, as a result, receive a great deal of public attention. In many popular articles the reasons for the problems are purported to be inadequate early teaching, faulty curricula with too much emphasis on nonacademic subjects, or coddling, which is believed to destroy a child's motivation to learn.

The etiology of reading problems, in fact, is complex. Children with reading problems do not form a homogeneous group: some are handicapped by limited intelligence; others lack biologic readiness; some have brain damage; and a large number do not learn to read because of psychogenic disturbances. Most children cannot learn to read until they reach a mental age of about six. A child with below average intelligence may be seven or eight years old chronologically before his mental age is high enough. By this time he may have experienced great frustration in his attempts to learn to read so that the problem becomes further complicated by the effects of his failure experiences. In addition to possessing the necessary intelligence, a certain level of biologic

readiness must be achieved by the child before he can learn to read with ease. Reading readiness tests have been designed to estimate whether or not the child has this readiness. For example, one series of Reading Aptitude Tests (Munroe, 1935) is comprised of visual tests designed to measure orientation of forms, oculomotor control and visual memory; auditory tests that include measures of pronunciation, discrimination of sounds and auditory memory; language tests; articulation tests; and tests of motor skills that include both speed and steadiness. The child's competence in these basic skills determines with considerable accuracy how well he will learn to read.

In some children minimal brain dysfunctioning affects the areas that govern language functioning so that they may have particular difficulty with concept formation, visual-auditory memory or association, resulting in a general reading problem. As knowledge in this area increases, it is becoming apparent that many children with reading problems are aphasic. Still other children cannot learn to read because they are incapacitated by anxiety, preoccupation with other matters or a limited attention span. For still others, reading failure is a means of expressing rebelliousness—for which no other outlets are psychologically possible—against parents and teachers. In summary, children with reading problems may fall into any of the diagnostic categories described previously. They may evidence transient adjustment problems, or they may be neurotic, psychotic, delinquent, or mentally subnormal or have brain damage. A child with a reading problem must be given a careful diagnostic examination in order to determine the nature and extent of his deficiency and the probable etiological factors involved.

CAUSATION, DEVELOPMENT AND DYNAMICS

Childhood disorders are essentially determined by the same etiological factors that determine the development in adults of neuroses, psychoses, character problems, psychophysiologic reactions, organic brain syndromes and mental subnormality. These factors and their complex interactions have been discussed fully in previous chapters and, therefore, are not included here. The content of this section, for the most part, is confined to material that is more applicable to children than adults and is not included elsewhere.

Heredity and Other Biological Factors

Very little information can be added to the discussions in previous chapters on the role of heredity in the causation of functional disorders. The two investigations presented here, however, are especially pertinent to the etiology of functional disorders in children.

Kallmann and Roth (1956), studying twins with "pre-adolescent schizophrenia," that is, schizophrenia developed before the age of 15, reported a much higher frequency of concordance among monozygotic than dizygotic co-twins of the same sex, an apparent indication of a hereditary etiology in childhood schizophrenia. Certain other disorders of childhood also appear to be strongly influenced by hereditary factors. Shields and Slater (1960) summarized the results of several twin studies of juvenile delinquency and behavior disorders or neurotic traits in childhood, and in each noted a higher frequency of concordance in MZ than in DZ co-twins of the same sex. Unfortunately, modern serological techniques for determining zygosity were not used in any of the preceding studies so that the findings are no more convincing than those of similar studies of adult twins. Furthermore, it is impossible to test specific hypotheses of the genetic transmission of specific disorders of childhood (except for mental subnormality), because the objective diagnostic criteria and family data necessary for statistical analysis are lacking.

The conclusions reached in previous chapters on the role of heredity in the etiology of functional disorders in adults are also valid for children.

Organic lesions of the brain have been clearly established as the basic cause of behavior disturbances associated with severe mental subnormality and brain syndromes developed after birth. Despite intensive investigations, comparable disorders of brain structure or function have not been found consistently or established definitely to be influential in other psychiatric disorders in children. A number of psychologists and psychiatrists (Bender, 1947; Goldfarb, 1961) have hypothesized that some children manifesting symptoms that lead to diagnoses of childhood schizophrenia do, in fact, have organic brain abnormalities, but the usual neurologic examination procedures are inadequate to uncover them. Similarly, Rimland (1964) attributes infantile autism to a single, highly specific type of cognitive defect, occurring on a neurophysiologic basis. Although these assumptions are still not verified, the histories of many such youngsters and the psychological test data accumulated on them are strongly suggestive of neurologic problems.

Stott (1959, 1962) believed that congenital defects were a major factor in the etiology of learning, reading and personality problems in children. He called attention not only to the academic problems of such children but also to a personality syndrome that was frequent among them. He summarized the characteristics — quietness, withdrawal, lack of self-confidence and poor motivation — with the term "unforthcomingness." He believed that prenatal stress in many of these children had made the fetus and then the infant especially susceptible to disease. In one study (1959), he followed up as school children a group of British infants who had been hospitalized for two weeks or longer very early in life. He found a higher incidence of the academic and personality problems in the group that had been hospitalized than in the control group. In a later study (1962), he surveyed the physical and emotional histories of 105 mentally subnormal children, some of whom had not received normal mothering. He was especially interested in these cases because of the opinions held by many investigators that maternal deprivation in one form or another is an important etiological factor in some cases of extreme retardation, which are sometimes labeled severe mental subnormality and sometimes schizophrenic disorders. He found, however, that in each child who had not had normal mothering there was an alternative factor — a suggestion of brain damage or prenatal stress — to which his disorder could be attributed and which might have contributed etiologically to his subnormality. Nor could maternal deprivation be considered the cause of academic retardation or "unforthcomingness," in his opinion, for he found no relation between the disturbances and length of early hospitalization to support the thesis.

In a similar investigation, Kawi and Pasamanick (1959) studied 372 boys with severe reading problems and the obstetric histories of 205 of them. The mothers of the subjects, when compared with matched controls, had a significantly higher incidence of obstetric complications; the more severe the reading problems were, the higher was the incidence of such complications. The most prominent complications were bleeding during pregnancy and toxemias.

Glueck and Glueck (1956) reported a much higher frequency of mesomorphic or "athletic" body build among persistent male delinquents than among matched nondelinquent controls. Unfortunately, the cause and effect relations responsible for such correlations are difficult to disentangle. Is the child delinquent because he is a mesomorph or is he a mesomorph because he is delinquent? (The confusions intrinsic to body-type studies were discussed in Chapter 6.) The higher frequency of delinquency and other behavior disorders among boys than girls (discussed in part in Chapter 16) may be attributed to inherent biologic differences, to differences in social learning and expectations, or to a combination of both factors. Certainly, Harlow (1962) has demonstrated differences in the behavior of male and female monkeys at a very early age that, presumably, are due to inherent biologic differences. The importance of social learning, however, is greater in humans than in subhuman species, and differences in the behavior of very young boys and girls may have been learned when they were even younger.

Psychological Determinants

In discussing learning theories in Chapter 7, a number of studies were reviewed that demonstrated the effects of the individual's early learning experiences on his development and later behavior. The kinds of learning found to have lasting effects on the individual included: (1) interoceptive conditioning, i.e., learning in which response patterns are set up within the internal organs of the body; (2) avoidance learning, i.e., learning by means of responses to stimuli that are consistently associated with very unpleasant experiences; and (3) operant learning that involves intermittent reinforcement —i.e., learning in which the organism becomes progressively more likely to respond in a situation with the same response that, in previous similar situations, sometimes brought him a reward. In addition, it was noted that bodily and emotional development may be affected adversely by either overstimulation or understimulation, as well as by isolation or deprivation— i.e., the lack of normal interaction with either parents or peers.

The human infant is completely dependent upon his parents and parent substitutes for stimulation and early learning experiences: they determine both the quantity and quality of what he receives. Great emphasis must be placed on the fact that much of a child's early learning is based on the nonverbal as well as verbal communications of affect and role-expectation which he receives from the significant persons in his immediate environment. This is true in preschool years as well as in infancy, for he is still dependent on parents during the preschool years: they determine his peer-relationships by their approval or disapproval, and, since the child generalizes from his family and early associates, they also contribute to his lifelong evaluations of himself and other people. A child's parents may be predictable or unpredictable; they may be consistent or inconsistent in the manner in which they gratify or frustrate his needs; they may be unexplainably absent or constantly with him; indifferent or excessively concerned; unconcerned for his welfare or overprotective or dominating. To a greater or lesser extent, the child internalizes his parents' instructions and prohibitions and identifies with their attitudes and ideals.

Because early experience is extremely varied and difficult to observe directly or reconstruct retrospectively in an objective manner, a direct causal relationship between early experiences and most forms of psychological disturbance has not yet been established. Everyone is very selective in remembering his childhood, no matter how inclusive he may try to be. In a similar fashion, parents are apparently selective in thinking about their children and themselves as parents. It has been discovered that mothers and fathers often describe their children differently and disagree on the nature of the disciplinary role that each plays. Although more direct observation of childhood relationships and experiences is encouraged, observers unwittingly select and interpret what they report. In addition, it is virtually impossible to infer with much accuracy the motivations that determine the actions of parents.

On the basis of our present knowledge, it appears that most manifestations of abnormal behavior are not the result of a single traumatic event, but of maladaptive learning that has occurred over a period of time. A change in the child's behavior, of course, may follow an event as traumatic as the death or permanent desertion of a parent. The loss of, or separation from, a parent may have profound adverse consequences for the child. The immediate visible effects are often diagnosed as reactive depressions. Some children may react to parental deprivation by longer lasting symptoms, such as vulnerability to depression, schizophrenia and delinquency. In most surveys of the child guidance clinic and child psychiatric hospital populations, and of juvenile delinquents, a higher percentage is found of parental absence in the home than in matched controls or in the general population (Glueck and Glueck, 1950; Kanner, 1957). Tuckman and Regan (1966) found that 33 per cent of 1767 children referred to guidance clinics come from broken homes, whereas only 10 per cent of children in the general population have broken home backgrounds. In Britain, Brown (1961) compared the records of adult outpatients diagnosed as depressives with general population data from the 1921 census and also with private practice patients, and discovered a significantly higher incidence of the loss of a parent before the age of 15 years in the depressive patients than in the others. Glueck and Glueck (1950) found a considerably higher frequency of all forms of parental loss in a group of 500 persistent delinquents than in a matched group of 500 nondelinquent controls.

Bowlby (1951) and others have suggested that a nonexistent or pathological relationship with the mother is more significant in the development of psychological disturbance than a nonexistent or pathological relationship with the father. This thesis, however, is based on evidence that largely associates the loss of both parents with ensuing delinquency. Andry (1960) found that when both parents were present in the home delinquent boys perceived greater defects in the roles of their fathers than in those of their mothers, whereas nondelinquents tended to perceive the roles of both parents as inadequate. Since many children tend to identify predominantly with the parent of the same sex, additional study may indicate that delinquent girls are more frequently exposed to the examples of delinquent mothers. The loss of either parent, however, or prolonged interaction with an abnormal parent of either sex, may precede the development of psychological disturbance in both boys or girls, although the predisposing significance of such factors remains largely a matter of conjecture.

For many years clinical workers have reported their impressions that the parents of patients in child psychiatric clinics and hospitals are often themselves psychologically disturbed and, therefore, unable to provide normal environments for their families. Not until recently, however, has this impression been investigated in any objective manner. Since 1959, several studies have been reported in which the MMPI was administered to such parents and compared with the MMPI's of parents whose children were not psychiatric patients (Hanvik and Byrum, 1959; Liverant, 1959; Goodstein and Rowley, 1961; Marks, 1961; Wolking et al., 1964). In general the results indicated that the parents of child psychiatric patients are a select group, measurably different from parents in the general population. The differences are markedly in the direction of personality deviation and maladjustment. According to these results, the parents of child psychiatric patients are maladjusted, but the maladjustment is a matter of degree: the parents are disturbed, but less so than persons who themselves seek help for personal psychological problems. Although it cannot be said with certainty that the problems of children are "caused" by the psychological disturbances of the parents (who may be, in part, reacting with more than usual anxiety, hostility and so forth to the burden of caring for difficult children), nevertheless, the studies indicate, at least, that the child is living in an environment in which considerable psychological disturbance is present. And, in view of the known stability of adult MMPI profiles over time, it is reasonable to suppose that, in many cases, the parents' maladjustment does have etiological significance for the problems of the child.

Some of the same authors have investigated the frequency with which various types of MMPI profiles occur among their parent populations in order to determine what types especially characterize this group. The next step, of course, is to determine whether certain kinds of child problems are associated with any particular types of parent profiles. Pioneers in this area are Hanvik and Byrum (1959), Marks (1961) and Wolking et al. (1964), who found that parents of patients in child psychiatric clinics and hospitals made significantly higher scores on a number of scales. The profiles seen most frequently were highest on the psychopathic deviate and hysteria scales. This is a profile often found in persons who, although frequently outwardly conforming, have hostile and rebellious feelings that are expressed indirectly. Many of them establish relationships with marginal, nonconforming, somewhat antisocial individuals, thereby, possibly, vicariously gratifying their own antisocial tendencies. The frequency of this type of profile among such parents appears to support the theories of Johnson. As a result of her clinical work with children and their parents, Johnson (1959) and

Johnson and Szurek (1952) hypothesized that antisocial acting out in children is unconsciously fostered and sanctioned by parents as a vicarious gratification of their own forbidden impulses. In turn, she postulated, the child's behavior stimulated an increased need in the parents for such satisfaction. Also, the child's acting out behavior unconsciously gratifies the destructive wishes of one or both parents toward the child who is repeatedly punished or "destroyed" for his behavior. Johnson described parents who experience obvious pleasure in describing their children's acting out behavior, and cited a number of examples of the verbalized evasions and deceptions of parents, such as "Here is an extra quarter, but don't tell your father," "You can get into the movie for half price, since you certainly don't look 12 years old," which subtly encourage the child in his antisocial activities.

Similarly, a neurotic child may be exposed to verbal reassurance but at the same time be given nonverbal reinforcement for his anxieties and fears. Conflicting communications have also been held responsible for the double-bind situation reported for some schizophrenics, in which they are required to act but meet with disapproval no matter what actions they take. Such formulations are all compatible with the theory that much maladaptive behavior is learned from inappropriate reinforcement.

Research on relationships between personality and behavior disorders of parents and children is still in its early phases. Wolking et al. (1964) report tentatively that the formal psychiatric diagnoses of children are easier to relate to the personalities of their parents than are the symptoms that the children manifest. They found that patients, particularly boys, with conversion reactions tend to have hypochondriacal fathers, and that patients with psychosomatic problems tend to have highly neurotic mothers with very similar problems. Symptoms, in general, are more related to age and sex than to either parent's personality characteristics. For example, adolescents are very often referred for psychiatric evaluation and treatment because of nonconforming behavior; children in middle childhood tend to be referred because of habit mannerisms, fears, anxiety and so forth; and in the preschool group, some difficulty in development, such as slowness, is perhaps the most common presenting complaint.

Relative social isolation has long been considered one of the possible determinants of schizophrenia in both adults and children.

Harlow (1962) raised in isolation infant monkeys of which some manifested autistic behavior, such as clutching their heads in both hands and rocking back and forth, and others manifested violent frenzies of rage (spontaneously or when approached), grasping and tearing at their legs in such fury that they sometimes required medical care. Equally interesting was his observation that normal adult social, sexual and maternal behavior depended on opportunities for early play contact with other young monkeys. Although comparable data for children are lacking, one might hypothesize from clinical experience that children who are deprived of interactions with other young children start life with a severe disadvantage that may result in persistent or progressively increasing isolation and excessive dependency on inner fantasy.

The significance of nonverbal communication has been explored by a number of authors. Stewart et al. (1954) studied excessive infant crying (colic) in relation to parental behavior, and reported that parents whose babies cried excessively responded inappropriately and inconsistently to their infants' needs with either overstimulation or relative neglect.

There is no question that the psychological climate of the child's home and his early interpersonal relations are crucial in determining many of his reactions, the defenses he learns and comes to use and the personality that he develops. However, much further research is required to establish the nature and specificity of various determinants of abnormal behavior.

Sociocultural Factors

It was noted earlier (Chapter 8) that some severe forms of adult psychological disturbance have been observed in all known cultures, although the manifestations of the disturbances may vary from one culture to another. The frequencies of the disorders may vary also, but since accurate transcultural incidence rates are not available, the amount of disturbance among adults in different cultures can only be inferred. Childhood psychological disturbance is even more difficult to compare across cultures, and even within cultures, because of its more amorphous nature and the greater variability in judging the behaviors of children. In our society, for example, there is a paucity of facts on the nature and frequency of different behaviors and symptoms in the children born into various social, economic and subcultural groups. In recent years investigators have become increasingly interested in observing the similarities and differences in the child-rearing practices found in these various groups, in the hope that new understandings of personality development would be gained from them.

One of the first detailed analyses of social-class differences in child rearing was compiled in Chicago by Davis and Havighurst (1946). Their findings, based on interview data gathered from middle and lower class mothers, indicated that middle class mothers were less permissive than lower class mothers. As a result of this and similar studies, social scientists began to picture lower class attitudes toward children as relaxed, expressive and generally undemanding. Subsequently, however, these interpretations were questioned and, largely as a result of more recent studies of class differences in child-rearing practices, have since been re-examined and reinterpreted. One such study, by Klatskin (1952), was based on data from 223 mothers at the New Haven Hospital rooming-in project; another, by Sears et al. (1957), was based on data obtained from structured interviews with 372 mothers from urban areas in New England. The results of both studies indicated that, contrary to the earlier findings, middle class mothers, by and large, are more gentle and less punitive toward their children. In the Sears study, the areas of socialization investigated included infant feeding, toilet training, dependency, sex training and aggression. Significant differences were not found between the classes in infant feeding but in the other four areas middle class mothers were generally more permissive than working class mothers. Physical punishment was employed less often, more vigorous activity was permitted in the houses, and the children were given more freedom to roam, visit and explore their neighborhoods. Middle class parents permitted more dependency, more expression of aggression against both themselves and other people, and were generally warmer and more demonstrative toward their children. Husbands and wives disagreed less on child-rearing attitudes and practices. It is true that the majority of mothers in both classes were affectionate and positive toward their children, but in a few cases a clear pattern of rejection emerged and these were found more often among the working class, less educated families.

Takala (1960) studied child-raising practices in the upper and lower classes in Finland and found many of the same differences as did Sears and his associates. Finnish upper class parents were less punitive and compulsive, and more democratic, in their relationships with children.

Kohn and Carroll (1960) investigated the attitudes of members of the middle and working classes toward support and constraint as part of the parental role. The mother was interviewed in each of the families and in every fourth family the father and a fifth-grade child as well. According to the results, middle class mothers expected their husbands to be primarily as supportive as they, and only secondarily to impose constraints. Working class mothers, on the other hand, wanted their husbands to be more directive and impose more constraints. Middle class fathers shared their wives' conceptions of the allocation of responsibilities toward sons, but seem to have been less supportive toward their daughters, apparently feeling that management of girls was more properly within the mothers' domains. Working class fathers, on the contrary, did not appear to assume either the directive role expected by their wives or the more highly supportive role seen in middle class fathers. To them, child rearing was completely the responsibility of their wives. The middle class boys who were interviewed seemed to identify with their fathers; they saw them as at least as supportive as their mothers who, in a sizable proportion of middle class families, took primary responsibilities for imposing constraints on the sons. Working class boys found it difficult to identify with their fathers; they associated support with their mothers and constraint with their fathers, although, in reality, both roles were assumed by the mothers.

TREATMENT

Kanner (1957) has traced, since the beginning of the century, various changes in attitudes toward the treatment of children's problems. In the early 1900's as part of a new cultural trend, people began to "think *about* children" and psychometry, dynamic psychiatry, juvenile courts and the mental hygiene movement were developed. In the next stage, leaders thought in terms of "doing things *to* children," and community facilities, such as special classes for the retarded and handicapped, probation for juvenile offenders and regulated foster home care, were organized to handle children with problems. The attitude then changed to "doing things *for* children," and the efforts of child guidance clinic personnel led to studies of family, school and community relationships, and to working with parents and teachers, to create more favorable emotional environments for children. In the 1940's and 1950's the emphasis turned to "working *with* children." Thus, at last, the child himself became the primary patient and directly involved in the therapeutic program. Implicit in these changes were the beliefs that not only should efforts be made to prevent maladjustment, improve social conditions and so forth, but that emotionally upset children also deserved direct treatment for their immediate problems. In current practice, evaluation and treatment of the child often takes place in the context of family membership so that not only he, but other members of his family, can be simultaneously involved in psychotherapy—both to minimize whatever contribution they are making to the child's problems and to help them with their own emotional problems. In any inclusive program of treatment for the disorders of childhood, however, all of these approaches must be combined and none emphasized to the exclusion of the others.

Effective treatment unlike successful techniques of prevention, is not always based on accurate knowledge of causation. This generalization applies to disorders of behavior as well as bodily function, and to disorders of childhood as well as to those of adults. The approach to treatment, therefore, is flexible and individualized; when the causation is known, such knowledge is utilized, otherwise, empirical methods that have proved effective are used. Working with children frequently requires a combination of approaches, such as interviews, psychotherapy with the parents, psychotherapy for the child, evaluation of school performance and remedial work in reading, spelling and so forth. Cooperation with welfare services may be necessary to ensure sufficient food and clothing for the child, or, in some cases, foster home placement. Environmental manipulation, such as providing household help for the mother to enable her to devote more time and interest to the child, may be indicated in some cases.

Speers and Lansing (1965) have described a rather successful group therapy program with autistic children. In this program children were seen regularly for over four years. Psychotherapists worked with the parents both individually and in groups. The authors also found it necessary to enlist the aid of remedial teaching specialists, school teachers and recreational therapists.

The same major approaches that are employed in psychotherapy with adults (discussed in Chapter 21) have also been used in working with children. They can be summarized as follows: (1) directive, authoritarian or suppressive therapy, involving a relationship of rapport and such techniques as advice, persuasion and suggestion; (2) nondirective relationship or release therapy, in which the therapeutic relationship is conceived as an immediate experience, and the therapist seeks to help the child draw on his own capacities toward a more creative acceptance and use of the self he has; (3) psychoanalytic therapy, in which the child's transference to the therapist (based on displacement of his unconscious emotions toward parents and other significant adults) is analyzed and interpreted; (4) psychotherapy that is based on learning theory and selectively reinforces adaptive behavior and extinguishes maladaptive behavior. Play therapy (described in Chapter 21) was especially designed for work with children.

Exponents of these various approaches are often quite critical of one another; nevertheless considerable overlap in the philosophies and techniques are frequently seen. Probably the most widespread approach to children's problems to date has been that of relationship therapy. Some of its implicit assumptions are expressed in the following passage from a pamphlet edited by the Jewish Board of Guardians and quoted by Bovet (1951):

Part of the treatment of many children consists of helping them to develop genuine affection for the worker (or for the educator, therapist, etc.). To love is to be vulnerable, whether it is between child and parents, between man and woman, between friends—or client and therapist. Poets have described it, scientists have proved it and everybody knows it. It is to place one's vital happiness at the mercy of another, to expose the most sensitive feelings to the possibility of abiding pain should this reaching out to another person be met with coolness or outright rebuff. Yet, without the capacity for affection, no permanent or deep happiness or contentment is possible. [Maladjusted children]. . . have had over and over again in their own lives the painful experience of being disappointed and frustrated in their close attachments, usually in their immediate family, and they fear to repeat this experience. Since such a child suffers from an inability to enter warm and satisfying relationships with other people, it becomes the task of the case worker to give him the experience of exchanging trust and affection with another person. The child is truly helped when he can permit himself to feel and to display affection once more and to find out that, although hurt may be in the offing, there is also potential happiness and growth in relinquishing the inward bitterness which had prevented a wholesome energetic approach to life; in its stead is substituted a readiness to like other people, a warmth and richness of feeling which are the essentials for a creative and happy life.

A number of child therapists would agree that this approach is most likely to be effective in repairing some of the damage resulting from prolonged emotional deprivation. Bettelheim (1950) and others, however, have rightly noted that love is not enough to remove all symptoms of emotional disturbance. Love, in its broadest sense, is not a process of unlimited giving without demands. On the contrary, emotional security results from unlimited affection with the imposition of consistent, firm limits on behavior so that the child may develop normal tolerance for frustration and respect for the rights of others. Thus, it is frequently considered desirable for both parents of the disturbed child to receive guidance, counseling or even individual psychotherapy.

Child psychiatrists were among the first to involve other family members in the treatment of disturbed behavior manifested by a child. One of the primary reasons, as has been pointed out earlier, is that emotional disorders in children are generally associated with the presence of emotional disorders in one or both parents, and treatment of the parents may result in improvement in the children's behavior. Howells (1961) and others, however, have emphasized that the child referred for psychological or psychiatric evaluation is not necessarily the most disturbed child in the family and that a child may have a considerable influence on a sibling. The involvement of siblings in therapy, therefore, may lead to improvement both in the child with the presenting problem and in other siblings who, otherwise, would not have been involved in therapy. It has also been observed (Ackerman, 1958) that treating one member of a family sometimes upsets a kind of balance within the family and may have a negative effect on other members and, therefore, other members should also become involved in psychotherapy for themselves.

Some disagreement has arisen over whether a single therapist can effectively treat both child and parents, and a usual pattern found in child guidance clinics is for a psychiatrist to treat the child and a social worker to counsel the parents. Because the demand for this type of

team therapy is great and the available personnel is limited; individuals in the field sometimes express the idea that only cases most likely to benefit from therapy should be accepted for treatment. (Such cases are also most likely to improve spontaneously.) These individuals would also impose additional restrictions on patients seeking help, such as accepting only cases in which both parents can be involved in the therapeutic process. This type of rigid thinking leads to the exclusion of many children who might benefit from psychotherapy to some degree.

Although the training and philosophy of the therapist often determines the treatment applied to the child, usually the type of therapy is determined largely by the child's age and the extent to which his attitudes and patterns of behavior—the initial responses to external situations—have become internalized and habitual. The young infant who is brought to the clinic by an overanxious or inadequate mother may benefit indirectly from counseling or psychotherapy undertaken with the mother alone. A preschool child may be helped by a single therapist interviewing both child and parents. The school-age child is more likely to require individual therapy but, at the same time, his parents and other significant adults are usually also involved in therapy with the same or a different therapist. The adolescent child may require prolonged individual psychotherapy and environmental manipulation, and other members of his family may or may not be involved.

When more than one therapist is concerned in the treatment of two or more members of a family, it is necessary for the therapists to confer with one another fairly often. These conferences, held in addition to the therapy sessions, are time-consuming and, thus, expensive. Consequently, the trend is for one therapist to see an entire family simultaneously. In addition, he is able to see at first hand the interactions among the various family members. Such sessions are an excellent source of information on family dynamics and interaction patterns. Bell (1961) has outlined a procedure for family-centered, rather than child-centered, treatment that, although directed toward helping the disturbed adolescent, is useful for children and adults as well. Family therapists have come to realize that many problems arise from crippling interaction patterns in the family. As family relationships and alliances are altered, changes in the child's behavior are more likely to occur and to receive the necessary support from the family. Family therapy is being used more and more in this country as the treatment of choice for many childhood disorders.

The attitudes and behavior of parents toward children may be dependent upon emotional factors that they cannot modify, even when they become aware of them. Making parents feel guilty for a child's behavior problems seldom improves matters; sometimes they become more emotionally disturbed and, hence, more disturbing to the child; sometimes parents with very disturbed children refuse to participate in therapy; and sometimes therapy involving both child and parents may be ineffectual in breaking the vicious cycle of hostile interaction between them. Under such circumstances a therapeutic separation may be desirable, and Howells (1963) has discussed various forms, such as complete or partial, temporary or permanent separation and even foster home or adoptive placement.

Ideally, placements are made with the understanding that in normal personality development stable long-term relationships with relatively well-adjusted parents or parent substitutes of each sex are essential. Unfortunately, the importance of this long-term stability is sometimes overlooked. It may even be preferable for a child to remain in a stable relationship with one or two somewhat inadequate parents than to experience the disturbance of making and breaking relationships which is implicit in short-term placements in one or more "good" foster home settings. When these considerations have been weighed carefully and therapeutic separation from parents is still considered mandatory,

every effort is made to place the child in a home with a well-adjusted and well-motivated parent substitute of each sex. The younger the child and the greater the psychological disturbance of his own parents, the more desirable it is that therapeutic separation be permanent and that it be followed by legal adoption rather than temporary foster home placement.

Hundreds of child guidance clinics, many hospitals, and residential treatment programs are now operated for children in the United States. Literally hundreds of thousands of children have been evaluated and treated for various disorders. In view of this, it is distressing that only a very few follow-up studies of such children are found in the literature. One of the best studies was conducted in St. Louis by O'Neal and Robins (1958). They found that patients of a child guidance clinic 30 years earlier manifested a high rate of psychiatric disorder as adults, in comparison with a matched group of normal controls. The patients differed little from the normal controls in rate of neurotic reactions but included many more cases with psychotic reactions, sociopathic personalities and alcoholism. Most of those with the diagnosis of sociopathic personality had been juvenile delinquents as children. Those rated psychiatrically normal had had, for the most part, neurotic problems as children. Neurotics, of course, are generally considered to have a more favorable prognosis than other diagnostic groups, whether or not they receive psychiatric treatment. The effectiveness of various treatment procedures, therefore, requires considerable further evaluation.

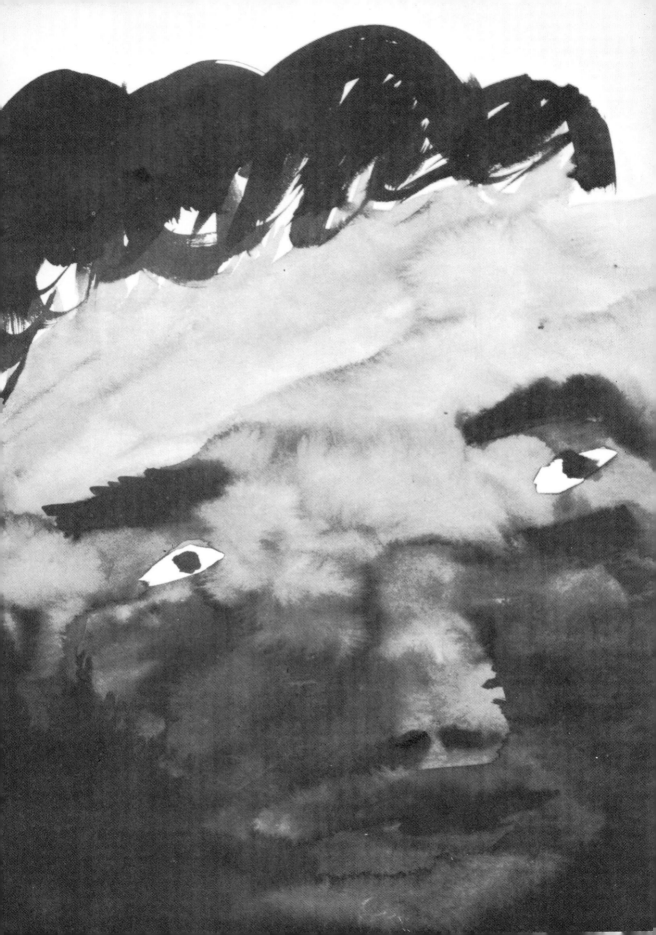

Speak of me as I am; nothing extenuate,
Nor set down aught in malice.

William Shakespeare, *Othello*

20

EVALUATION

In the preceding chapters we surveyed the classification, development, dynamics and multiple causes of psychological disorders as well as some specific syndromes; in the next chapter we shall discuss methods of treatment. The bridge between the earlier topics and treatment is evaluation of the individual patient and his difficulties.

One might suppose that patients would freely provide the information needed to evaluate them. Unfortunately this is often not the case. Patients may hold back much of what must be known. They disguise, completely disown or are unaware of thoughts, attitudes, motivations, fantasies and goals which may be important to the diagnostician. The behavior of a typical emotionally disturbed patient may be compared to that of an imaginary medical patient who appears in a doctor's office complaining of a severe pain but is unable to reveal where or how it hurts. The psychiatric patient, like everyone else, has a history of trained privacy. He has strong habits of dissembling shameful thoughts or feelings and concealing, both from himself and others, traits that might make an unfavorable impression. His self-perceptions and his social interactions — including interactions with a psychiatric or psychological interviewer — are largely governed by a defensive attempt to preserve and enhance his self-esteem.

To bypass this difficulty, the process of evaluation employs several technical methods, each of which contributes to an integrated formulation of a patient's disorder and recommendations for treatment. In addition to obtaining information from records of previous hospitalization or treatment and family members or other informants, the major methods of evaluating a patient are physical examination and laboratory tests, interviews, observation of behavior and psychological tests. Some methods contribute data that a patient could not supply through self-report; e.g., physical examination and laboratory tests. Other methods, such as interviews or personality tests, provide information that the patient could supply if he were insightful and free of defensiveness. A comprehensive understanding of the dynamics and etiology of a case is often not achieved until therapy is well under way, but a useful, tentative formulation may be made on the basis of the standard methods of evaluation.

Another function of evaluation is to provide an accurate description of the patient so that the best form of treatment can be employed. Diagnostic evaluations often provide important clues to the patient's likely behavior in psychotherapy, and the likelihood of his benefiting from it. Also, it is important to determine whether a disorder is primarily organic and should be treated medically. Unfortunately, two

413

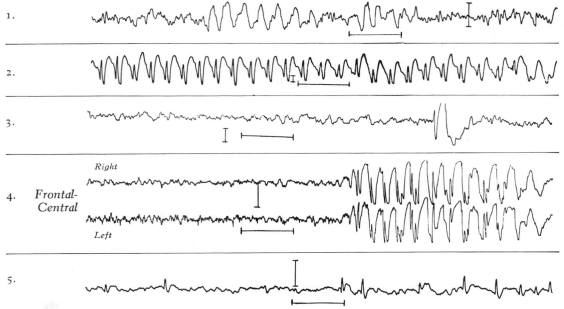

Figure 20–1. *"Some electroencephalographic abnormalities seen in epilepsy. The horizontal markings denote one second; the vertical markings indicate 100 microvolts." (From Strauss, H. 1959. Epileptic Disorders.* In *Arieti, S. (Editor), American Handbook of Psychiatry. New York, Basic Books.)*

types of errors often occur in distinguishing organic from functional disorders. Patients with emotional problems may be treated by unnecessary surgery or other purely medical procedures when psychological ameliorative techniques would be more appropriate. Some women, for example, who experience functional pelvic difficulties shop around from one physician to another until one is found who agrees to perform a hysterectomy. The reverse error may also occur: a patient may be treated by psychotherapy when his symptoms are caused by an organic ailment. George Gershwin, the composer, spent some time in psychoanalysis for the treatment of various somatic complaints; an autopsy showed he had a brain tumor of considerable size. In the absence of a careful physical examination it is all too easy to conclude that a patient's confusing symptoms stem from a neurotic disorder.

The best method of assessing possible physiological disorders is through the physical examination. Some physiological disorders, such as peptic ulcers, can have serious consequences if the proper medical care is not instituted with regular monitoring during the course of psychotherapy. Another function of the physical

examination is to identify any medical factors that aggravate a primarily functional disorder. Neurotics, depressives, schizophrenics and other functional patients have as many or more toothaches, visual difficulties and allergies as anyone else, and their physical ailments often exacerbate their emotional ills.

A physical examination of psychiatric patients includes a routine check of the major bodily organs and systems and several specialized neurological procedures. These include tests of reflexes, sensory difficulties, motor difficulties and the functioning of the central nervous system. Among the last, a frequently used procedure is electroencephalography, the graphic recording of the electrical activity of the brain (so-called "brain waves"). Fine electrodes are attached at various points in the patient's scalp and an elaborate device transforms the brain's electrical activity into a continuous record on a moving strip of paper; the record is called an electroencephalogram or EEG. A brain affected by tumors, epilepsy or some other pathological condition usually yields one of several recognizable abnormal EEG patterns; the particular pattern often helps to determine the specific type of pathology. The particular areas of the scalp from which the deviant EEG's are obtained help to determine the specific location of lesions. In Figure 20–1, adapted from Strauss (1959), several epileptic EEG's are shown; they are characterized by sudden bursts of electrical activity, irregular waves and "spikes" (sharp peaks indicating rapid and large changes in voltage). The normal EEG varies from person to person but is usually fairly regular and smooth. (Functional disturbances are also sometimes accompanied by EEG peculiarities; deviant EEG's have been reported in some cases of obsessive-compulsive reaction, antisocial behavior disorder and schizophrenia.)

THE INTERVIEW

Life for the clinician would be easier if the patient was both willing and able to provide the information needed for an adequate evaluation. However, much of what bothers the patient, just as what bothers most of us, is frequently beyond understanding. The patient may know that he feels extremely low or worthless, but he may not know that these feelings are related to his inability to acknowledge and handle his own anger and resentment. Or he may be aware of important feelings but still be unwilling to discuss these with the clinician who is a total stranger to him. The patient, like most persons reading this page, has a history of trained privacy. For example, all of us are taught early and well that hostility toward loved ones is wicked, that sexual feelings are not to be discussed in polite company, that some body parts are to be concealed so carefully that they are referred to as "privates."

In an encounter with a stranger, whether a professional person or not, the patient is likely to avoid or deny those thoughts and actions he has been taught he should not have. The denial may be conscious, so as to avoid looking ridiculous to the clinician, or it may be unconscious, the patient believing absolutely that not for one fleeting moment has he experienced the shameful impulse in question. He is afraid that what he says will be held against him and he does not understand how revealing unpleasant thoughts will be of any help. It is the clinician's task to help the patient know why and how he avoids unacceptable feelings and how this avoidance or defensiveness affects those with whom he interacts.

The initial interview with a patient is aimed at acquiring information of his recent difficulties,

his family and social relationships and his major personality characteristics. The patient's statements are not taken at face value but are used as pieces of verbal behavior from which inferences are made. A patient's statement, "I get along fine with everybody" may mean that he is truly on excellent terms with everyone, or that he is on fairly good terms with some people or that he dislikes his family, acquaintances and coworkers so much that he excludes them from "everybody." Which of these meanings should be inferred from his statement depends on how he says it and on his other statements.

A skilled interviewer maximizes a patient's readiness to communicate. To overcome the patient's reluctance to talk freely, the interviewer must be interested in the patient and accept him. Acceptance is not approval: an interviewer may communicate a nonjudgmental attitude even when he does not approve of a patient's behavior. He neither endorses nor censures, but listens sympathetically and tries to understand why the patient behaves as he does.

An intake interview usually probes sensitive areas of the patient's life, for example, suicidal thoughts or attempts, past episodes of disorganized behavior, relationships with various family members and sexual behavior. To elicit this information without causing the patient to feel more anxious and guilty than he already does requires skill. It cannot—or should not—be done by fixing him with a steely eye and frightening him into self-revelations. Rather, the interviewer's manner should establish an atmosphere in which the patient feels that no harm will come to him no matter what he says. In a permissive atmosphere and with only a little encouragement he may discuss intimate or threatening topics. If encouragement does not help the patient talk, he can be urged on by judicious questioning.

There are a number of techniques for questioning that can be very productive when employed by a trained interviewer. First, as a rule, the sequence of questions should move from the general to the specific. Second, the questions should move from less intimate to more intimate matters; for example, it is usually best for inquiries into interests or work history to precede an inquiry into suicidal urges, sexual history or interpersonal problems. Once embarked on a sensitive area, the inquiry may move progressively closer to the central aspects of the area. For example, suspected suicidal tendencies in a depressed individual may be ex-

plored by successively asking as many of the
following questions as necessary:
What are your thoughts when you are upset or
   feel blue?
Do you ever feel life is just not worth while?
Has the thought of killing yourself ever
   crossed your mind?
How were you going to kill yourself?

However, people vary considerably in what
threatens them. A particular patient may speak
freely of sexual matters but freeze up if vocational aspirations are mentioned, or he may
reveal bizarre fantasies readily and in detail but
refuse to say a word about his financial situation. The interviewer must guard against
assuming that all patients are alike, or—worse
yet—that they are all like him.

Another technique consists of embedding a
significant question, asked in a casual voice, in
the middle of a sequence of routine and affectively neutral questions. The aim is not to trap
the patient but to neutralize a threatening area
and thus make it easier for him to talk about it.

Still another technique uses leading questions,
e.g., "What do you usually do when you get
angry with your wife?" Again, the aim is not to
entrap but to facilitate a response by implying
that every husband is sometimes angry with his
wife. The technique may backfire, however, if
the interview atmosphere is not permissive and
sympathetic.

If emotionally charged material causes a patient to block early in the interview, the material
can be ignored and brought up later in another
context. Sometimes indirect questions are useful, e.g., "What do you think might lead a
person to commit suicide?" or "What kind of a
relationship do you think there should be between a husband and wife?" The answers to
these questions may be followed up in detail.

In contrast to techniques for probing sensitive areas, some aspects of the patient's functioning are best explored by very direct and
simple questions. For example, memory can be
assessed by asking the patient when he was
born, when he graduated from school, when he
was married or when well-known historical
events occurred. Recent memory can be tested
by asking what the patient ate for breakfast or
what he did the day before. Hallucinations may
be revealed by asking the patient if he ever had
a vision or a dream-like experience while
awake or if he ever heard people when no one
else was present. Orientation for time, place and

person is easily appraised by asking the patient to give the day and date, his address, the
name of the place he is now in and his own and
the interviewer's names.

Skilled interviewing, however, does not consist of the mechanica use of a list of "good"
questions. In fact, concentrating on the questions instead of on the patient will result in
poor interviewing; interviewing technique is secondary to the interviewer's *attitude*. The best
way to convey warmth or interest is to feel it.
Supervised practice in diagnostic and therapeutic interviewing—an important part of the
training of a psychiatrist or clinical psychologist
—usually focuses on the feelings and attitudes
of the trainee more than on his words.

In the following excerpt from the middle of
an unproductive interview by a neophyte interviewer, the trouble was deeper than the overly
specific and staccato nature of the questions.
The real difficulty was that the interviewer felt
very uncomfortable in the situation and consequently fired point-blank questions which
were unconsciously designed to keep the inter-
viewee from talking.

Do you have any brothers or sisters?
A brother.

How old is he?
Thirty.

What does he do?
He's a supervisor in a box factory.

Do you see him often?
No, about once every four months.

Do you correspond?
No.

What does your father do?
He's a policeman.

The entire interview resembled the quoted
excerpt; the interviewer was concerned entirely
with facts and never with feelings. He did not
say, "Tell me about your family" or "How do
you feel about your family?" because he was
afraid he would be unable to handle the emotional material that would emerge. Purely
factual responses may provide useful, biographical information, but it is information that
can just as well be obtained from a routine
admission form.

Sometimes a patient may withhold pertinent
information due to marked emotional blocking,
amnesia or muteness. In these circumstances,
he may become much more accessible and

open under hypnosis or under the influence of certain sedative or stimulant drugs. Two sedative drugs administered by intravenous injection prior to interviews—Sodium Amytal and Pentothal—have been especially widely used and have at times led to dramatic increases in verbalization. Each one has been called a "truth serum." They are particularly helpful when it is diagnostically or therapeutically desirable for a patient to recapture and experience the emotions of a traumatic and repressed episode. Such drugs are frequently used in combat situations, for example, where it is important to deal with conflictual traumatic material quickly before more fixed symptoms have a chance to develop. Still there is no guarantee that a patient will tell all or even a significant part of the truth under the influence of any known drug; in general, hypnotic or drug techniques do not take the place of interviewing skills.

BEHAVIORAL OBSERVATIONS

There is a limit to the information which even the most skilled interviewer can obtain from a cooperative patient. The interview setting is rather formal, the interaction is limited to verbal behavior, and the time sample is brief, usually not longer than one hour. Friends and colleagues, however, know each other far better than an interviewer can know any of them. Further, they know each other informally, when neither is on guard, and have a chance to observe each other in a variety of situations over a period of time.

While friends may not be able to conceptualize their observations in psychological terms, they can bear witness to many important aspects of the patient's behavior. The problem is in quantifying such observations. A commonly used form of peer rating is to ask members of a particular group to nominate members for specific functions. For example, children have been asked to name their best friends or to name the best readers and spellers. The relationship between such choices and an external measure of performance is usually quite high (Cronback, 1960). Peer ratings are part of the battery of assessment techniques used in the Peace Corps. It has been found that the answer to such questions as "Name five trainees who will be the most successful volunteers overseas" is the best single predictor of overseas

performance, better than any other test or interview procedure. Since the trainees see each other many hours a day in a variety of circumstances it is little wonder that they know more about each other than the psychologists and psychiatrists do.

Another form of behavioral rating frequently employed is derived from information recorded from observations of behavior in the hospital. A perceptive hospital nurse or ward aide may learn a great deal about a patient by observing his behavior during the course of daily activities. To organize and record both interview and hospital-ward observations, a number of rating scales have been constructed. One such scale (Lorr, 1953) includes 40 items to summarize interview observations or inferences and 22 items to cover ward observations. The items comprise a broad sample of symptoms characteristic of the functional psychoses. The following three items are based on the interview:*

Are his thoughts and feelings consistent, or is there a discernible lack of harmony between them? (Reports, smiling, that he was tortured with blow torches all night.)

1	2	3	4
Consistent	A little disharmonious	Distinctly disharmonious	Appear totally unrelated

Does he tend to feel or to believe on slight evidence or without good reason that he is unworthy, sinful, evil, or guilty?

1	2	3	4
No feelings or ideas of sinfulness	Unwarranted feelings of sinfulness	Conviction of unusual sinfulness and guilt	Conviction of unpardonable sins and crimes

To what degree is he concerned or preoccupied with his health and the functioning of his bodily organs?

1	2	3	4
No concern	A little concerned	Moderately concerned	Extremely concerned and preoccupied

The following three items are based on ward observations:

*From Lorr, M. 1953. Multidimensional Scale for Rating Psychiatric Patients. Hospital Form. Washington, D.C., Veterans Administration Technical Bulletin TB 10-507.

Does he ever talk to himself or to no one in particular?

1	2	3	4
Never	Only occasionally	Rather frequently	Almost continually

When in action (walking, talking, dressing, eating), does he move slower, faster, or at about the same rate of speed as the average person?

1	2	3	4	5
Markedly slower	A little slower	At an average rate	A little faster	Distinctly faster

Does he tear up papers, magazines, clothing or damage objects such as furniture?

1	2	3
Damages nothing	Occasionally	Fairly often. Must be watched

The ratings of the items may be combined into scores for several dimensions of psychopathology, such as paranoid projection, exaggerated activity level, perceptual distortion, withdrawal and so forth, in order to provide an overall summary of the patient's symptomatology. In addition to their usefulness in patient evaluation, ratings of this kind are of great importance in gathering objective and quantifiable data on disturbed behavior for research purposes.

PSYCHOLOGICAL TESTS

In contrast to the other professional persons who work with emotional disturbance, a clinical psychologist is specially trained to administer and interpret psychological tests. A psychological test may be defined as an instrument for obtaining controlled observations of an individual's behavior in a standard situation. It is a sample of behavior from which inferences may be made with regard to other behaviors. For example, from a subject's responses to a brief, standardized vocabulary test one may, with some confidence, make inferences as to the precision and logic of his thinking, his alertness, the probability of his succeeding in school or in various occupations, and many other aspects of behavior.

The number of tests in existence is very large. Three types are particularly important for abnormal psychology: intelligence tests, tests of intellectual impairment primarily due to organic brain disorders, and personality tests. Intelligence tests are, of course, essential for assessing mental deficiency; they are also helpful for many other purposes. For example, since the likelihood that a patient will benefit from intensive psychotherapy seems to be greater if he is superior rather than average in intelligence, the determination of his I.Q. may affect recommendations for treatment. Tests of intellectual impairment aid in diagnosing the existence and extent of disturbance due to brain damage, although the major diagnostic tools in organic cases are medical. Personality tests assist in diagnosis, help determine whether a patient should be closely supervised, treated psychotherapeutically or discharged, and also give the therapist some advance knowledge of what to expect in psychotherapy so that it may be planned intelligently. In addition to these three types of tests, others are sometimes used in evaluation, particularly tests to measure interests, special aptitudes and achievement.

Intelligence. The intelligence tests in widest clinical use are the Wechsler scales (1944, 1949, 1955). These include the *Wechsler-Bellevue Scale* for adolescents and adults, a revision known as the Wechsler Adult Intelligence Scale (WAIS), the Wechsler Intelligence Scale for Children (WISC), and the Wechsler Preschool and Primary Scale of Intelligence (WPPSI). Both the adults' and children's tests cover verbal and nonverbal (performance) components of intelligence. Representative of the verbal subtests are general information items (e.g., How many pints make a quart? How far is it from Paris to New York?); items asking for the similarity between two objects (e.g., praise and punishment; a fly and a tree); and vocabulary items (definitions). Some of the performance subtests require the subject to arrange scrambled pictures into a logical story sequence, to assemble jigsaw puzzle pieces and to reproduce printed designs by manipulating several blocks, each of which has a part of the design on one of its faces.

The trained psychologist can often draw useful inferences other than an I.Q. score from the patterning of responses to the test. For example, schizophrenic subjects often show a great deal of variability from subtest to subtest. Easy items may be missed because of a personalized interpretation while more difficult items are answered correctly. School underachievers will often perform more poorly on verbal portions of the test than on the performance scales since many of the verbal tests (i.e., arithmetic, vocabulary) are highly loaded with subjects covered in school. Of course, there may be many reasons for the underachievement but the patterning of test results can lead to the inference that the child has not obtained the benefits from formal education that one might expect based on his general level of performance on other portions of the test.

Intellectual Impairment. The purpose of tests of intellectual impairment is to estimate the extent to which the intellectual functioning of a disturbed individual has fallen below his earlier level. Intellectual deterioration is most marked in patients with organic disorders, but many functional psychotics seem also to manifest an intellectual decline. (As mentioned in an earlier chapter, however, the apparent intellectual deterioration in a functional psychosis such as schizophrenia may actually reflect a loss in test-taking motivation.)

The most direct way to evaluate a mental deficit is to compare test scores before and after the onset of a disorder. Unfortunately, reliable pre-illness test scores are usually not available. A substitute method consists of comparing current I.Q. with an estimate of past I.Q. based on school or other achievements, but the estimate is obviously open to many errors. Consequently, much effort has been expended in attempts to identify two kinds of test items: those tapping intellectual abilities that decline relatively little during the course of a disorder and those tapping abilities that decline markedly. There is considerable evidence that vocabulary items decline less than scores on items involving speed, abstract reasoning and use of concepts. Vocabulary is therefore taken to be a measure of past intellectual level; the discrepancy between vocabulary and other tests indicates the amount of decline.

The *Shipley-Hartford Scale* (1940) is the most widely used of several such devices. The vocabulary part of the scale consists of 40 multiple-choice items (e.g., MOLLIFY: mitigate, direct, pertain, abuse). The abstract, conceptual part consists of 20 completion items, in each of which the patient is to discover a general rule and apply it (e.g., tam tan rib rid rat raw hip---). (These illustrative vocabulary and abstract items are among the most difficult in the test.) The abstract score is divided by the vocabulary score to yield a Conceptual Quotient score; a very low Conceptual Quotient is presumed to indicate impairment. Unfortunately the Shipley-Hartford Scale, like other tests of impairment, has sharp limitations. It does not successfully discriminate between functional and organic psychotics and it is inaccurate for patients whose pre-illness mental

ability is quite low. It is useful for detection of brain damage only in combination with other methods of assessment; by itself, it is not dependable enough.

An interesting and quite different approach to testing organic intellectual impairment is embodied in the *Goldstein-Scheerer Tests* (1941). The basic assumption of these tests is that the normal individual can function on both an abstract and concrete level, whereas the individual with brain pathology is limited to concrete behavior. To evaluate concreteness of behavior, Goldstein and Scheerer devised several sorting tests. In the object-sorting test the patient is presented with 33 small objects of various form, color, material and use. He is asked to group the ones that belong together and to state the basis of his grouping; he is also asked to explain the basis of various groups presented to him by the tester and then to shift to new bases of grouping. An inability to take the abstract approach may be manifested in various ways. The patient may be incapable of abstracting a common aspect of the objects, resulting in failure to sort them at all. Or he may group only two or three objects, or group a larger number on the concrete basis of their use (e.g., he may put all eating utensils together) but not on a conceptual basis (e.g., he is unable to combine tools for eating with carpentry tools to form a broader category of "tools").

A second test in the Goldstein-Scheerer battery, the color form test, requires the patient to sort four triangles, four circles and four squares—each set containing a red, yellow, blue and green figure—according to color; and then to shift to form as the principle of classification (or to sort according to form and then to shift to color). Other Goldstein-Scheerer tests require grouping woolen skeins according to colors and shades, and reproduction of abstract geometrical designs. The concrete thinking of mental defectives, brain-damaged patients or severe schizophrenics may be manifested on only one or two of the tests or it may result in poor performance on all of them.

One of the most frequently used tests of organic brain impairment is the Bender Visual-Motor Gestalt. The test consists of nine simple geometric designs. The designs are presented one at a time and the subject is asked to make free-hand copies on blank white paper. Persons with certain organic brain impairments may incorrectly rotate designs, be unable to copy angles correctly, perseverate in copying certain dot patterns, or may show any of a variety of other signs. A developmental scoring system developed by Koppitz (1964) has enabled the test to be used with young children in order to identify neurologically underdeveloped children who are in need of special instructional services.

Personality. There are two major types of personality tests, structured and projective. Structured tests include questionnaires, inventories and devices for self-rating. The subject responds to pretested and standardized items by indicating agreement or disagreement, or by choosing a position on a rating scale.

The most carefully constructed and widely used of existing personality inventories is the *Minnesota Multiphasic Personality Inventory* or *MMPI* (1943). It consists of 556 items covering a wide variety of areas such as worry over physical functioning, antisocial attitudes, bizarre thinking, overactivity, masculinity or femininity of interests and many others. The subject responds "True," "False" or "Cannot Say" to each item. His responses are grouped into scales for different behavioral tendencies (for example, defensiveness and intraversion) and different syndromes (for example, hypochondriasis, depression, hysteria, paranoia and schizophrenia). Each scale was constructed and validated with psychiatric patients.

The important feature of this test is that it is empirically derived. Items were selected for each scale on a strictly empirical basis. For example, if most schizophrenics answered "True" to the item "I like mechanics magazines," while other persons answered the same question "False," then this item was placed on the schizophrenic scale even though the content of the item has little obvious relevance to schizophrenia. The greater the number of items a patient answers in the same direction as schizophrenics the greater the likelihood he is himself a schizophrenic. Naturally, everyone will answer some questions in the same direction as schizophrenics. Scores on each of the scales are tabulated and a profile is drawn indicating the extent to which the subject resembles each of the diagnostic categories which appear on the test. The profile of scale scores, as well as the individual scales themselves, also provides diagnostic information. In addition to classification, the MMPI is a tool for personality description. An individual frequently manifests the personality characteristics of persons who have profiles similar to his own.

His profile may indicate dependency, rebelliousness, mistrust, impulsiveness, compulsiveness, fearfulness, a tendency to repression or many other traits.

Some sample MMPI items are the following:

My daily life is full of things that keep me interested.
I have had very peculiar and strange experiences.
I am easily embarrassed.
I am afraid of using a knife or anything very sharp or pointed.
A large number of people are guilty of bad sexual conduct.

In projective tests or techniques the individual is presented with stimuli and tasks sufficiently unstructured and ambiguous to permit maximal projection of his motives, defenses and attitudes. For example, he tells what he sees in ink blots, makes up stories to fit somewhat vague pictures, draws or completes pictures, or finishes incomplete sentences.

The basis of such tests is that since there are no "correct" or "right" answers to the materials, the individual must draw on his own inner resources in order to respond. In so doing, he reveals characteristic modes of viewing the world and his individual approach to vaguely defined situations. It is difficult for the individual to falsify projective responses since he does not know what one "should" do and since he does not know what inferences will be made from his responses. Hence, projective responses are less easily colored by efforts to present a favorable picture of oneself. Compared to inventories or highly structured tests, projective tests are more subtle. The ambiguity and subtlety of projective tests afford an opportunity to tap fairly deep levels of personality—fantasies, private attitudes and unconscious motivations. On the other hand, projective tests are complex and difficult to validate empirically. Most clinical psychologists feel that both structured and projective tests have strengths and limitations.

The most widely used projective test in clinical practice is the *Rorschach ink-blot test,* devised by the Swiss psychiatrist Herman Rorschach, in which the subject looks at 10 symmetrical ink blots in succession and tells what he sees in each. The Rorschach test is scored for the particular blot areas utilized by the subject, the adequacy of form of his responses, his use of color and shading, his projection of movement and depth into the blots, the qualitative content of his responses, the language he uses to describe what he sees and

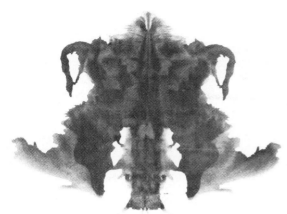

Figure 20–2. Rorschach Card #4. *(By permission from Hans Huber, Medical Publisher, Berne, Switzerland.)*

objective warrant for the stories; the storyteller must draw on his own thoughts, fantasies, attitudes to people, values and motivations.

The following story was told in response to the TAT card shown in Figure 20–3 by a 42-year-old mother of three who was hospitalized with severe headaches for which there was no apparent organic basis:

> This woman, the younger one, is worried about her husband or someone in the family—let's say her husband. He is away on a trip and she just learned that he is ill. She is worried about him, for they are very close. She wants to go see him at once but the old woman is telling her not to go. She's saying that she is sick and old, and that there will be no one to look after her if the younger woman goes to her husband. The young woman is torn apart. She wants to go to her husband but she is afraid of hurting her mother—this old woman—who needs her so much. It is an impossible situation. [Question: How will it turn out?] There is no end. It will just go on that way.

This patient told a number of stories with the theme of someone being unable to resolve the conflicting demands of others. This theme seems particularly significant in view of the fact that the patient's father had been living

many other interrelated response characteristics. Responses can be scored and interpreted only by a trained clinician. The following illustrative responses were given by several patients to the blot reproduced in Figure 20–2.

A depressed patient with feelings of anxiety and guilt:

> I see a tired old woman in the middle and it looks like something up here is about to fall on her.

A conversion reaction patient who relied on the defense mechanisms of denial and repression to handle anxiety:

> It's a very pretty dancer who is a great favorite among the people. She's quite graceful. It is a lovely picture.

A disorganized patient in the midst of an acute paranoid schizophrenic episode gave the following response:

> That's a person personified. It's a man who in the larger scheme of things must conceal these feminine interests which others affix to him. This is symbolized by the female hips which someone has painted on his garment. He is continually bothered by the petty tricks of little men.

The *Thematic Apperception Test (TAT)* consists of a number of pictures, some realistic and some symbolic, for each of which the patient tells a story. He is instructed to tell what led up to the situation in each picture, what is happening, what the characters are thinking and feeling and what the outcome will be. Obviously, the pictures themselves do not provide a sufficient,

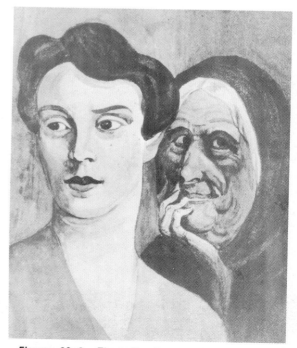

Figure 20–3. Thematic Apperception Test #12F. *(Courtesy of Harvard University Press.)*

with her and her husband for several years. He was a demanding person who frequently placed the patient in the position of having to choose between her father and her husband. This led to considerable marital discord. The patient began developing severe headaches shortly after the first major argument with her husband following her father's move into the house. The tension she feels and the definition of the problem as an insoluble one, as well as her sense of helplessness in coping, were clearly revealed in this and other stories.

The Rorschach, TAT and sentence completion tests are examples of verbal projective techniques. Many projective devices are non-verbal; an example is the *Test of Masculinity-Femininity* by Franck and Rosen (1949). In this test, the subject completes simple drawings in any way he wishes. Figure 20–4 shows a number of the stimulus drawings (S30, S27 and so forth) and typical drawing completions by male college students, female college students, relatively masculine women and relatively feminine men. The completions made by different groups differ in content and in "style"—elongation of the stimuli, expansion, closure, internal elaboration and so forth.

Other Tests. In recent years there has been an increasing tendency to discharge from mental hospitals patients who were formerly considered incurable. Prior to discharge they are helped to prepare for posthospital adjustment by educational or vocational evaluation and counseling. Aptitude and achievement tests are widely used in hospitals and outpatient clinics for this type of evaluation. Among the most popular tests are the Strong Vocational Interest Blank and the Kuder Preference Record for measuring interests, the Minnesota Clerical Test, the O'Rourke Mechanical Aptitude Test and the Stanford Achievement Tests. Data from these tests may be supplemented by records of past vocational and educational achievement and interview information.

SOME PROBLEMS OF EVALUATION

From the vast number of available procedures for evaluation, the clinician must select the best possible ones. Selection may be guided by the criteria of reliability, validity, objectivity, minimum time expenditure, breadth and depth, and relevance to the particular evaluative problem. The more reliable a test or other pro-

cedure is—that is, the more consistent and stable—the better. If a test yields radically different results at different times and if these differences have no systematic relation to

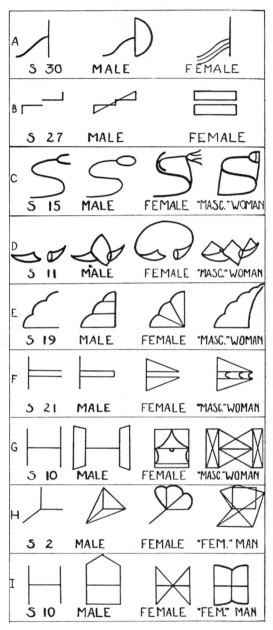

Figure 20–4. Examples of stimulus drawings and their completions by different persons, from the Test of Masculinity-Femininity. Franck, K., and Rosen, E. 1949. A projective test of masculinity-femininity. J. Consult. Psychol., 13:252. Copyright 1949 by the American Psychological Assn., Inc.

identifiable external or internal events, then the test is as useless as a yardstick made of elastic.

Second, the more valid a method—that is, the more successful in measuring what it purports to measure—the better. Of course, it may be valid for one purpose but not another. For example, interviews and many personality tests are reasonably valid for estimating how depressed a patient is at a given time, but no procedure is very successful in predicting the likelihood of emerging from a depression in the future. The descriptive and diagnostic validity of most procedures is stronger than their prognostic validity.

Third, the more objective the administration and interpretation of a test, the better. Intelligence tests are quite objective (as well as highly reliable and reasonably valid). Structured personality tests also tend to be objective. Interviews, projective tests and behavior observations are much more subjective; the processes of gathering and interpreting data through these procedures are dependent on the skills, theoretical biases and beliefs of the clinician.

Fourth, the less time-consuming an evaluative procedure, the better. Many projective tests take so much time to score and interpret properly that they do not leave enough time for other important activities.

Fifth, the criteria of breadth and depth suggest that a method is particularly valuable if it examines behavior comprehensively and deeply rather than narrowly and superficially, even if the price paid for breadth and depth is a partial loss of reliability, validity, objectivity and time. Good projective tests and skilled interviews both draw their strength from their flexible breadth and their capacity for exploring personality in depth. Most clinicians feel that if only one hour (or less) is available for evaluating a patient, the time is best spent in a wide-ranging interview. If more time is available, other procedures may be added to supplement the interview, rather than interviewing at greater length, for every procedure makes a unique contribution.

Finally, methods must be chosen with reference to the particular purposes of the evaluation. For example, the Rorschach test may be used, among other tests, to evaluate suitability of a neurotic patient for psychotherapy; it helps assess motives, defenses, ego-strength and other relevant variables. On the other hand, a patient with suspected brain damage needs medical examination and tests of intellectual

impairment more than a Rorschach test. The criteria of reliability, validity, objectivity, minimum-time expenditure, breadth and depth cannot yield a standard battery of tests to be used routinely with all patients.

A major problem is that of integrating evaluative information. It often happens that the results of different procedures are contradictory and one must decide what to give most weight to. Here again, there are several guiding criteria. Procedures with proved reliability and validity naturally are most heavily weighted. Where objective, empirical evidence of validity is lacking, the clinician's past experience with the procedures guides his integration of evaluative data. The criterion of internal consistency is also helpful: it is assumed that an individual is self-consistent even when there are surface contradictions, and the clinician's evaluation is therefore guided by the need to draw a self-consistent picture of the patient's personality. For example, in one particular case the score for schizophrenia on the MMPI may be in the normal range, whereas the indicators of schizophrenic thought processes in the Rorschach test or TAT may be quite definite. Neither test is necessarily "wrong": the criterion of consistency suggests that the patient does have bizarre, schizoid thoughts but defends himself against them by denial and therefore answers "False" to all items directly suggesting their presence. At one level he has psychotic tendencies; at the more public level he has learned how to appear relatively normal. The two tests together may thus be integrated to yield much more information than either test alone, for in tapping different levels of personality they suggest how processes at different levels interact with each other.

A comprehensive and integrated evaluation usually covers developmental factors plus the five symptom types discussed in an earlier chapter—disturbances of sensation and perception, intelligence and thought, affect, motivation, and verbal and motor behavior—although not necessarily in this order. In addition, the patient's appearance is usually described (posture, clothing, degree of tension or relaxation, tendency to physical withdrawal or dejection, smiling or frozen and unchanging expression and so forth. Most important, the strength of his ego and superego, the nature of his conflicts and defenses, and his degree of insight are assessed.

In the following illustrative case, several methods of evaluation proved to be productive and useful:

Mrs. L., a neat, conventionally dressed 30-year-old married woman with three children, was referred to an outpatient clinic by her physician. She complained of feelings of depression, headaches, inability to sleep and various other symptoms which the physician believed were due to anxiety. A physical examination was completely negative.

The patient was of superior intelligence. A Wechsler-Bellevue Test administered several years earlier had yielded an I.Q. of 125. Her school record was excellent. After graduation from high school she attended a business school and then did secretarial work. She was reported to be efficient and well-liked on the job.

Mrs. L.'s husband was a sick man. He had a chronic heart condition and was also subject to recurrent psychotic episodes which had necessitated several hospitalizations. A psychiatrist who had been treating him reported that he was full of impractical ideas and plans which kept his wife and children in a constant state of turmoil. He had difficulty supporting his family because of his physical and emotional condition.

From this background information it seemed that several questions needed consideration. To what extent were Mrs. L.'s psychological difficulties a response to reality—her difficult family situation—and to what extent did they reflect longstanding personality problems? Was she a suitable candidate for outpatient psychotherapy? Was she depressed enough to warrant hospitalization? Given her family problems, how much could therapy achieve? If psychotherapy were undertaken, what should its aims be? To help answer these questions, both Mrs. L. and her husband were interviewed and she was given the MMPI, Rorschach and sentence completion tests. (The diagnostic interviews with Mrs. L. merged into therapy, and it would be impossible to say where evaluation ended and treatment began.)

Her husband reported that her parents had preferred their two sons to her and that they adored her own children, who were all boys. They had always felt it important not to spoil her and they minimized her abilities and constantly criticized her. She had wanted to attend college but they had talked her out of it although they were well-to-do. Her husband believed that his own condition added to her difficulties, but that her disturbed emotional state stemmed primarily from her family background. This statement turned out to be quite accurate; his emotional problems did not prevent him from being a discriminating source of information. He did not blame her for any part of his own disturbance and he was strongly in favor of psychotherapy for her.

Mrs. L.'s MMPI profile was severely neurotic. Her scores were extremely high on depression and psychasthenia (fears and compulsions), and fairly high on the scales measuring hypochondriacal worries, hysteroid tendencies, femininity and strong intraversion. She was afraid of people and would not find it easy to start talking freely in a psychotherapeutic situation. On the other hand, the pressure of her variegated symptoms, as evidenced by the MMPI

peaks, might be expected to overcome her initial resistance to talking, provided she were given a little encouragement.

The Rorschach responses were those of a potentially creative and imaginative person in whom paralyzing fears had resulted in achievement far short of capacity. She saw guns, hungry wolves, claws, fires and a dragon with an open mouth; these are all anxiety-laden responses. Her attitudes to other people were striking: male figures in the ink blots were perceived vaguely, or were seen as clowns or as messy and inept creatures; female figures fought each other. Her self concept was poor: she showed a great deal of conflict over sex and femininity and a fear of her own aggressive flareups. She was very detail-minded and compulsively sought safety in absorption by many little blot details. Although her responses were neurotic, most were well-organized; a few times she gave childish or disorganized responses but she then recovered quickly and returned to her usual level. Her Rorschach was consistent with the hypothesis that her defenses were beginning to fail in her efforts to cope with increasing internal and external stress. The Rorschach did not corroborate the severe depression suggested by the MMPI.

The sentence completions revealed fear, tension and discouragement. A few representative responses were the following:

When I was young . . . I needed companionship and didn't get it.
I like people who . . . don't hurt my feelings.
Sometimes it's hard for me . . . to keep going.
I could never . . . relax and enjoy myself thoroughly.

Her handwriting in the completions was unusually neat, even and conventional, pointing to a striking degree of overcontrol.

In interview, Mrs. L. looked tense and fearful. She was apparently holding her emotions under tight control; she understood this and used the expression, "I'm sitting on a powder keg." Her speech was clear and completely rational. She talked evenly, a little rapidly, sometimes with a touch of apathy and a little less expression than one would expect. She frequently smiled in a self-deprecatory manner as if apologizing for her "silly symptoms." Several times she began to weep, then recovered and continued to talk; she was clearly ashamed of what she had to say but kept trying to fight her sense of shame. (As the interview progressed, she talked more freely and experienced considerable relief in doing so.)

She reported being quite religious and in general manifested various signs of a strong, even rigid, superego. She described herself as too sensitive, jittery, unable to concentrate, hostile to her husband and guilty over her hostility, and afraid that she was "losing her mind." She feared insanity, death and working with other people; she was sure others were secretly critical of her. The future sometimes looked pretty grim but she had never felt suicidal: her depressive tendencies were real but they seemed to be more a reaction to her reality situation than the central feature of her case. Anxiety was much more central and she manifested many different signs of it. Sometimes she would feel mildly apprehensive for an entire day, and sometimes she suffered brief and very severe anxiety attacks for part of a day. In the severe attacks she would shake all over, feel that something nameless but horrible was about to happen and be certain that she was losing her mind.

She felt very inferior and inadequate. In a recurrent dream, she was a little girl again and her parents abandoned her. She also had a recurrent dream in which she killed her parents. She could admit to her feelings of inadequacy but her aggressive wishes provoked too much guilt to be admitted. Thus she could see that the first dream indicated inadequacy feelings but she could not "see any sense" in the second dream.

Corroborating the Rorschach, a major problem area revealed in interview with Mrs. L. was that of sex. She found it hard to accept her femininity and unsuccessfully fought against the feeling that sex was "bad"; her mother had taught her to regard anything sexual as evil.

The evaluative procedures used with Mrs. L. led to certain clear conclusions:

First, the tests and interviews pointed to a diagnosis of severe mixed neurosis, predominantly of the anxiety-reaction type but with secondary compulsive and depressive features.

Second, her difficulties resulted both from her family situation and from within herself. Treatment could not alter reality but it might modify her personality and behavior.

Third, she was definitely suited for psychotherapy. She was intelligent, communicated well, could be encouraged to open up in therapy, and had a fairly strong ego and considerable capacity for insight. Along with psychotherapy, sedatives or minor tranquilizing drugs could be used to help control her anxiety symptoms. There was no need for hospitalization.

Fourth, several psychotherapeutic goals were feasible. She could be helped to accept herself, to realize that she had talents and strengths that she had learned to decry or deny, and to be better prepared to cope with her reality difficulties. With an increasing acceptance of herself—including her aggressive traits—one could expect a diminution of her guilt, anxiety and inferiority feelings, a reduction of energy expended on defenses and fewer headaches and other symptoms of anxiety. To achieve these aims would take a long time and she could be told not to expect a quick and miraculous change.

Finally, on the basis of the evaluation the therapist could expect the material relevant to her sexual problems would be brought up as soon as she felt enough confidence in him. This expectation proved correct. During therapy she remembered childhood sexual events she had long before pushed out of mind: sleeping in a room adjoining that of her parents, she had more than once been awakened when they engaged in sexual intercourse. She had

been frightened and disgusted and had felt uncomfortable with sex ever since. As a sensitive, intelligent child of parents who preferred boys, she had early become involved in intense and complex affectional and competitive relationships with them. The childhood sexual incidents had further complicated these relationships and resulted in ambivalence to her parents, her children and people in general.

The childhood sexuality, parental rejection and severe emotional conflict foreshadowed by the evaluation proved to be the crucial areas in the psychotherapeutic sessions. Although the nature of Mrs. L.'s neurosis would have been understood eventually without the evaluative procedures, the evaluation accelerated the discovery of the roots of her problems and increased the effectiveness of the therapeutic sessions.

A different example is provided in the following evaluation of a 20-year-old, single college drop-out who was seen in a state hospital. A week prior to admission he had attempted to hang himself in the city jail following his arrest for the possession and selling of illegal drugs (LSD and mescaline). He was referred for diagnostic evaluation and for recommendations concerning further treatment. The psychologist interviewed the patient and administered the following tests: the Shipley-Hartford, the Rorschach, a Wechsler Memory Scale, and the MMPI. Excerpts from the psychologist's report follow:

The patient states that at the time of his arrest he was under the influence of LSD and had become convinced that his friends were engaged in an elaborate trick to drive him crazy by acting out his life before his eyes. He felt that the whole world was cooperating with them and that everyone was out to "get him" for his past mistakes. He called the police himself in order to get the expected punishment over with. In jail he did not "clear" as the drug effects wore off. In fact, he became more convinced that he was the object of a diabolical plot. He felt that he had caused a flood and other natural disasters. He believed that the police wanted him dead because of the misery he had caused. He attempted to hang himself because he believed himself to be guilty and in order to forestall an even worse fate at the hands of his captors. In the hospital he was placed on tranquilizers and while his persecutory delusions have begun to fade, they are still detectable. The patient is able to state that some of his beliefs were clearly imaginary but about others he says "they seemed so real at the time that I still can't quite convince myself that they did not happen."

According to the patient's account of his family history, he was the only child of lower middle class parents. His father was a postal clerk who is described as a kind, gentle, easy-going man with many friends. His mother was seen as somewhat cool and aloof, with little to offer emotionally. "She leaned on my father and on her own mother and gave little to anyone herself." The patient was close to his father as a child but describes himself as a shy, introverted person with few friends. He read a great deal, practiced his music, made average grades, and confined his social contacts mostly to members of the extended family. When he was 15 years of age, his father became bedridden with terminal cancer. The patient, knowing of the impending death, was unable to face his father. He avoided the house as much as possible until the death and then felt extremely guilty over not having provided more emotional support and closeness to his father during a long and painful illness. His guilt became so great that he wished himself dead. His mother had been totally dependent on the father and after his death turned to her mother for emotional support. She was preoccupied with her own grief and ignored her son. The patient withdrew even more at this time. He was afraid to see anyone other than his mother and grandmother and feared hurting inanimate objects. The bulk of his time was spent in reading religious writings, contemplating the cruelty of society and the meaning of life, and in various fantasies. This pattern has continued largely unchanged up to the present. The patient let his hair grow (and refused to cut it again until five years later) and adopted bizarre forms of dress. These latter behaviors led to his being expelled from high school. After completing high school through correspondence courses, the patient enrolled in college to avoid the draft and because he "couldn't face having to make some kind of job choice."

In college he had no friends and little social life. Most of his time was spent in studying or in solitary contemplation. His grades were quite modest. After three quarters he left the state to enroll in a college in Oregon. It was there that he made his first friends in almost three years. He became very attached to a girl who was also emotionally involved with another young man. The patient had had almost no dates prior to meeting this girl. He says "it was a crazy triangular relationship which the three of us had going and when she finally chose him instead of me it was almost more than I could bear." It was while going with this girl that the patient was introduced to LSD, "pot," mescaline and "anything else we could think of to blow our minds." The patient says that he was obsessed with the cruelty and harshness of the world. He also describes himself as quite depressed. He engaged in potentially self-destructive behavior such as driving his motorcycle recklessly in the hope that he would have a fatal accident. While in Oregon, the patient entered a mental hospital in order to "cop a plea as a nut and get out of the draft." The doctors there learned of his plan but still felt that he had what they described to him as "serious emotional problems." The suggestion that he had any emotional problems was offensive to the patient at the time, so he withdrew from the hospital and returned to his home state. He lived with a "hippie" group on the edge of campus but did not enroll in college. He withdrew from drugs "except for an occasional joint"

until taking the LSD last month which apparently precipitated the present difficulty.

On interview the patient was found to be cooperative and fully compliant. Speech was voluble and goal-directed. Thought was clear and coherent but seemed somewhat slow and deliberate. His affect was shallow except when discussing his father's death, when he became tearful and was unable to continue talking for a few minutes. He appeared slightly retarded in his movements.

Personality testing in general suggests that this is an emotionally unstable person with a longstanding schizoid personality disorder. His MMPI profile is in keeping with such a diagnosis. His elevated scores conform without exception to a syndrome characterized by the following therapist descriptive statements for patients of this profile type: "Ambivalent. Unable to love. Most frequently unmarried and with history of poor heterosexual adjustment. Pan-anxiety, shy, quiet, withdrawn, obsessive, ruminative, sensitive. Thinking may be bizarre at times. Flat affect, severe depression, fatigue, weakness, insomnia, apathy. Perpetual student. Strong feelings of inadequacy and inferiority. Indecisive. Interest in reading and ruminating about obscure subjects or religion. Ideas of reference and brief acute psychotic episodes sometimes occur." His Rorschach responses tend to confirm the presence of preoccupation with guilt and some autistic thinking. Thus, from interview material and from test results, it is evident that this is a person of borderline psychotic adjustment with a great deal of guilt, self-destructive behavior, marked interpersonal aversiveness, and some peculiarity of thought.

The patient has superior intellectual skills but is unable to perform up to capacity because of his emotional problems. He is sufficiently anxious at present that his concentration and some immediate memory functions are impaired.

Finally, there is some evidence in the literature that suggests that there may be some permanent spatial-perceptual disturbances as a result of prolonged LSD use. This is difficult to assess in the patient's present condition. A complete neuro-psychological examination might be in order once the patient has sufficiently improved that he can be safely withdrawn from all medications.

This then looks like a patient who may have been emotionally deprived in early life as a result of a non-giving, distant mother. As long as the father lived, the patient received some oral gratification and was able to maintain an adequate though somewhat marginal adjustment. With the father's death he was left without emotional support and withdrew into a frankly schizoid life with few social contacts. In an undemanding setting which allowed minimal social skills and maximal self-indulgence through fantasy, he was able to maintain a marginal adjustment until the drug-induced psychotic episodes.

At the present time the psychosis appears to be clearing. He is left with a severe personality disorder and strong unremitting guilt feelings which still have the potential for precipitating self-destructive acts. He appears never to have adequately dealt with the guilt feelings surrounding the events of his father's death.

The psychologist recommended that the patient be kept busy with physical activities to discourage withdrawal into fantasy preoccupations. For similar reasons, gradually increasing social participation was recommended. It was felt best to avoid any evocative or uncovering type of treatment since the patient was already excessively introspective and ruminative and since his hold on reality was tenuous. It was recommended that the patient be provided with a long-term supportive therapy relationship which would be active in nature and oriented toward realistic adaptation to external demands.

Finally, the psychologist suggested that the patient should not be pressured into making career choices at that time since his interpersonal skills were minimal, his guilt was too great, and his intellectual capacities too impaired. It was felt best that he work out specific career plans over a period of time in the context of an ongoing therapeutic relationship where he could receive emotional support.

Treatment—the topic of the next chapter—is an art as well as a science, and its course and outcome are often unpredictable; a major goal of evaluation is to help make treatment more predictable and effective.

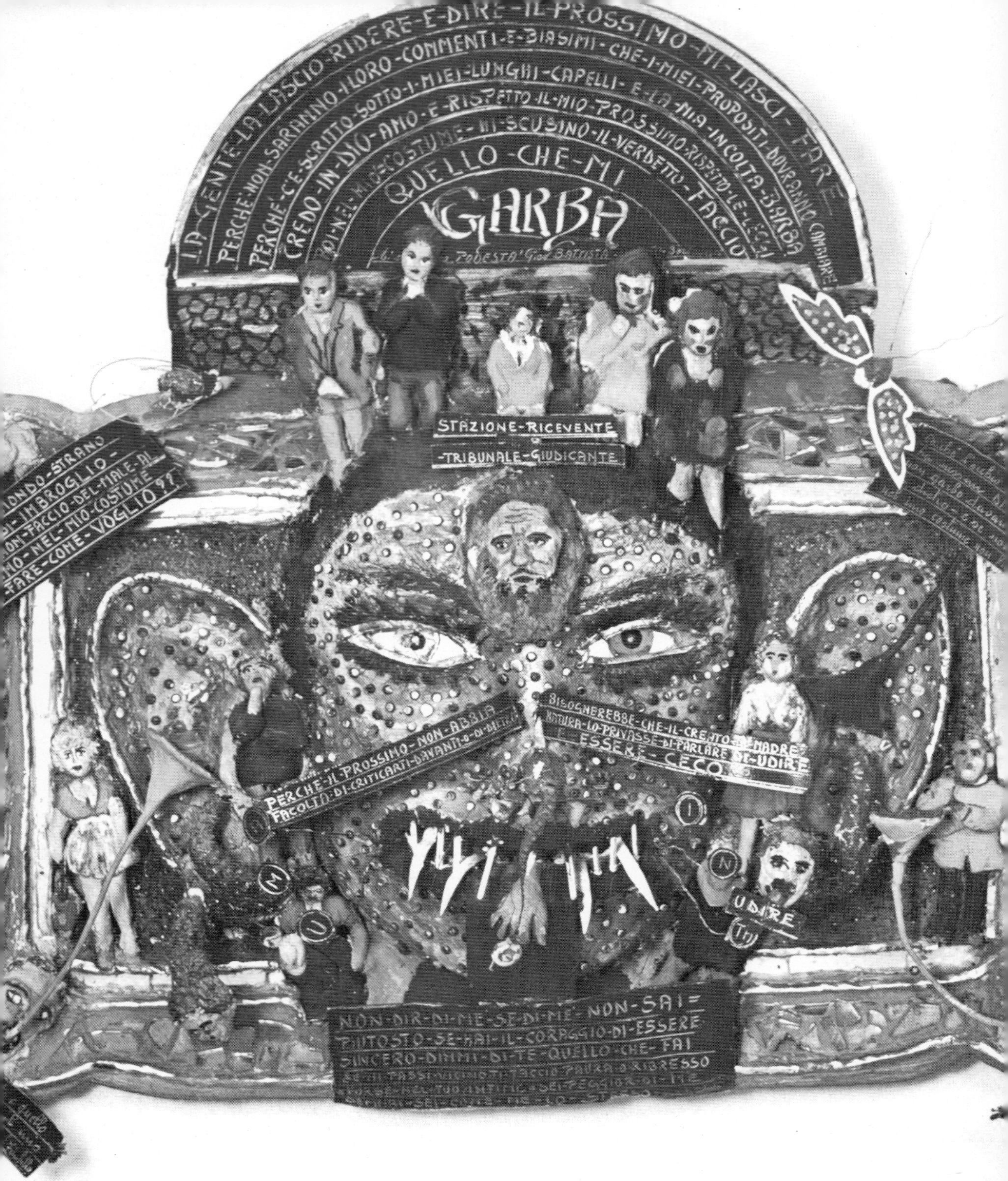

LA-GENTE-LA-LASCIO-RIDERE-E-DIRE-IL-PROSSIMO-MI-LASCI-FARE
PERCHE-NON-SARANNO-I-LORO-COMMENTI-E-BIASIMI-CHE-I-MIEI-
PERCHE-C'E-SCRITTO-SOTTO-I-MIEI-LUNGHI-CAPELLI-E-LA-MIA-
CREDO-IN-DIO-AMO-E-RISPETTO-IL-MIO-PROSSIMO
QUELLO-CHE-MI
GARBA
STAZIONE-RICEVENTE
-TRIBUNALE-GIUDICANTE
PERCHE-IL-PROSSIMO-NON-ABBIA
FACOLTA-DI-CRITICARTI-DAVANTI-O-DI-DIETRO
BISOGNEREBBE-CHE-IL-CREATO
E-ESSERE-CECO
UDIRE
NON-DIR-DI-ME-SE-DI-ME-NON-SAI=
PIUTOSTO-SE-HAI-IL-CORAGGIO-DI-ESSERE
SINCERO-DIMMI-DI-TE-QUELLO-CHE-FAI

21

TREATMENT

[handwritten annotations:]
1) SOMATIC - bio
2) PSY. - psy
3) ENVIORNMENT - socio
   MILIEU

It is an axiom of our society that suffering, maladjustment and interpersonal friction are undesirable, whereas comfort, peace of mind, personal productiveness and good relations with people are desirable. The basic purposes of therapy—another term for treatment—are to help the sick, unhappy or unproductive individual and to make life smoother for him and the people around him. Therapy is also a source of knowledge of behavior, for much of what we know about the dynamics of emotional disturbance is based on discoveries made by Freud and other leading psychotherapists.

There are three broad approaches to the treatment of a disturbed individual: somatic therapy, psychotherapy and environmental manipulation. Somatic therapy treats the patient by drugs, electroconvulsive procedures, brain surgery and other such methods. Obviously, these procedures should be employed only by a specially trained physician. Psychotherapy is based on psychological principles; the therapist may be a psychiatrist, a psychologist or some other professionally trained person. Environmental manipulation alters behavior by procedures such as modifying a patient's housing conditions, guiding him into appropriate work or other activities or organizing the

structure of a hospital to benefit him maximally. Several different professions may be involved—psychiatrists, psychologists, social workers, occupational therapists and others.

Each of the three therapeutic approaches corresponds to an etiological category. Somatic therapy manipulates the organism biologically; psychotherapy modifies psychological factors by helping the patient to learn new and adaptive, emotional responses in place of old and maladaptive ones; and milieu therapy largely works to modify the sociocultural factors in psychological disturbance.

SOMATIC THERAPY

The somatic treatments currently used in psychiatric practice have been developed for the most part by empirical trial and error. The attitude of the originators usually was "Let's try it and see" and the theoretical bases of the treatments were frequently incorrect or inadequately tested. Nevertheless, out of this relatively crude approach a number of useful methods have emerged. We will concentrate on the major methods; for each of these, we will discuss the kind of patient for whom it is most suitable, how it is applied and its effects.

Drug Therapy

The outstanding therapeutic development in recent years has been the discovery of the *ataractic drugs* (from "ataraxy," meaning freedom from confusion), often also referred to as the *major tranquilizers*. They have become the primary means of treatment in our mental hospitals. Prior to the use of ataractic drugs, the number of hospitalized patients increased uninterruptedly from year to year. With the introduction of the drugs, the average length of hospital stay has been shortened so markedly that despite an overall increase in the general population the pre-drug increase in patient population has been halted and even reversed.

The major tranquilizers help to control various symptoms of disturbance without impairing intelligence or clarity of consciousness. They diminish anxiety, agitation, aggressive behavior, hallucinations and delusions. The tranquilized patient becomes more docile and cooperative, no longer needs physical restraints and becomes more accessible for psychotherapy. Ataractic drugs have made it possible to unlock many previously locked wards; the patient's resultant freedom to come and go is itself believed to have a therapeutic effect. Hospital wards have become more manageable since tranquilized patients are less likely to excite other patients and, in consequence, the attitudes of hospital aides and nurses toward patients have become more positive.

The major tranquilizers are used primarily with schizophrenics and manics but are also helpful in controlling the excitement displayed by some alcoholic and senile patients. Basically, the major tranquilizers are anti-psychotic; the so-called "minor tranquilizers," to be discussed later, are more appropriate for the alleviation of neurotic tension and anxiety.

The first of the ataractic drugs to be used on a wide scale was *chlorpromazine*, a drug derived from a chemical substance known as *phenothiazine.* Ataractic drugs are administered in pill form, usually several times daily, the dosage varying from patient to patient. The drugs require close medical supervision since in many patients they produce undesirable side effects such as drowsiness, dryness of the mouth, blurred vision, lowered blood pressure, jaundice, a disorder of the white blood cells, extreme skin sensitivity or severe muscular tremor. Since there are great individual differences in reactions to the drugs, they must first be used on a trial basis with each patient; the

physician observes the beneficial and side effects and determines whether to continue the treatment and, if so, the dosage to prescribe.

The ataractic drugs suppress rather than eradicate emotional disturbance. The schizophrenic patient's anxiety, delusions and excitement may be diminished by drug treatment, but his personality conflicts, disordered affects and distortion of reality remain much the same. However, the suppression of anxiety and concomitant symptoms is itself a great gain. Apart from making both the patient and the people around him more comfortable, it enables him to interact better with other persons in or out of the hospital; the improvement in social interaction may then become the source of other improvements in his condition.

Pritchard (1967a) compared two groups of 50 schizophrenics each who were hospitalized before and after the introduction of phenothiazines. The group treated with phenothiazines was found to have a better short-term prognosis than the group hospitalized before such drugs were available. However, on a three-year follow-up of these same patients, Pritchard (1967b) found that the patients treated with phenothiazines were rehospitalized at the same rate as those who were treated by other methods. Pritchard pointed out that at the time these data were gathered it was not yet common practice to keep patients on drugs after discharge from the hospital, and, had such maintenance medications been provided, many patients may have been able to remain out of the hospital longer.

Most professional hospital personnel thoroughly believe in the great value of ataractic drugs, but it is no simple matter to confirm this belief by well-designed, objective research. The major problem is that of finding research methods that will eliminate the effects of suggestion on both the patient and the investigator who evaluates the patient's responses. If either believes strongly enough that a drug is beneficial, he is more likely to report the occurrence of desirable effects. Research on the treatment of the common cold has demonstrated the importance of suggestion in drug studies. Hundreds of subjects reported fewer, briefer and less severe colds after they took inactive pills that were effective only by suggestion.

To correct for the effects of suggestion, a *placebo* (a substance that superficially resembles an active medication but contains nothing medicinal, so that it benefits the patient only by "pleasing" him) is administered to a control group while the test drug is administered to an experimental group. The effects of the test drug are then compared with those reported for the placebo. In well-controlled studies, a *double-blind* design is used: the patient does not know whether he is receiving a test drug or a placebo, and neither does the evaluator. Furthermore, the patient does not know the exact purpose of the drug study, or that more than one medication is being studied, and in an ideal study he is even ignorant of the fact that a study is in progress.

However, placebos and double-blind designs do not completely eliminate the problems of testing ataractic drugs. The evaluator may see through the blind and know which patients are being treated by the real medication because the test drug and the placebo have different side effects; in such a case, suggestion will still operate. To circumvent this difficulty, one of three procedures may be followed. First, an "active" rather than an inert placebo may be used, that is, a drug lacking in medical benefits but mimicking the side effects of the test drug. In research on ataractics, phenobarbital may be used as an active placebo since it mimics ataractics by producing drowsiness. Second, the beneficial effects of two different ataractics may be compared if the two have similar side effects. In a study discussed below (Casey et al., 1960) four substances—two tranquilizers, phenobarbital and an inert placebo—were all tested in one design. Third, patients may be put on a tranquilizing regimen and then taken off it to study the effects of withdrawal.

A large number of studies, employing these procedures, have demonstrated the effectiveness of the major tranquilizers. The following are illustrative studies. Olson and Peterson (1962) administered chlorpromazine in a double-blind study to three groups of chronic schizophrenic patients for one month. The following month one group received an inert placebo, a second group received no treatment at all and a third was treated by a tranquilizer similar to chlorpromazine. The percentage of patients who showed no behavior upset as a result of the change of regimen in the second month was 15 for the no-treatment group, 71 for the inert placebo and 92 for the substitute tranquilizer. In other words, the ataractic was somewhat superior to the placebo but the placebo was far superior to no treatment at all; both the test drug and the process of suggestion produced real results. Three additional groups in the same study were treated in the first

month by another major tranquilizer (thioridazine, also a phenothiazine derivative) instead of chlorpromazine. The two tranquilizers proved to be equally superior to the placebo and to the complete cessation of treatment.

In a double-blind study, Good, Sterling and Holtzman (1958) discontinued chlorpromazine therapy for 112 schizophrenic patients for three months or longer and substituted a placebo. Ratings of behavior on the hospital ward, intellectual tests and personality tests showed a definite regression in a number of patients when the drug was withdrawn. The patients manifested an increase in hallucinations, delusions and incoherence and confusion. Resumption of chlorpromazine treatment after the withdrawal period eliminated these symptoms.

In an impressive and well-designed double-blind study, Casey and his associates (1960) administered chlorpromazine, promazine (another phenothiazine derivative), phenobarbital and a placebo to 629 schizophrenic patients. Some of the patients were put on one drug for 12 weeks and another for 12 more weeks, and some continued on the same medication for 24 weeks. The effects were evaluated by a team of observers who rated the patient's behavior and by tests of anxiety. Chlorpromazine was significantly superior and promazine second best in reducing the total amount of rated psychopathology. Chlorpromazine decreased withdrawal, conceptual disorganization, perceptual distortion and violent behavior. The inert placebo and phenobarbital were significantly less effective than both ataractics and not significantly different from each other.

The precise physiological action of ataractic drugs is uncertain. There is reason to believe that they affect subcortical rather than cortical brain centers and exert a sedative influence on the midbrain in particular. One speculative explanation is that slowing down the activity of the midbrain (where the neural centers that control the organism's vegetative functions are located) increases the ability of the nervous system to cope with external stress and internal stimulation (Hoch, 1959).

In addition to the major tranquilizers, three other kinds of drugs—minor tranquilizers, antidepressives and sedatives—are important in current therapeutic practice. The use of minor tranquilizers and antidepressives is a recent development, but sedatives have been known for many decades.

The *minor tranquilizers* have no effect on psychotic symptoms but are widely used to reduce neurotic anxiety. Although they produce fewer side effects than the major tranquilizers, they have a stronger tendency to become habitual. The minor tranquilizer in greatest use is *meprobamate*, marketed under the trade names Equanil and Miltown. There is no convincing evidence that the minor tranquilizers reduce anxiety more effectively than a number of sedatives such as phenobarbital (see below), but they do not interfere with clarity of consciousness and cause sleepiness as the sedatives do and they are therefore useful in situations in which sedatives are undesirable. Some of the minor tranquilizers are muscle relaxants and reduce tension by acting directly on the muscular apparatus rather than on the central nervous system. Minor tranquilizers are used more in outpatient therapy than in hospital treatment.

In the last decade a number of drugs have been found useful in combating depression. Some of the *anti-depressives* speed up the physiological functioning of the organism, as shown by the fact that they increase heart rate, blood pressure and associated processes, while others act directly on the central nervous system without these physiological concomitants. The anti-depressives diminish apathy and lethargy. The "bogged down" patient becomes more active, interested in reality and amenable to other, nonsomatic treatment measures. Some of the anti-depressives have severe side effects and some reduce apathy at the cost of so great an increase of anxiety and agitation that they cannot be used for the agitated depressive states found in involutional melancholia. In melancholia, a combination of chlorpromazine to reduce anxiety and an anti-depressive to stimulate the patient has often proved effective. One of the most widely used anti-depressives has been *imipramine* (marketed under the name Tofranil). Although some depressives and melancholics do not respond favorably to it, others improve within one to three weeks. Generally speaking, the anti-depressives are more experimental than the major tranquilizers and their usefulness has not been as clearly demonstrated.

Sedative drugs—phenobarbital and many others—act directly on the cerebral cortex and have long been used to combat anxiety, overactivity and insomnia. The effects of phenobarbital tend to be cumulative and the patient may become addicted to it; in large doses it may induce an unwanted depression of mood. With adequate medical supervision, however, phenobarbital and the other sedatives are useful for purely symptomatic relief. The advent of the tranquilizers has cut down on widespread sedative treatment but has not eliminated it.

Electroconvulsive Therapy *ELECTROSHOCK*

Prior to the discovery of the ataractic and anti-depressive drugs, ECT (electroconvulsive therapy, often also referred to as electroshock therapy or EST) was used perhaps twice as much as it has been since. More recently, it has been second among the somatic treatment measures in total frequency of usage. It is particularly helpful for depression and involutional melancholia, of some help for mania and occasionally useful for schizophrenic and other reactions. It is valuable for patients who do not respond favorably to drugs or who suffer too severe side effects, although it is sometimes used without first trying drugs.

ECT was preceded by other types of convulsive therapy. In 1933, Meduna, a Hungarian psychiatrist, initiated convulsive therapy on the basis of a belief that epileptic convulsions were less frequent among schizophrenics than in the general population. Meduna reasoned that a "biological antagonism" existed between epilepsy and schizophrenia and that schizophrenics might therefore be cured by deliberately inducing epileptic-like convulsions in them. At first he used injections of camphor in oil to produce the convulsions, but soon turned to the use of a drug known as *Metrazol* or *Cardiazol*. When injected intravenously, this substance quickly caused the patient to become rigid, lose consciousness and undergo a severe convulsive seizure lasting about one minute. Following the seizure, the patient was confused, dizzy and often very anxious and fearful. A full course of treatment consisted of 10 to 20 seizures.

For several reasons the use of Metrazol was abandoned within a few years. The convulsions were so violent that fractures often occurred, the patients experienced very unpleasant sensations between the moment of injection and the loss of consciousness, and the minimum necessary dosage for each patient was difficult to determine. Metrazol was replaced by electroconvulsive therapy, introduced by Bini and Cerletti in Italy in 1938.

In the typical administration of ECT the patient lies on his back with a rubber gag between his teeth to prevent injury to the tongue during

BINI + CERLETTI 1938

the seizure. Electrodes are fastened to the temples and an alternating current, usually between 100 and 200 volts, is passed through the cortex for half a second or less. Since electricity travels faster than nerve impulses, the patient loses consciousness before he can feel any pain. The loss of consciousness is accompanied by a sudden jerk of the body and occasionally by a loud cry. Thereafter, for about 10 seconds, the patient is in a tonic phase of muscular rigidity, followed by a half minute clonic phase consisting of spasmodic contractions of various muscles and jerking of the arms and legs. The patient then becomes quiet and remains unconscious for up to half an hour, following which he awakes and experiences a state of drowsiness, confusion and disorientation for a brief while. A few patients manifest excitement and combativeness in this stage. There is a danger of fractures during the convulsions; administration of relaxant drugs prior to each treatment greatly minimizes the strength of the muscle contractions and reduces the frequency of fractures. Patients with cardiac difficulties may be treated by ECT only with great caution, for it may be too violent and stressful for them.

A standard schedule for ECT consists of three treatments per week. Involutional melancholics and manic-depressives usually improve dramatically with about 6 treatments, but they may be given up to 10 or 12 in order to consolidate their gains. In the pre-ataractic era, many schizophrenic patients received as many as 50 ECT's. Neurotics may show a marked improvement after one treatment, probably due to suggestibility, but they then relapse quickly; it is generally believed that ECT is inappropriate for the treatment of neurosis, except perhaps for neurotic depression. ECT may diminish neurotic depressive symptoms and it sometimes even eliminates the depressive component present in a number of organic patients, although it cannot of course eliminate the organic pathology itself.

The attitude of patients to ECT is variable. Some are indifferent, some seem to enjoy the attention they receive and some interpret the therapy as a punishment for their sins and welcome it masochistically, but most regard it with apprehension and fear, despite the absence of pain. (On the average, however, ECT arouses less fear than Metrazol or insulin coma therapy.) A mental hospital has a culture of its own, with a complex social structure; a frequent component of this structure consists of older patients "hazing" new arrivals by describing the supposed horrors of ECT to them. To minimize patient apprehension, Sodium Amytal may be administered before each treatment. In any case, the patient's attitude seems to have no effect whatever on whether he will benefit from the treatment.

ECT has both short- and long-term effects. In the short run, manics become quieter and depressives more cheerful, resulting in a marked change of mood for the better in both cases. After a treatment, most patients are amnesic for the events that immediately preceded it, but with time the amnesia tends to dissipate. However, after a series of treatments some patients become amnesic for large blocks of past events and remain amnesic long after the series is concluded. The age of the patient is a relevant variable: older patients are likely to become confused and amnesic after a short series of only two or three treatments, while young adults usually show little or no amnesia after as many as 20 treatments. The spacing of treatments is another relevant variable: the more closely massed they are, the greater the likelihood of amnesia. Cameron (1960) reported that schizophrenics treated by ECT were more amnesic for past episodes of disorganized, schizophrenic behavior than for episodes in which they had functioned normally. He suggested that the greater the discrepancy between these two sets of memories, the more stable the patient's recovery. This hypothesis implies that ECT is beneficial because it helps the patient to preserve adaptive responses while making it difficult to remember maladaptive ones.

The evidence bearing on the overall effectiveness of ECT with the affective disorders is clear and impressive. It causes quick and dramatic improvement in as many as 90 per cent of manic-depressives in a depressed phase and involutional melancholics. The proportion of manic patients who improve is almost as large. However, this figure is for improvement, not for complete recovery.

In ECT treatment of the manic-depressive type of depression, a complete disappearance of symptoms shortly after treatment has been reported for 40 to 80 per cent of the patients in different studies. For involutional melancholia, the percentages reported have been even higher, but for manics somewhat lower. Among catatonic schizophrenics, a remission figure as high as 68 per cent has been reported (Kalinowsky and Hoch, 1952), but the results usually reported are much lower than this. Paranoid schizophrenics respond less well than catatonics, and both simple and hebephrenic schizophrenics yield remission figures as low as 10 per cent. Taking all the evidence together, most observers have concluded that ECT is extremely effective with involutional melancholics, almost as effective with depressives, somewhat less with manics, of limited use with catatonics and quite ineffective with all other schizophrenics. With the first three groups, ECT increases the probability of improvement or remission and causes it to occur sooner. An involutional melancholic, for example, has 9 chances in 10 of improving in less than one month if treated by ECT, whereas spontaneous improvement occurs in half or fewer of the patients and may take years. To some extent the results may be due to the extra attention often accompanying ECT, for the patient perceives that he is an object of concern to the staff. But the primary factor must be the somatic treatment itself, for attention alone without ECT does not produce impressive results.

ECT has some negative aspects. Despite precautions, some fractures and dislocations occur, especially with muscular, young, male patients. Fatalities have been reported about once in 5000 treatments. In addition, experiments with monkeys, dogs, cats and mice have proved that brain damage can result from a long series of treatments. In humans, brain damage has not been proved to occur, but the long-range amnesia found in some patients suggests that it *can.*

ECT does not alter the basic personality of the patient nor does it decrease the probability of recurrence of a manic or depressive episode. In fact, there is some evidence that it tends to increase this probability slightly (Salzman, 1947).

Given these negative aspects and limitations, plus the fear of electric "shock," it is not surprising that some professional persons as well as the general public should mistrust ECT. Many experts feel that ECT and other somatic procedures for the treatment of functional disorders are barbarous and sadistic. Somatic therapy has been described as a despairing effort to blast the patient's symptoms out of existence instead of trying to understand him and help him to understand and change himself. On the other hand, it is an objectively demonstrable fact that several types of somatic therapy decrease symptoms and make patients more comfortable. Furthermore, a diminution of symptoms and discomfort itself sometimes leads to deeper personality changes as effectively as psychotherapy does.

The reasons for the effectiveness of ECT with the affective disorders are unclear. Both psychological and physiological explanations have been offered. Various theorists have hypothesized that the really important psychological aspect of ECT is the attention given the patient, or the amnesia ECT induces, or the opportunity to "rest" during the brief periods of unconsciousness or the patient's perception of the treatment as a symbolic death that expiates his sins. None of these hypotheses is adequate: attention without ECT is not very effective, some patients improve without experiencing amnesia, unconsciousness induced by means other than an electric current through the brain is therapeutically useless, and there is no reason to believe that most patients perceive the treatment as a symbolic death. Furthermore, none of these hypotheses explains why melancholics and depressives respond better than others.

Some physiological explanations that have been suggested are also untenable. Meduna's theory of a biological antagonism between schizophrenia and epilepsy does not explain ECT, since these disorders may occur in the same individual more frequently than he believed. Another physiological theory is that ECT works because it temporarily deprives the brain of oxygen. It is not clear, however, why anoxia should be beneficial for any type of functional psychosis, or why it should be more beneficial for affective than schizophrenic reactions, or why it is necessary to induce anoxia by electricity rather than by any other method.

Still another physiological theory is highly speculative but plausible. It is possible that the electric current acts as a biological stressor and arouses the brain to mobilize some defensive chemical substance not as yet identified. If such a substance were to persist for a period after the termination of ECT treatment, it could temporarily increase the ability of the nervous system to withstand internal and external pressures; when the substance dissipates, the psychosis recurs. The speculative nature of this explanation must be emphasized, however.

Insulin Coma Therapy

The technique of insulin coma therapy was devised by a Polish psychiatrist, Manfred Sakel, in Vienna in 1932, several years before ECT. Insulin coma therapy is time-consuming, expensive and dangerous, and since the introduction of ataractic drugs has been used less and less. Nevertheless, it is somtimes helpful

HYPOGLYCEMIA — low Bl. sugar
INSULIN blots out glucose !! which give us 90% of our energy.

with schizophrenics who do not benefit from drug treatment.

Insulin in a large enough dose to induce hypoglycemia—low blood sugar level—is injected into the patient intramuscularly. For about an hour after the injection, the patient feels weak, hungry and drowsy and he perspires freely. He then becomes unconscious and manifests signs of physiological shock; he trembles and twitches convulsively and eventually goes into a coma in which he does not respond to a pinprick or other painful stimulation. After about an hour in the coma stage the patient's blood sugar level is raised and he is aroused by feeding him orange juice through a tube. The time from the initial injection to the termination of each treatment is four or five hours. A total of 50 to 60 treatments is administered on a schedule of five or six mornings a week. To find the proper dosage for each patient's tolerance level, it is customary to inject a small amount of insulin the first day and rapidly increase the dosage on successive days until a deep coma is produced. In a variation of the treatment, referred to as "subshock," a smaller amount of insulin is injected and the patient's reaction stops short of the coma stage. Insulin subshock treatment is sometimes used to quiet anxious or excitable patients, but it is of little help with schizophrenics.

On arousal from an insulin treatment, a schizophrenic is likely to be temporarily amnesic but also more rational and less withdrawn than he was prior to the treatment. In the early course of the treatments this improvement tends to fade and be dissipated by the next day, but in a successfully treated case the lucid, socially responsive intervals lengthen from day to day and begin to hold into the next day so that further treatments eventually become unnecessary. In a large scale study, Malzberg (1938) reported recovery for 13 per cent and improvement for 54 per cent of treated schizophrenics. The rates for a control group of untreated cases were 3.5 per cent for recovery and 19 per cent for improvement. Kalinowsky and Hoch, in their survey of somatic treatments (1952), conclude that a remission rate of 40 to 50 per cent is the best one can hope for from insulin treatment of schizophrenia; the rate usually attained is considerably lower. On the average, catatonics and paranoids respond to insulin treatments better than simple and hebephrenic schizophrenics. Improvement is not always maintained over a long period. In one study of schizophrenics, Hinko and Lipschutz (1947) reported that five years after insulin

treatment and hospital discharge the percentage of discharged patients who did not need hospital readmission was only 4 per cent greater than for an untreated control group.

In insulin treatments the stress on the cardiovascular and nervous systems is much greater than in ECT and the therapy is therefore usually limited to healthy adults aged 15 to 45. It cannot be used for patients who have severe cardiac difficulties, hypertension, tuberculosis, diabetes or chronic respiratory diseases. In somewhat less than 1 per cent of cases, the patient goes into an irreversible, stuporous shock and the outcome is fatal. Insulin treatment is obviously a calculated risk to be used with severely ill patients when less strenuous methods have failed.

Like ECT, insulin does not alter the patient's basic personality makeup. As yet no one has discovered the mechanism to which insulin therapy owes its effectiveness with some patients.

Psychosurgery

Here again we are dealing with a type of therapy that was widely adopted a few decades ago and then decreased in usage as the major tranquilizers were developed. Psychosurgery is used today only when all other methods have failed, and even then with reluctance. It was foreshadowed thousands of years ago in the practice of trephining. Much later, in medieval Rome, when it was observed that disordered behavior sometimes improved following an injury to the brain by a sword blow, some attempts were apparently made to let out the evil humors of psychotic individuals by boring into their skulls. In 1888, a Swiss psychiatrist, Burkhardt, operated on the brain of an extremely disturbed woman who had been in his asylum for 15 years and hallucinated continually. In the belief that her hallucinations were caused by localized disease of the cerebral cortex, Burkhardt therefore performed four successive operations at intervals of several weeks to remove some of the cortical tissue. Considerable improvement occurred, but the results of surgery on five additional patients were not spectacular. In reporting his success with his first patient, Burkhardt commented that although some physicians held fast to the precept, "above all do not injure the patient," others were guided by the principle, "better a doubtful remedy than none." "I belong, naturally, to the second category," he wrote.

It remained for a Portuguese physician, Egas Moniz, to recommend the surgical interruption of the frontal association pathways as a treatment for psychotics. The first such operation was carried out under his direction in 1935. The basis of the procedure was Moniz's unwarranted belief that psychotics had fixed arrangements of cellular connections in the frontal lobes which were responsible for their persistent delusions and that destruction of these connections would eliminate the delusions.

Psychosurgery is occasionally used today for agitated depressions, schizophrenic reactions and particularly severe and stubborn obsessive reactions. It has also proved useful for relieving the intractable pain that sometimes occurs in such diseases as inoperable cancer. It should not be used for impulsive and irresponsible patients since it is likely to make them even more irresponsible.

A number of specific surgical techniques have been worked out. In the most frequent procedure—lobotomy, also known as prefrontal lobotomy or leucotomy—some of the nerve connections are severed between the frontal lobes and the thalamus. The operation can be performed painlessly with a local anesthetic. Among the alternative procedures are topectomy, in which parts of the frontal lobes are removed, and thalectomy, in which an electric needle severs nerve tracts in the thalamus.

Immediately after the surgery, the patient is confused, but he recovers from this state in a few days. About one in every three patients undergoes marked improvement and another one-third improves sufficiently to leave the hospital. Most of the rest improve a little and a small number show no change or worsen. It must be remembered that psychosurgery tends to be restricted to patients with whom everything else has been tried and has failed, so that any improvement at all may be considered a great gain. Jenkins et al. (1954) found twice the improvement in lobotomized than in untreated chronic schizophrenics, and other studies have produced comparable results. In a successful case, a decrease is noted in anxiety, paralyzing inhibitions, self-consciousness, rumination over the past and worry over the future, and an increase occurs in extraversion and cheerfulness. The loss of intellectual ability in the average case is insignificant.

There are also negative consequences. Brain surgery is a serious matter and results in death in 1 to 4 per cent of patients, the rates varying for different procedures. The weakening of inhibitions may be accompanied by an increase in tactlessness and aggressiveness and affect may become more shallow as it becomes more positive. Following brain surgery, many patients live so much in the present and take so little thought for the future that they can be described as having lost the ability to plan. Porteus and Peters (1947) found a deficit in the ability of lobotomized patients to succeed on the Porteus Mazes, a test calling for a considerable degree of planning and foresight. The patient's ability to generalize and think in abstract terms may also be impaired; his thinking becomes more concrete and rigid. Another danger is that partial amnesia for pre-operative events may persist permanently. In some cases, appetite increases inordinately and in others the patient loses his drive and becomes extremely passive and content to do nothing. A particularly unfortunate consequence in a few cases is the loss of the ability to control urination or defecation.

Like drugs, ECT, insulin coma and other somatic approaches, psychosurgery works best for patients whose illness is of recent origin, but it tends instead to be prescribed for patients who have been ill a long time. Relatives are often very reluctant to give permission for the operation unless the patient's condition is quite deteriorated. It has been remarked that the more reluctant the physician is to recommend psychosurgery the better the end result is likely to be. Many dynamically oriented psychiatrists regard it as barbarous and inhuman; their attitude is well expressed in the following statement (Group for the Advancement of Psychiatry, 1948):

. . . It represents a mechanistic attitude toward psychiatry which is a throwback to our prepsychodynamic days, which in itself would not be of great concern if it were successful and did not harm the patient. It is a man-made, self-destructive procedure that specifically destroys several human functions which have been slowly evolved and that especially separate us from other animals. If the operation is of importance as a therapeutic procedure in certain selected cases, it becomes all the more important for us to establish definite clinical indications and controls so that its usefulness will not be diluted by utilization in situations where it can do little good and much harm.

Granted—as even this statement seems to do—that psychosurgery is sometimes useful, its effectiveness calls for explanation. The explanation seems to lie in the fact that the frontal and prefrontal lobes are involved in foresight and planning whereas the thalamus and hypothalamus mediate affective behavior. Cutting some of the connections between the two areas reduces their interaction so that the patient's thinking becomes less anxiety-laden and emotionally distorted, and his emotional responses become less freighted with rumination. Irrational ideas and persecutory delusions may survive a lobotomy, but the individual becomes less troubled by the ideas and less fearful of being persecuted.

PSYCHOTHERAPY

Most troubled people have an urge to talk to someone—a relative, friend, minister, physician, colleague or even a casual acquaintance. Psychotherapy is a special way of talking with an especially qualified person—the therapist—to achieve a better adjustment. It may take place in a variety of settings such as private offices, outpatient clinics, hospitals, schools and welfare agencies. A comprehensive definition of psychotherapy is the following statement by Wolberg (1954):

Psychotherapy is a form of treatment for problems of an emotional nature in which a trained person deliberately establishes a professional relationship with a patient with the object of removing, modifying or retarding existing symptoms, of mediating disturbed patterns of behavior, and of promoting positive personality growth and development.

Depending on the particular patient and on the personality, skill and theoretical orientation of the therapist, there are variations in the specific relationship that is established, the specific goals that are sought and the techniques employed. There are a number of systems or "schools" of psychotherapy; psychoanalysis, client-centered therapy, and learning theory approaches are three prominent examples. Although there are some common factors in the various systems, each is grounded in a different theory of personality maladjustment, each has its own concepts of the therapeutic process and each employs techniques compatible with its concepts.

One of the difficulties in discussing psychotherapy is in the very nature of the terms applied as well as in the whole concept of emotional disorders. Words such as "patient" and "treatment" imply a medical procedure designed to cure an illness. Yet, as we saw in the early discussion on definitions of abnormal

behavior (see Chapter 1), the illness model is only one of several acceptable ways of conceptualizing emotional problems. A person who compulsively strives for achievement in order to compensate for his private belief that he is an inadequate human being can scarcely be said to be ill in the usual sense of the word. Nor can the establishment of a special human relationship designed to provide him with a corrective emotional experience be properly thought of as a treatment. What the client is exhibiting is one kind of problem in living, which, as it happens, can often be alleviated through certain kinds of special human relationships (such as psychotherapy).

Another feature of psychotherapy which separates it from other forms of "treatment" is the emphasis which is placed on the patient-therapist relationship. With the possible exception of behavior modification or learning theory approaches, all theories of psychotherapy emphasize the special nature of this relationship and the vital role it plays in the patient's subsequent change or growth. A physician can remove an appendix from a person he scarcely knows without untoward effects. But a psychotherapist who does not hold the trust, respect and confidence of his client is almost certainly doomed to failure. The uniqueness of a significant, interpersonal relationship seems essential to patient change and development, though many experts differ about the necessary ingredients of the relationship.

In the following discussion, the terms "patient," "treatment" and the like will be used because they are so prevalent in current literature but the reservations just delineated should be kept in mind.

The Goals of Psychotherapy

Depending on the patient's need and suitability for psychotherapy, a therapist may seek to attain relatively ambitious or relatively limited goals. Or he may decide that the patient is unlikely to benefit from psychotherapy and dissuade him from embarking on it.

The most suitable candidate for psychotherapy—particularly the more intensive varieties—is somewhere between late adolescence and the forties. (Special therapeutic techniques for children will be discussed later in this chapter.) With age, people become more rigid and their behavior is less easily modified. The ideal candidate is also at least average in intelligence and verbal fluency, is willing to discuss his feelings and behavior and is neither psychotic nor sociopathic. A patient who seeks psychotherapy of his own volition and genuinely wishes to modify his behavior, attitudes or personality traits is more suited for therapy than a patient who has been forced into it by a relative or other person. Another characteristic of the ideal patient is that he is not at the mercy of a hopeless reality situation. Finally, middle and upper class patients usually respond better than lower class patients to psychotherapy.

Of course, such statements about patient suitability are only general statements, which are more often correct when applied to a random sample of people who present themselves for psychotherapy as it is typically practiced. In fact, there are many variations and modifications of psychotherapeutic approaches which have been used successfully with older people, with psychotics, with sociopaths and with persons from the lower socioeconomic levels.

The choice of therapeutic goals depends on the patient's assets and liabilities, on the amount of time, effort (and often money) he is willing to invest, and on the available therapeutic resources. The amount of time and energy required of both therapist and patient may be considerable. Some centers offer "crisis intervention" services which are aimed at providing brief psychotherapy to persons in a state of acute emotional crisis. The purpose is to help people readjust to the level of adaption which they had attained prior to the emotional crisis. Such efforts typically consist of one to six interviews spread over a few days or weeks.

Other therapists prefer to work with the patient on a once or twice weekly basis over a period of months or years. Typically these approaches emphasize the current patient-therapist relationship as a way of showing the patient his interpersonal strengths and weaknesses as well as more adaptive alternatives to previously fixed maladaptive behaviors. Behavior modification techniques tend to be somewhat briefer, as the primary focus is on learning adaptive techniques and unlearning maladaptive ones. Here the focus is on the symptom rather than on either the patient-therapist relationship or the patient's phenomenological world. Treatment terminates when the symptom is alleviated. Whether or not the patient understands himself better as a result is usually not a matter of concern to the behavior therapist. At the opposite extreme is the psychoanalytic approach developed by Freud.

The patient usually is seen three to five times per week for two to five years. The emphasis here is to make the patient's unconscious strivings conscious through analyzing the patient's dreams, fantasies and free associations. Insight or self understanding is important if the patient is to gain control over the unconscious strivings and defenses which previously affected his behavior.

Which of these general approaches is used in a given instance depends upon many factors, some of which will be discussed later in this chapter. One factor is the goal of the therapist. If his goal is symptom removal, he may employ a behavior modification approach. If his goal is personality reorganization or increased self-awareness and flexibility, he may employ a psychoanalytic approach, or some modification. In the following sections we will examine three different psychotherapeutic approaches which employ differing techniques to achieve what is in each instance considered to be the most desirable goals. While these theories are representative of current views, they are not exhaustive. The list of approaches is extensive. In effect, since each psychotherapist is different, there may be as many systems of psychotherapy as there are practitioners. The systems described here are intended only as an introduction to alternative methods of conceptualizing the psychotherapeutic process.

Systematic Approaches to Psychotherapy

The scientific basis of psychotherapy is imperfect and incomplete. We do not know the precise nature of the processes at work in the complex psychotherapeutic situation, or just which patients will be helped in therapy and which will not, or why some patients are helped and some not. Psychotherapy is thus more of an art than a science, and it is not surprising that many systems of psychotherapy have developed and gathered adherents. A convinced follower of a system who finds emotional and intellectual security in it is likely to be a more effective therapist than the skeptic who must constantly question the validity of his procedures. Just as the research scientist needs to avoid dogmatism, the therapeutic practitioner needs to avoid continual self-doubt.

Psychoanalysis. Most psychoanalytic patients fall into the diagnostic categories of psychoneurosis, disorders of personality and psychophysiologic disorders; with some exceptions, psychotics are not amenable to standard psychoanalytic treatment. Although psychoanalysis is usually carried out in private offices, many patients have been successfully analyzed in hospitals. To determine if a patient is amenable to psychoanalysis, a trial analysis is first conducted for a few weeks. In this period the analyst determines if the patient can learn to free associate and whether his problems can be helped in analysis or are due to insurmountable environmental obstacles.

The fundamental rule of psychoanalysis is that the patient, lying on a couch, must free associate, that is, he must say whatever is on his mind. He must not hold back past or present events, attitudes toward the therapist or fantasies, no matter how unpleasant, unflattering or embarrassing they may be. It is easier for the patient to do this when lying on a couch than when facing the analyst; the use of the couch also keeps the patient's thoughts free of influence by the therapist's facial expression and it maximizes the transference (that is, the patient's tendency to attribute to the therapist or transfer onto him, those attitudes and feelings which were previously attributed to significant others, such as parents). Freud stated another reason for preferring the couch: he disliked being stared at hour after hour.

The basis for the fundamental rule is the belief that neurotic conflicts can be exposed by this method. Intrapsychic conflicts with their roots in early childhood are exposed by the nature of the unedited ideas, affects and associations which are produced in connection with current life experiences. It will be recalled that Freud believed that earlier conflicts, though repressed and unconscious, continue to exert influence on the patient's adult life and are directly responsible for symptoms such as anxiety, depression, phobias and the like. Through his free associations and, more importantly, through his difficulties in submitting to the fundamental rule to say whatever comes to mind, the patient's neurotic conflicts become apparent. For although free association is an easy task on the face of it, in practice it turns out to be exceedingly difficult. The difficulties are of two types: (1) the patient soon encounters material or feelings which he does not wish to share with the therapist and which he decides to withhold; (2) even though desiring to cooperate, the patient finds that he becomes "blocked," that "nothing comes to mind," or that he cannot get his mind off an insignificant detail. These difficulties are called *resistances* and are the

means by which a patient protects himself from acknowledging unacceptable or painful affects. The resistances themselves provide clues to the patient's conflicts. For example, a patient who fell silent while discussing a sexually tinged subject and later in the same hour went blank while engaging in free association about his mother was later discovered to be still struggling against the acceptance of erotic feelings toward his mother. His resistance provided an early clue to this conflict as well as to his fear of ridicule and rejection should the therapist learn of his primitive fantasies.

Resistances are overcome by the therapist's interpretations. Interpretations are communications designed to identify and call to the patient's attention the presence of resistances. An additional function of interpretations is to suggest reasonable hypotheses concerning the nature of the conflict underlying the resistance. More interpretations tend to be directed at the exposure of resistances than toward the explanation of how and why they came into being. Fenichel (1941) summarizes the process of psychoanalytic interpretation as follows:

(1) What is interpreted is first isolated . . . (2) The patient's attention is drawn to his own activity; he himself has been bringing about that which up to now he has thought he was experiencing passively. (3) He comprehends that he had motives for this activity which hitherto he did not know of. (4) He comes to note that at some other point too, he harbors something similar, or something that is in some way associatively connected. (5) With the help of these observations he becomes able to produce less distorted "derivatives" and through these the origins of this behavior gradually becomes clear.

The following example of free association from Wolberg (1954)* demonstrates how verbalizing one's kaleidoscopic thoughts produces a meaningful communication. The patient was female, 38 years old, suffering from a phobic disorder. Prior to the quoted excerpt, she had been talking about her sexual fears and then about her father.

Pt. I just thought of something. When father died, he was nude. I looked at him, but I couldn't see anything, I couldn't think clearly. I was brought up not to be aware of the difference between

---

*Reprinted by permission from Wolberg, L. R., 1954. The Technique of Psychotherapy, New York, Grune & Stratton, Inc., pp. 392–395.

a man and a woman. I feared my father, and yet I loved him. I slept with him when I was very little, on Saturdays and Sundays. A wonderful sense of warmth and security. There was nothing warmer or more secure. A lot of pleasure. I tingle all over now. It was a wonderful holiday when I was allowed to sleep with father. I can't seem to remember anything now. There's a blur in my mind. I feel tense and afraid.

The analyst's interpretation of her "blur" as resistance and as a manifestation of fear, motivated her to move closer to her unconscious conflicts in the rest of the session.

The analysis of dreams, which Freud termed the "royal road to the unconscious," is an important part of psychoanalysis. The following illustration (Wolberg, 1954) demonstrates the recurrent themes in a series of dreams and the manner in which dream analysis may lead to insight. The patient's major symptom was sexual impotence. In the session from which the excerpt is quoted, he had been describing how far short most women were of his standards and ideals.

Th. What about dreams; have you had any since our last visit?

Pt. Yes, quite a few. On Tuesday night I dreamed I was in some sort of a revolutionary turmoil, and some dictator had his arm torn off. Then I became the dictator, and my arm is attached. As I proceed somewhere, each time someone touches my arm, I feel it's going to be torn off. This is followed by a dream in which I and a girl are going somewhere, and running to catch a bus, and my hand begins to bleed. I'm becoming covered with blood, and she says, "Look what's happening." I say, "It doesn't matter; let's get there in a hurry." Then I exclude from an appointment I had arranged with people, this girl.

Th. Exclude her?

Pt. Yes, she was excluded in some way.

Th. By whom?

Pt. By me.

Th. Mm hmm.

Pt. I was in considerable turmoil. And then I dreamed of my cousin, my young cousin at school. He reports that a number of children at school have succumbed to some epidemic, to some disease. Following this, I help him conceal a knife that he's to use illegally in fights with other boys, and I instruct him how to use it. Then I walk along a dark street alone and see adults discussing something. Then these adults transform into a group of children. I walk along in imminent fear of attack. I pass a boy with a large hound. At first the dog jumps on me and seizes me by the arm, and, oh, I had a painful sensation in my arm. (Pause)

Th. Is that all?

Pt. Yes.

Th. What do you make of it, the dreams, I mean?

Pt. I suppose I am upset and afraid. I must be the dictator whose arm is hurt.

Th. Yes, as if you are in jeopardy of being attacked as a dictator and physically hurt.

Pt. Yes.

Th. What about being a dictator?

Pt. That's what some girls call me, when they fall in love with me and get angry. This dream followed this date with the girl.

Th. I see. Perhaps your feelings about this girl touched off the dreams. It's significant that in the dream you are running with the girl to catch a bus and your arm is bleeding.

Pt. Yes, we are going somewhere and I want to get there in a hurry.

Th. Where do you think you want to go in a hurry?

Pt. (Pause) To get sex I suppose. I am in a rush to get this thing settled.

Th. But perhaps this dream tells us why it's difficult to get things done in a hurry. After all, your arm is mutilated. Could it be that in rushing into sex you feel you might be mutilated in some way?

Pt. (Emotionally) There must be something that scares me. I feel anxious as I talk now.

Th. In what way could you be mutilated? Who would mutilate you and why?

Pt. I don't know. In the dream I help my cousin fight off an attack. This must be an aspect of me. Then I am attacked by a boy and a dog who jumps me.

Th. And you get a painful sensation in your arm. The arm that bled in the other part of the dream?

Pt. Yes.

Th. But what about the part of the dream where you exclude her?

Pt. I don't know.

Th. Why should she be excluded?

Pt. I might want to exclude her, I suppose, from myself.

Th. That's what you actually did in your feelings toward her during the date.

Pt. Yes.

Th. And is that what you do with other women?

Pt. I suppose so.

Th. Is it possible that you exclude her because of feelings, indicated by the dream, of fear, of bloody mutilation?

Pt. If I were to expect attack from this source I can see that.

Th. One way to escape attack is to give up the sex object, remove yourself from her, become impotent and apathetic. [Interpretation]

Pt. I just remembered. I had a dream the day before I saw the girl.

Th. Mm hmm.

Pt. A series of two dreams, not entirely clear. There's a small girl who demonstrates strong friendship feelings towards me and offers something valuable which, in the dream, is a source of energy which she tells me to take from a series of intangible columns of materials. Later in the dream a small girl is very friendly to me. However, she transforms into a small boy who then picks up my pack of cigarettes and throws it out of the window, despite my protests. Then I'm with a police officer and he hides a pearl necklace in the files. I'm interested in it, but tell him I'm not, and I just want to go to some town. I go to the railway station, check my suitcase and enter the train car. Then some woman rushes out with a suitcase that looks like mine. I follow her, but we investigate and find the suitcase is hers. I return to the car and find my suitcase. The contents are all female articles, and I think to myself it will be difficult to prove that this is my suitcase. (*Pause*) And that's all.

Th. I see. What do you think of that?

Pt. (*Laughs*) Well, I suppose my impending date got me to dream of this girl. I think of this treasure, the pearl necklace.

Th. The treasure being hidden by a police officer?

Pt. Yes, keeping it from me.

Th. What is the most precious treasure you can think of?

Pt. What I want here. To have sex with a woman. Sex must be locked away from me, if we are to believe the dream, by some authority.

Th. Mm hmm.

Pt. The recognition of that by the woman—the suitcase—is rather more puzzling. It apparently involves some uncertainty in my, uh, virility and masculine qualities, as much as the woman had the same suitcase as I.

Th. As if she's a counterpart of you, as if you don't know your identity—male or female. [*Interpretation*]

Pt. Yes, I can see something now; it occurs to me that the arm in the dreams is a symbol of my genitals.

Th. Mm hmm.

Pt. And the dictator, being in the position of dominance like a male, can have his genitals hurt and not be a man. If I try to be a man, I may be hurt—my superiority and power torn off so to speak.

Th. And sexually mutilated.

Pt. Yes, undoubtedly.

Th. And in a sexual role with a woman?

Pt. I'll be sexually hurt, hurt.

Th. Now, if it's true that you could be hurt for trying to be a man, what defense would you use?

Pt. To get away, run away, or to be a woman and not have to face it.

Th. What about fighting back?

Pt. Yes, yes. The aggression. Like in the dream, the attacking with a knife.

Th. Your dreams seem to bring out mechanisms of why you act the way you do.

Pt. I can definitely see that, but it's so peculiar. I know it's true. I feel it. But it's so strange.

Th. It would explain your coldness with women, the impotence. If you expect to be castrated, that's no fun.

Pt. (*Laughs*) Gosh, uh, yeah, uh, I had one reaction of this sort, which I became conscious of, and that is that in playing with my girl friend, the old one, she accidentally hurt me very slightly around the genital region, but it was very slight. And nonetheless it, for a while, caused a complete disappearance of sexual desire.

Th. When did this happen?

Pt. A number of days ago.

Th. Before or after the dream?

Pt. Before.

As seen in the illustration, the analyst may take a very active therapeutic role. In fact, psychoanalysts have been accused of first convincing patients by repeated suggestions and persuasion that they teem with sexual and aggressive impulses and conflicts, and then citing the patients' verbalizations as proof of the existence of these very impulses and conflicts. In other words, the method of psychoanalysis has been criticized for creating what it claims to discover in nature. On the basis of present evidence, it is not clear how valid this criticism is.

The interpretation of free associations and dreams is based on the assumption of *psychic determinism,* the postulate that mental processes are never accidental but are completely determined by their antecedents. Thoughts and symptoms, in fact, are believed to be overdetermined, that is, to have a number of converging, causal antecedents. As a guide to disentangling the antecedents in each case, the analyst makes use of the Freudian concepts discussed in Chapter 4: the conflict among the id, ego and superego, the individual's pregenital development through the oral, anal and phallic stages dominated by the erogenous zones, the Oedipal triangle, the defense mechanisms and so on. To the analyst, the patient's associations mean something quite different from what the patient thinks they mean, for they are assumed to be derivatives of repressed instincts whose roots lie in childhood.

One of the principal concepts of psychoanalytic therapy is *transference.* Essentially the concept refers to the patient's tendency to transfer to contemporaries feelings that at one time were experienced toward significant figures of his childhood, particularly his parents. While regarded as a universal phenomenon, transference tendencies are particularly pronounced in neurotics and emerge in a particularly powerful way when the therapist assumes a passive, neutral role while encouraging the patient to free associate. That is to say, transference feelings are more likely to emerge when the therapist deliberately de-emphasizes his own emergence as a real person while encouraging the patient to indulge in fantasies, reveries and dreams. In response to this ambiguous situation the patient unwittingly re-creates the conflict which he had failed to resolve with his parents.

For example, the patient may come to hold the therapist in high esteem and idealize him far out of proportion to any help that has been forthcoming. He may become jealous of the therapist's other patients and desire to be the therapist's favorite or best patient. These and other needs and the conflicts which go with them thus reproduce affects the patient previously experienced toward his parents and have little to do with the therapist's feelings or behavior in the current situation. In a manner of speaking, the patient suffers from what was, in childhood, an interpersonal conflict. This conflict was internalized and made into an intrapsychic conflict because of the patient's inability to resolve it with the other person(s) involved. The analytic situation reverses the process so that the conflict is once again made into an interpersonal one, this time between the patient and the therapist. The patient comes to see that his relation as an adult to the therapist often has elements of a child relating to his parents and is helped to achieve new and more adaptive modes of relating. Thus the conflicts of the past are relived in the present and resolved in the context of the current interpersonal relationship.

The following case (Wolberg, 1954) demonstrates the role of a transference in the growth of insight:*

Sporadic backaches (lumbago) were among the patient's most disturbing symptoms. From time to time, backaches became exaggerated during a treatment session. Observing the content of his conversations when this happened, it was determined that backaches developed whenever the patient bragged or boasted about himself, whenever he voiced comments that might be construed as criticisms of me, whenever he expressed demands which I might possibly reject, or whenever he mentioned circumstances in which he had behaved in a selfish or intolerant manner. On one occasion, when these facts were brought to his attention, the patient stiffened with severe back pain which became so intense that he winced. This was coupled with pain in

---

*Reprinted by permission from Wolberg, L. R. 1954. The Technique of Psychotherapy. New York, Grune & Stratton, Inc.

his scrotum and drawing sensations in the perineum [lower part of the trunk]. Asked to tell me what was on his mind, he expostulated that he could never express himself frankly with his father. A stern puritanical man, his father had subjected him to severe discipline whenever the patient deviated in the least from the righteous path of moral, unpretentious living. Even childish pranks were forbidden. When questioned about the form of punishment his father employed, the patient said, "He would beat me across the back with a stick," The area of attack coincided precisely with the zone of his present backaches.

At this point I mentioned that it was rather significant that in talking to me about certain topics, he had symptoms of backache. This sounded as if he were being punished for his thoughts. Seemingly, no impression was made on the patient by the interpretation. However, when he appeared for the next session, he was manifestly disturbed. Hitherto gentle and courteous, he stormed into my office and launched into a verbal attack on me. A fragment of this session follows:

Pt. I haven't wanted to say this, but it's bothered me for some time. Your attitude, I mean. (*The patient is quite anxious as he talks.*)
Th. My attitude?
Pt. You remember when I first came to see you and told you about my flight instruction and taking my instructor's test?
Th. Yes. (*This incident was a minor one I had almost forgotten.*)
Pt. Well, you acted very flippant and disinterested.
Th. In what way?
Pt. The way you talked and looked.
Th. I wonder. Why didn't you mention this at the time?
Pt. (*pause*) Well, I thought that I was wrong to boast about it. And I felt you resented my boasting, blowing my horn. I know I feel this, and you'll say it's my imagination, but I feel I'm right that you cut me off from talking. I felt you were contemptuous of me.
Th. If this were true, I certainly wouldn't blame you for feeling the way you do. But searching into myself, and trying to recapitulate what happened, I don't remember wanting to cut you off, or feeling flippant, or deriding you in any way or acting contemptuous toward you. Is it possible that you see in what I did or said, something that wasn't there?
Pt. (*angrily*) I don't believe you. I think you're saying that to be therapeutic. I feel that.
Th. As if I'm saying this to reassure you?
Pt. Yes, because I feel this is what you did.
Th. Cut you off and acted contemptuous on the basis that you were boasting?
Pt. Yes. It's confusing to me.
Th. Say, how come you bring that up now? This happened five months ago.
Pt. Something you said last time I was here made me mad. I don't know what it is now. (*Apparently*

my pointing out the possibilities of a transference reaction, removed his repression and released hostility.) I still feel you don't want to admit what you did.

Th. Well, I'll try to examine my feelings about you, and see if I really did cut you off and deride you. As far as I know right now, this isn't how I felt. As far as I can see right now, I don't feel at all contemptuous toward you.

Pt. It's hard for me to believe that. I mean it's hard to see why you shouldn't be annoyed.

Th. Why should I be annoyed at you?

Pt. Look at the crazy things I did, I told you about. That episode with that woman and everything else that followed.

Th. Maybe you feel I ought to look down on you for what you've done?

At the next session the patient was again accusatory. He said that I acted detached and unfriendly. I didn't give him an opportunity to attend my lectures or to socialize with me. He recalled that he had recently met me at a restaurant and that I had nodded, but did not offer to share my table with him. Again I assured him that if it were true that I had willfully rejected him, he had a right to be angry. However, the nature of the therapeutic situation was such that any social contact might interfere with an opportunity to work out his problems.

For several sessions, we talked back and forth in this manner. I was aware of the fact that the patient was trying to goad me into acting in an angry, recriminatory way, paralleling his father's reactions. Were I to have responded in this way, he probably would have left therapy, convinced that I was an arbitrary, hostile person. Or he would have submitted himself and then developed a dependent, compliant attitude with a continuance of his symptoms. The upshot of our talks was a recognition of his projection into our relationship of attitudes he had about his father which had conditioned his general feeling toward authority. His ability to challenge my reaction, to vent his hostility, to understand that his reactions were carry-overs of earlier patterns, without encountering counter-hostility enabled him successfully to work through his problems in therapy.

The lengthy nature of psychoanalysis is in part due to the phenomenon of *working through:* If lasting insight into an impulse or conflict is to be gained, each of its many derivatives and connections must be traced, including the patient's transference reactions. Each impulse or conflict is examined again and again. The major goals of psychoanalysis—deep insight and substitution of sublimation for unsatisfactory defenses—are achieved only slowly and with difficulty.

The patient, like everyone else, desires to change but does not like to be hurt. Yet the very process of analysis often requires probing sensitive areas and the unleasing of powerful unpleasant affects. In addition, much of the neurotic pattern of behavior is learned early in childhood before full biological and emotional maturation and thus is deeply ingrained and overlearned. It is difficult to re-create that early state of malleability. The task is somewhat analogous to inducing a patient to give up his mother tongue while attempting to teach him a foreign language. The subject becomes frustrated, angry and often despairing and it requires great skill to insist on change while pointing out failures and yet maintain hope.

Finally, analysis takes time because psychoanalysis is committed to helping the patient achieve independence and autonomy. As a result direct advice or persuasion are minimized while the patient is encouraged to find his own solutions. This requires restraint and patience from the therapist and perseverance from the patient. False starts, blind alleys and mistakes are common as the patient struggles with new adaptive techniques, but they are necessary if the patient is to come to have real confidence in his own abilities. Such learning requires time. Time to act, to make mistakes, to be discouraged, and to try again.

Various technical modifications of the traditional psychoanalytic procedures have been suggested by Jung, Adler, Horney, Sullivan and others who have revised Freudian theory. Adlerians, for example, put more emphasis on conscious material and tend to complete treatment more rapidly than do traditional analysts. Alexander and French (1946), while adhering to psychoanalytic *theory,* advocate the use of a briefer and more flexible type of analytic therapy for many patients. These theorists recommend that a decision be made on the basis of an initial evaluation of each patient whether to employ the classical procedures of psychoanalysis or to adopt a schedule of only one or two interviews a week with periodic interruptions of treatment to test out therapeutic gains in real life. The therapist may decide to use face to face interviewing instead of the couch, to minimize the transference and so forth.

Freud's contributions to psychotherapy have not been confined to the psychoanalytic approach. Many of his concepts and ideas are incorporated and accepted by theorists who have little in common with the psychoanalyst. Concepts such as the unconscious, transference, resistance, defensiveness, interpretation and the like have become a part of the very warp and woof of the fabric of psychotherapy as it is practiced by the majority of experts in this country today.

Client-Centered Therapy. The aims of client-centered therapy, devised by Rogers (1951, 1957), are similar in a general sense to those of psychoanalysis: a decrease in internal conflict, a better integrated and more mature personality and an increase in the energy available for effective living. Rogers (1957) believes that certain therapeutic conditions are crucial for the achievement of these goals. First, at the beginning of therapy, the client must perceive and feel threatened by a discrepancy between his self concept and his actual experiences. (Proponents of client-centered therapy prefer the term "client" to "patient" because of the medical connotations of the latter). Second, the therapist must not present a facade to the client but must be geniuinely himself in the therapeutic hour. Contrary to the doctrines of many other therapeutic approaches, he must not play a special role. Third, unless the therapist feels "unconditional positive regard" for the client and accepts him completely as he is, there will be no progress. The therapist must *care* for the client. Fourth, the therapist must experience "an empathetic understanding of the client's internal frame of reference and [he] endeavors to communicate this experience to the client." Finally, the therapist must succeed in communicating his feelings to the client so that the latter will perceive the therapist's positive regard and understanding.

Rogers disagrees with a number of widely held assumptions about therapy. For example, he does not believe that the client's diagnostic category is relevant to success in treatment, or that psychotherapy involves a special kind of relationship in which one party is an expert (it is simply a good human interaction such as one finds between two very close friends), or that a special kind of intellectual and professional knowledge of human behavior is needed to be a therapist. The only crucial therapeutic trait is the capacity for empathy and acceptance. These are usually communicated to the client by the techniques of reflection and clarification.

The following example (Rogers, 1951) vividly illustrates how far a client-centered therapist may be willing to go in respecting the client's right to make decisions. The client threatens suicide or psychotic withdrawal and the therapist makes no attempt to dissuade her but, with two exceptions ("It's up to you," and "I believe you are able to make your own decision"),

he reflects her threats as he would other material.*

S [*Subject* or *Client*]: I've never said this before to anyone—but I've thought for such a long time—This is a terrible thing to say, but if I could just—well (*short, bitter laugh; pause*), if I could just find some glorious cause that I could give my life for I would be happy. I cannot be the kind of a person I want to be. I guess maybe I haven't the guts—or the strength—to kill myself—and if someone else would relieve me of the responsibility—or I would be in an accident—I—I—just don't want to live.

C [*Counselor*]: At the present time things look so black to you that you can't see much point in living—

S: Yes—I wish I'd never started this therapy. I was happy when I was living in my dream world. There I could be the kind of person I wanted to be—But now—There is such a wide, wide gap—between my ideal—and what I am. I wish people hated me. I try to make them hate me. Because then I could turn away from them and could blame them—but no—It is all in my hands—Here is my life—and I either accept the fact that I am absolutely worthless—or I fight whatever it is that holds me in this terrible conflict. And I suppose if I accepted the fact that I am worthless, then I could go away someplace—and get a little room someplace—get a mechanical job someplace—and retreat clear back to the security of my dream world where I could do things, have clever friends, be a pretty wonderful sort of person—

C: It's really a tough struggle—digging into this like you are—and at times the shelter of your dream world looks more attractive and comfortable.

S: My dream world or suicide.

C: Your dream world or something more permanent than dreams—

S: Yes. (*A long pause. Complete change of voice.*) So I don't see why I should waste your time—coming in twice a week—I'm not worth it—What do you think?

C: It's up to you, Gil—It isn't wasting my time—I'd be glad to see you—whenever you come—but it's how you feel about it—if you don't want to come twice a week—or if you do want to come twice a week?—once a week?—It's up to you. (*Long pause.*)

S: You're not going to suggest that I come in oftener? You're not alarmed and think I ought to come in—every day—until I get out of this?

C: I believe you are able to make your own decision. I'll see you whenever you want to come.

S: (*Note of awe in her voice.*) I don't believe you are alarmed about—I see—I may be afraid of myself—

---

*From Rogers, C. 1951. Client-Centered Therapy. New York, Houghton Mifflin Co., 1951.

but you aren't afraid of me— (*She stands up—a strange look on her face.*)

C: You say you may be afraid of yourself—and are wondering why I don't seem to be afraid for you?

S: (*Another short laugh.*) You have more confidence in me than I have. . . . I'll see you next week —(*that short laugh*) maybe. (*Her attitude seemed tense, depressed, bitter, completely beaten. She walked slowly away.*)

A conviction of the individual's worth is implicit in client-centered therapy. Each client is assumed to have within himself resources for healthy adjustment and he needs only a deep affectional relationship with the therapist to learn how to use his resources.

Rogers (1961) has described the essence of psychotherapy as a process in which the client comes to reciprocate the attitudes of the therapist. As the client finds acceptance in the therapist for his thought and feelings he becomes able to acknowledge and accept them himself. Feelings which were previously so frightening or disorganizing that they were shut off from awareness are shared with the therapist and accepted by him with no diminution in this regard for the client. Gradually the client moves toward adopting the same attitude toward himself and his feelings. As the client is better able to know, and experience, and express all of himself as he really is, he becomes more internally congruent, and there is less discrepancy between himself and his idealized self-image.

The client-centered approach has been criticized on many grounds. Many observers believe that it is more effective with mildly maladjusted individuals than with severe neurotics. Its assumption that every individual has a healthy core is ethically and emotionally appealing, but it is not clear what this assumption means scientifically. The insistence that the therapist need not be an expert strikes many psychiatrists and psychologists as an unwise abdication of the therapist's professional role. Finally, its hostility to diagnostic procedures ignores the fact that in some cases diagnostic information prevents therapeutic errors. But despite these criticisms, Rogers has influenced the thinking and practice of many contemporary psychotherapists and he and his colleagues have also made important contributions to research on therapeutic processes and outcome.

Behavior Modification. This approach is a relatively recent development which has achieved increasing prominence over the past two decades. All behavioral therapists do not espouse a single theoretical approach or set of techniques but they share an emphasis on observable behavior and the application of the principles of learning to clinical problems. They draw heavily on the theories of Pavlov, Thorndike, Hull and Skinner. A preference for one theorist or another leads to some variation in their conceptions of how the symptomatic behavior was learned and the best techniques for therapy. However, they are united in the belief that all behavior is learned (including so-called abnormal behavior) and that the symptom is the problem. Removal of the symptom constitutes the cure and thus there is no need to analyze or postulate an underlying conflict (see Chapter 4).

In some respects the emergence of behavior therapy may be viewed as a reaction to traditional, particularly psychoanalytic, techniques for effecting therapeutic change. The dissatisfaction with traditional conceptualization came from several quarters. First, the research evidence on the results of psychoanalytic treatment was unimpressive to many. There are many difficulties with respect to research on psychotherapeutic results and most of the earlier studies contain defects which make their conclusions highly questionable. (This problem is discussed later in this chapter). Nonetheless, the data available were particularly unfavorable to those who espoused a dynamic approach. Secondly, many clinicians were uncomfortable with Freud's conception of a neurotic symptom as merely a representation of an unconscious conflict. They felt that his principles were insufficiently supported by empirical evidence, vague in conceptualization, and incapable of being proved or disproved. Finally, because of its time-consuming demands and highly verbal format, psychoanalysis tended to be limited to the intelligent, educated, well-motivated, affluent neurotic. Techniques which had wider applicability and which gave promise of greater returns for less investment of time and money were in urgent demand.

Behavior therapists fall into two major groups: (1) those favoring the classical learning theory of Pavlov, and (2) those who have adapted the operant conditioning model of Skinner. An example of one technique derived from each type of learning theory is presented in the following paragraphs for illustrative purposes.

Wolpe has made use of Pavlov's theory in developing his technique of systematic desensitization. According to Pavlov an originally innocuous stimulus with no power to provoke a particular response may, through fortuitous circumstances, become associated with a stimulus which does evoke the response. The simultaneous pairing of such stimuli leads to a conditioned response which is maintained through reinforcement.

Applying this formula to phobias, such unrealistic fears may be seen as conditioned fear responses. Thus a child frightened by a dog may begin to show anxiety at the sight of a dog when, prior to the traumatic event, the visual stimulus of a dog would not have evoked a fear response. The fear becomes generalized so that the child is afraid not only of a particular dog but of all dogs, and possibly, of all four-legged animals. A phobia is thus formed. This formula is somewhat oversimplified in that the learning sequence is often more complex, but the principle is the same. Wolpe developed the technique of systematic desensitization to treat phobias, although it has been applied to other symptoms as well. Essentially the task is to re-create a facsimile of the original anxiety situation and then to evoke a different, usually antagonistic, response. The subject is conditioned to respond differently to the anxiety stimulus by repeated pairings of a different response to that stimulus.

Wolpe uses the first interview to determine the exact nature of the anxiety or phobia responses and the events surrounding the response. Typically patients report intense anxiety in some situations and milder reactions in others. After detailed inquiry the therapist and patient construct an anxiety hierarchy consisting of a graduated list of anxiety-prone situations ranging from most to least frightening. In the following excerpt from an initial interview, Wolpe (1969) is developing an anxiety hierarchy by helping the patient specify differences in the frightening aspects of particular situations having to do with her fear of being watched.*

Therapist: Well, is it correct to say that you are sort of scared of being watched?
Miss G.: Yes. I think everybody is always watching me.
Therapist: Now, that is at work. What other circumstances scare you when you are away from work?
Miss G.: Just going out. I am afraid, you know, that they'll see the way I am. I am afraid to pick

something up, because I am afraid that I am going to shake, and my mouth is all tightened up. I am afraid to look at people directly in the eye.
Therapist: Are you only afraid of looking at your escort in the eye, or afraid of anybody?
Miss G.: Anybody.
Therapist: So looking at a person face to face increases your nervousness?
Miss G.: Yes.
Therapist: Suppose that you were walking down the street and there was a bench across the road with some people waiting for a bus. Now those people would be sort of vaguely looking across the street. Would you be aware of their presence?
Miss G.: Yes, definitely.
Therapist: Even though they might not be particularly looking at you?
Miss G.: Yes.
Therapist: Now, supposing we take people away altogether. Suppose that you are just walking all by yourself, say in a park. There is no one else at all there. Are you then completely comfortable?
Miss G.: Yes.
Therapist: I must be quite certain of this.
Miss G.: Yes.
Therapist: If you are completely by yourself, are you absolutely calm and comfortable?
Miss G.: Yes, I am. The same way I am at home. I feel all right.
Therapist: Well, that means there are some people who can look at you and not bother you.
Miss G.: Yes, at times. But I don't know why this happens.
Therapist: Well, what about your mother?
Miss G.: No, it doesn't bother me at home.
Therapist: Your mother can look at you as much as she likes?
Miss G.: Yes. It's silly but . . .
Therapist: Well, that's not silly. I mean this is just the way things have developed.
Miss G.: I know.
Therapist: And who else can look at your without bothering you?
Miss G.: My whole family.
Therapist: Who is in your family?
Miss G.: My father, my mother, my sister, my grandmother.
Therapist: Besides these people, are there any others at all who can look at you without disturbing you?
Miss G.: No.
Therapist: What about a little baby?
Miss G.: No, that doesn't disturb me, and an older person who is senile or something. That doesn't bother me.
Therapist: What about a little boy of four?
Miss G.: No.
Therapist: Six?
Miss G.: No.
Therapist: Eight?

*Wolpe, J. 1969. The Practice of Behavior Therapy. New York, Pergamon Press, Inc. pp. 46–48.

Miss G.: No. It's when they get older, I get nervous.
Therapist: Twelve?
Miss G.: Around in their teens.
Therapist: About twelve? They sort of begin to bother you?
Miss G.: Yes.
Therapist: I take it that a boy of twelve wouldn't be as bad as one of eighteen?
Miss G.: No.

From the beginning of therapy the patient also receives instruction in deep muscle relaxation. The patient relaxes in a comfortable lounging chair and progressively learns to relax the various voluntary muscle groups. Once the patient has mastered the relaxation technique, systematic desensitization begins. The patient is asked to imagine as vividly as possible the least anxiety-producing scene from the previously constructed anxiety hierarchy. If he can do this without anxiety while relaxed, he is asked to imagine the next most anxiety-laden situation and so on. If at any point the patient feels anxious he signals the therapist who then asks him to abandon the scene and return to the relaxed state. This procedure is repeated through subsequent sessions until the patient is able to imagine even the most acutely anxiety-producing situation without experiencing the original discomfort. In this manner the patient becomes desensitized to the phobic object. He has learned to associate relaxation responses rather than anxiety-laden ones to the originally frightening stimulus. If successful, the gains achieved in therapy will generalize to the real life situation.

In a study of 39 patients treated in this manner, Wolpe reports complete or marked improvement in 91 per cent of the hierarchies. Sometimes it is necessary to construct several hierarchies of a single patient since he may have several types of phobic fears and responses. The mean number of sessions required per phobia is 11.2—a very brief course of treatment when compared to the typical time required of other techniques.

Skinner's learning theory has provided the basis for other behavioral approaches to treatment. Skinner is more concerned with the consequences of a response than with the stimulus for that response. Essentially, this approach takes the view that all behaviors have certain consequences on the environment and these consequences either tend to reinforce the response (and thus make the response likely to recur) or not. If a response is not reinforced it will extinguish. In clinical application, the therapist looks at a behavior or symptom and asks what effect the behavior has on the environment. By control of the effects (rewards), he can achieve control over the response.

A case report by Bachrach, Erwin and Mohr (1965) shows a successful application of this principle in treating a female patient suffering from anorexia nervosa (severe refusal to eat or regurgitating food, a condition sometimes so extreme as to produce life-threatening weight loss). The patient was admitted to the hospital at the age of 37 following a gradual but persistent weight loss over the preceding 17 years. During that time she had gone from a weight of 118 pounds to only 47 pounds at the time of admission (see Figure 21–1, *A*). She was completely debilitated and could stand only with assistance. A thorough medical and endocrinological evaluation failed to reveal any lesion or disease process which could account for the patient's reduced food intake and the severe malnutrition bordering on death. The treatment program involved placing the patient in a bare room and depriving her of all previous sources of pleasure including television, magazines, record player, radio and social contacts. These rewards were now made contingent on eating. When the patient ate she was allowed to watch television briefly or talk to a staff person or patient or to listen to music. Gradually she was required to consume increasing amounts of food in order to obtain the rewards which relieved the bleak boredom of her room. Later, actual gains in weight were substituted for eating and the reinforcers were made contingent upon weight gain. At the time treatment was terminated the patient weighed 88 pounds (see Figure 21–1, *B*).

The behavior modification procedures provide powerful therapeutic leverage for many types of emotional problems. Positive results have been reported with cases ranging in severity from mild phobias to childhood autism. Whether these procedures are ultimately superior to other techniques is unproved despite many such claims. What is clear is that behavior modification techniques have broad applicability, require less training of therapists, and often achieve good results at a far lower cost in time and money than many other therapies.

There are many approaches to psychotherapy. Some theorists place great emphasis on the nature of the therapeutic relationship while others see the relationship as relatively unimportant. Some therapists rely heavily on techniques which are largely condemned by others.

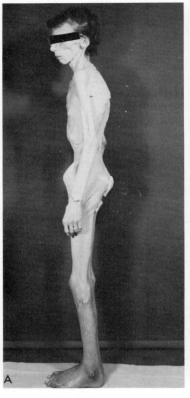
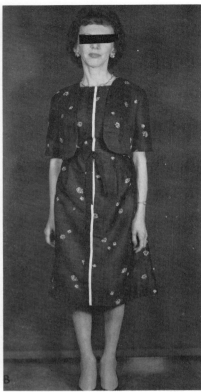

Figure 21–1. A, At admission this patient suffering from anorexia nervosa weighed only 47 pounds. B, At the termination of treatment the patient weighed 88 pounds. (Reprinted by permission from Bachrach, A. J., Erwin, W. J., and Mohr, J. P. The control of eating behavior in an anorexic by operant conditioning techniques. In L. Ullmann and L. Krasner, Editors: Case Studies in Behavior Modification, 1965, Holt, Rinehart and Winston, Inc., New York.)

Differences also exist concerning the nature of psychotherapeutic change and obstacles to progress. Before turning to the question of effectiveness of psychotherapy, we will present some generally accepted views concerning the psychotherapeutic relationship and the techniques of psychotherapy, although there are many legitimate exceptions to these views.

The Psychotherapeutic Relationship

The therapist-patient relationship is a significant factor in most psychotherapies. With some exceptions, treatment is effective only in a warm and permissive atmosphere and only if the patient feels that the therapist is genuinely interested in him as a person. For most patients, the psychotherapeutic relationship is different from anything previously experienced with friends, relatives or other persons. In a good relationship, the patient feels that it is safe for him to say what he wishes without fear of censure. To quote Levine (1952), the therapist tries to be ''nonjudgmental, noncondemning, nonsubmissive, nonanxious, noncontrolling, firm, consistent and realistic.'' Further, the

therapist's basic role is that of ''a firm, helpful friend, who wants to help and be sustaining but expects the patient to be as self-reliant and independent as he can be.'' A relationship that combines all these traits is unique and difficult to establish and maintain. The ideal therapist has been described by various writers as perceptive and sensitive in human relationships, insightful into his own behaviors and motives, relatively nondefensive, tactful and controlled, tolerant and respectful of the integrity and freedom of others, objective and realistic, likeable, warm, responsible and technically knowledgeable about others' motivations and behavior. Of course, all therapists fall short of being such paragons of perfection, some more so and some less, but the description of the ideal indicates how therapists feel they should *try* to behave with patients.

A good therapeutic relationship has two major consequences. First, the human context within which the specific, moment-by-moment, treatment techniques are employed determines how effective the techniques will be. To take an example: a female patient who, as a child, had competed intensely with her brothers expresses an aggressive and critical attitude toward her husband but sees no connection between her present and childhood behavior. The therapist interprets the connection: "Could it be that you're acting toward your husband as you did toward your brothers?" If the patient feels safe in the relationship, she is almost certain to pick up the interpretation and start to explore her feelings toward her brothers and husband. (She need *not agree* with the interpretation; its major function is to uncover motivations, not to provide a formula to be parroted by the patient.) If the relationship is poor, however, the patient may feel that the therapist really means, "What a ridiculously childish way to behave!", and she may defensively inhibit expressions of her attitudes to men.

In a good relationship, the patient is likely to accept suggestions and reassurances. In a poor relationship, he rejects suggestions and perceives as threats comments that are intended to reassure. On one occasion, to reassure a patient who had improved but who voiced a fear that he would not be able to maintain his gains, the therapist commented, "You might slide back again but it would probably be temporary and you will pick up again. You're improving as fast as can be expected." The patient, who was somewhat paranoid, was not comfortable in the therapeutic situation and he interpreted the comment to mean, "When you slide back maybe you will pick up and maybe not. You're doing as well as I expect, but I don't expect very much."

The second consequence of the therapeutic relationship is a deeper one. Many patients have a history of severe interpersonal difficulties which are the source, arena and end result of their disturbances. A good therapeutic relationship may become the model for a crucial improvement in interpersonal interactions and the improvement may become the starting point from which generalizations to extra-therapeutic situations begin. The patient learns to feel safe with others as well as with the therapist, manifests less anxiety and more positive feelings in interaction with others and in turn elicits positive attitudes from them. As a result, he begins to experience the feeling that he is a worthwhile person. Allen (1942) describes the importance of the relationship in the following quote:

While maintaining an interest in understanding what has been wrong, the therapeutic focus is on what the individual can begin to do about what was, and, more important, still is wrong. Therapy emerges, then, from

an experience in living, not in isolation but within a relationship with another from whom the patient can eventually differentiate himself as he comes to perceive and accept his own self as separate and distinct.

The Techniques of Psychotherapy

By and large, the techniques of psychotherapy are divisible into two categories: *directive* and *nondirective*. The directive therapist behaves as an expert qualified to guide the patient. Verbalizations during the therapeutic session or extra-therapeutic behavior are guided by such directive techniques as reconditioning, advice, task setting, persuasion, suggestion, reassurance, selective focusing and interpretation. (These vary in the *degree* to which they are directive. Advice, for example, is far more directive than interpretation.) The major nondirective techniques, utilized primarily in client-centered therapy but to some extent also in other types of therapy, are reflection and clarification. They are predicated on the assumption that the patient must find his own paths to his own goals, both within and without therapy; the therapist can only provide a permissive atmosphere that will give the patient the freedom and courage to guide himself.

Advice and Task Setting. In the third century A.D., the Roman writer Diogenes Laertius wrote in his *Lives and Opinions of Celebrated Men,* "When Thales was asked what was difficult, he said, 'To know one's self.' And what was easy? 'To give advice.'" Most patients beginning therapy want advice and they repeatedly appeal to the therapist, "Tell me what to do." However, for a number of reasons, advice—easy as it is to give—may not only fail to help the patient but may be therapeutically harmful. First, many patients have sought and received advice from friends and relatives prior to psychotherapy. If a therapist behaves no differently from the previous advisers, the patient will not perceive the therapeutic relationship as special and different from his other relationships, most of which have been unsatisfactory. Second, people who request advice, often want a particular kind of advice and they distort or reject whatever does not fit their expectations. Unwelcome advice may be carried out in such a manner as to guarantee that it will fail. For example, a mother who had a neurotic need to overfeed an obese, demanding five-year-old child followed a physician's advice to feed him less by reducing his portion at meals, but she compensated by giving him large snacks between meals when no other family members were present. The child's weight continued to increase and the mother called on the family to witness that she had followed the advice given and that it was obviously no good. Still another difficulty with advice is that too often it is a counsel of perfection which the patient cannot possibly carry out successfully because of his emotional state. He tries, fails and then feels more guilty and anxious than ever.

Advice is therapeutically beneficial only if these difficulties have been circumvented. It should not be given until the therapist understands the patient well, until a solid relationship has been established and until there is reason to believe that the advice can be carried out successfully.

Persuasion. The therapeutic use of persuasion was first advocated in modern times by DuBois (1909) who attempted to persuade his patients to substitute thoughts of health for their preoccupations with disease and discomfort. Patients were shown how they used symptoms as a means of escaping from responsibilities and then proper thoughts and attitudes were vigorously hammered into them. Insomniacs were to say to themselves, "If I sleep, good; if I don't, it doesn't matter." Patients were told to ignore symptoms, cultivate the belief that they were going to get well and substitute altruistic and religious sentiments for selfish and immoral ones.

More recent adaptations of persuasion in therapy are somewhat less crude. Depending on the patient, the therapist may try to persuade him to want to get well, control impulsiveness, tolerate frustrations and anxiety or behave responsibly. Persuasion appeals to the conscious, rational part of the patient's ego; it tends to ignore the unconscious and irrational determinants of behavior. A patient who has failed to recognize the maladaptive nature of his behavior may be persuaded to face psychological reality and attack his problems, either in therapy or outside of it. An excitable, impulsive patient may be persuaded not to make major changes in his life—not to quit his job, or leave his family or start a new business venture —until he has talked over the proposed change with the therapist. A succinct statement by Thorne (1950) summarizes and evaluates the therapeutic role of persuasive techniques:

Persuasion consists of making appeals to the client's intellect, trying to convince him of the desirability of accepting an idea or plan of action.

Persuasion works most effectively in the presence of good rapport and positive transference. The object of persuasion is psychotherapeutic re-education in which the client is directed toward better adjustment. Persuasion operates primarily on supportive or symptomatic levels to secure limited objectives. It is usually ineffective in modifying deep emotional factors. . . . Although persuasion methods have been largely abandoned by adherents of psychoanalysis and nondirective methods, it has definite indications and may be used effectively in limited situations.

Suggestion. Either in the ordinary, waking state or by use of hypnosis, suggestion may be used to induce thoughts, attitudes, feelings or actions. The aims of suggestion are similar to those of persuasion.

Nonhypnotic suggestions are ordinarily couched in such tentative language as "Have you thought of the possibility of . . .," or, "Could it be that . . .," or, "Another way of approaching your problem might perhaps be. . . ." The therapist avoids telling the patient, "What you must do is . . .," or, "The right way is . . ." and thus permits the patient to share in making decisions. A great variety of changes may be induced by waking suggestions. To cite a few examples, a homosexual female patient who wishes to change her sexual pattern may accept the suggestion that she dress, wear her hair and talk in a more conventionally feminine manner; an immature patient may give up baby talk or begin to avoid overdependence on other persons; and a patient who tends to become extremely angry in discussions of religion may accept the suggestion that he explore the internal source of his anger or that he avoid religious discussion and argument.

The usual procedures for induction of a hypnotic state consist of having the subject relax physically, shut out extraneous physical stimuli as well as all ideas except those of the hypnotist and concentrate visually by "looking through" a designated point of fixation. Except for a minority of patients who cannot be hypnotized, these procedures result in a state of heightened suggestibility. A deeply hypnotized subject will accept the suggestions that a painful stimulus such as a sharp pinprick is pleasant, that an empty room contains furniture or people, that he is someone else and so forth.

In therapy, hypnosis may be used in two different ways, both capitalizing on heightened suggestibility. One procedure, known as posthypnotic suggestion, consists of giving the patient suggestions to be carried out after the hypnotic session is over. A patient suffering from a hysterical paralysis may be induced to walk in the hypnotic state and told that he will continue to be able to walk later. An insomniac may be given the post-hypnotic suggestion that he will fall asleep more easily. Suggestion may be used to help a fearful individual feel calm at an impending social occasion. Students have sometimes been helped by post-hypnotic suggestion to concentrate better in studies and be less anxious when taking tests. When a post-hypnotic suggestion is successfully carried out, the individual's confidence is built up and he may find he can cope with his problems with no further therapeutic help. One hypnotic session is rarely adequate for this purpose and the procedure may have to be repeated again and again.

In the popular mind, hypnosis has a mysterious and magic aura that makes people in difficulties both afraid of and attracted to it. Many patients make the request, "Can't you hypnotize me and get all these terrible thoughts out of my mind?", or, "I know what to do but I just don't do it—can't you hypnotize me and *make* me do it?" In actuality, hypnosis does not have the extraordinary power often attributed to it. It is one of a number of directive techniques, sometimes successful and sometimes not. Like other directive techniques, it suppresses difficulties or supports defensive and other behavior patterns without uncovering motivations or modifying personality radically.

A second use of hypnosis consists of recovering memories that have been repressed or lost in amnesic episodes. Hypnotic probing of this type may be combined with psychoanalysis in *hypnoanalysis*. In this approach, material uncovered during hypnotic sessions is analyzed in subsequent psychoanalytic sessions in the waking state. The hypnotic sessions may also be used to stimulate free associations—since the patient's resistance to free association may be lower when hypnotized—and sometimes to induce dreams which, like dreams during sleep, may then be analyzed.

Reassurance. Patients commence therapy with certain fears about the therapy itself. They may be afraid that they cannot be helped or that they will be told they are "crazy," basically homosexual or hopelessly evil. Some patients fear that they will become too dependent on the therapist and others or that the therapy will change them so completely they will lose their talents and capabilities or even their special identities. The professional writer fears he will no longer want to write and the businessman that he will lose his assertive competitiveness.

Fundamentally and unconsciously, what all patients are afraid of is losing their neurotic or otherwise deviant habits. They are dissatisfied with themselves but they fear new and untried behaviors that will rob them of their present gratifications, limited as these may be.

Reassurance is a supportive technique which attempts to overcome fears and thus remove the obstacles to proceeding with therapy. A patient may be reassured that his case is not at all unusual (many patients think their problems are unique), that his condition is well understood, that he can be helped or that his symptoms are a nuisance to him but not dangerous. Emphasizing that he is unhappy and upset rather than blameful or sinful may be very reassuring. He may be assured that therapy is likely to make him more independent and that it does not destroy talents nor the motivation to use them productively. However, reassurance is ineffective unless it is based on fact, is used sparingly and judiciously and is given within a good relationship. Telling a psychotic patient that he is really all right is a deception that he is likely to see through and that may do him harm. Apart from deception, if a patient's problems are repeatedly met by nothing but reassurance, the technique will defeat its own purpose.

Even when the therapist does not use reassurance as a deliberate technique, his behavior may reassure the patient. As he follows the patient's train of thought and feelings he may occasionally smile, nod and encourage him to keep talking, and these evidences of interest reassure the patient that he is being taken seriously.

Interpretation. An interpretation is a statement or question in which the therapist formulates the meaning or significance of the patient's behavior. There are many types of interpretation; the following examples illustrate a few. In the first example, a cause is connected with a symptom; in the second, the past with the present; and in the third, an unconscious motive with a defense.

In previous interviews, a patient had discussed her frequent headaches and her anger with her husband. She had never connected the two. On the basis of other material, it was clear to the therapist that her somatic symptoms were precipitated by disturbing emotions.

Pt. I got sore at Jim yesterday for practically no reason at all. I had no right to be angry—he hadn't done anything to make me angry. I remember I had a headache yesterday evening. Maybe that's why I was mad.

Th. Could it be the other way—could the headache come from the anger instead of the anger from the headache?

A highly intelligent male patient began therapy because his career was not progressing as fast as he felt it should.

Pt. I like my boss. He's a fine man but lately I feel that I don't really trust him. I don't understand it—I don't understand why—he's wonderful to work for, and for no reason at all I just don't trust him. Somehow I hold back and sort of watch him. I don't put everything into working for him the way I myself want to—crazy, isn't it?

Th. You told me before how you didn't trust your father when you were a child and how you still don't trust him. You always expected him to pull a fast one, you said.

Pt. You mean I'm acting to my boss like to my father?

A female patient who often felt hostile to her children was only dimly aware of her hostility, and did not connect it with the fact that she worried about them excessively.

Pt. I worry and worry about my children. I imagine the most dreadful things happening to them. I even dreamed that one of them got killed. What a terrible thing! (*Patient beings to weep.*)

Th. Do you ever get angry with them?

(The tentative nature of this last interpretation should be noted. It is a preparatory invitation to the patient to undertake the anxiety-provoking task of exploring her hostility to her children and her reaction-formation against hostility. Interpretations often distress patients and arouse immediate anxiety, although one of the objectives of interpretations is eventual reduction of anxiety.)

The earlier the stage of therapy, the more limited the objectives of interpretation are. The objective may be as simple as the demonstration to the patient that a symptom exists, or that he is defensive; for example, the patient who dreamed that her child was killed had been told early in therapy that her worries had *some* kind of motivation. Later, in the fragment quoted, the connection with hostility was barely suggested; still later, the connection was explored more fully as the roots of her hostility became the new focus of therapy. An excerpt from Colby (1951) illustrates how a deep interpretation may be made too soon; the therapist turned the interpretation to good use, however, by immediately saving face for the patient.

Th. Did you feel some hostility toward your mother?

Pt. (*Indignantly recoiling*) Oh, of course not! I love my mother very much. How could you suggest such a thing?

Th. (*Affably*) It occurred to me, but don't take everything I say as necessarily true. I'm often wrong. My comments are meant only as trial balloons to see what thought they bring to your mind. In this case you feel that hostility was out of the question, that you have only friendly feelings toward your mother.

Pt. That's right. We do have little squabbles at times, but they never amount to very much.

Th. (*Moving on*) What other things do you squabble about?

Interpretation is the major technique of psychoanalysis and of many types of psychotherapy that have been influenced by psychoanalysis. Although therapeutic gains often occur without interpretation, with many patients it is more potent than any other technique.

Reflection and Clarification of Feeling. This technique consists of apprehending the patient's emotions and feelings with as little distortion as possible and reflecting them back, preferably in the patient's own language, in order to clarify them. It is important to realize that the therapist reflects the patient's emotions and feelings and not the ideational content of what he says. The technique often helps a patient to go below the level of his conscious affective reactions and become aware of hitherto obscure, repressed emotions. Both negative and positive feelings are reflected; frequently the reflection of negative feelings is sufficient to prevent the patient from acting them out antisocially. Properly utilized, the technique helps the individual to feel deeply understood, makes it clear to him that his emotions influence the rest of his behavior, and—since the technique is nondirective—demonstrates to him that he is responsible for his own decisions and actions. In the following example of reflection and clarification, the patient—whose first marriage had terminated in divorce—brings up his fears in connection with his current, second marriage. The patient's movement from negative to positive feelings at the end of the interview excerpt, after his worries, dislikes and self-hate had been reflected, is a frequent occurrence in psychotherapy.

Pt. Joan [the second wife] is different from what Alice [the first wife] was like. I never got along with Alice. We fought all the time. (*Pause*) Sometimes I wonder why she married me—I don't think she really liked me. (*Pause*) I guess with Joan—I have arguments with her and I wonder if the whole thing is starting over, like with Alice.

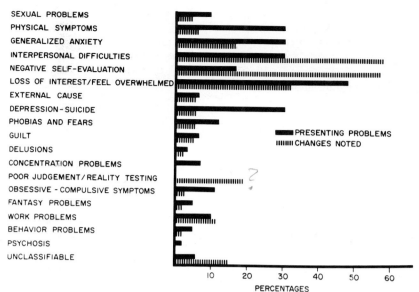

Figure 21–2. *Comparison of most important changes experienced and presenting problems, as reported by former psychotherapy patients. (From Strupp, H., Fox, R., and Lessler, K., 1969. Patients View Their Psychotherapy. Baltimore, Johns Hopkins Press.)*

Th. You feel Joan is different but you're worried this marriage will go bad too.

Pt. (*Spoken with heat.*) That's right. We argue and argue and I think maybe it's my fault. I just can't get along with anybody—I hate Joan's father, I - I - I can't stand my stepfather—I get jealous when anybody so much as looks at Joan, and I get mad at myself when I get jealous. I guess I just wreck things—spoil them. (*Tears appear in his eyes.*)

Th. You hate other people and you hate yourself—*nothing* is any good.

Pt. I don't like having to come here either—I ought to be able to manage things better. I'm the boy who always louses things up. (*Said in a sarcastic and bitter tone.*)

Th. You feel you always were a failure and still are.

Pt. Yes—well—maybe some things I manage better. (*Pause*) For instance. . . .

The Nature of Psychotherapeutic Change

Personality change is a complex matter and difficult to measure (see Chapter 20). The problems in constructing adequate personality measures make the evaluation of psychotherapy hazardous since the aim of most psychotherapy is personality change. At present there is no such thing as an emotional thermometer with which we can measure exact changes or shifts. However, Berenson and Carkhuff (1967), after reviewing the research on counseling and

psychotherapy, did feel that some generalized statements about psychotherapeutic change were possible from the weight of available evidence. Their points are paraphrased below:

1. Therapists with different orientations seem to be about equally effective.
2. Changes in patients appear to be on a broad front and are not restricted to symptom alleviation. Such changes are independent of the therapist's theoretical approach or professional affiliation.
3. Psychotherapy provides a core of facilitative conditions which seem essential for patient change: (a) an emotional experience, (b) a didactic experience, (c) the role model of the therapist.
4. These facilitative conditions are likely to characterize all effective human encounters whether or not they are labeled "psychotherapy" or "counseling."
5. Psychotherapy, like all interpersonal encounters, may have constructive or deteriorative consequences.
6. Effective psychotherapy seems to provide the patient with experiences which are the reverse of experiences which were associated with the onset of difficulties.
7. In effective psychotherapy, the patient incorporates into his own life style the facilitative conditions which were provided in therapy. He learns new techniques of effective living—namely, openness, understanding, and respect for self and others.

Strupp, Fox and Lessler (1969) asked 122 former psychotherapy outpatients to describe the problems for which they sought help and to list the most important changes they had experienced (see Figure 21–2). Almost 50 per cent of all patients reported feeling overwhelmed by their problems and disinterested in much of their daily lives when they came for therapy. The next most frequently mentioned complaints were physical symptoms, depression, interpersonal difficulties and generalized anxiety. The most important changes experienced as a result of therapy were improved interpersonal relationships, increased self-esteem and an increased interest in day-to-day activities. It is noteworthy that in their reports of change patients placed relatively minor emphasis on the alleviation of common neurotic symptoms, such as anxiety, depression and physical disturbances. Change was described as occurring in a broader front and affecting a wide spectrum of life experiences. These results seem to support some of the conclusions of Berenson and Carkhuff, listed above.

Some therapists aim at broadly defined personality changes from the outset while others concentrate only on alleviation of a particular symptom, such as a phobia. But regardless of the therapist's intention, change is difficult to confine to a specific area of functioning. For example, a patient who is freed of a phobia of crowds is also likely to have, as a result, greater sense of competence and increased self-confidence. He is not simply a person without a phobia. He is a person who has a different view of himself, who reacts differently to others and who probably gets different feedback as a result.

Therapy With Children

A child does not have a mature ego or superego, cannot think or talk at an adult level and cannot control his life situation. For these reasons, therapy with children differs radically from therapy with adults.

In child therapy, play is used to a considerable extent as a substitute for verbal interaction. Toys, water paints, drawing materials, guns, blocks and clay are made available to the child. The manner in which they are used differs in different approaches to child therapy, for, as in adult therapy, there are a multitude of theoretical and practical systems.

Levy (1938) developed an approach known as "release therapy." The therapist selects appropriate toys—for example, detachable dolls to represent the family of a child who is hostile to family members—and encourages the child to release his aggressions and express his anxieties in play. The child who is experiencing sibling rivalry may stamp on or dismember a doll representing a new baby. The angry child may throw clay, spill water, smear finger paints or violently bump toy cars together. In release therapy, the therapist does little verbal interpretation of play activities. Rather, as with verbal catharsis for adult patients, the release itself is presumed to be therapeutically valuable because it occurs in the framework of a permissive relationship. Levy believes that release therapy is useful only for children less than 10 years old whose symptoms have been precipitated by a quite recent, specific event such as the birth of another child in the family. Furthermore, the symptoms should be definite and circumscribed—temper tantrums, nightmares, speech disturbances and so forth—and the child's family relationships should be essentially stable. For children whose difficulties are severe and long-standing, and whose family situation is highly deviant, Levy believes more complex therapeutic approaches are advisable.

Procedures for the psychoanalytic treatment of children have been formulated by Melanie Klein (1949) and Anna Freud (1946). Melanie Klein assumed that childhood play activity is the equivalent of adult free association and interpreted play in Freudian terms. Turning over a car might be interpreted to mean unconscious hostility against the father, thrusting a pencil at the therapist might be taken to represent an unconscious sexual impulse directed at her, probably due to transference, and so forth. Klein reported that direct and deep interpretation of the child's basic, unconscious conflicts reduces his anxiety level, but her approach has been rejected by most child psychologists and psychiatrists.

In Anna Freud's approach, the therapist first motivates the child for therapy by being helpful or interesting to him. Following this, the child's play, drawings, dreams and day-dreams are analyzed. Interpretations do not go deeply into unconscious levels, for Anna Freud believes that the child's immaturity and dependence on parents preclude deep analysis. Child analysis, in her view, has an educational as well as therapeutic function and can accomplish much at the level of consciousness and overt behavior.

Client-centered therapy has been adapted for work with children, primarily using the medium of play with no interpretation. Some limits are necessarily set on the child's behavior; for example, he may not assault the therapist or destroy physical equipment and he must keep the scheduled appointments. For the rest, he is completely free to play or not, as he wishes, and to talk or be silent. Therapeutic acceptance of the child is presumed to be the only agent necessary for progress.

An important type of therapy with children is Allen's "relationship therapy" (1942). The therapist interprets the child's play in terms of the concept of individuation: each individual, it is assumed, matures by becoming progressively separated and differentiated from others. Interpretations are aimed at encouraging the child to separate himself psychologically from persons on whom he is too dependent, most commonly a demanding and overly possessive mother. The child may become dependent on the therapist, but he is then helped by interpretations to free himself of this dependent relationship also. The focus of interpretations is the present rather than the past, and the child is aided to become aware of his current feelings and to make his own decisions. Meanwhile, the parents are seen in a series of interviews by another therapist; the procedure of employing two separate therapists further encourages differentiation of the child from the parents.

Group and Family Therapy

In *group therapy*—a major development of the last few decades—a single therapist works with a group of patients or the relatives of patients or both. The group usually consists of six to twelve members who meet one or more times a week. Different groups have been led by psychiatrists, psychologists, psychoanalysts, social workers, clergymen, nurses and hospital aides, and the setting has varied widely from private practice to outpatient clinics, mental hospitals and prisons. The patients who compose a group have in some cases been homogeneous with respect to age, sex and diagnosis, and in others have been quite heterogeneous. It is generally unwise to mix patients who are enormously different, for example, teen agers with elderly persons or intellectually dull with very bright individuals. Patients sometimes receive both group and individual therapy at the same time, usually with different therapists.

The motivation for the development of group therapy has been twofold. First, the shortage of professional personnel makes it impossible to treat all patients by individual means. Second, some patients may benefit more from group than individual treatment, for example, those who have lacked adequate social relationships or who find an individual psychotherapeutic relationship too threatening; some patients, for example, perceive it as potentially homosexual. The major advantages of group therapy are the opportunities it affords the patient to test social reality when he reports actual or contemplated changes in behavior, or when he expresses his feelings and attitudes toward himself and the other group members. The others' reactions vividly demonstrate to the patient how he affects people and how they perceive him; in a sense, every group member is a therapist for every other.

The theoretical groundwork of group therapy is as variable as that of individual therapy. There are supportive and expressive group leaders, inspirational leaders, persuasive leaders whose major technique is that of lecturing, group leaders who have adapted Wolpe's reconditioning procedures to group work, as well as client-centered, psychoanalytic and eclectic group therapists. Most group therapists maintain a permissive atmosphere, keep the group from wandering too far from its therapeutic tasks, promote a certain degree of group unity, reflect group and individual attitudes and occasionally make interpretations.

An example from Frank (1961a) demonstrates the complex give and take of group therapy.* In the fragment quoted, Mr. K. is a 33-year-old single man who has a pathological fear of women, in particular a female cousin; Mrs. B. is a dominating, anxious 33-year-old housewife; and Dr. F. is the group leader. Earlier in the session, Mr. K. had accused Mrs. B. of being overbearing; she had defended herself against this charge, and Mr. K.'s head began to ache (one of his frequent symptoms). Two other group members had earlier discussed whether they felt Mrs. B. was overbearing, but they are silent in the following interchange in which Mr. K. reevaluates Mrs. B. and thus finally faces up to his fear of women, and Dr. F. interprets Mrs. B.'s behavior:

Mr. K. On the subject of overbearing, well, a woman has a right to be overbearing if she wants.
Mrs. B. Well, with my own children—
Mr. K. That's what hit me Saturday with my cousin. I kept her husband out; he was supposed to

*From Frank, J. D. 1961. Therapy in a group setting. *In* Stein, M. I. (Editor). Contemporary Psychotherapies. Glencoe, Ill., The Free Press, pp. 55–56.

come home to go to the store [*laughs*]. I was the one!

Dr. F.   She gave you the devil?

Mr. K.   No, but I could see she wanted to jump on me, see? And, boy, that headache really got terrific.

Dr. F.   And here it is again.

Mr. K.   Right here again.

Dr. F.   Was it the word [i.e. "overbearing"] rather than what she was saying or the way she was saying it?

Mr. K.   Just maybe the word or what she was saying—I don't believe I could accept that, that a woman could be aggressive.

Dr. F.   Without being dangerous?

Mr. K.   Being dangerous, passive—They have a right to be—I mean, they're human. [*Laughter*] I don't know, maybe that—that struck me funny there in a way—just the way she was talking and the word "overbearing."

Mrs. B. About what I said about my own children, I didn't actually realize. . . .

Dr. F.   I think the problem, Mrs. B., as I see it now, is that you feel you've got to be liked all the time. At the same time, you're a strong person.

Mrs. B. Yes, and it's a conflict.

Dr. F.   Well, maybe it's a soluble one. Maybe you're not using your strength in the right way in trying to be liked.

A variation of group therapy is *family therapy*. In this approach (Jackson, 1961), a patient and his family are treated together on the theory that unhealthy intrafamilial relationships are determinants of the patient's emotional disturbance. In turn, the patient's disturbance further strains family relationships, thus setting up a vicious circle that the therapy is intended to break. The family members discuss their attitudes to each other, take a fresh look at each other, acquire insights that may serve to modify unhealthy family patterns, and learn more effective means of communicating. The whole family is the patient, so to speak, in family therapy.

Treating the family as a unit is a recent innovation which grew out of the realization that emotional disturbance occurs in an interpersonal context, the most important part of which is the family. It was frequently observed that patients who improved in the hospital manifested a reappearance of symptoms when they returned to their families. When the patient was studied along with his family it became apparent that his symptoms seemed to serve an adaptive function in maintaining the family's emotional equilibrium. If the patient changed, some other family member often showed symptoms of emo-

tional disturbance. Thus, it became necessary to change the family relationships.

The marital relationship is typically seen as the axis around which all other relationships in the family are formed. The parents are, so to speak, the emotional architects of the family. Difficulties in the marital relationship lead to difficulties in parenting. The identified patient is the family member who is most obviously affected by the pained marital relationship. An example can help illustrate the principles involved.

A ten-year-old boy was referred to a psychologist by his teacher because of his extreme fearfulness of getting hurt while playing and his poor school achievement. An interview with the family revealed that the parents had been emotionally distant from each other for many years and had slept in separate bedrooms for the last five years. During this time the mother slept in her son's bedroom. The father was an aloof, emotionally distant person who had great difficulty in forming close relationships. His wife had finally dispaired of a meaningful relationship with him and had become increasingly attached to her son. Her overprotection was an attempt to bind her son to her and thus make up for some of what she could not get from her husband. The son became overly dependent, unassertive, and unsure of his own abilities. His whining, dependent attitude infuriated the father, who often punished him for his lack of aggressiveness, but this only made the boy more timid and drove him further into the mother's arms. By working with the family together the psychologist was able to help the husband to be more demonstrative toward his wife and the wife to be more receptive and accepting of him. As the marital relationship improved the father was better able to help the mother to give up her overprotection of the boy and both began to insist firmly on greater autonomy and independent behavior. Improvement in the family relationships led to a rapid improvement in the boy's behavior at school.

In the following excerpts of another family in therapy, the therapist has excused the children so as to help the parents focus on their own sexual problems and attitudes.*

*From Ackerman, N. A family therapy session. In Ackerman, Beatman and Sherman (Eds.). Expanding Theory and Practice in Family Therapy, 1967. Family Service Association of America. Reprinted by permission.

Therapist: Tell me, are you married to your wife?

Father: I think so.

Therapist: You think. You're not sure of anything.

Father: No, I'm married to her.

Therapist: You don't say you think. You're not united as parents and you haven't been; so I wonder whether you are united as man and wife. Are you?

Father: Yes.

Therapist: How well joined are you as man and wife? Is it very good now?

Father: Yes.

Therapist (to mother): Do you love your husband?

Mother: Yes.

Therapist: And so the loving between you now is better than it was?

Father: Yes.

Therapist: Well, what did it used to be?

Father: Well, up to a certain time it wasn't a normal situation in the respect that you'd call normal.

Therapist (sarcastically): Well, now, I understand perfectly exactly what he means. Speak English.

Father: I find it difficult to discuss.

Therapist: In these circumstances?

Father: In any circumstances.

Therapist: Like your sexual life together?

Father: I'm not talking about only under these circumstances; I'm talking about any circumstances.

Therapist: Do you feel very sensitive about sexual matters?

Father: I think we both are.

Therapist: Are you, Mother? You too?

Father: When we hear people talk about their sexual life—I'm talking about friends and so forth—well, we tell them it's none of their business.

Therapist: Are you telling me now it's none of my business?

Father: No, no, because if there is an answer in that then we have to bring it out.

Therapist: Well, I think there might be. I'd like to know what trouble you've had in your sexual life together.

Father: Well, while we kept company, while we were going together—we went together about a year, over a year—I think we were very much in love. We had no premarital relations. We liked to go out with each other; we enjoyed each other's company. The night that we got married, it was like a shade was drawn, and sexual life was very poor.

Therapist: Can you be a little more specific? I might understand.

Father: Well, I just couldn't get to my wife.

Therapist: She closed the gates on you completely on your honeymoon night. Pulled down the curtain, wouldn't let you in?

Father: On the altar they pulled the shade.

Therapist: How did you do that, Mother?

Mother: I just couldn't——

Therapist: Tell me, how did you close him out? You married him and then——

Mother: I know, something snapped in me and I just couldn't——

Therapist: I'd like to understand that.

Mother: I would have liked to, too.

Therapist: What did it feel like?

Mother: Well, I felt very jumpy.

Therapist: You got panicky.

Mother: Yes.

Therapist: Were you afraid of sex?

Mother: I never thought I was until that time.

After discussing their courtship and honeymoon the couple return to the topic of their attitudes toward sex.

Mother: We actually didn't have a happy married life until we moved into our own apartment.

Therapist: So you took flight from your parents. Were you brought up by them so you should never think of doing anything dirty like sex?

Mother: Yes.

Therapist: Sex is dirty?

Mother: It was never spoken about.

Therapist: Did you feel it was clean, Pop?

Father: Yes. I was brought up that way. My father was very open.

Therapist: About sexual matters. Was your mother too?

Father: Yes, my mother never frowned upon it. We used to discuss certain things; it was never dirty.

Therapist: Well, now, did you then really culminate your marriage? Did you have full intercourse after four or five weeks, or something?

Father: Yes, then——

Therapist: She let you in.

Father: Then it slackened down again after her parents came back, but when we moved to our own apartment——

Therapist: When Ma and Pa came in, you went out?

Mother: Yes.

Therapist: Let's say she shoved you out. She was married to her parents, not to you, is that right?

Father: I think she was having relations with me while listening.

Therapist: What kind of marriage was this with your parents?

Mother: Well, their advice or their thoughts actually were more important to me then. It took me a long time to divorce myself from that.

Therapist: I see, and as long as you were married to your parents you couldn't be married to your husband—either/or? They come home; you lock him out. How long did you live with your parents?

Mother: Well, my mother died. She died nine months after we were married.

Therapist: I see. So did you have to wait the nine months to get in again, Pop?

Father: No, but as I was saying it was like . . . she was looking to her. . . . She was with me but listening to them.

Therapist: That's very interesting, what you just said. Can you guess what I'm thinking? You can't—can you guess?

Mother: Yes.

Therapist: What?

Mother: I didn't want them to walk in on us or to be aware or——

Therapist: Of course, she is smart. You didn't want your parents to catch you in the act, the dirty act. Now you treat your children like you treated your parents; you don't want them to walk in on you. What are the sleeping arrangements?

Father: Now they have their own room.

Therapist: Do you worry now, Mom, about the kids walking in on you while you're having intercourse, making love? You shook your head yes. (*To father*) Was she worried about that?

Father: Was she? Oh, yes!

Therapist: Worried about the kids walking into the bedroom?

Father: Yes.

Therapist: Did you ever walk in on your parents?

Mother: No, not that I ever remember. No,

Therapist: You never caught them in the act?

Mother: No. I don't think I ever thought of them that way.

Therapist: You mean in your mind your parents couldn't do such a thing; they're pure.

Mother: Yes. Even after I learned all about it, I don't think it ever entered my mind.

Is Psychotherapy Effective?

Almost all psychiatrists, clinical psychologists and other professional personnel believe that psychotherapy works, i.e., that it is an effective means of helping emotionally disturbed individuals. Yet it is very difficult to prove the validity of this belief. Pointing to individual cases of dramatic improvement does not constitute proof, for the improvement could have occurred spontaneously or been caused by concurrent environmental changes. It is even more meaningless to try to prove that one psychotherapeutic system is superior to another by pointing to individual successes; a fundamental rule is that *all types of psychotherapy help some patients.* If the most outrageous kind of treatment that could be devised were applied to enough patients a few would improve markedly.

Obviously, the need is for careful controlled research on psychotherapeutic effectiveness. The research performed to date is extensive but difficult to interpret, primarily due to deficiencies of control in the design of the research.

Strupp and Bergin (1969) compiled an exhaustive, critical review of psychotherapy research which called attention to some of the deficiencies and difficulties with research efforts to date. They pointed out that therapists vary

widely in skill, technique, personality and experience, even within the same theoretical school. Thus, they cannot be regarded as interchangeable units by researchers. Similarly, patients come with differing problems, differing personalities and varied socioeconomic backgrounds. Finally, therapeutic techniques cannot be examined in isolation but must be viewed in the context of the many patient and therapist variables already enumerated. Research efforts thus far have too often compared patients in therapy with patients not in therapy, or patients in treatment with client-centered therapists with patients being seen by psychoanalysts. However, since such investigations fail to control for the numerous patient, therapist and technique variables which have been identified, it is difficult to draw firm conclusions concerning the effectiveness of psychotherapy or of particular forms of psychotherapy.

As Strupp and Bergin observe, psychotherapy is not a unitary process applied in the same fashion to all patients or to all problems. This being the case, the question "Is psychotherapy effective?" seems inappropriate. Instead attention must be given to the question of which specific kind of therapist, using which technique, will produce specific changes in which patient? Unfortunately, personality measures and research sophistication are not yet capable of producing precise answers. In the following paragraphs some of the major variables in psychotherapy research are discussed.

Therapist Variables. Many writers have described the personality attributes which a therapist should possess in order to be effective. The "ideal" therapist, according to these descriptions, is warm, empathic, accepting, objective, mature, genuine, open, self-understanding, and free of neurotic conflicts. Obviously, few human beings are capable of being such paragons of virtue. Additionally, it has been difficult to demonstrate that these general personality traits are causally linked to better outcomes. It has been possible to show that certain therapist personality variables are related to the nature of the interaction or relationship which is established with the patient. For example, Truax and Carkhuff (1967) found that more empathic behavior on the part of the therapist was associated with a greater tendency toward self-exploration in the patient. These authors also found that empathy, warmth and acceptance are created by the therapist and are largely independent of the personality of the patient. Thus, it seems that therapist warmth and acceptance are necessary and helpful in the therapeutic undertaking, but by themselves such therapist attributes are not sufficient to produce change. The therapist, it appears, must create the proper climate for growth but whether or not the patient will actually change is dependent on other variables.

Other studies concerning the therapist's contribution to the treatment process have focused on therapist types, therapist styles and therapist values. Some therapists have been found to be more effective with schizophrenic patients but exactly why this is so is still largely a mystery (Whitehorn and Betz, 1960). Rice (1965) found that therapists with a fresh connotative language and expressive voice quality tended to have more favorable treatment outcomes. Finally, Bandura (1965) has shown rather clearly that part of therapeutic influence involves modeling and imitation of the therapist by the patient. It follows that the therapist's values will influence the nature of the results he obtains.

This discussion has touched on only a few of the highlights of findings concerning the therapist variable. The evidence to date leaves little doubt that the person of the therapist, in both a positive and negative sense, represents an important force in shaping the process and outcome of psychotherapy. The precise nature of his influence and the specific consequences of particular attitudes or actions remain to be discovered.

Technique Variables. Apart from his style or personality, the therapist may make use of a variety of techniques to help the patient toward greater integration and autonomy. Since such technical interventions are largely embedded in the therapist's verbalizations, studies of the effects of various techniques have tended to focus on the ongoing interaction between the participants. A representative study of technique variables is that of Strupp (1960), who asked therapists to view a therapy film and at certain points to indicate what they would say or do if they were that therapist. It was found that therapists' verbal interventions varied as a function of their level of experience, theoretical orientation, professional affiliation, and whether they had had analysis. Other investigations have obtained similar results from studies of actual interviews.

While such studies are useful in demonstrating differences in technical interventions among therapists they have been of limited value in helping to specify which techniques are useful in achieving specific goals. A possible exception to this generalization is provided by certain behavior modification investigators. Much of this body of research has focused on the effects of a variety of technical operations with highly suggestive results (see earlier discussion in this chapter on Behavior Modification). For example, systematic desensitization is a technique which has been found to be highly effective in the alleviation of phobias (Paul, 1966).

No form of psychotherapy relies exclusively on the use of a single technique. Schools of therapy differ in their emphasis of particular techniques but the emphasis is relative rather than exclusive. Most therapists make use of a variety of techniques in their daily work. It remains for the researcher to make further refinements in the comparison of different techniques in specified situations and the assessment of different effects.

Patient Variables. Every therapist has ideas about the kind of patient who is most likely to benefit from psychotherapy and many such formulations have been experimentally verified. A few of the many patient characteristics which have been linked to successful outcome are verbal fluency, motivation for change, ability for self-scrutiny, low overt disturbance, recent onset of disturbance, being married, being employed, middle or upper social class membership, and capacity for empathy. Some observers have taken such findings to mean that only patients who are not too disturbed and thus in little need of help can benefit from therapy. However, it is probably more correct to say that patients who still manage to meet life's responsibilities while struggling with severe psychological conflicts are the better therapeutic risks.

A recent trend in psychotherapy research has been to examine the similarity between patient and therapist and its effects on remaining in treatment and outcome. Strupp and Bergin (1969) summarized a number of studies showing that similarity in socioeconomic background, in values, and in expectations about what therapy will be like are closely associated with positive outcomes.

Outcome. As already indicated the question of outcome, or psychotherapeutic effectiveness, is too broad to be answered simply. A well-known attempt to do so is the following study by Eysenck.

Eysenck (1952) reviewed a number of previous studies of psychotherapeutic outcome for three groups of neurotic patients. One group

NB

had been treated psychoanalytically, a second by nonanalytic psychotherapy and a third had received no psychotherapy but had either been hospitalized or treated by nonpsychiatric physicians. The proportion who improved was very similar in the three groups, and Eysenck arrived at the drastic conclusion that psychotherapy, psychoanalytic or other, is valueless. Few psychologists have accepted this conclusion, however, for it is questionable whether the patients in the three groups were comparable in severity of disorder, personality or socioeconomic backgrounds, whether the therapists were similar in experience, style or personality, and also whether the outcome criteria were equivalent. In a reply to Eysenck, Rosenzweig (1954) pointed out that the criterion of success for hospitalized patients consists of sufficient symptomatic improvement to enable the patient to return to the community, whereas in psychoanalysis the outcome is not considered successful unless a reorganization of personality occurs. This criterion is more stringent than that of return to the community.

Strupp, Fox and Lessler (1969) contacted 122 former patients who had been in psychotherapy, to secure their impressions of the effectiveness of treatment. Of the group 78 per cent felt that they had benefited either a fair amount or a great deal from their therapy. Similarly, 79 per cent reported being moderately to extremely satisfied with the results of their experience. Conversely, only 11 per cent of the patients reported no improvement or a worsening of their initial symptoms and 12 per cent felt that they had changed very little as a result of therapy. While these data are subjective impressions and constitute no final proof of the effectiveness of psychotherapy, they do support similar data from other investigators. By and large, patients feel they benefit from psychotherapy, but isolating objective indices of such benefits has remained difficult to date.

Meaningful research on therapeutic effectiveness requires that the patients in the experimental and control groups be equated for diagnosis, severity of disturbance, age, socioeconomic status and intelligence. One procedure for obtaining a nontreatment control group consists of interviewing potential patients to assess their status on the variables that must be controlled, dividing them into two subgroups matched for these variables and then treating one subgroup while withholding treatment from the other. Unfortunately this procedure is tantamount to a positive rejection of the control

groups and therefore itself constitutes a variable that affects the outcome of the study. To quote Frank (1959), "Psychotherapy is one form of interpersonal relationship, refusal of psychotherapy is another; it cannot be regarded as neutral."

Since no research so far performed has succeeded in the difficult, and perhaps impossible, task of controlling all the relevant patient and therapist variables while conducting a study of adequate size, there is to date no definitive proof or disproof of the effectiveness of psychotherapy. On theoretical grounds, it seems reasonable to assume that a patient who is anxious and bewildered and has lacked good human relationships will benefit from a relationship with an understanding therapist. Meanwhile, efforts to improve the methodology of research on the outcome and also on the processes of psychotherapy—the sequence of changes in patients' feelings, perceptions and attitudes—are being undertaken by many psychologists. Process research is closely related to efforts to increase the effectiveness of therapy, for the more completely we understand the processes through which behavior changes occur the more effective psychotherapy should be.

ENVIRONMENTAL MANIPULATION AND MILIEU THERAPY

Manipulation of the patient's environment may take many forms. Children may be removed from intolerable home conditions by court order and placed in foster homes. A social worker may aid a disturbed adult to find a job or better housing or join a social or recreational group. Milieu therapy—often also termed social or situational therapy—is an attempt to modify the patient's social setting. Family and group therapy are in a sense special forms of milieu therapy that make use of psychotherapeutic principles.

The most widely recognized type of milieu therapy occurs within those modern mental hospitals that have broken with tradition. Although the social structure of mental hospitals has been rapidly changing since World War II, many still have an organization well described by Frank (1961b) in which milieu therapy plays no part:*

---

*From Frank, J. D. 1961. Persuasion and Healing. Baltimore, The Johns Hopkins Press, pp. 192–193.

The basic assumption underlying its [the traditional mental hospital] structure and organization is that mental patients are irresponsible and therefore liable to harm themselves or others. Furthermore, most patients are viewed as suffering from chronic illnesses that are unlikely to improve, so that they will require lifelong care. These assumptions have led to the building of mental hospitals in rural settings at a distance from the communities they serve, where patients are cared for behind locked doors, economically and out of harm's way.

. . . The treatment staff forms a complex hierarchy, with physicians at the apex, professionally trained ancillary personnel such as nurses and social workers next, and aides or attendants at the bottom. The patient's role is to submit to treatment and take orders without question. Since he is presumed to be irresponsible, he does not know what is good for him and must therefore accept the judgment of the staff. Thus patients tend to be treated as objects rather than persons. Their communications with treatment personnel are strictly limited, and the nature of the communications is chiefly determined by the staff.

Because of the very small ratio of physicians to patients, the physicians spend most of their time with those newly admitted patients who seem most likely to respond to treatment. Others, such as senile patients, are placed immediately in custodial wards, to be joined by those who, failing to respond promptly to therapy, must make room for newcomers. Thus the hospital becomes an end station for most of its inmates, where they are expected to spend the rest of their lives. It shelters, feeds, clothes, and protects them, but they are no longer regarded as objects of treatment or candidates for return to the community, and they receive minimal attention from the treatment personnel. They pass their lives under conditions of extreme monotony in an atmosphere of hopelessness.

We may add that in the traditional mental hospital the patient is stripped of his self-esteem and even of part of his identity. His personal belongings are taken away and his mail is censored.

Despite—or perhaps because of—its authoritarianism, the structure of the traditional hospital is beneficial for some patients. Its lack of ambiguity and its simplicity tax the resources of patients less than the outside world does and permit mobilization of their recuperative forces. Sullivan (1947) felt that ". . . the severity of any mental disorder is to an important degree a result of insecurity about one's status. . . . This part of the problem could be solved by removing the patient to a society in which vertical mobility is not possible. Just this, in effect, is achieved by his admission to the custodial institution." Even the unpleasantness of the traditional hospital may exert an ameliorative effect if it increases the patient's motivation to recover and leave the hospital.

Since World War II, however, the primary goal of mental hospitals has begun to change from that of custody to planned, rather than incidental, treatment. The *therapeutic community* is a term frequently used to designate the modern mental hospital that employs milieu therapy. The goals of milieu therapy are to help patients identify with a social group and to modify their social attitudes and behavior. The patients are urged to join recreational and occupational as well as more strictly therapeutic groups. In some hospitals, patients share responsibility for the daily program through decisions arrived at by parliamentary discussion.

The whole social structure of the hospital changes with the introduction of such a program. Patients are no longer expected to follow all staff orders blindly; they have the right to ask questions and receive explanations. The shift from autocracy to some degree of democracy arouses anxiety in many staff personnel and a training program is usually necessary before personnel will accept the new principles and relationships.

Wards in the best modern hospitals are attractively furnished—within the limits of available funds—as contrasted with the barrack-like wards in the old-fashioned mental hospital. Fewer doors are locked and most patients may come and go freely in what has come to be designated as "the open hospital." The majority of units built for mental patients in the last few years have been attached to general hospitals in urban centers instead of being isolated at a distance from the communities they serve. Community members are often brought into the modern hospital to help develop recreational programs and to aid in finding jobs for discharged patients. One consequence of these interactions with the community is that members of the population at large develop more positive attitudes toward mental hospitals. In turn, a consequence of this attitudinal change is an increase in the proportion of voluntary admissions and a decrease in involuntary commitments.

One other aspect of the therapeutic community is the development of programs for the systematic care of patients after discharge. The programs make use of outpatient departments attached to the hospital, "halfway houses" where patients may live until they become reestablished in the community, and foster homes.

It was stated earlier that ataractic drugs have

been a major cause of the recent increase in hospital discharges. Many professional persons believe that the changed social atmosphere of modern mental hospitals has had an equally important effect on patients. The two factors are connected, for tranquilizing makes it possible for patients to cooperate in the various programs of the best hospitals. In the pre-tranquilizer era it would have been very difficult to apply the principles of the therapeutic community, the open hospital and milieu therapy on a mass scale. The experience of one state (Minnesota) is illustrative: from 1960 to 1962 the number of patients in mental hospitals declined 11 per cent, the percentage of open hospital wards increased from 52 to 76 per cent, voluntary admissions increased from 25 to 48 per cent and several new community clinics were established. Each of these changes is an enormous gain for mental health.

MODERN TRENDS IN TREATMENT: COMMUNITY MENTAL HEALTH

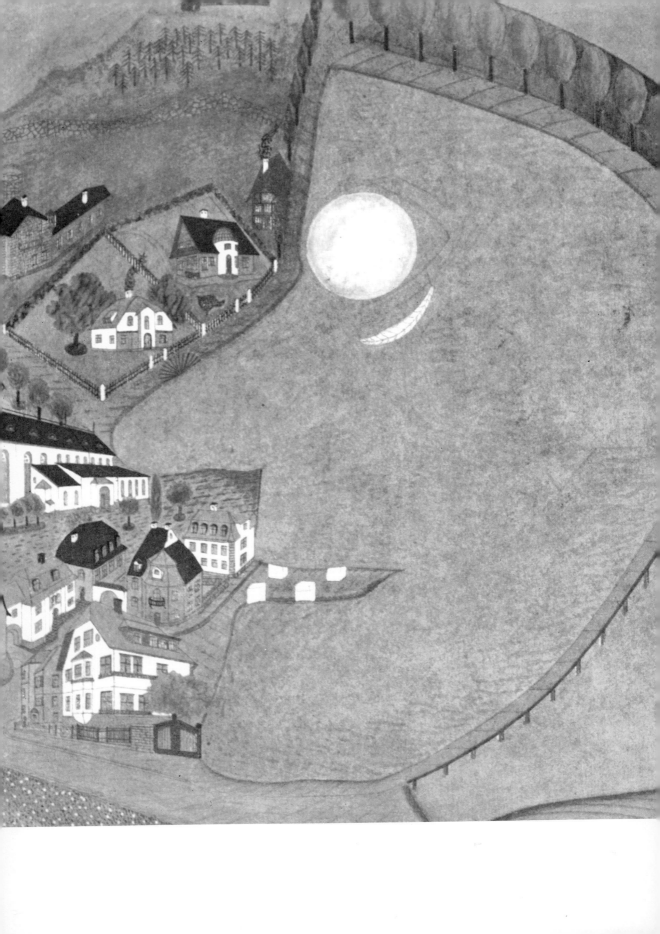

The only freedom which deserves the name is that
of pursuing our own good in our own way, so long as we
do not attempt to deprive others of theirs, or impede
their efforts to obtain it. Each is the proper guardian
of his own health, whether bodily, or mental and spiritual.
Mankind are greater gainers by suffering each
other to live as seems good to themselves, than by compelling
each to live as seems good to the rest.

John Stuart Mill

MODERN TRENDS IN TREATMENT: COMMUNITY MENTAL HEALTH

In the last 20 years, we have seen the emergence of a rapidly expanding series of new approaches to the understanding and alleviation of emotional disorders. In part, the changes reflect increased scientific understanding of mental disturbances, but the major portion of the impetus for change has come from current social, political and economic pressures. The public is demanding more rapid treatment, a greater variety of treatment approaches, and increased accessibility to treatment facilities.

The mass media and public education programs have resulted in a population which is increasingly sophisticated about mental health problems. Mental disturbance is less a stigma than it was only a generation ago. Many kinds of behavior are now easily recognized by most persons as symptoms of emotional problems for which help is available. As awareness and tolerance expanded, the demand for treatment services increased dramatically. Some have speculated that the increased demand reflects a greater incidence of emotional disorders but such assumptions are very difficult to prove.

In addition to their response to the increased sophistication of the general public, the changes in the mental health movement appear to be, in part, a reflection of the broad changes which are overtaking the delivery of all health-related services. Increasingly the public looks to government to provide and support health services. Just as we were busy building hospitals in small communities all over the country several years ago, we are now establishing mental health services. As of 1970, funds had been allocated for the establishment of over 2000 community mental health centers.

As man has struggled with the vast scientific and cultural changes which have occurred since World War II, it has become obvious that we live increasingly in a complex, interrelated social world. Such a world is not only shaped by man but also acts as an active agent affecting man's behavior in numerous ways. Many individual psychological dispositions are now seen as related to systematic differences in the environment. Many studies have led to this conclusion. Berry (1966, 1967), for example, compared the cultures of the Temne of Sierra Leone and the Eskimos of Baffin Island on certain perceptual scales and in a social conformity situation. He was able to demonstrate that the Eskimos' tendency to show less closure and less field dependence on perceptual tests, as well as less conformity in the social situation, was related to social, cultural and topographic differences in their environment. With respect to psychopathology, such studies lend support to a concept of etiology which emphasizes the importance of the environment or community. As Lehmann (1971) put it:

> . . . the quantity and quality of behavioral pathology are related to the community from whence it comes. The community can no longer be viewed as an uncompromising set of conditions to which everyone must adjust. Instead it is an active participant in molding behavior and establishing demands and limitations on it.

Thus, one of the major changes in the mental health movement in recent years has been the tendency to define mental illness in broad social terms which implicate the community at large in the cause and cure. Mental illness is seen no longer as simply an illness with which someone is afflicted. Rather, it is seen as a symptom which may reflect problems in living with others in the environment or problems in coping with an increasingly alienated, mechanized world. As the definition of illness has broadened to include the individual's community or context, it has been necessary to alter our ideas of intervention. Until recently, treatment was, in a sense, aimed at adjusting the patient to his environment. If a person required hospitalization, he was removed from his community, family and job, sent to a distant hospital and returned when he was capable of functioning in the original setting. Now experts are turning attention to the need for alterations in the environment as well as in the patient. A good example of this viewpoint is found in family therapy where it is recognized that changes in the emotional life of a family are often necessary in order for the identified patient to be maintained outside the mental hospital.

CHANGES IN MENTAL HOSPITALS

Another factor in the pressures for changes in mental health care came from accumulated experiences with the effects of prolonged hospitalization. Some of the difficulties with traditional hospital programs were discussed in the previous chapter. Here we will look more explicitly at studies of the untoward effects of hospitalization and some of the revisions in treatment which are now available.

Institutionalism

Institutionalism or "hospitalitis" is the term used to describe patients who become overly dependent on the hospital for emotional support. Some patients adapt to the protected environment of the hospital and find a niche for themselves within that social order. When the added stresses of discharge and adaptation to the outside environment threaten, there may be a reappearance of symptoms. The longer a person is hospitalized, the greater the risk of his becoming dependent on the hospital and the greater the stress of readjustment to the normal environment. Wing (1962) studied mental symptoms, word behavior and attitude toward discharge in randomly selected chronic male schizophrenic patients in two London hospitals. He found that "patients gradually develop an attitude of indifference toward events outside the hospital which is part of a syndrome of "institutionalism." Table 22–1 clearly shows how the wish to leave the hospital decreases as the length of hospitalization increases.

Lehrman (1961) used three criteria in investigating the effects of hospitalization on patients in three hospitals in different states: (1) the percentage of patients (of a particular age and diagnosis) who were eventually discharged; (2) the percentage of those discharged and not readmitted; and (3) the percentage of those who were out of the hospital at the time of the follow-up study, whether or not they had been readmitted previously. With Wing, Lehrman concluded that "prolonged hospitalization in itself may be harmful to psychiatric patients and the longer they are exposed to the hospital, the more adversely they sometimes seem to be affected." He recommended that alternatives to long-term hospital care be developed and that greater emphasis be placed on short-term hospital programs

TABLE 22–1. Influence of Length of Stay in Hospital on Attitude to Discharge

N = ?

Rating of attitude to discharge	Length of stay in hospital				
	2 yrs.	2 to 5 yrs.	5 to 10 yrs.	10 to 20 yrs.	Over 20 years.
	Number (Percentage)	Number (Percentage)	Number (Percentage)	Number (Percentage)	Number (Percentage)
Definite wish to leave	36 (50.7)	12 (29.3)	13 (23.6)	6 (11.3)	1 (2.8)
Vague wish to leave	17 (23.9)	15 (36.6)	14 (25.5)	6 (11.3)	5 (13.9)
Indifferent or wish to stay	18 (25.4)	14 (34.2)	28 (50.9)	41 (77.4)	30 (83.3)

Adapted from Wing, J. K. 1962. Institutionalism in mental hospitals. Brit. J. Soc. Clin. Psychol. *1*:38–51.

aimed at reintegrating the patient into the community as soon as possible.

Some critics have gone so far as to advocate doing away with hospitals altogether except for the care of acute problems. Such a view seems too extreme to most authorities. It is true that hospitalization sometimes has untoward effects. Mahrer (1963), for example, recorded patients' symptoms on admission and again 8.25 weeks later and found that "psychiatric hospitalization is accompanied by the appearance of psychological symptoms not present at the point of admission." However, removal from a stressful environment and a sheltered milieu appear beneficial for many disturbed persons. Ryan (1962) interviewed 100 mental patients at the time of discharge concerning various aspects of their hospital experience. Forty-five per cent of the group indicated that protection from the community and superimposed control of their lives were the two factors most significant in their recovery. What is required is the provision of a protected, simplified environment for the patient while he needs it, and the initiation of a process of readjustment to the community as soon as the acute phase subsides.

Decentralization of Hospitals

Faced with an increasing patient population and inadequate resources, the large mental hospital gradually evolved an organizational model marked by selective deployment of resources in favor of acutely ill patients to the detriment of long-term sufferers. Patients failing to respond after brief treatment are transferred to "long-term patient" wards where there are fewer professional personnel, poorer physical facilities and little chance of constructive efforts for change. Hospital decentralization prevents such organizational shifts by arranging the hospital into small, autonomous units responsible for all patients assigned to the unit. Often each hospital unit serves a particular geographic region and is responsible for the care of all mental patients from that area. Having no chronic ward to which some patients can be transferred, the unit personnel are inclined to be more innovative in their efforts to care for difficult patients.

The benefits of unitization are numerous. Since all the patients come from a restricted geographical area, coordinated care for the patient becomes more feasible. The unit staff can develop consulting arrangements with agencies and resources in the community to ease the patients' transition in and out of the hospital. Pre- and post-hospital care which is coordinated rather than discontinuous becomes more likely. The patient benefits from having a specific staff who maintain continuous responsibility for him. He will not be transferred to another ward requiring another adjustment, and when he is discharged he will have professional personnel who are already familiar with his case involved in his outpatient treatment. A further benefit of decentralization is that greater responsibility and autonomy are given to the unit staff. This necessitates the constructive involvement of many more staff members in patient care. Nurses and attendants become more than custodians or medicine dispensers. They become involved directly in patient care and realistic after-care planning, or as therapists (Schulberg and Baker, 1969).

Decentralization has had striking success in reducing inpatient populations by as much as 50 per cent over a period of three to five years. Smith et al. (1965) found that five years of usage of modern drugs had little effect on the size of the patient population at a mental hospital in Colorado. However, an abrupt administrative change due to unitization was followed by a significant patient population decrement.

Partial Hospitalization

Another trend in hospital care is the more flexible use of hospital facilities to meet the needs of patients who do not require 24-hour supervision. Many patients can participate in various hospital programs while continuing to live at home. Important social ties can thereby be preserved. The kinds of programs which may be offered under a partial hospitalization format are too numerous to list here, but examples of such activities include vocational counseling, group therapy, job training and cooperative group efforts designed to increase socialization skills.

Some hospitals have established halfway house programs for long-term patients, who often experience difficulty in readjusting to normal life. In such programs groups of patients live in the now familiar routine of the hospital while working in the community. Group meetings and gradually increasing responsibilities for running the halfway house help the patients cope with the stress of adjustment to a new routine and new way of life.

Home Treatment

Several hospitals have begun active treatment of certain patients in their home as an alternative to hospital care. The first program of this type in the United States was the Home Treatment Service of Boston State Hospital (Meyer et al., 1967). Begun in 1957, the service makes use of home visits by psychiatric nurses, consultation with caretaker personnel (welfare workers, family physicians) who are involved with the patient, and involvement of the family in the treatment goals, to maintain psychotic patients in the community. Of the first 154 patients referred to this service, only 38 per cent were hospitalized and some of these required relatively brief inpatient care. Pittman, et al. (1965) worked intensively with randomly selected psychotic patients who had been recommended for hospitalization in Denver. In this program the patient's family was made an integral part of the treatment and planning process. The patient's problem was interpreted to the family as a family crisis rather than as an illness. By use of family therapy and an active, goal-oriented approach, it was possible to avert hospitalization in 24 of the first 25 patients in this program. Early evidence suggests that patients treated in this fashion function as well in the community as patients who are provided with traditional hospitalization treatment.

COMPREHENSIVE COMMUNITY MENTAL HEALTH SERVICES

Mental Health Acts

Public demand, professional advancements, and various social-political pressures led to the passage of the Mental Health Study Act in 1955. This act resulted in the establishment of a Joint Commission on Mental Illness and Health which was given a mandate from Congress to survey the resources and to make recommendations for combating mental illness in the United States. The studies and reports of this commission provided the springboard for sweeping changes in the delivery of mental health services, in the training and thinking of mental health workers, and in the passage of the necessary enabling legislation.

It was the report of this commission which helped accelerate the changes in mental hospital care described previously. The need for change was apparent and had already begun in some hospitals, but the findings of the commission lent added sanction and impetus to programs which had been resisted by some. The words of the commission were quite specific. Two samples from their final report on hospitals capture the main thrust of their thinking on the topic (Joint Commission on Mental Illness and Health, 1961):

No more state hospitals of more than 1000 beds should be built, and not one patient should be added to any existing mental hospital already housing 1000 or more patients.

The objective of modern treatment of persons with major mental illness is to enable the patient to maintain himself in the community in a normal manner. To do so, it is necessary (1) to save the patient from the debilitating effects of institutionalization as much as possible, (2) if the patient requires hospitalization, to return him to home and community life as soon as possible, and (3) thereafter to maintain him in the community as long as possible. Therefore, after-care and rehabilitation are essential parts of all service to mental patients, and the various methods of achieving rehabilitation should be integrated in all forms of services, among them day hospitals, night hospitals, after-care clinics, public health nursing homes, rehabilitation centers, work services, and ex-patient groups.

50,000

The commission also recommended that one fully staffed, full-time clinic be established for each 50,000 of population. Such clinics were seen as the main line of defense in reducing the need of many persons for prolonged or repeated hospitalization. This would be accomplished by identifying problems sooner and intervening promptly. Clinics' main functions were seen as: (1) providing treatment by experts for persons with acute disturbances; (2) caring for incompletely recovered patients, either short of admission to a hospital or following discharge; and (3) providing a headquarters for mental health consultants working with mental health counselors.

The third function listed above was a major one. Here the commission addressed itself to the fact that there was a severe shortage of mental health professionals which was not likely to be rectified in the foreseeable future. It was further recognized that many persons in the community (such as clergymen, family physicians, teachers, public health nurses, and the like) were already trying to help and to treat the mentally ill in the absence of professional help. It was recommended that experts trained in mental health work devote a major portion of their time to consulting with such community helpers with the aim of increasing their skills and thereby indirectly helping a greater number of persons than any expert could see by himself.

Subsequent to the final report and recommendations of the commission, Congress passed enabling legislation providing funds for the construction and staffing of Comprehensive Community Mental Health Centers throughout the country. By 1967, 256 centers had been funded, and it was hoped that the total would be close to 2000 by 1970. The idea of a community mental health center is not a new one. Querido (1969) has described one which he helped establish in Amsterdam in the 1930's. However, such programs were not widespread and the action by Congress in the mid-1960's has resulted in a virtual revolution in mental health care in this country.

The Essential Services /5 ESSENTIALS

In order to qualify for federal support a comprehensive community mental health center must provide five essential services for its clients: inpatient, outpatient, partial hospitalization, 24-hour emergency, and consultation and education services. This range of services

I O P E C

offered by a single organization provides for the continuity of care of local mental patients. The emergency service enables a patient to seek help at any time, day or night, without delay, referral, or a trip to a distant center. He can receive help immediately and in his own community. An emergency service may function as a crisis intervention center with a suicide prevention function (see Chapter 11). This is a method for dealing with a crisis while it is in progress. Operating 24 hours a day, the service is always available to the desperate person. Trained lay persons or professionals attempt to find out what is bothering the caller or visitor, provide reassurance that solutions are possible, and make referrals to appropriate agencies. The goal in the crisis phase of a problem is not to provide a ready-made solution but rather to provide immediate relief and hope, since the suicidal mood is typically a temporary one. The crisis intervention center is directed toward averting the immediate crisis (whether it be suicide or some other acute difficulty) so as to allow time for working out long-term solutions to the person's problems.

If a patient does not require hospitalization, he can be seen in the outpatient clinic while continuing to work and live at home. Should hospitalization be required, the patient is placed in an inpatient unit in the local hospital, close to friends, relatives and his familiar world. After hospitalization, the patient may be seen on an outpatient basis by the same staff which has been responsible for his care from the beginning. Some patients may need certain benefits of hospitalization without 24-hour care and may be placed in a day-care or partial hospitalization program (see Chapter 21).

In addition to providing continuity of care in the patient's community, the center strives to improve the level of mental health care in its area through its consultation program. Studies of the Joint Commission on Mental Illness and Health showed that 71 per cent of persons with emotional problems first seek help from their family physician or their clergyman. It is only later that they turn to a mental health professional. Many persons receive the help, advice and support they need at this level and never go further. Obviously, if such front-line helpers can be helped to be more expert in their handling of emotional problems, everyone benefits. More patients are reached, since ministers and family physicians see many more persons than the average psychologist or psychiatrist in private practice. Patients who need to be seen by an expert can be referred more promptly if the person they see first is aware of when to refer and when to attempt to alleviate the situation himself. The first-line professional is helped by becoming more effective in work he is already doing. The mental health worker benefits by influencing many more persons than he could reach alone. When a school teacher learns to deal more effectively with some emotional problems in the classroom, it not only benefits current students but future students as well. Many school consultation programs are directed toward helping teachers in identifying emotional problems and in learning more effective means of preventing or treating them. An understanding teacher who can spot the insecurity behind a child's quiet shyness and early withdrawal can go a long way toward preventing the development of more severe problems later.

The forms of the consultation and education services provided by centers may be many and varied. They have included such progressive steps as training selected police officers to be specialists in family crisis situations (Bard, 1970) and the use of indigenous lay people as therapeutic agents in the rehabilitation of disadvantaged psychotic adults (Christmas, 1967).

The Joint Commission report called for the training of mental health counselors and workers for specific roles without their undergoing the lengthy study required of a professional. The roles vary widely, but many programs are involved in training lay persons for specific mental health worker roles. Some high school graduates have been trained in the administration of certain psychological tests, thus freeing the psychologist for other needed activities. In one of the bolder programs growing out of the move to train lay persons, Margaret Rioch and her co-workers trained carefully selected housewives to do counseling and psychotherapy, under supervision, with selected types of patients. The housewives selected were typically college graduates whose children were grown and who were interested in reentering the job market. This program has demonstrated to many skeptics that a mature person with reasonable judgment can be trained relatively quickly to handle many of the counseling and psychotherapeutic functions now restricted exclusively to professionals. Such lay workers need to be supervised but a single professional can oversee the treatment of many more patients than he could ever see himself.

The problem of individual psychotherapy has been a vexing one in the community mental

health movement. The emphases of the movement have been on rapid treatment, consultation and environmental manipulation. The realization that there will never be enough therapists to provide a long-term, one-to-one relationship for all who need it has led many to emphasize other alternatives to treatment and to conclude that the need for individual psychotherapy will be thereby reduced. In this regard Wallerstein (1968) correctly observes:

Rather than diminishing the requirement for individual psychotherapy, the successfully operating community mental health program will, I am convinced, widen and deepen it . . . all of our experience to date has been that as intensive mental health services are rendered available on understandable and acceptable terms, the more demand is generated, the more individual treatment cases can be found.

EFFECTIVENESS OF COMMUNITY APPROACHES

The effectiveness of the community mental health program is a matter of debate, although the balance of the evidence seems to suggest that the results have been worth the vast expenditures of time and money. A few of the arguments and counterarguments are summarized in the remainder of this chapter.

It is a fact that by the end of 1968 the number of resident hospital patients in the United States had dropped to one-half of the number who would have required hospitalization if the trend prior to 1955 had not been reversed. This downward trend from early projections still continues, so that the National Institute of Mental Health now estimates that by 1973 the total resident population will drop to 186,000 (Yolles, 1969). While this trend is a fact, its cause is a matter of debate. Some experts credit the decline to the introduction of tranquilizers in the early 1950's. Others believe that the decline in hospitalization rates is due to the changes in hospital organization (such as unitization) and the establishment of a better continuity of care through partial hospitalization, home treatment services, follow-up clinics and the like. Since the community mental health programs and tranquilizers both arrived on the scene relatively recently, and both are widely used, it is virtually impossible to isolate their specific effects.

It is also true that the effect of drugs on the treatment of mental disorders was broader than a mere chemical effect. By making patients more manageable, more accessible and amenable to influence, the drugs had the effect of changing the attitudes of both staff and patients toward the treatability of mental disturbances. With less need for physical restraints, locked doors and constant surveillance, the staff was free to explore other approaches and to deal with its charges more humanely. Such changes in attitude, with their attendant sense of hope, may have produced benefits equal to, if not exceeding, the actual pharmacological effects of the drugs. Some of the available data seem to support such a conclusion. Statistics from the Office of Biometry of the National Institute of Mental Health show that the chronic schizophrenic population in this country did not begin to decline until five years after the widespread availability of tranquilizers. Such a delay may be a measure of the time necessary for changes in attitudes on the part of patients and staff to take effect. Mosher (1970) reviewed data in numerous studies conducted in the United States and Europe and concluded that the decline in the number of chronically hospitalized patients "appears to be as much a reflection of changing attitudes as it is of the direct pharmacologic effects of the drugs."

Some critics have pointed out that comprehensive community mental health centers have no significant effect on reducing the number of hospital admissions from areas they serve. All that the new programs have created, so the argument goes, is a hospital with a revolving door through which patients pass quickly after superficial treatment of a crisis-oriented nature (Shatan, 1969). Such critics point to the high readmission rates which generally accompany high discharge rates. It may be that patients are merely being shuffled from one place to another without really being helped. However, several studies have shown that an effective after-care program can reduce the readmission rate from 45 per cent to 12 per cent (Boyles and Waldrop, 1967). An important datum missing from these studies is the level of adjustment of the patient to the community.

One of the most innovative attempts to compare alternative types of hospital care is a study conducted by Fairweather and his associates (1969). In this study, a group of chronic mental patients was first organized in the hospital and later moved into a community lodge as a unit after already having lived and worked together in the hospital for several weeks. The lodge group served as a subsociety to help sustain patients in the community. The group formed a janitorial business to produce income and were given increasing autonomy in conducting their own routine affairs. This group was contrasted with a control group (which was in a hospital small-group treatment program) on the reduction of the hospital recidivism rate and the reduction of continuous hospitalization. Matched patients participated in the two programs. Compared to the control group, a greater percentage of the lodge group was able to remain out of the hospital and to assume employment. Sixty-five per cent of the lodge group and only 24 per cent of the control group remained out of the hospital for the first six months. While all of the lodge group left the hospital (to live in the lodge), 35 per cent of the control group never left the hospital. Members of the lodge group not only were more likely to stay out of the hospital, but also had a better employment record. Fifty per cent of the lodge group, but only 3 per cent of the matched control group, were employed full time for a six-month follow-up period. These same results obtained over the next three and one-half years of follow-up. The daily cost of keeping patients in the lodge program was less than half that required for their matched controls.

The enormous cost of funding new programs, new centers and new hospitals has diverted needed money from other, more traditional services, which still have demonstrable utility. Many patients still need, and benefit from, long-term custodial care. But such hospitals today are in a poor competitive position for funds and staff compared with the newly glamorous community mental health programs. More research is needed to better identify exactly which patients benefit from which types of care. Many approaches have a place in mental health treatment but experts are still often uncertain as to which kind of program is most suitable in a given instance.

GLOSSARY

abreaction. Emotional release or catharsis associated with conscious recollection of previously forgotten (repressed) unpleasant experiences.

abulia. Loss of the ability to perform voluntary actions or make decisions.

acrophobia. Morbid fear of heights.

acting out. A pattern of defense in which unconscious emotional conflicts are expressed (acted out) in behavior that tends to be maladaptive or antisocial.

acute disorder. Disorder with sudden onset and of short duration. An acute brain syndrome is reversible.

addiction. Emotional and physiological dependence on alcohol or drugs.

adjustment reaction. Transient situational personality disorder, especially in children.

affect. Emotional feeling tone or mood. The term affect is frequently used as synonymous with emotion.

affective disorders or reactions. Those syndromes in which the predominant feature is a disorder of affect or mood, as in manic depressive or psychotic depressive reactions.

agoraphobia. Morbid fear of open spaces.

agraphia. Inability to translate language into appropriate written symbols. A form of motor aphasia.

alarm reaction. First and defensive stage of the stress reaction.

alexia. Inability to understand written language. A form of sensory aphasia.

allergy. Hypersensitivity of tissues to a physical or chemical agent.

Alzheimer's disease. Progressive, widespread deterioration of the cerebral cortex accompanied by deterioration of intellect, in the presenile period.

amaurotic family idiocy. A group of disorders characterized by blindness occurring without apparent lesion of the eye and associated with severe mental subnormality.

ambivalence. Simultaneous existence of conflicting feelings or attitudes toward an object, person or goal.

amentia. Mental deficiency. Lifelong intellectual retardation or subnormality.

amnesia, anterograde. Loss of memory for events occurring after a precipitating event, usually trauma.

amnesia, retrograde. Loss of memory for events that occurred prior to a precipitating event.

amok. Frenzied emotional outburst, frequently homicidal.

Amytal. A sedative drug (like Pentothal) used to help patients recapture and describe past experiences. Popularly known as a "truth serum."

anal stage. Period in which anal sensations preoccupy the child and yield pleasure.

anal triad. Obstinacy, stinginess and orderliness, attributed by Freud to fixations during the anal stage.

anesthesia. Loss of sensitivity to stimuli.

anhedonia. Inability to experience pleasure.

anorexia. Loss of appetite.

anorexia nervosa. Loss of appetite for emotional reasons.

anoxia. Deficiency in oxygen supply.

anti-depressive drugs. Drugs used to diminish an affect or mood of depression.

antisocial reaction (antisocial sociopathy). Reaction marked by impulsiveness, pleasure-seeking, lack of loyalty, weak superego and absence of anxiety.

anxiety. Exaggerated state of fear that motivates a variety of behaviors, especially defensive behaviors. The presence of anxiety may be indicated by physical signs (e.g., sweating, tremors, nausea), by a conscious apprehensiveness or by disorganization of overt behavior.

anxiety reaction. Neurotic reaction with diffuse anxiety and physiological anxiety indicators (sweating, palpitation, etc.).

apathy. Lack of feeling or response. Indifference.

aphasia. Impaired ability to communicate by language or speech, due to organic brain disease.

May be predominantly *sensory* (impressive) or predominantly *motor* (expressive).

aphonia. Loss of ability to speak.

apnoea. Breathlessness caused by an excess of oxygen in the blood or forced respiration.

apoplexy. Sudden loss of consciousness and motor control. A stroke.

archetype. Term used by Jung to denote a universal unconscious image.

arteriosclerosis. Thickening and loss of elasticity of the walls of the arteries.

astasia-abasia. Symptom in which the person can perform complex movements of the legs but cannot stand or walk.

asthenic (leptosomatic). Slender physique characterized by poor muscular development.

ataractic drugs. Tranquilizing drugs, used to reduce anxiety, confusion and over-activity, without producing excessive sedation and somnolence.

ataxia. Loss of coordination with inability to maintain balance in standing or walking.

aura. Premonitory sensations or hallucinations that may warn an epileptic patient of an impending convulsion.

autism (early infantile). Disorder characterized by extreme withdrawal, inaccessibility, inability to relate to other persons, and language difficulties.

autistic thinking (dereistic, magical or prelogical thinking). Highly subjective thinking controlled by unrealistic gratification of drives in fantasy.

autoeroticism. Sexual arousal or gratification without the participation of another person. Masturbation is one form of autoeroticism.

automatic writing. More or less meaningful material written without conscious intent or control.

automatism. Mechanical, repetitive motor behavior, carried out unconsciously.

autonomic nervous system. Part of the nervous system that is not subject to voluntary control but regulates glands, smooth muscles and viscera. It consists of sympathetic and parasympathetic divisions.

autosome. Chromosome that does not affect the individual's sex.

basic anxiety. Child's feeling of helplessness in an environment perceived as hostile (according to Horney).

basic personality structure. Kardiner's term for the modal traits and behaviors shared by members of a culture.

behavior disorder (conduct disorder). Type of behavior deviation characterized by impulsive, antisocial acts. Sometimes used for any type of abnormal behavior.

blocking. Stoppage in train of thinking or speech, particularly due to emotional factors.

bulimia. Insatiable hunger.

cardiovascular. Pertaining to the circulatory system.

castration anxiety. Boy's fear that the father will punish him by injuring or depriving him of his genitals.

catatonic schizophrenia. Schizophrenic reaction in which motor disturbances, especially stupor or excitement, are conspicuous.

catharsis. Release of tension and anxiety by emotional reliving of past events, especially repressed events.

central nervous system. The brain and spinal cord.

cerebral arteriosclerosis. Thickening of the walls of the arteries to the brain, that may result in symptoms of an organic brain syndrome.

cerebrotonia. Temperament corresponding to ectomorphy.

chlorpromazine. A major tranquilizer.

chorea. Involuntary spasmodic movement.

chromosome. Body in the nucleus of a cell which contains the genes.

chronic disorder. A disorder that is long-lasting and tends to be irreversible.

circumstantiality. Thinking or conversation in which many trivial details are unnecessarily elaborated.

clang association. Association of words or ideas by similarity in sound.

classical conditioning. Process whereby a previously neutral stimulus, on being paired with an unconditioned stimulus (UCS), acquires the potentiality of evoking a response similar to the one previously evoked by the UCS.

claustrophobia. Morbid fear of closed places.

clinical psychology. Branch of psychology that employs psychological knowledge and techniques to help persons in emotional difficulties.

clonic phase. The stage of an epileptic convulsion in which there are spasmodic muscle contractions with jerking of the limbs.

clouding of consciousness. State of confusion characterized by lack of perceptual clarity.

coitus. Sexual intercourse.

coma. State of maximal stupor and unconsciousness.

combat neurosis. Traumatic neurosis originating from battle experiences and the conditions of military life.

compensation neurosis. Traumatic neurosis partly motivated by prospects of financial compensation.

compulsion. Overwhelming urge to perform an irrational act or ritual.

concordance. Occurrence of a trait in both members of a twin pair.

concrete thinking. Inability to generalize or think abstractly; thinking controlled by an immediate stimulus.

confabulation. Distortion of memory in which the patient fills amnesic gaps with imaginary experiences.

congenital. Present at birth.

conscience. The morally self-critical aspects of the personality, fulfilling the conscious inhibitory functions of the superego or internal control system.

constitution. (1) Vulnerability or predisposition. (2) The momentary product of all past physical and psychological processes. (3) The relatively enduring biological characteristics of the organism which influence responses. (Definition 3 is preferred.)

conversion reaction. Neurotic reaction in which anxiety is converted into a loss or alteration of a sensory or motor function.

countertransference. Therapist's displacement of feelings and projection of needs and conflicts onto the patient.

cretinism. A type of mental deficiency resulting from hypothyroidism in infancy or earlier.

cunnilingus. Apposition of the mouth to the female genitals.

cyclothymia. Personality tending to alternating moods of elation and dejection.

defense mechanism. Response, typically unconscious, by which the ego is protected from anxiety, guilt, shame or loss of pride.

delirium. Confused and excited state of organic origin characterized by incoherence, illusions, hallucinations and disorientation.

delirium tremens. Delirium associated with muscular tremors, occurring in some cases of alcoholism.

delusion. False belief, inconsistent with individual's own knowledge and experience and not shared by the cultural group. Major types are delusions of reference, influence, persecution and grandeur; the depressive delusions (guilt, self-accusation, etc.) and somatic delusions.

dementia. Progressive mental deterioration (contrast with amentia).

dementia praecox. Largely obsolete term for schizophrenia. The term implies that mental deterioration is inevitable (dementia) and that the disorder occurs in youth or "precociously" (praecox).

denial. Defensive refusal to recognize external reality, emotional reactions or motives.

depersonalization. Loss of feeling of one's own and others' reality.

depression. (1) Mood of morbid sadness. (2) Group of disorders (including psychotic depression and neurotic depression) in which there are several symptoms, including a depressed mood.

depressive reaction. Neurotic or psychotic depression occurring in reaction to environmental loss or stress.

diagnosis. Determination of the nature of a disease or abnormality by consideration of descriptive symptoms, dynamic defenses and factors involved in its causation.

differential diagnosis. Considering all possible diagnostic categories that might be compatible with what is known about an individual's abnormality and its development.

diplopia. Double vision.

discordance. Occurrence of a trait in only one member of a twin pair.

disorientation. Inability to identify time, place or persons accurately, accompanied by perplexity and confusion.

displacement. The unconscious transferring of an affect or emotion from its original source onto a more acceptable substitute.

dissociative reaction. Neurotic reaction in which amnesia, fugue, somnambulism or multiple personality occurs.

dizygotic twins. Twins developed from two separate ova. Also known as binovular, dizygous, DZ or fraternal twins.

dominant gene. A gene that produces an observable effect on the offspring even when paired with a recessive gene.

double bind. A pattern of communication consisting of contradictory messages.

double blind design. A research design in which both subjects and evaluators do not know which subjects are in the experimental group and which are in the control group.

downward drift hypothesis. The hypothesis that disturbed individuals are mobile downward and drift to disorganized neighborhoods.

dynamics. The study of forces in action, and hence the study of defense mechanisms and changing factors in the causation of human behavior. Frequently contrasted with the static or descriptive study of symptoms and their classification.

dysplastic. Physique characterized by lack of harmony in development of body parts (dysplasia).

dyssocial reaction (dyssocial sociopathy). Disregard for social codes in individuals reared in an abnormal social environment. May be loyal to own socially deviant group.

echolalia. Echo-like, automatic repetition by a patient of what is said to him.

echopraxia. Automatic repetition of another's movements.

ectomorphy. Sheldon's body component of thinness; linearity of physique.

ego. One of the three major divisions of personality proposed by Freud. The ego has evaluative and executive functions, and serves to mediate between the demands of primitive instinctual drives (the id), internalized prohibitions and ideals (the superego), and external reality.

ego-ideal. The part of the superego that motivates the personality toward positive ideals and values, developed through identification with significant persons whom the individual emulates.

ego-strength. Ability of ego to mediate among id, superego and reality effectively and flexibly.

electroconvulsive therapy (ECT) (electroshock therapy, EST). Treatment by passing an electric current through the brain. Widest use is for affective disorders.

electroencephalogram (EEG). Graphic record of changes in the electric potential of the brain.

encopresis. Involuntary defecation that is not caused by organic defect or illness.

endocrine gland. Gland that secretes hormones into the lymph or blood stream.

endogenous. Referring to causal factors within the body or within the system in which the morbid condition exists.

endomorphy. Sheldon's body component in which viscera are highly developed.

enuresis. Nocturnal bed-wetting after the age of three.

epilepsy. Disorder characterized by convulsive seizures, disturbances of consciousness, or both.

epinephrine (Adrenalin). Substance secreted by adrenal glands. Increases blood pressure, accelerates heart rate and facilitates muscular activity.

erogenous zones. Parts of the body that respond erotically to stimulation, especially the oral, anal and genital areas.

etiology. Causation.

euphoria. Exaggerated feeling of well-being and lack of inhibition.

exhibitionism. Exposure of male genitals to females, usually in order to obtain sexual gratification.

exogenous. Referring to causal factors outside the body or outside the system in which the morbid condition exists.

expectancy. Probability that an individual will develop a disorder over a given period of time.

experimental neurosis. Maladaptive behavior or symptoms resembling those of neurosis, produced experimentally by means of biological or psychological stress.

extroversion. Characterizing the direction of one's energy and interests toward external environmental and social phenomena. Opposite of introversion.

fantasy. (1) A daydream. (2) Process of daydreaming. (3) Defensive gratification of drives in imagination.

fellatio. Apposition of the mouth to the male genital.

fetishism. Sexual excitement or gratification obtained habitually from an inanimate object or a part of the body.

fever therapy. Induction of fever by malaria or other means, usually for the treatment of general paresis (syphilis of the brain).

fictive goal. Adler's term for the individual's unrealistic, compensatory aspirations.

fixation. Defensive persistence of a pattern of behavior or stage of development with failure to move to a more advanced level.

flight of ideas. A series of rapid jumps from one idea to another. The ideas are loosely connected or fragmentary.

folie à deux. Psychosis shared by two people in an intimate relationship.

free association. Uninhibited expression by patient in therapy of all his thoughts as they occur.

frigidity. Partial or complete inability of the female to be aroused sexually or achieve orgasm.

fugue. Dissociative reaction in which amnesia and physical flight occur.

functional autonomy. Hypothesis that behavior becomes independent of the drive from which it originated.

functional disorders. Abnormalities of behavior without clearly defined physical cause or structural change in the brain.

gamete. Sex cell (ovum or spermatozoon).

gene. Units of inheritance consisting of submicroscopic particles arranged along chromosomes.

general adaptation syndrome. Selye's term for the reaction to stress, consisting of three stages.

genital stage. The culminating stage of psychosexual development in which heterosexual interests are dominant.

glove anesthesia. Anesthetic area on hand and wrist. Functional in origin.

grand mal. A generalized convulsive seizure that is accompanied by loss of consciousness.

hallucination. Visual, tactile, auditory, olfactory, gustatory or other perception that has no basis in external stimulation.

hallucinogen (psychotomimetic substance). A substance capable of producing hallucinations in an experimental subject.

hebephilia. A consistent preference for sexual relations with young adolescents up to the age of sixteen years.

hebephrenic schizophrenia. Schizophrenic reactions, usually developing during adolescence and characterized by inappropriate affect, unpredictable giggling, silly behavior and mannerisms, and profound regression.

hemiplegia. Paralysis of one side of the body.

heterozygous. Characterizing an individual who carries both a dominant and recessive gene for a given trait.

homeostasis. Maintenance of constancy in physiological processes.

homosexuality (overt). Sexual activity with a member of the same sex.

hormone. Substance that is secreted into the blood stream by an endocrine gland and acts to regulate physiological activity.

Huntington's chorea. An organic brain syndrome caused by a single dominant gene.

hydrocephaly. A condition characterized by an increased volume of cerebrospinal fluid within the skull and consequent damage to the brain, resulting in mental subnormality.

hyperesthesia. Excessive sensitivity to stimuli.

hypertension. High blood pressure.

hypnoanalysis. Use of hypnosis in psychoanalytic therapy to facilitate uncovering of unconscious material.

hypnosis. Highly suggestible state induced by an artificial process (hypnotism).

hypochondria (hypochondriasis). Exaggerated concern with health or physical functioning. Occurs in conjunction with many disorders, particularly depression.

hypoesthesia. Decreased sensitivity to stimuli.

hypomania. Mild degree of mania.

hypothyroidism. Insufficient thyroid activity.

hysteria. Neurotic syndrome that comprises conversion reactions and dissociative reactions.

id. One of the three major divisions of personality proposed by Freud. The id consists of the unconscious instinctive drives.

identification. The unconscious emulation and adoption of personality characteristics and values of another person.

idiopathic. Of unknown causation.

idiot. Individual with severe mental subnormality, i.e., I.Q. below 20.

illusion. Misinterpretation of a stimulus or pattern of stimuli.

imbecile. Individual with moderate mental subnormality, i.e., I.Q. between 20 and 49.

impotence. Partial or complete failure of the male to achieve orgasm or experience sexual pleasure.

incest. Culturally prohibited sexual activity between persons of close blood relationship.

incidence. Rate of occurrence of new cases of a given condition in a given time period.

index cases. Individuals who manifest a particular trait and are, therefore, the starting point of a genetic or other study of the trait.

insanity. Legal term for mental illness, roughly equivalent to psychosis. Implies inability to be responsible for one's acts. The term is rarely used in current psychiatry or psychology.

instrumental learning. Type of learning in which the subject is reinforced only when he makes the required response in the presence of a given stimulus; thereafter the subject is more likely to make that response when presented with the stimulus.

insulin therapy (insulin coma therapy). Treatment by insulin injections to induce hypoglycemia (deficiency of sugar in the blood) and loss of consciousness (coma).

introjection. Defensive process of internalizing the attributes of others into oneself.

introversion. Characterizing the direction of one's energy and interests toward oneself and the inner world of experience. Opposite of extroversion.

inversion. Adoption of feminine attitudes and behavior by men, or of masculine attitudes and behavior by women. May be associated with overt homosexuality, trans-sexualism or transvestism.

involutional psychotic reaction. A psychotic reaction occurring in late middle life, usually characterized by severe depression (involutional melancholia) and somtimes by paranoid thinking.

isolation. (1) Defensive failure to connect behavior with its motives. (2) Defensive failure to connect contradictory attitudes or behaviors with each other.

Korsakoff's psychosis. Organic syndrome characterized by amnesia, confabulation and peripheral neuritis. Usually associated with alcoholism and vitamin deficiencies.

lability. Instability and variability.

latency stage. Pre-adolescent stage in which sexuality is dormant.

lesbianism (sapphism). Homosexual behavior in females.

lesion. A tissue change due to injury or disease.

libido. Energy of the id instincts, especially the sexual ones. (The term is often also used as a synonym for the id or for sexuality.)

lobotomy (prefrontal lobotomy, leucotomy). Form of psychosurgery that involves the cutting of nerve fibers that connect the frontal lobes with the thalamus.

logorrhea. Excessive speech, often incoherent.

LSD 25 (lysergic acid diethylamide). A widely used hallucinogen.

macropsia. Perceptual distortion in which objects seem larger than they are.

malingerer. Individual who feigns an illness or disability.

mania. (1) Excitement, e.g., the manic phase of manic-depressive reaction. (2) Compulsion or preoccupation, e.g., pyromania (compulsion to set fires), kleptomania (compulsion to steal), monomania (preoccupation with a single idea or activity) or megalomania (preoccupation with a grandiose delusion).

manic-depressive reaction. Recurrent episodes of elation, depression or both in alternation.

marasmus. Wasting of the tissues.

masculine protest. Adler's term for the female's compensatory attempts to deny her femininity and compete with men.

masochism. (1) Obtaining sexual gratification through suffering pain. (2) More broadly, acceptance of any type of pain.

masturbation. Sexual pleasure obtained by manual or mechanical stimulation of an erogenous zone.

mecholyl (acetylcholine). Substance producing similar effects to stimulation of parasympathic nervous system, including a drop in blood pressure.

megalomania. Grandiose delusions.

melancholia. Severe depression.

mental deficiency. Used interchangeably with mental subnormality.

mental retardation Used interchangeably with mental subnormality.

mental subnormality. Below normal intelligence, usually considered to be between I.Q.'s of 0 and 69. May result from any of a variety of causes.

meprobamate (Equanil, Miltown). A minor tranquilizer, used to reduce anxiety.

mescaline. A hallucinogen derived from a variety of cactus plants.

mesomorphy. Sheldon's body component in which muscles are highly developed.

Metrazol therapy (cardiazol therapy). Treatment by induction of seizures through administration of the drug Metrazol. Has been replaced by electroconvulsive therapy.

microcephaly. An abnormally small size of head and brain, associated with subnormal intellectual development (mental subnormality).

micropsia. Perceptual distortion in which objects seem smaller than they are.

milieu therapy. Treatment by modification of the patient's life circumstances or immediate environment.

mongolian idiot. An individual of moderate to severe mental subnormality, with facial characteristics of a mongolian cast, as a result of chromosomal anomaly.

monogenic. Characterizing hereditary variation due to a single major gene. (Also known as simple, or mendelian inheritance.)

monomania. Logical system of delusions based on a single false premise.

monozygotic twins. Twins developed from a single ovum. Also known as monovular, monozygous, MZ or identical twins.

mood. Prevailing affect or emotional tone.

moron. Individual with mild mental subnormality, i.e., I.Q. between 50 and 69.

multiple personality. Dissociative reaction in which two or more relatively complete systems of emotional and cognitive reactions are manifested by one individual.

mutism. Inability or refusal to speak.

myxedema. Hypothyroidism, sometimes severe enough to produce an organic brain syndrome.

narcissism. Excessive love of self.

narcoanalysis. Psychotherapy conducted under the influence of sedative drugs such as Amytal or Pentothal.

narcosis. A sleep-like state similar to hypnosis, but induced by a sedative drug.

negativism. Refusal to cooperate with a request, or performance of behavior opposite to that requested.

neologism. A new word or condensed combination of several words, the meaning of which may be known only to the patient who coined it. Commonly associated with schizophrenic thought disorder.

neurasthenia. Excessive fatigue of neurotic origin.

neuritis. Inflammation of a nerve.

neurodermatitis. Inflammation of the skin, emotional in origin.

neurosis. (neurotic reaction, psychoneurosis). Emotional disturbance characterized by severe anxiety or exaggerated defenses. Personality is not grossly disorganized and contact with reality is good.

nihilistic delusion. Belief that the self and external reality have ceased to exist.

nosology. Systematic classification of disease.

nuclear schizophrenia. Characterized by poor pre-morbid personality, early and insidious onset, and poor prognosis.

nymphomania. Insatiable impulse to sexual gratification in women.

obsession. Persistent intrusion into consciousness of an unwanted idea or impulse.

obsessive-compulsive reaction. Psychoneurotic reaction marked by persistent obsessional thoughts, compulsions or both.

occupational neurosis. Neurosis in which symptoms are related to the individual's occupation and interfere with its pursuit.

Oedipus situation. Incestuous impulses of the boy to the mother, accompanied by hostility to the father. The corresponding triangle of girl, father and mother is sometimes referred to as the Electra situation.

oligophrenia (small mind). Mental subnormality.

open hospital. Psychiatric hospital without restraints or confinement enforced by locked doors.

oral stage. Earliest period of life in which the mouth and lips are major sources of pleasurable sensation.

organic brain syndrome. Neurotic, psychotic or other disturbances of behavior associated with brain pathology.

overcompensation. A conscious or unconscious process involving exaggerated correction of a real or imagined physical or psychological defect.

paralogical thinking. Involuntary false reasoning.

paranoid reaction. Disorder with well systematized delusions. Affect and overt activity are consistent with delusions, intelligence is not impaired, hallucinations are absent and personality is not disorganized.

paranoid schizophrenia. Schizophrenic reaction marked by illogical and relatively fragmentary delusions, usually accompanied by auditory hallucinations.

paraphilia. Sexual deviation or perversion.

paraplegia. Paralysis of both legs.

parasympathetic nervous system. Division of the autonomic nervous system that is generally inhibitory in function.

paresis. Chronic brain syndrome caused by syphilitic infection.

paresthesia. Distorted perception of stimuli.

pathology. The study of disease, particularly of changes in bodily structure, their development and causation. Sometimes used to refer to any manifestations of disease or abnormality.

pederasty. Anal intercourse with boys.

pedophilia. Sexual activity with a child.

pellagra. Disease resulting from vitamin B deficiency, which may cause an organic brain syndrome.

penis envy. Desire on the part of the female to possess male genitals.

Pentothal. A sedative drug. *See* Amytal.

perceptual selectivity. Selective effect of motivation on attention and perception of stimuli.

peripheral schizophrenia. Characterized by good premorbid personality, late and acute onset, and favorable prognosis.

persona. Jung's term for the protective mask the individual wears.

petit mal. Momentary loss of consciousness without motor convulsions.

phallic stage. Period in which genital sensations, masturbation and Oedipal involvements are dominant, roughly between three and six years of age.

phenobarbital. A widely used sedative drug.

phenothiazine. A chemical substance from which a number of tranquilizers, e.g., chlorpromazine, have been derived.

phenylketonuria (PKU). A metabolic disorder of hereditary nature that causes severe mental subnormality.

phobia. An irrational, obsessive fear.

phobic reaction. Psychoneurotic reaction with irrational fears.

pica. A craving to eat unnatural substances, such as hair, sand or plaster. Found in mentally subnormal or disturbed children.

Pick's disease. Presenile psychosis caused by atrophy of the cerebral cortex.

placebo. An inactive substance resembling medication, but having no pharmacological effects, that may be given for therapeutic or experimental reasons because of its potential psychological effects.

polygenic. Characterizing hereditary variation resulting from many minor genes.

polyneuritis. Inflammation of peripheral nerves.

post-partum reaction. Emotional disturbance after childbirth.

precipitating cause. An event occurring immediately or shortly before its effects.

preconscious. Not imagined or verbalized at a given time, but capable of being imagined or verbalized.

predisposing cause. A cause that is relatively remote in time from its effects.

pregenital sexuality. Dominance of any form of sexuality—oral, anal, etc.—that precedes adult sexuality.

presbyophrenia. Senile brain disorder with severe memory defects.

prevalence. The total frequency of a given condition at a particular moment in time.

primary process. Psychoanalytic term for the nature of unconscious activity. The primary process is unrealistic, illogical and infantile.

process schizophrenia. Characterized by social inadequacy, gradual onset, poor prognosis, and possibly a basis that is fundamentally biologic.

prognosis. Prediction of the course and outcome of a disorder.

projection. Defensive attribution of blame or of an unacceptable trait or impulse to others instead of to oneself.

projective technique. Personality test consisting of ambiguous stimuli or ambiguous tasks to which the subject may respond in a wide variety of ways which are presumed to reflect his fantasies, private attitudes and unconscious motivations.

promiscuity. Nonselective sexual intercourse with a variety of partners.

pseudo-neurotic schizophrenia. Symptoms of a severe, mixed neurosis overlaying latent or incipient schizophrenia.

pseudo-psychopathic schizophrenia. Antisocial symptoms overlaying latent or incipient schizophrenia.

psychasthenia. Phobic and obsessive-compulsive reactions.

psychiatrist. A medical doctor with further special training in the diagnosis and treatment of mental disorders.

psychiatry. Branch of medicine that deals with mental disorders.

psychoanalysis. A theory of abnormality (especially neurosis), a general theory of personality, and a method of psychotherapy formulated by Freud and modified by many other investigators.

psychoneurosis. *See* neurosis.

psychopathic personality. *See* sociopathic personality disturbance.

psychopathology (behavior pathology). The study of abnormal behavior, its manifestations, development and causation. Sometimes used to refer to any manifestations of abnormal behavior.

psychophysiologic disorder (psychosomatic disorder). Pathological change in the structure or functioning of an organ innervated by the autonomic nervous system. The pathological change may originate in exaggerated physiological accompaniments of emotional states.

psychosexual stages. Series of developmental stages hypothesized by Freud to be universal. In order: oral, anal, phallic, latency and genital.

psychosis. A major mental disorder involving misinterpretation of reality and obvious departure from normal patterns of thinking, feeling and acting.

psychosomatic. (1) *See* psychophysiologic disorder. (2) Holistic approach to disturbances of the organism which pays attention to both "psyche" and "soma," i.e., to emotional and physical aspects.

psychosurgery. Brain surgery performed to treat mental disorders.

psychotherapy. Treatment by psychological techniques.

psychotic depressive reaction. Severe nonrecurrent depression of psychotic intensity.

pyknic. Stocky, plump, rounded physique.

pyknolepsy. A form of epilepsy commonly seen in children. It is characterized by frequent and short periods of loss of consciousness.

rationalization. Explanation and justification by the conscious mind of attitudes and behavior that have been determined by unacceptable unconscious emotions and motives.

reaction-formation. Defensive reinforcement of a repression by behavior that is directly opposed to an unconscious trend, e.g., kindness instead of cruelty.

reactive depression. Neurotic or psychotic depression occurring in reaction to environmental loss or stress.

reactive schizophrenia. Characterized by basically adequate personality that breaks down in response to stress. Onset is acute and prognosis is favorable.

recessive gene. A gene that produces no observable effect on the offspring except when paired with another recessive gene.

regression. Defensive retreat to an earlier pattern of behavior or stage of development.

regressive shock therapy. Electroconvulsive therapy administered on a schedule of two or three treatments per day up to a total of approximately 50 treatments. Produces amnesia, confusion and regression.

remission. Temporary improvement or long-term abatement of symptoms of a disease.

repetition-compulsion. Tendency to reexperience a trauma in nightmares, ruminations, etc., or to repeat any maladjustive behavior over and over.

repression. Defense mechanism consisting of expulsion of ego-threatening experiences and impulses from consciousness.

resistance. Patient's defensive opposition to the therapist's efforts, especially opposition to uncovering unconscious material.

retardation. (1) Slowing down of thinking and overt activity. Common in depressions. (2) The term is also used as a synonym for mental subnormality.

role. Organized and interrelated set of attitudes and responses prescribed by the social environment.

role-taking. Expression in fantasy, play or other behavior of the behaviors constituting a role.

rubella. German measles.

sadism. (1) Attaining sexual gratification through infliction of pain. (2) More broadly, any kind of cruelty; extreme aggression.

sadomasochism. Sadism and masochism coexisting in an individual.

satyriasis. Insatiable impulse to sexual gratification in men.

schizo-affective reaction. Mixture of schizophrenic and affective (manic or depressive) reactions.

schizoid. Schizophrenic-like "shut in" personality.

schizophrenia (schizophrenic reactions). Group of psychotic reactions characterized by marked distortion of reality. Major symptoms are loosening of associations, autistic withdrawal, ambivalence and inappropriate affect. Major types are simple, paranoid, catatonic and hebephrenic.

scoptophilia (scopophilia). Voyeurism.

secondary gain. Advantage accruing from a neurosis that is secondary to an original illness.

secondary process. Conscious, rational activity guided by reality.

senile brain disease. In the aged, a chronic disorder characterized by impairment of the brain tissue and dementia.

sex-linked. Characteristic transmitted by genes located on sex chromosomes (X or Y chromosomes).

sex-typing. Imitative or modeling activity in which child practices appropriate sex-role behavior.

sexual deviation. Persistent preference for sexual object or mode other than genital, heterosexual behavior with an adult.

simple schizophrenia. Schizophrenic reaction marked by apathy, lack of initiative and withdrawal.

sociopathic personality disturbance (sociopathy). Failure to conform to prevailing social and ethical standards.

sodomy. Anal-genital intercourse between males. (The term is sometimes used to mean any type of "unnatural" sexual relations.)

somatic. Bodily.

somatic vulnerability. The hypothesis that an autonomically unstable individual breaks down in his weakest organ as a response to stress.

somatotonia. Temperament corresponding to mesomorphy.

somatotype. Physique; bodily habitus.

somnambulism. Complex activity, especially walking, in a sleep-like state, followed by amnesia for the activity.

statutory rape. Sexual relations outside of marriage with a female below the legal "age of consent."

stereotyped mannerism. Conscious grimace, gesture or movement of the whole body.

stimulus generalization. The tendency—after the individual learns to make a certain response to a certain stimulus—to make that response to similar stimuli.

stress. Stimulus conditions—biological or psychological, external or internal, noxious or depriving—that demand very difficult adjustments.

stress reaction. Severe disturbance, on exposure to stress stimuli, of balance and regulation of functioning.

stressor. A stress condition (in Selye's terminology).

structured personality test. Questionnaire, inventory or self-rating device consisting of standardized items for personality measurement.

stupor. State of lethargy and immobility.

stuttering (stammering). Interruption of speech by hesitations, repetition of sounds and breathing spasms.

sublimation. An unconscious defense mechanism whereby unacceptable instinctual drives (e.g., sexual and aggressive) are diverted into personally and socially acceptable channels.

superego. One of the three major divisions of personality proposed by Freud. Superego functions involve conscious and unconscious self-criticism and control, and include both negative prohibitions and positive striving. (*See also* conscience and ego-ideal.)

suppression. Conscious exclusion of desires or inhibition of impulses.

sympathectomy. Severing of certain autonomic nerves to control psychophysiologic symptoms.

sympathetic nervous system. Branch of the autonomic nervous system that prepares the organism for emergency action.

symptom. A manifestation of an illness or emotional disturbance.

syndrome. Constellation or pattern of symptoms typical of a disorder.

therapeutic community. Term for a modern mental

hospital that employs group and milieu therapy and gives patients considerable responsibility.

therapy. Treatment.

tic. Periodic muscular twitch, especially facial.

tonic phase. Muscular rigidity. Precedes clonic phase in electroconvulsive therapy and in grand mal epilepsy.

tpmo. Murray's term for the allowable time, place, mode and object for need satisfaction.

transference. A displacement in which unconscious attitudes originally felt toward an important childhood figure are directed toward the therapist.

trans-sexualism. Conscious desire for anatomical change of sex.

transvestism. Dressing in clothing appropriate to the opposite sex, usually for the purpose of obtaining sexual gratification.

trauma. A bodily or emotional injury.

traumatic neurosis. Neurotic reaction that develops shortly after a traumatic stress.

tremor. Continuous, involuntary, spasmodic contraction or trembling in a small group of muscles.

unconscious. Incapable of being imagined or verbalized, except by special techniques, such as hypnosis.

undoing. Defensive and magical attempt to wipe out or atone for guilt.

verbigeration. Monotonous repetitions of words or sentences, often without apparent meaning.

viscerotonia. Temperament corresponding to endomorphy.

voyeurism (scoptophilia). Sexual gratification obtained from observing the genitals or sexual behavior of others.

waxy flexibility. State in which the patient permits his limbs to be molded into various positions.

Wernicke's syndrome. Organic psychosis marked by ataxia, clouding of consciousness and paralysis of eye muscles.

word salad. Unintelligible mixture of meaningful words and phrases with neologisms.

working through. Process of facing an impulse or conflict over and over in psychotherapy by exploring the various derivatives and corrections of the impulse or conflict.

zoophilia (bestiality). Sexual relations with an animal.

zygote. Fertilized ovum.

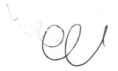

SELECTED REFERENCES

Abraham, K. 1926. The psychological relations between sexuality and alcoholism. Int. J. Psychoanal. 7:2–10.

Ackerman, N. W. 1958. The Psychodynamics of Family Life. New York, Basic Books.

Ackerman, N. W., and Behrens, M. L. 1956. A study of family diagnosis. Amer. J. Orthopsychiat., 26:66–78.

Ackerman, N., Beatman, F., and Sherman, S. (Editors). 1967. Expanding Theory and Practice in Family Therapy. New York, Family Service Association of America.

Adler, A. 1941. The individual psychology of the alcoholic patient. J. Crim. Psychopathol., 3:74–77.

Adler, A. 1924. The Practice and Theory of Individual Psychology. New York, Harcourt, Brace and Co.

Aichhorn, A. 1935. Wayward Youth. New York, Viking Press.

Akesson, H. O. 1961. Epidemiology and Genetics of Mental Deficiency in a South Swedish Population, translated by R. N. Elston. Uppsala, Sweden, Almqvist & Wiksell.

Alexander, F. 1943. Fundamental concepts of psychosomatic research: psychogenesis, conversion, specificity. Psychosom. Med., 5:205–209.

Alexander, F., 1944. The indications for psychoanalytic therapy. Bull. N.Y. Acad. Med., 20:319–334.

Alexander, F. 1950. Psychosomatic Medicine: Its Principles and Application. New York, W. W. Norton & Co.

Alexander, F., and French, I. 1946. Psychoanalytic Therapy. New York, The Ronald Press Co.

Alexander, F., and French, T. (Editors). 1948. Studies in Psychosomatic Medicine. New York, The Ronald Press Co.

Alexander, F., and Szasz, T. S. 1952. The psychosomatic approach in medicine. In Alexander, F., and Ross, H. (Editors). Dynamic Psychiatry. Chicago, The University of Chicago Press.

Allen, C. 1949. Modern Discoveries in Medical Psychology, 2nd Ed. London, Macmillan & Co., Ltd.

Allen, C. 1962. A Textbook of Psychosexual Disorders. London, Oxford University Press.

Allen, F. H. 1942. Psychotherapy with Children. New York, W. W. Norton & Co.

Allport, G. W. 1961. Pattern and Growth in Personality. New York, Holt, Rinehart and Winston.

Amark, C. 1951. A Study in Alcoholism. Clinical, Social Psychiatry and Genetic Investigations. Acta Psychiatrica Supplementum, 70.

American Psychiatric Association. 1968. Diagnostic and Statistical Manual of Mental Disorders, 2nd Ed. Washington, D.C., American Psychiatric Association.

Anastasi, A. 1958. Differential Psychology. New York, The Macmillan Co.

Anastasi, A. 1961. Psychological Testing. 2nd Ed. New York, The Macmillan Co.

Anderson, H., and Anderson, G. (Editors). 1951. An Introduction to Projective Techniques. New York, Prentice-Hall, Inc.

Andry, R. G. 1960. Delinquency and Parental Pathology. London, Methuen and Co., Ltd.

Angus, L. R. 1948. Schizophrenics and schizoid conditions in students in a special school. Amer. J. Ment. Defic., 53:227–238.

Apperson, L., and McAdoo, W. 1968. Parental factors in the childhood of homosexuals. J. Abnorm. Psychol. 73:201–206.

Arieti, S. (Editor). 1959. American Handbook of Psychiatry, Chapters 11–21. New York, Basic Books.

Arieti, S. (Editor). 1959. American Handbook of Psychiatry, Chapters 32–39. New York, Basic Books.

Arieti, S. 1960. Etiological considerations of schizophrenia. In Sher, S. C., and Davis, H. R. (Editors). The Outpatient Treatment of Schizophrenia. New York, Grune & Stratton, Inc.

Arieti, S. 1955. Interpretation of Schizophrenia. New York, Robert Brunner.

Arieti, S. 1959. Schizophrenia. In Arieti, S. (Editor). American Handbook of Psychiatry. New York, Basic Books.

Arieti, S. 1961. Volition and value: A study based on catatonic schizophrenia. Compr. Psychiat., 2:74–82.

Arieti, S., and Meth, J. M. 1959. Rare, unclassifiable, collective, and exotic psychotic syndromes. In Arieti, S. (Editor). American Handbook of Psychiatry. New York, Basic Books.

Armstrong, J. D. 1961. Psychiatric theories of alcoholism. Canad. Psychiat. Assoc. J., 6:140–149.

Armstrong, J. D. 1958. The search for the alcoholic personality. Ann. Amer. Acad. Polit. Soc. Sci., 315:40–47.

Ascher, E. 1949. Folie à deux. A. M. A. Arch. Neurol. Psychiat., 61:177–182.

Asher, E. J. 1935. The inadequacy of current intelligence tests for testing Kentucky mountain children. J. Genet. Psychol., 46:480–486.

Association for Research in Nervous and Mental Disease. 1950. Life Stress and Bodily Disease. Research Publications of the Association for Research in Nervous and Mental Disease, Vol. XXIV. Baltimore, The Williams & Wilkins Co.

Auerbach, A. H., Scheflen, A. E., Reinhart, R. B., and Scholz, C. K. 1960. The psychophysiologic sequelae of head injuries. Amer. J. Psychiat., 17:499–505.

Babigian, H., et al. 1965. Diagnostic consistency and change in a follow-up study of 1215 patients. Amer. J. Psychiat., *121*:895–901.

Bachrach, A., Erwin, W., and Mohr, J. 1965. The control of eating behavior in an anorexic by operant conditioning techniques. *In* Ullman, L., and Krasner, L. (Editors). Case studies in Behavior Modification. New York, Holt, Rinehart and Winston.

Bachrack, A. J. (Editor). 1962. Experimental Foundations of Clinical Psychology. New York, Basic Books.

Bacon, M. K., Child, I., and Barry, H. 1963. A cross-cultural study of correlates of crime. J. Abnorm. Soc. Psychol., *66:* 291–300.

Bacon, S. D. 1958. Alcoholics do not drink. Ann. Amer. Acad. Polit. Soc. Sci., *315*:55–64.

Baker, A. B. 1958. An Outline of Clinical Neurology, Dubuque, Iowa, Brown Book Co. Chapters 7–18.

Baldwin, A., Kalhorn, J., and Breese, F. 1945. Patterns of parent behavior. Psychol. Monogr., 58, #268.

Bales, R. F. 1946. Cultural differences in rates of alcoholism. Quart. J. Stud. Alcohol, 6:480–499.

Baller, W. R. 1936. A study of the present social status of adults who, when they were in elementary schools, were classified as mentally deficient. Genet. Psychol. Monogr., *18*:165–244.

Bandura, A. 1965. Influence of models' reinforcement contingencies on the acquisition of imitative responses. J. Personality Soc. Psychol. *1*:589–595.

Bandura, A., and Walters, R. 1959. Adolescent Aggression. New York, The Ronald Press Co.

Bard, M. 1970. Training Police as Specialists in Family Crises Intervention. U.S. Department of Justice. Washington, U.S. Government Printing Office.

Barry, H., and Lindemann, E. 1960. Critical ages for maternal bereavement in psychoneurosis. Psychosom. Med., *22*:166–181.

Barry, M. J., and Johnson, A. 1958. The incest barrier. Psychoanal. Quart. 27:485–500.

Barthell, C., and Holmes, D. 1968. High school yearbooks: a nonreactive measure of social isolation in graduates who later became schizophrenic. J. Abnorm. Psychol., 73:313–316.

Bateson, G., Jackson, D. D., Haley, J., and Weakland, J. 1956. Toward a theory of schizophrenia. Behav., Sci., *1*:251–264.

Beach, F. A. 1948. Hormones and Behavior. New York, Hoeber-Harper. Reprinted 1961 by Cooper Square Publishers, Inc.

Becker, W. C., Peterson, D. R., Hellmer, L. A., Shoemaker, D. J., and Quay, H. C. 1959. Factors in parental behavior and personality as related to problem behavior in children. J. Consult. Psychol., 23:107–118.

Beckett, P. G. S., Frohman, C. E., Gottlieb, J. S., Mowbray, J. B., and Wolf, R. C. 1962. Schizophrenic-like mechanisms in monkeys. Paper presented at annual meeting of the American Psychiatric Association. May, 1962.

Beckett, P. G. S., Frohman, C. E., Senf, R., Tourney, G., and Gottlieb, J. S. 1963. Energy production and premorbid history in schizophrenia. A.M.A. Arch. Gen. Psychiat. 8: 155–162.

Beers, C. W. 1908. A Mind That Found Itself. New York, Longmans, Green and Co.

Beier, E. G., Gorlow, L., and Stacey, C. L. 1951. The fantasy life of the mental defective. Amer. J. Ment. Defic., 55:582–589.

Bell, J. 1948. Projective Techniques. New York, Longmans, Green and Co.

Bell, J. E. 1961. Family Group Therapy. Public Health Monograph No. 64. Washington, U.S. Printing Office.

Bellak, L. 1948. Dementia Praecox. New York, Grune & Stratton, Inc.

Bellak, L. 1958. Schizophrenia: A Review of the Syndrome. New York, Logos Press.

Bena, C. E. 1960. The Child with Mongolism. New York, Grune & Stratton, Inc.

Bender, L. 1947. Childhood schizophrenia: clinical study of 100 schizophrenic children. Amer. J. Orthopsychiat. *17:* 40–56.

Bender, L. 1954. A Dynamic Psychopathology of Childhood. Springfield, Ill., Charles C Thomas.

Bender, L. 1963. Mental illness in childhood and heredity. Eugen. Quart., *10*:1–11.

Bender, L., and Blau, A. 1937. Reaction of children to sex relations with adults. Amer. J. Orthopsychiat., 7:500–518.

Bender, L., and Paster, S. 1941. Homosexual trends in children. Amer. J. Orthopsychiat., *11*:730–744.

Benedict, P. K., and Jacks, I. 1954. Mental illness in primitive societies. Psychiatry, 17:377–389.

Benedict, R. 1934. Patterns of Culture. New York, Houghton Mifflin Co.

Benson, W. M., and Schiele, B. C. 1960. Current status of tranquilizing and anti-depressant drugs. J. Lancet (Minneapolis), *80*:579–592.

Berenson, B. G., and Carkhuff, R. (Editors.) 1967. Sources of Gain in Counseling and Psychotherapy. New York, Holt, Rinehart and Winston.

Berg, J. M., and Kirman, B. H. 1959. Some aetiological problems in mental deficiency. Brit. Med. J., 2(2):848–852.

Berry, J. 1967. Independence and conformity in subsistence-level societies. J. Personality Soc. Psychol., 7:415–418.

Berry, J. 1966. Temne and Eskinn perceptual skills. Int. J. Psychol., *1*:207–229.

Bettelheim, B. 1950. Love is Not Enough. Glencoe, Ill., The Free Press.

Bexton, W. H., Heron, W., and Scott, T. H. 1954. Effects of decreased variation in the sensory environment. Canad. J. Psychol. 8:70–76.

Bieber, I., Dain, H., Dince, P., Drellich, M., Grand, H., Gundlach, R., Kremer, J., Rifkin, A., Wilbur, C., and Bieber, T. 1962. Homosexuality: A Psychoanalytic Study. New York, Basic Books.

Bigelow, N., Roizin, L., and Kaufman, M. A. 1959. Psychoses with Huntington's chorea. *In* Arieti, S. (Editor). American Handbook of Psychiatry. New York, Basic Books, pp. 1248–1259.

Bijou, S. W., and Baer, D. M. 1961. Child Development. New York, Appleton-Century-Crofts.

Blacker, C. P. 1952. Problem Families: Five Inquiries. London, Eugenics Society.

Blacker, K. 1969. Drug and setting. Clin. Toxicol., 2:201.

Bleuler, E. 1911. Dementia Praecox or the Group of Schizophrenias. Translated by J. Zinkin, 1950. New York, International Universities Press.

Bleuler, M. 1955. A comparative study of the constitutions of Swiss and American alcoholic patients. *In* Diethelem, O. (Editor). Etiology of Chronic Alcoholism, Springfield, Ill., Charles C Thomas, pp. 167–178.

Bluemel, C. S. 1948. War, Politics, and Insanity. Denver, The World Press.

Blum, R. 1969. Students and Drugs. San Francisco, Jossey-Boss.

Boatman, M. J., and Szurek, S. A. 1960. A clinical study of childhood schizophrenia. *In* Jackson, D. D. (Editor). The Etiology of Schizophrenia. New York, Basic Books, pp. 389–440.

Bonner, C. D. 1959. Prognostic evaluation for rehabilitation of patients with strokes. Geriatrics, *14*:424–428.

Book, J. A. 1953. A genetic and neuropsychiatric investigation of a North Swedish population. Acta Genet. *4*:1–100, 345–414.

Bovet, L. 1951. Psychiatric Aspects of Juvenile Delinquency. Geneva, World Health Organization, Monograph Series No. 1.

Bowen, M., Dysinger, R. H., and Bassamania, B. 1959. The role of the father in families with a schizophrenic patient. Amer. J. Psychiat., *115*:1017–1020.

Bowlby, J. 1951. Maternal Care and Mental Health. Geneva, World Health Organization, Monograph, Series No. 2.

Boyles, P. D., and Waldrop, G. S. 1967. Development of a community-oriented program in a large state hospital of limited resources. Amer. J. Psychiat., *124*:29–31.

Bradley, C., and Bowen, M. 1941. Behavior characteristics of schizophrenic children. Psychiat. Quart., *15*:296–315.

Bradway, K. P. 1935. Paternal occupational intelligence and mental deficiency. J. Appl. Psychol., *19*:527–542.

Brady, J. V. 1958. Ulcers in "executive" monkeys. Sci. Amer., *199*:95–100.

Brancale, R., Ellis, A., and Doorbar, R. 1952. Psychiatric and psychological investigations of convicted sex offenders: A summary report. Amer. J. Psychiat., *109*:17–21.

Brandon, M. W. G. 1957. The intellectual and social status of children of mental defectives. J. Ment. Sci., *103*:710–738.

Breger, L., and McGaugh, J. 1965. Critique and reformulation of "learning theory" approaches to psychotherapy and neurosis. Psychol. Bull., *63*:338–358.

Breuer, J., and Freud, S. 1895. Studies of Hysteria. New York, Basic Books.

Brill, H. 1963. Misapprehensions about drug addiction—some origins and repercussions. Compr. Psychiat., *4*:150–159.

Brill, H. 1959. Postencephalitic psychiatric conditions. *In* Arieti, S. (Editor). American Handbook of Psychiatry. New York, Basic Books, pp. 1163–1174.

Bromberg, W. 1937. The Mind of Man: The Story of Man's Conquest of Mental Illness. New York, Harper and Bros.

Bromberg, W., and Thompson, C. B. 1937. The relation of psychosis, mental defect and personality types to crime. J. Criminal Law, Criminology and Police Science, *28*:70–89.

Bronson, W. C. 1959. Dimensions of ego and infantile identification. J. Personality, *27*:532–545.

Brosin, H. W. 1959. Psychiatric conditions following head injury. *In* Arieti, S. (Editor). American Handbook of Psychiatry. New York, Basic Books, pp. 1175–1202.

Brown, F. 1961. Depression and childhood bereavement. J. Ment. Sci., *107*:754–777.

Brown, F., Epps, P., and McGlashan, A. 1961. The remote and immediate effects of orphanhood. Proceedings of the Third World Congress of Psychiatry. Montreal, McGill University Press, Vol. II:1316–1319.

Brown, F. W. 1942. Heredity in Psychoneuroses. Proc. Roy. Soc. Med., *35*:785–790.

Brown, W. 1953. Monkey on My Back. Philadelphia, Chilton Co.

Browne, W. A. F. 1873. What Asylums Were, Are, and Ought To Be: Being the Substance of Five Lectures Delivered before the Managers of the Montrose Royal Lunatic Asylum. Edinburgh, Adam and Charles Black.

Bruetsch, W. L. 1952. Mental disorders arising from organic disease. *In* The Biology of Mental Health and Disease, Twenty-seventh Annual Conference of the Milbank Memorial Fund. New York, Hoeber-Harper, pp. 303–322.

Bruetsch, W. L. 1959. Neurosyphilitic conditions. *In* Arieti, S. (Editor). American Handbook of Psychiatry. New York, Basic Books, pp. 1003–1020.

Bruhn, J. G. 1953. Manic-Depressive Disease. Philadelphia, J. B. Lippincott Co.

Buck, C., and Hobbs, G. E. 1959. The problem of specificity in psychosomatic illness. J. Psychosom. Res., *3*:227–233.

Buckle, D., and Lebovici, S. 1960. Child Guidance Centres. Geneva, World Health Organization, Monograph Series No. 40.

Buell, B., 1955. Preventing and controlling disordered behavior. Ment. Hyg., *39*:365–375.

Burgess, E. W. 1955. Mental health in modern society. *In* Rose, A. M. (Editor). Mental Health and Mental Disorder. New York, W. W. Norton & Co.

Burks, B. S. 1928. The Relative Influence of Nature and Nurture Upon Mental Development. 27th Yearbook, Nat. Soc. Stud. Educ., Part I.

Burney, C. 1952. Solitary Confinement. New York, Coward-McCann, Inc.

Burrows, G. M. 1828. Commentaries on the Causes, Forms, Symptoms and Treatment, Moral and Medical, of Insanity. London, Thomas and George Underwood.

Burt, C., and Howard, M. 1956. The multifactorial theory of inheritance and its application to intelligence. Brit. J. Statis. Psycho., *9*:95–131.

Busse, E. W. 1961. Psychoneurotic reactions and defense mechanisms in the aged. *In* Hoch, P. H., and Zubin, J. (Editors). Psychopathology of Aging. New York, Grune & Stratton, Inc., pp. 274–284.

Byrd, R. D. 1938. Alone. New York, G. P. Putnam's Sons.

Cabeen, C. W., and Coleman, J. C. 1961. Group therapy with sex offenders: Description and evaluation of group therapy program. J. Clin. Psychol., *17*:122–129.

Cameron, D. E. 1960. Production of differential amnesia as a factor in the treatment of schizophrenia. Compr. Psychiat., *1*:26–34.

Cameron, N. 1959. Paranoid conditions and paranoia. *In* Arieti, S. (Editor). American Handbook of Psychiatry. New York, Basic Books, Inc.

Cameron, N. 1963. Personality Development and Psychopathology. Boston, Houghton Mifflin Co.

Cameron, N. 1947. The Psychology of Behavior Disorders. Boston, Houghton Mifflin Co.

Cameron, N. 1938. Reasoning, Regression and Communication in Schizophrenics. Psychol. Monogr., Vol. 50, No. 1.

Cameron, N., and Cameron, M. A. 1951. Behavior Pathology. Boston, Houghton Mifflin Co.

Camus, A. 1946. The Stranger. New York, Alfred A. Knopf.

Cannon, W. B. 1929. Bodily Changes in Pain, Hunger, Fear and Rage. 2nd Ed. New York, Appleton-Century-Crofts.

Cannon, W. B. 1932. The Wisdom of the Body. New York, W. W. Norton & Co.

Caplan, G. 1961. Prevention of Mental Disorders in Children. New York, Basic Books.

Carothers, J. C. 1953. The African Mind in Health and Disease. Geneva, World Health Organization, Monograph Series No. 17.

Carrier, N. A., Orton, K. D., and Malpass, L. F. 1962. Responses of bright, normal, and EMH children to an orally-administered manifest anxiety scale. J. Educ. Psychol., *53*(6):271–274.

Carter, M. P., and Jephcott, P. 1952–1954. The Social Background of Delinquency. (Typescript available on loan from the University Librarian, Nottingham, England.)

Casey, J. F., Bennett, I. F., Lindley, C. J., Hollister, L. E., Gordon, M. H., and Springer, N. N. 1960. Drug therapy in schizophrenia. A.M.A. Arch. Gen. Psychiat., *2*:210–220.

Castaneda, A., McCandless, B. R., and Palermo, D. 1956. The children's form of the manifest anxiety scale, Child Develop., *27*:317–326.

Caveness, W. F. 1955. Emotional and psychological factors in epilepsy. Amer. J. Psychiat., *112*:190–193.

Celsus, Aurelius Cornelius. De Medicina. (With an English translation by W. G. Spencer, 1935.) Cambridge, Harvard University Press.

Chafetz, M. E., and Demone, H. W. 1962. Alcoholism and Society. New York, Oxord University Press.

Chapanis, A., and Williams, W. C. 1945. Results of a mental survey with the Kuhlmann-Anderson Intelligence Tests in Williamson County, Tennessee. J. Genet. Psychol., *67*:27–55.

Chapman, L. F., and Wolff, H. G. 1959. The cerebral hemispheres and the highest integrative functions of man. Arch. Neurol., *1*:357–424.

Charles, D. C. 1953. Ability and accomplishment of persons earlier judged mentally deficient. Genet. Psychol. Monogr., *47*:3–71.

Chein, I., et al. 1964. The Road to H: Narcotics, Delinquency, and Social Policy. New York, Basic Books.

Chess, S. 1959. An Introduction to Child Psychiatry. New York, Grune & Stratton, Inc.

Child, I. L. 1954. Socialization. *In* Lindzey, G. (Editor). Handbook of Social Psychology. Cambridge, Addison-Wesley.

Christmas, J. 1967. Sociopsychiatric treatment of disadvantaged adults. Amer. J. Orthopsychiat. *37*:93–100.

Christoffel, H. 1956. Male genital exhibitionism. *In* Lorand, S., and Balint, M. (Editors). Perversions: Psychodynamics and Therapy. New York, Random House, Inc.

Clausen, J. A. 1957. Social patterns, personality and adolescent drug use. *In* Leighton, A. H., Clausen, J. A., and Wilson, R. N. (Editors). Explorations in Social Psychiatry. New York, Basic Books.

Cleckley, H. 1955. The Mask of Sanity, 3rd Ed. St. Louis, The C. V. Mosby Co.

Cleckley, H. 1959. Psychopathic states. *In* Arieti, S. (Editor). American Handbook of Psychiatry. New York, Basic Books.

Cochran, I. L., and Cleland, C. C. 1963. Manifest anxiety of retardates and normals matched as to academic achievement. Amer. J. Ment. Defic., *67*:539–542.

Cohen, A. K. 1955. Delinquent Boys: The Culture of the Gang. Glencoe, Ill., The Free Press.

Cohen, G. B., Cohen, R. A., Fromm-Reichmann, F., and Weigert, E. 1954. An intensive study of twelve cases of manic-depressive psychosis. Psychiatry, *17*:103–137.

Cohen, S., Allen, M., and Pollin, W. 1971. Schizophrenia in veteran twins: A follow-up report. Presented at the annual meeting of the American Psychiatric Association.

Conger, J. J. 1951. The effects of alcohol on conflict behavior in the albino rat. Quart. J. Stud. Alcohol, *12*:1–21.

Connell, P. H. 1956. Amphetamine Psychosis. Maudsley Monograph No. 5. New York, Oxford University Press.

Conrad, K. 1935. Erbanlage und Epilepsie. Z. ges. Neurol. Psychiat., *153*:271–326.

Coppen, A. J. 1959. Body-build of male homosexuals. Brit. Med. J. *2*:1443–1445.

Cormier, B. M., Kennedy, M., and Sangowiczy, J. 1962. Psychodynamics of father-daughter incest. Canad. Psychiat. Assoc. J. *7*:203–217.

Cowen, E. L. 1955. Psychotherapy and play techniques with the exceptional child and youth. *In* Cruickshank, W. M. (Editor). Psychology of Exceptional Children and Youth. Englewood Cliffs, N.J., Prentice-Hall.

Cowie, V., and Slater, E. 1959. Psychiatric genetics. *In* Fleming, G. W. T. H., and Walk, A. (Editors). Recent Progress in Psychiatry, Vol. 3. New York, Grove Press Inc.

Cramer, J. B. 1959. Common neuroses of childhood. *In* Arieti, S. (Editor). American Handbook of Psychiatry. New York, Basic Books, pp. 797–815.

Crawshaw, R. S., and Peterson, L. V. 1961. Supportive psychotherapy with an aged transient. Geriatrics, *16*:454–458.

Cronback, L. J. 1960. Essentials of Psychological Testing. New York, Harper.

Darling, H. F., and Sanddal, J. W. 1952. A psychopathologic concept of psychopathic personality. J. Clin. Exper. Psychopathol., *13*:175–180.

David, P. R., and Snyder, L. S. 1954. Genetics and disease. *In* Proceedings of the Second National Cancer Conference. New York, American Cancer Society.

Davis, W. A., and Havighurst, R. J. 1946. Social class and color differences in child rearing. Amer. Sociol. Rev., *II*:698–710.

Dekaban, A. S. 1962. Cerebral birth injury: pathology of hemorrhagic lesions. In Kolb, L. C., Masland, R. L., and Cooke, R. E. (Editors). Mental Retardation. Baltimore, The Williams & Wilkins Co. Research Publications, Ass. Res. Nerv. Ment. Dis., *39*:196–227.

DeSanctis, S. 1925. Neuropsychiatria Infantile. Rome, Stock.

Despert, J. L. 1952. Diagnostic criteria of schizophrenia in children. Amer. J. Psychother., *6*:148–159.

Despert, J. 1942. Prophylactic aspect of schizophrenia in childhood. Nerv. Child, *1*:199–236.

Despert, J. L. 1954. Treatment in child schizophrenia: presentation of case. *In* Murphy, G., and Bachrach, A. J. (Editors). An Outline of Abnormal Psychology. New York, Modern Library, pp. 120–149.

Deutsch, A. 1949. The Mentally Ill in America, 2nd Ed. New York, Doubleday, Doran & Co.

Deutsch, F., and Murphy, W. F. 1955. The Clinical Interview, Vol. 1: Diagnosis. New York, International Universities Press.

Dewan, J. G., and Spaulding, W. B. 1958. The Organic Psychoses. Toronto, The University of Toronto Press.

Dews, P. B. 1962. Psychopharmacology. *In* Bachrach, A. J. (Editor). Experimental Foundations of Clinical Psychology. New York, Basic Books.

DiMichael, S. G. 1956. Proposals on a federal program of action in 1956–57 for America's mentally retarded children and adults. Mimeographed manuscript quoted by Doll, E. E. 1962. The mentally deficient. *In* Trapp, E. P., and Himelstein, P. (Editors). Readings on the Exceptional Child. New York, Appleton-Century-Crofts.

Diven, K. 1937. Certain determinants in the conditioning of anxiety reactions. J. Psychol., *3*:291–308.

Doane, B. K., Mahatoo, W., Heron, W., and Scott, T. H. 1959. Changes in perceptual function after isolation. Canad. J. Psychol. *13*:210–219.

Dollard, J., and Miller, N. E. 1950. Personality and Psychotherapy. New York, McGraw-Hill Book Co., Inc.

Dorcus, R. M., and Shaffer, G. W. 1950. Textbook of Abnormal Psychology. 4th Ed. Baltimore, The Williams & Wilkins Co.

Doust, J. W. L. 1952a. Dysplastic growth differentials in patients with psychiatric disorders. Brit. J. Soc. Med., *6*:169–177.

Doust, J. W. L. 1952. Psychiatric aspects of somatic immunity. Brit. J. Soc. Med., *6*:39–67.

DuBois, P. 1909. The Psychic Treatment of Mental Disorders. New York, Funk and Wagnalls.

Dunaif, S. L., and Hoch, P. 1955. Pseudopsychopathic schizophrenia. *In* Hoch, P. H., and Zubin, J. (Editors). Psychiatry and the Law. New York, Grune & Stratton, Inc.

Dunbar, F. 1954. Emotions and Bodily Changes, 4th Ed. New York, Columbia University Press.

Dunbar, F. 1939. Psychosomatic histories and techniques of examination. Amer. J. Psychiat., *95*:1277–1304.

Dunn, W. L., Jr. 1954. Visual discrimination of schizophrenic subjects as a function of stimulus meaning. J. Personality, 23:48–64.

Eaton, J. W., and Weil, R. J. 1955. Culture and Mental Disorders. Glencoe, Ill., The Free Press.

Ebaugh, F. G., and Tiffany, W. J., Jr. 1959. Infective-exhaustive psychoses. In Arieti, S. (Editor). American Handbook of Psychiatry. New York, Basic Books, pp. 1231–1247.

Edwards, A. S., and Jones, L. 1938. An experimental and field study of North Georgia mountaineers. J. Soc. Psychol., 9:317–333.

Ehrenberg, R., and Gullingsrud, M. J. O. 1955. Electroconvulsive therapy in elderly patients. Amer. J. Psychiat., 111:743–747.

Eisenberg, L., and Kanner, L. 1956. Early infantile autism, 1943–1955. Amer. J. Orthopsychiat., 26:556–564.

Ellis, A. 1963. Reason and Emotion in Psychotherapy. New York, Lyle Stuart.

Ellis, A., and Abarbanel, A. (Editors). 1961. The Encyclopedia of Sexual Behavior, Vols. I and II. New York, Random House, Inc.

Engel, G. L. 1962. Psychological Development in Health and Disease. Philadelphia, W. B. Saunders Co.

Engel, G. L. 1956. Studies of ulcerative colitis, IV. The significance of headaches. Psychosom. Med., 18:334–336.

Engel, G. L., and Romano, J. 1959. Delirium—a syndrome of cerebral insufficiency. J. Chron. Dis., 9:260–277.

Erikson, E. H. 1950. Childhood and Society. New York, W. W. Norton & Co.

Erlenmeyer-Kimling, L., and Jarvik, L. F. 1963. Genetics and intelligence: a review. Science, 142:1477–1479.

Estes, H. R., Haylett, C. H., and Johnson, A. M. 1956. Separation anxiety. Amer. J. Psychother., 10:682–695.

Ewing, J., and Fox, R. Family therapy of alcoholism. In Masserman, J. (Ed.) Current Psychiatric Therapies, Vol. 8. New York, Grune & Stratton, Inc., pp. 86–91.

Eysenck, H. J. 1959. Learning theory and behavior therapy. J. Ment. Sci., 105:61–75.

Eysenck, H. J. 1952. The effects of psychotherapy: an evaluation. J. Consult. Psychol., 16:319–324.

Eysenck, H. J., and Prell, D. B. 1951. The inheritance of neuroticism. J. Ment. Sci., 97:441–465.

Fairweather, G., Sanders, D., Maynard, H., and Cressler, L. 1969. Community Life for the Mentally Ill: An Alternative to Institutional Care. Chicago, Aldine.

Farber, I. E., Harlow, H. F., and West, L. J. 1957. Brain washing, conditioning and D. D. D. (debility, dependency and dread). Sociometry, 20:271–285.

Farina, A. 1960. Patterns of role dominance and conflict in parents of schizophrenic patients. J. Abnorm. Soc. Psychol., 61:31–38.

Faris, E. 1937. The Nature of Human Nature. New York, McGraw-Hill Book Co., Inc.

Faris, R. E. L., and Dunham, H. W. 1939. Mental Disorders in Urban Areas. Reprinted 1960. New York, Hafner Publishing Co.

Feffer, M. H. 1961. The influence of affective factors on conceptualization in schizophrenia. J. Abnorm. Soc. Psychol. 63:588–596.

Feldhausen, J. F., and Klausmeier, H. J. 1962. Anxiety, intelligence and achievement in children of low, average and high intelligence. Child Develop., 33:403–409.

Fenichel, O. 1941. Problems of Psychoanalytic Technique. Albany, Psychoanal. Quart.

Fenichel, O. 1945. The Psychoanalytic Theory of Neurosis. New York, W. W. Norton & Co.

Ferraro, A. 1959. Senile psychoses, presenile psychoses, and psychoses with cerebral arteriosclerosis. In Arieti, S. (Editor). American Handbook of Psychiatry. New York, Basic Books, pp. 1021–1108.

Finch, S. M. 1960. Fundamentals of Child Psychiatry. New York, W. W. Norton & Co.

Fisher, C. 1965. Psychoanalytic implications of recent research on sleep and dreaming: Part I, Empirical findings. J. Amer. Psychol. Assoc., 13:197–270.

Fleck, S., Lidz, R., and Cornelison, A. 1963. Comparison of parent-child relationships of male and female schizophrenic patients. A.M.A. Arch. Gen. Psychiat., 8:1–7.

Fontana, A., Klein, E., and Cicchetti, D., 1967. Censure sensitivity in schizophrenia. J. Abnorm. Psychol., 72:294–302.

Ford, C. S., and Beach, F. A. 1951. Patterns of Sexual Behavior. New York, Hoeber-Harper.

Fotheringham, J. B. 1957. Psychopathic personality—a review. Canad. Psychiat., Assoc. J., 2:25–70.

Foucault, M. 1965. Madness and Civilization. New York, New American Library.

Fouls, L. B., and Smith, W. D. 1956. Sex-role learning of five year olds. J. Genet. Psychol., 53:105–116.

Fowler, E. P., Jr., and Kastein, S. 1962. Hypoacusis, dysacusis and retardation. In Kolb, L. C., Masland, R. L., and Cooke, R. E. (Editors). Baltimore, The Williams & Wilkins Co. Research Publication, Ass. Res. Nerv. Ment. Dis., 39:270–288.

Franck, K., and Rosen, E. 1949. A projective test of masculinity–femininity. J. Consult. Psychol., 13:247–256.

Frank, J. D. 1959. Problems of controls in psychotherapy as exemplified by the psychotherapy research project of the Phipps Psychiatric Clinic. In Rubinstein, E. A., and Parloff, M. B. (Editors). Research in Psychotherapy, Washington, D.C., American Psychological Association.

Frank, J. D. 1961b. Persuasion and Healing. Baltimore, The Johns Hopkins Press.

Frank, J. D. 1961a. Therapy in a group setting. In Stein, M. I. (Editor). Contemporary Psychotherapies. Glencoe, Ill., The Free Press.

Frank, L. K. 1936. Society as the patient. Amer. J. Sociol., 42:335–344.

Frankl, V. 1955. The Doctor and the Soul. (Trans. by Winston), New York, Alfred A. Knopf.

Franks, C. 1960. Conditioning and abnormal behaviour. In Eysenck, H. J. (Editor). Handbook of Abnormal Psychology. London, Pitman Medical Publishing Co.

Franks, J., et al. 1959. The role of anxiety in psychophysiological reactions. A.M.A. Arch. Neurol. Psychiat., 81:227–232.

Freedman, A. M. 1962. Long-range anterospective study of premature infants. Wld. Ment. Hlth., 14:9–15.

Freeman, D. 1959. Rehabilitation of the mentally ill aging. Soc. Wk., 4(4):65–71.

Freeman, F. N., Holzinger, K. J., and Mitchell, B. C. 1928. The influence of environment on the intelligence, school achievement and conduct of foster children. Yearbook Nat. Soc. Stud. Educ., 27(I):101–217.

Freeman, R. V., and Grayson, H. M. 1955. Maternal attitudes in schizophrenia. J. Abnorm. Soc. Psychol., 50:45–52.

Freeman, W., and Watts, J. W. 1942. Psychosurgery. Springfield, Ill., Charles C Thomas.

Fremming, K. H. 1951. The Expectation of Mental Infirmity in a Sample of the Danish Population. Occasional Papers on Eugenics, No. 7. London, Eugenics Society and Cassell & Co.

Freud, A. 1937. The Ego and the Mechanisms of Defense. London, Hogarth Press.

Freud, A. 1946. The Ego and the Mechanisms of Defence. New York, International Universities Press.

Freud, A. 1946. The Psycho-analytic Treatment of Children. London, Imago Publishing Co., Ltd.

Freud, A. 1928. The Technique of Child Analysis. Nervous and Mental Disease Monograph No. 48. New York, Nervous and Mental Disease Publishing Company.

Freud, A., and Burlingham, D. T. 1943. War and Children. New York, Medical War Books.

Freud, S. 1937. Analysis terminable and interminable. Int. J. Psychoanal., 18:373–405.

Freud, S. 1935. Autobiography. New York, W. W. Norton & Co.

Freud, S. 1938. The Basic Writings of Sigmund Freud. New York, Modern Library.

Freud, S. 1930. Civilization and its Discontents. New York, Cape and Smith.

Freud, S. 1912. Contributions to the psychology of love: The most prevalent form of degradation in erotic life. In Collected Papers, Vol. 4. London, Hogarth Press.

Freud, S. 1933b. Fragment of an Analysis of a Case of Hysteria (Collected Papers, Vol. III). London, Hogarth Press.

Freud, S. 1896. Further remarks on the defense neuro-psychoses. In Collected Papers, Vol. 1. New York, Basic Books.

Freud, S. 1949. A General Introduction to Psychoanalysis. New York, Garden City Publishing Co.

Freud, S. 1916. The History of the Psychoanalytic Movement. Nervous and Mental Disease Monograph No. 25. New York, Nervous and Mental Disease Publishing Company.

Freud, S. 1938. The interpretation of dreams. In The Basic Writings of Sigmund Freud. New York, Modern Library.

Freud, S. 1920. Introductory Lectures on Psychoanalysis. Reprinted 1953. Permabooks M-5001.

Freud, S. 1917. Mourning and Melancholia. In Collected Papers, Vol. 4. London, Hogarth Press.

Freud, S. 1924. Neurosis and psychosis. In Strachey, J., (Editor). 1959. Collected Papers, Vol. 11. New York, Basic Books.

Freud, S. 1933a. New Introductory Lectures on Psychoanalysis. New York, W. W. Norton & Co.

Freud, S. 1904. On psychotherapy. In Collected Papers, Vol. 1. London, Hogarth Press.

Freud, S. 1911. Psychoanalytic notes upon an autobiographical account of a case of paranoia (dementia paranoides). In Collected Papers, Vol. III. New York, Basic Books, Inc., 1959.

Freud, S. 1930. Three Contributions to the Theory of Sex, 4th Ed. Washington, D.C., Nervous and Mental Diseases Publishing Company.

Freund, K. 1960. Some problems in the treatment of homosexuality. In Eysenck, H. J. (Editor). Behaviour Therapy and the Neuroses. London, Pergamon Press.

Friedman, A. 1964. Minimal effects of severe depression on cognitive functioning. J. Abnorm. Soc. Psychol., 69:237–243.

Friedman, P. 1959. Sexual deviations, In Arieti, S. (Editor). American Handbook of Psychiatry. New York, Basic Books.

Fromm, E. 1955. The Sane Society. New York, Holt, Rinehart and Winston.

Fromm-Reichmann, F. 1950. Principles of Intensive Psychotherapy. Chicago, The University of Chicago Press.

Fromm-Reichmann, F. 1954. Psychoanalytic and general dynamic conceptions of theory and of therapy. J. Amer. Psychoanal. Assoc., 2:718.

Fromm-Reichmann, Frieda. 1949. Recent advances in psychoanalysis. J. Amer. Med. Wom. Assoc. 4:320–326.

Frumkin, R. 1955. Occupation and major mental disorders. In Rose, A. M. (Editor). Mental Health and Mental Disorder. New York, W. W. Norton & Co.

Fuller, J. L., and Thompson, W. R. 1960. Behavior Genetics. New York, John Wiley & Sons, Inc.

Funkenstein, D. H., Greenblatt, M., and Solomon, H. C. 1951. Autonomic changes paralleling psychologic changes in mentally ill patients. J. Nerv. Ment. Dis., 114:1–18.

Funkenstein, D. W. 1954. Psychophysiologic studies of depression: some experimental work. In Hoch, P. H., and Zubin, J. (Editors). Depression. New York, Grune & Stratton, Inc.

Galdston, I. (Editor). 1954. Beyond the Germ Theory. New York, New York Academy of Medicine, Health Education Council.

Gallagher, J. J. 1957. A comparison of brain-injured and non-brain-injured mentally retarded children on general psychological variables. Monogr. Soc. Res. Child. Develop., 22, No. 2.

Gallinek, A. 1948. The nature of affective and paranoid disorders during the senium in the light of electric convulsive therapy. J. Nerv. Ment. Dis., 108:293–303.

Gardner, G. E. 1959. Psychiatric problems of adolescence. In Arieti, S. (Editor). American Handbook of Psychiatry. New York, Basic Books, pp. 870–892.

Gardner, G. E. 1956. Separation of the parent and the emotional life of the child. Ment. Hyg. 40:53–57.

Garfield, S. 1957. Introductory Clinical Psychology. New York, The Macmillan Co.

Garmezy, N. 1952. Stimulus differentiation by schizophrenic and normal subjects under conditions of reward and punishment. J. Personality, 20:253–276.

Garmezy, N., and Rodnick, E. H. 1959. Premorbid adjustment and performance in schizophrenia: implications for interpreting heterogeneity in schizophrenia. J. Nerv. Ment. Dis., 129:450–466.

Gedda, L. 1951. Studio Dei Gemelli. Rome, Edizioni Orizzonte Medico.

Gellhorn, E. 1943. Autonomic Regulation. New York, Interscience Publishers.

Gerard, D. L., and Houston, L. G. 1953. Family setting and the ecology of schizophrenia. Psychiat. Quart., 27:90–101.

Gerard, D. L., and Kornetsky, C. 1954. A social and psychiatric study of adolescent opiate addicts. Psychiat. Quart., 28:113–125.

Gerard, D. L., Saenger, G., and Wile, R. 1962. The abstinent alcoholic. Arch. Gen. Psychiat., 6:83–95.

Gesell, A. 1925. Mental Growth of the Preschool Child. New York, The Macmillan Co.

Gesell, A., and Thompson, H. 1929. Learning and Growth in Identical Infant Twins. Genet. Psychol. Monogr. 6:5–120.

Gibbons, R. J. 1953. Chronic Alcoholism and Alcohol Addiction. Brookside Monograph No. 1. Toronto, Alcoholism Research Foundation and University of Toronto Press.

Gibson, R. W. 1958. The family background and early life experience of the manic-depressive patient. Psychiatry, 21:71–90.

Gillies, H. 1956. Acute delirious states. Brit. Med. J., 1(1): 623–625.

Ginzberg, E., and Bray, D. W. 1953. The Uneducated. New York, Columbia University Press.

Glueck, S., and Glueck, E. 1934. One Thousand Juvenile Delinquents. Cambridge, Harvard University Press.

Glueck, S., and Glueck, E. 1956. Physique and Delinquency. New York, Harper & Brothers.

Glueck, S., and Glueck, E. 1950. Unraveling Juvenile Delinquency. Cambridge, Mass., Commonwealth Fund and Harvard University Press.

Gluenck, B. C., Jr. 1956. Final Report, Research Project for the Study and Treatment of Persons Convicted of Crime Involving Sexual Aberrations. New York State Department of Mental Hygiene.

Goddard, H. H. 1912. The Kallikak Family. New York, The Macmillan Co.

Goldberg, E., and Morrison, S. 1963. Schizophrenia and social class. Brit. J. Psychiat., 109:785–802.

Goldberg, T. B. 1953. Factors in the development of school phobia. Smith Coll. Stud. Soc. Work, 23:227–248.

Goldfarb, A. I. 1957. Contributions of psychiatry to the institutional care of aged and chronically ill persons. J. Chron. Dis., 6:483–496.

Goldfarb, A. I., and Sheps, J. 1954. Psychotherapy of the aged ill. Psychosom. Med., 16:209–219.

Goldfarb, H. 1945. Effects of psychological privation in infancy and subsequent stimulation. Amer. J. Psychiat., 102:18–33.

Goldfarb, W. 1961. Childhood Schizophrenia. Cambridge, Harvard University Press.

Goldfarb, W. 1962. Families of schizophrenic children. In Kolb, L. C., Masland, R. L., and Cooke, R. E. (Editors). Mental Retardation. Baltimore, The Williams & Wilkins Co. Research Publication, Ass. Res. Nerv. Ment. Dis., 39:256–269.

Goldfarb, W. 1943. Infant rearing and problem behavior. Amer. J. Orthopsychiat., 13:249–266.

Goldfarb, W. 1945. Psychological privation in infancy and subsequent adjustment. Amer. J. Orthopsychiat., 15:247–255.

Goldhamer, H., and Marshall, A. W. 1953. Psychosis and Civilization. Glencoe, Ill., The Free Press.

Goldman-Eisler, F. 1953. Breastfeeding and character formation. In Kluckholn, C., Murray, H. A., and Schneider, D. M. Personality in Nature, Society, and Culture, 2nd Ed. New York, Alfred A. Knopf.

Goldstein, K. 1939. The Organism. New York, American Book Co.

Goldstein, K., and Scheerer, M. 1941. Abstract and Concrete Behavior: An Experimental Study with Special Tests. Psychol. Monogr., No. 239, Vol. 53.

Goldstein, M., Kant, H., Judd, L., Rice, C., and Green, R. 1971. Exposure to pornography and sexual behavior in deviant and normal groups. In Technical Reports of the Commission on Obscenity and Pornography, Vol. 7, U.S. Government Printing Office, Washington, D.C.

Good, W. W., Sterling, M., and Holtzman, W. 1958. Termination of chlorpromazine with schizophrenic patients. Amer. J. Psychiat., 115:443–448.

Goodstein, L. D., and Rowley, V. N. 1961. A further study of MMPI differences between parents of disturbed and nondisturbed children. J. Consult. Psychol., 25:460.

Gordon, H. 1923. Mental and scholastic tests among retarded children. London, Bd. Educ., Educ. Pamphlet No. 44.

Gottesman, I. I. 1961. The efficiency of several combinations of discrete and continuous variables for the diagnosis of zygosity. Paper read at the Second International Conference of Human Genetics. Rome, Italy. September, 1961.

Gottesman, I. 1966. Genetic variance in adaptive personality traits. J. Child Psychol. Psychiat. 7:199–208.

Gottesman, I., and Shields, J. 1967. A polygenic theory of schizophrenia. Proceed. Nat. Acad. Sci., 58:199–205.

Gottesman, I., and Shields, J. 1966. Schizophrenia in twins: 16 years' consecutive admissions to a psychiatric clinic. Brit. J. Psychiat., 112:809–818.

Gottlieb, J. S. 1962. Biochemistry and schizophrenia: implications for the future. In Hoch, P. H., and Zubin, J. (Editors). Future of Psychiatry. New York, Grune & Stratton, Inc.

Gottlieb, J. S., et al. 1956. Research in Psychosomatic Medicine. Washington, D.C., American Psychiatric Association, Psychiatric Research Reports No. 3.

Grainick, A. 1942. Folie à deux: the psychosis of association. Psychiat. Quart., 16:230–260.

Grayson, H. M., and Olinger, L. B. 1957. Simulation of "normalcy" by psychiatric patients on the MMPI. J. Consult. Psychol., 21:73–77.

Green, E., Silverman, D., and Geil, G. 1943. Petit mal electroshock therapy of criminal psychopaths. J. Crim. Psychopathol., 5:667–673.

Greenacre, P. 1953. Affective Disorder. New York, International Universities Press.

Greenacre, P. 1945. Conscience in the psychopath. Amer. J. Orthopsychiat., 15:495–509.

Greenblatt, M., Arnot, R., and Solomon, H. C. (Editors). 1950. Studies in Lobotomy. New York, Grune & Stratton, Inc.

Greenfield, N. S. 1959. The relationship between recalled forms of childhood discipline and psychopathology. J. Consult. Psychol., 23:139–142.

Greenwald, H. 1968. The Active Psychotherapies. New York, Atherton Press.

Gregory, I. 1959. An analysis of family data on 1000 patients admitted to a Canadian mental hospital. Acta Genet., 9:54–96.

Gregory, I. 1960. Genetic factors in schizophrenia. Amer. J. Psychiat., 116:961–972.

Gregory, I. 1956. Mental disorder associated with thyroid dysfunction. Canad. Med. Assoc. J., 75:489–492.

Gregory, I. 1961. Psychiatry: Biological and Social. Philadelphia, W. B. Saunders Co.

Gregory, I. 1955. The role of nicotinic acid (niacin) in mental health and disease. J. Ment. Sci., 101:85–109.

Gregory, I. 1958. Studies of parental deprivation in psychiatric patients. Amer. J. Psychiat. 115:432–442.

Griesinger, W. 1845. Mental Pathology and Therapeutics, 2nd Ed. London, The New Sydenham Society.

Grinker, R. R., and Spiegel, J. P. 1945. War Neuroses, Philadelphia, The Blakiston Company.

Group for the Advancement of Psychiatry. 1959. Basic Considerations in Mental Retardation: A Preliminary Report. New York, G. A. P. Report No. 43.

Group for the Advancement of Psychiatry. 1954. Collaborative Research in Psychopathology. New York, G.A.P. Report No. 25.

Group for the Advancement of Psychiatry. 1961. Problems of Estimating Changes in Frequency of Mental Disorder. New York, G.A.P. Report No. 50.

Group for the Advancement of Psychiatry. 1948. Research in Prefrontal Lobotomy. G.A.P. Report No. 6, pp. 1–9.

Group for the Advancement of Psychiatry. 1959. Some Observations on Controls in Psychiatric Research. New York, G.A.P. Report No. 42.

Guilleband Report. 1956. Committee on Enquiry into the Cost of the National Health Service. London, H.M.S.O.

Gunzberg, H. C. 1958. Psychotherapy with the feebleminded. In Clark, A. M., and Clarke, A. D. B. (Editors). Mental Deficiency: The Changing Outlook. New York, The Free Press, pp. 365–392.

Gutheil, E. 1959. Reactive depressions. In Arieti, S. (Editor). American Handbook of Psychiatry, New York, Basic Books.

Guttmacher, M. S. 1951. Sex Offenses: The Problem, Causes and Prevention. New York, W. W. Norton & Co.

Hafemeister, N. R. 1951. Development of a curriculum for the trainable child. Amer. J. Ment. Defic., 55:495–501.

Halliday, A. 1828. A General View of the Present State of Lunatics and Lunatic Asylums, in Great Britain and Ireland,

and in Some Other Kingdoms. London, Thomas and George Underwood.

Halliday, J. L. 1948. Psychosocial Medicine: A Study of the Sick Society. New York, W. W. Norton & Co.

Halperin, S. L. 1945. A clinico-genetical study of mental defect. Amer. J. Ment. Defic., 50:8–26.

Hamilton, M., Pickering, G. W., Roberts, J. A. F., and Sowry, G. S. C. 1954. The aetiology of essential hypertension. 4: The role of inheritance. Clin. Sci., 13:273–304.

Hammer, E. F., and Glueck, B. C., Jr. 1955. Psychodynamic patterns in the sex offender. In Hoch, P. H., and Zubin, J. (Editors). Psychiatry and the Law. New York, Grune & Stratton, Inc.

Hampson, J. L. 1963. Determinants of psychosexual orientation (gender role) in humans. Canad. Psychiat. Assoc. J., 8:24–34.

Hanvik, L. J., and Byrum, M. 1959. MMPI profiles of parents of child psychiatric patients. J. Clin. Psychol., 15:427–431.

Hare, E. H. 1956. Family setting and the urban distribution of schizophrenia. J. Ment. Sci., 102:753–760.

Harlow, H. F. 1962. The heterosexual affectional system in monkeys. Amer. Psychol., 17:1–9.

Harlow, H. F., and Woolsey, C. N. (Editors). 1958. Biological and Biochemical Bases of Behavior. Madison, University of Wisconsin Press.

Harlow, H. F., and Zimmermann, R. R. 1959. Affectional responses in the infant monkey. Science, 130:421–430.

Harlow, H. F., and Zimmermann, R. R. 1958. The development of affectional responses in infant monkeys. Proc. Amer. Phil. Soc. 102:501–509.

Harrell, R. F., Woodyard, E., and Gates, A. I. 1955. The Effect of Mothers' Diets on the Intelligence of Offspring: A Study of the Influence of Vitamin Supplementation on the Diet of Pregnant and Lactating Women on the Intelligence of Their Children. New York, Bureau of Publications, Teachers College.

Hartman, A., and Nicolay, R. 1966. Sexually deviant behavior in expectant fathers. J. Abnorm. Psychol. 71:232–234.

Hartmann, H. 1958. Ego Psychology and the Problem of Adaptation. New York, International Universities Press.

Hathaway, S. R., and McKinley, J. C. 1943. The Minnesota Multiphasic Personality Inventory. New York, The Psychological Corporation.

Hathaway, S. R., and Monachesi, E. D. 1963. Adolescent Personality and Behavior: MMPI Patterns of Normal, Delinquent, Drop-Out and Other Outcomes. Minneapolis, University of Minnesota Press.

Havighurst, R. J., and Davis, A. 1955. A comparison of the Chicago and Harvard studies of social class differences in child rearing. Amer. Sociol. Rev., 20:438–442.

Hazell, K. 1960. Social and Medical Problems of the Elderly. London, Hutchinson Medical Publications.

Healy, W., and Bronner, A. 1926. Delinquents and Criminals. New York, The Macmillan Co.

Heath, R. G., Martens, S. Leach, B. E., Cohen, M., and Angel, C. 1957. Effect on behavior in humans with the administration of taraxein. Amer. J. Psychiat., 114:14–24.

Hebb, D. O. 1947. Spontaneous neurosis in chimpanzees: theoretical relations with clinical and experimental phenomena. Psychosomat. Med., 9:3–16.

Helfand, I. 1956. Role taking in schizophrenia. J. Consult. Psychol., 20:37–41.

Hellbrun, A. B., Jr. 1960. Perception of maternal child rearing attitudes in schizophrenics. J. Consult. Psychol., 24:169–173.

Henderson, D., and Batchelor, I. R. C. 1962. Henderson and Gillespie's Textbook of Psychiatry, 9th Ed. London, Oxford University Press, pp. 355–442.

Henderson, D. K. 1939. Psychopathic States. New York, W. W. Norton & Co.

Hendrick, I. 1958. Facts and Theories of Psychoanalysis. 3rd Ed. New York, Alfred A. Knopf.

Heron, W., Bexton, W. H., and Hebb, D. O. 1953. Cognitive effects of a decreased variation in the sensory environment. Amer. Psychol., 8:366.

Herron, W. G. 1962. The process-reactive classification of schizophrenia. Psychol. Bull., 59:329–343.

Herskovitz, H. H., Levine, M., and Spivak, G. 1959. Anti-social behavior of adolescents from higher socio-economic groups. J. Nerv. Ment. Dis., 129:467–476.

Hess, E., Seltzer, A., and Shlien, J. 1965. Pupil response of hetero- and homosexual males to pictures of men and women. J. Abnorm. Psychol. 70:165–168.

Heston, L. 1966. Psychiatric disorders in foster home reared children of schizophrenic mothers. Brit. J. Psychiat., 112:819–825.

Hetherington, E. M., and Banta, T. J. 1962. Incidental and intentional learning in normal and mentally retarded children. J. Comp. Physiol. Psychol., 55:402–404.

Higgins, J. V., Reed, E. W., and Reed, S. C. 1962. Intelligence and family size: a paradox resolved. Eugen. Quart., 9(2):84–90.

Hilgard, E. R. 1956. Theories of Learning. 2nd Ed. New York, Appleton-Century-Crofts.

Hill, D., and Watterson, D. 1942. Electroencephalographic studies of the psychopathic personality. J. Neurol. Psychiat., 5:47–65.

Himwich, H. E. (Editor). 1957. Alcoholism, Basic Aspects and Treatment. Washington, D.C., Amer. Assoc. Adv. Sci., Publication No. 47.

Hinko, E., and Lipschutz, L. 1947. Five years after shock therapy. Amer. J. Psychiat., 104:387–390.

Hippocrates. Medical Works. Translated by J. Chadwick and W. N. Mann, 1950. Oxford, Blackwell Scientific Publications.

Hirschfeld, M. 1944. Sexual Anomalies and Perversions. London, Francis Adlor Publisher. Reprinted 1948. New York, Emerson Books, Inc.

Hirsh, J. 1959–1960. Suicide (Parts 1 to 4). Ment. Hyg., 43:516–524; 44:3–10, 44:274–280; 44:382–388.

Hobson, W., and Pemberton, J. 1955. The Health of the Elderly at Home. London, Butterworth, pp. 481–482.

Hoch, P. H. 1963. Comments on narcotics addiction. Compr. Psychiat., 4:140–144.

Hoch, P. H. 1959. Drug therapy. In Arieti, S. (Editor). American Handbook of Psychiatry. New York, Basic Books.

Hoch, P. H. 1957. The problem of schizophrenia in the light of experimental psychiatry. In Hoch, P. H., and Zubin, J. (Editors). Experimental Psychopathology, New York, Grune & Stratton, Inc.

Hoch, P. H., and Polatin, P. 1949. Pseudoneurotic forms of schizophrenia. Psychiat. Quart., 23:248–276.

Hoch, P. H., and Zubin, J. (Editors). 1953. Current Problems in Psychiatric Diagnosis. New York, Grune & Stratton, Inc.

Hoch, P. H., and Zubin, J. (Editors). 1954. Depression. New York, Grune & Stratton, Inc.

Hoch, P. H., and Zubin, J. (Editors). 1957. Experimental Psychopathology. New York, Grune & Stratton, Inc.

Hoch, P. H., and Zubin, J. (Editors). 1961. Psychopathology of Aging. New York, Grune & Stratton, Inc.

Hoch, P. H., and Zubin, J. (Editors). 1955. Psychopathology of Childhood. New York, Grune & Stratton, Inc.

Hoch, P. H., and Zubin, J. (Editors). 1949. Psychosexual Development. New York, Grune & Stratton, Inc.

Hoff, H. 1959. Indications for electro-shock, Tofranil and psychotherapy in the treatment of depressions. Canad. Psychiat. Assoc., 4, Special Supplement: S55–S64.

Hollingshead, A. B., and Redlich, F. C. 1958. Social Class and Mental Illness. New York, John Wiley & Sons, Inc.

Holmes, O. W. 1927. Buck v. Bell. 274 U.S. 200, p. 207.

Holway, A. R. 1959. Early self-regulation of infants and later behavior in play interviews. Amer. J. Orthopsychiat., 19:612–623.

Holzinger, K. 1929. The relative effect of nature and nurture on twin differences. J. Educ. Psychol., 20:241–248.

Hood, A. 1963. A study of the relationship between physique and personality variables measured by the MMPI. J. Personality, 31:97–107.

Hooker, D., and Hare, C. C. (Editors). 1954. Genetics and the Inheritance of Integrated Neurological and Psychiatric Patterns. Res. Pub., Assoc. Res. Nerv. Ment. Dis., Vol. 33. Baltimore, The Williams and Wilkins Co.

Horney, K. 1937. The Neurotic Personality of Our Time. New York, W. W. Norton & Co.

Horton, D. 1943. The functions of alcohol in primitive societies: a cross-cultural study. Quart. J. Stud. Alcohol, 4:199–320.

Horwitt, M. K. 1956. Fact and artifact in the biology of schizophrenia. Science, 124:429–430.

Hoskins, R. G. 1946. The Biology of Schizophrenia. New York, W. W. Norton & Co.

Howells, J. G. 1961. From Child to Family Psychiatry. Proceedings of the Third World Congress of Psychiatry, Montreal, Canada, McGill University Press, pp. 472–475.

Howells, J. G. 1963. Child-parent separation as a therapeutic procedure. Amer. J. Psychiat., 119:922–926.

Huff, D. 1954. How to Live with Statistics. New York, W. W. Norton & Co.

Hull, C. L. 1951. Essentials of Behavior. New Haven, Yale University Press.

Huschka, M. 1942. The child's response to coercive bowel training. Psychosom. Med., 4:301–308.

Huschka, M. 1943. A study of training in voluntary control of urination in a group of problem children. Psychosom. Med. 5:254–265.

Hutt, M. L., and Gibby, R. B. 1958. The Mentally Retarded Child. Boston, Allyn & Bacon, Inc.

Inouye, E. 1961. Similarity and dissimilarity of schizophrenia in twins. In Proceedings of the Third World Congress of Psychiatry, Vol. 1. Montreal, Canada, McGill University Press.

Jackson, C. R. 1944. The Lost Weekend. J. J. Little & Ives Co.

Jackson, D. 1961. Family therapy in the family of the schizophrenic. In Stein, M. I. (Editor). Contemporary Psychotherapies. Glencoe, Ill. The Free Press.

Jackson, D. D. (Editor). 1960. The Etiology of Schizophrenia. New York, Basic Books.

James, I., and Levin, S. 1964. Suicide following discharge from psychiatric hospital. Arch. Gen. Psychiat., 10:43–46.

Janet, P. 1920. The Major Symptoms of Hysteria, 2nd Ed. New York, The Macmillan Co.

Jarvie, H. F., and Hood, M. C. 1952. Acute Delirious Mania. Amer. J. Psychiat., 108:758–763.

Jellinek, E. M. 1951, 1952. In World Health Organization Technical Report Series Nos. 42 and 48.

Jenkins, R. 1950. Nature of the schizophrenic process. Arch. Neurol. Psychiat., 64:243–262.

Jenkins, R., and Glickman, S. 1946. Common syndromes in child psychiatry: II. The schizoid child. Amer. J. Orthopsychiat., 16:255–261.

Jenkins, R., Holsopple, J., and Lorr, M. 1954. Effects of prefrontal lobotomy on patients with severe chronic schizophrenia. Amer. J. Psychiat., 111:84–90.

Jenness, A. R. 1962. Personality dynamics. In Farnsworth, P. R., McNemar, O., and McNemar, Q. (Editors). Annual Review of Psychology, Vol. 13. Palo Alto. Annual Review Inc.

Jervis, G. A. 1959. The mental deficiencies. In Arieti, S. (Editor). American Handbook of Psychiatry. New York, Basic Books, pp. 1289–1314.

Johnson, A. M. 1959. Juvenile delinquency. In Arieti, S. (Editor). American Handbook of Psychiatry. New York, Basic Books.

Johnson, A. M., Falstein, E. I., Szurek, S. A., and Svendsen, N. 1941. School phobia. Amer. J. Orthopsychiat., 11:702–711.

Johnson, A. M., and Szurek, S. A. 1952. The genesis of antisocial acting out in children and adults. Psychoanal. Quart., 21:323–342.

Johnson, L. C. 1969. Physiological and psychological changes following total sleep deprivation. In Kales, A. (Editor) Sleep: Physiological Pathology. Philadelphia, J. B. Lippincott.

Johnston, N., Savitz, L., and Wolfgand, M. E. (Editors). 1962. The Sociology of Punishment and Correction. New York, John Wiley & Sons, Inc.

Joint Commission on Mental Illness and Health. 1961. Action for Mental Health. New York, Basic Books.

Jones, D., and Hall, S. B. 1963. Significance of somatic complaints in patients suffering from psychotic depression. Acta Psychother. et Psychosom., 11:193–199.

Jones, E. 1957. The Life and Work of Sigmund Freud (three volumes). New York, Basic Books.

Jones, M. 1953. The Therapeutic Community—A New Treatment Method in Psychiatry. New York, Basic Books.

Juda, A. 1939. Quoted by Shields, J., and Slater, E. 1961. Heredity and psychological abnormality. In Eysenck, H. J. (Editor). Handbook of Abnormal Psychology. New York, Basic Books, pp. 326–328.

Jung, C. G. 1936. The Psychology of Dementia Praecox. New York, Nervous and Mental Disease Publishing Co. Monograph No. 3.

Jung, C. G. 1916. Psychology of the Unconscious. New York, Moffat, Yard and Co.

Kahn, E. 1931. Psychopathic Personalities. New Haven, Yale University Press.

Kaij, L. 1957. Drinking habits in twins. Acta Genet. 7:437–441.

Kaines, S. H., 1957. Mental Depressions and Their Treatment. New York, The Macmillan Co.

Kalinowsky, L. B. 1958. Withdrawal convulsions and withdrawal psychoses. In Hoch, P. H., and Zubin, J. (Editors). Problems of Addiction and Habituation. New York, Grune & Stratton, Inc.

Kalinowsky, L. B., and Hoch, P. H. 1952. Shock Treatments, Psychosurgery and Other Somatic Procedures in Psychiatry, 2nd Ed. New York, Grune & Stratton, Inc.

Kallmann, F. J. 1959. The genetics of mental illness. In Arieti, S. (Editor). American Handbook of Psychiatry. New York, Basic Books.

Kallmann, F. J. 1950. The genetics of psychoses, In Congrès International de Psychiatrie, Paris, 1950. VI. Psychiatrie Sociale. Paris, Hermann and Cie.

Kallmann, F. J. 1953. Heredity in Health and Mental Disorders. New York, W. W. Norton & Co.

Kallmann, F. J., and Jarvik, L. F. 1961. Individual differences in constitution and genetic background. *In* Birren, J. E. (Editor). Handbook of Aging and the Individual. Chicago, The University of Chicago Press.

Kallmann, F. J., and Roth, B. 1956. Genetic aspects of pre-adolescent schizophrenia. Amer. J. Psychiat., *112:*599–606.

Kanner, L. 1957. Child Psychiatry. 3rd Ed. Springfield, Ill., Charles C Thomas.

Kanner, L. 1944. Early infantile autism. J. Pediat., *25:*211–217.

Kanner, L. 1953. Parents' feelings about retarded children. Amer. J. Ment. Defic. *57:*375–383.

Kanner, L. 1949. Problems of nosology and psychodynamics of early infantile autism. Amer. J. Orthopsychiat., *19:*416–423.

Kanner, L. 1959. The thirty-third Maudsley lecture: Trends in child psychiatry. J. Ment. Sci., *105:*581–593.

Kaplan, B. (Editor). 1961. Studying Personality Cross-Culturally. Evanston, Ill., Row, Peterson and Co.

Kaplan, J. 1970. Marijuana—The New Prohibition. New York, World Publishing Co.

Kaplan, S. D. 1960. Autonomic visual regulation, Part II, Differential spectral centralization to autonomic drugs in depression. *In* West, L. J., and Greenblatt, M. (Editors). Explorations in the Physiology of Emotions. Washington, D.C., American Psychiatric Research Reports No. *12:*115–118.

Kardiner, A. 1945. The Psychological Frontiers of Society. New York, Columbia University Press.

Kardiner, A. 1959. Traumatic neuroses of war. *In* Arieti, S. (Editor). American Handbook of Psychiatry. New York, Basic Books.

Karpman, B. 1954. The Sexual Offender and His Offenses. New York, Julian Press.

Kasanin, J., Knight, E., and Sage, P. 1934. The parent-child relationship in schizophrenia. J. Nerv. Ment. Dis., *79:*249–263.

Katz, S. 1953. My twelve hours as a madman. Toronto, Maclean's Magazine, Oct. 1, p. 9.

Kawi, A. A., and Pasamanick, B. 1959. Prenatal and paranatal factors in the development of childhood reading disorders. Monographs of the Society for Research in Child Development, *24:*1–80.

Kay, D. W. K., and Roth, M. 1961. Environmental and hereditary factors in the schizophrenias of old age ("late paraphrenia") and their bearing on the general problems of causation in schizophrenia. J. Ment. Sci., *107:*649–686.

Kay, D. W. K., and Roth, M. 1955. Physical accompaniments of mental disorder in old age. Lancet, *259:*740–745.

Kemeny, J. G., Snell, J. L., and Thompson, G. L. 1956. Introduction to Finite Mathematics. Englewood Cliffs, N.J., Prentice-Hall, Inc.

Kemp, T. 1957. Genetic-Hygienic experiences in Denmark in recent years. Eugen. Rev., *49:*11–18.

Kennedy, R. J. R. 1948. The Social Adjustment of Morons in a Connecticut City. Hartford, Conn., Mansfield-Southbury Social Service.

Kennedy, W. 1965. School phobia: rapid treatment of fifty cases. J. Abnorm. Psychol., *70:*285–289.

Kestenberg, J. S. 1954. The history of an autistic child. J. Child Psychiat., *3:*5–35.

Kety, S. S. 1959. Biochemical theories of schizophrenia. Science, *129:*1528–1532.

Kety, S. S. 1952. Cerebral circulation and metabolism. *In* The Biology of Mental Health and Disease, Twenty-seventh Annual Conference of the Milbank Memorial Fund. New York, Hoeber-Harper, pp. 20–31.

Keyes, A. 1952. Experimental induction of psychoneuroses by starvation. *In* The Biology of Mental Health and Disease. New York, Hoeber-Harper.

Kierkegaard, S. 1954. The Sickness Unto Death. (Translated by W. Lowrie.) New York, Doubleday.

Kiernan, I., and Porter, M. 1963. A study of behavior disorder correlations between parents and children. Amer. J. Orthopsychiat., *33:*539–541.

King, G. F. 1958. Differential autonomic responsiveness in the process-reactive classification of schizophrenia. J. Abnorm. Soc. Psychol., *56:*160–164.

Kinsey, A. C., Pomeroy, W. B., and Martin, C. E. 1948. Sexual Behavior in the Human Male. Philadelphia, W. B. Saunders Co.

Kirsner, J. 1961. Peptic ulcer. Worldwide Abst. Gen. Med., *4:*8–16.

Klaber, M. M. 1960. Manifestations of hostility in neuro-dermatitis. J. Consult. Psychol., *24:*116–120.

Klatskin, E. H. 1952. Shifts in child-care practices in three social classes under an infant care program of flexible methodology. Amer. J. Orthopsychiat., *22:*52–61.

Klein, E., Sophn, H., and Cicchetti, D. 1967. A test of the censure-deficit model and its relation to premorbidity in the performance of schizophrenics. J. Abnorm. Psychol., *72:*174–181.

Klein, M. 1961. Narrative of a Child Analysis. New York, Basic Books.

Klein, M. 1949. The Psychoanalysis of Children, 3rd Ed. London, Hogarth Press.

Kline, N. S. 1961. On the relationship between neuro-physiology, psychophysiology, psychopharmacology and other disciplines. *In* Pavlovian Conference on Higher Nervous Activity. Ann. N.Y. Acad. Sci., *92:*1004–1016.

Kline, N. S., et al. (Editors). 1957. Research in Affects. Washington, D.C., American Psychiatric Association, Psychiatric Research Reports No. 8.

Kline, N. S., and Gerard, D. L. 1953. Taxonomy of mental disease, J. Gen. Psychol., *49:*201–207.

Klopfer, B., Ainsworth, M., Klopfer, W. G., and Holt, R. 1954. Developments in the Rorschach Technique, Vol. 1. Yonkers, World Book Co.

Kluckhohn, C., Murray, H. A., and Schneider, D. M. (Editors). 1953. Personality in Nature, Society, and Culture. 2nd Ed. New York, Alfred A. Knopf.

Knapp, P. H., and Nemetz, S. J. 1960. Acute bronchial asthma. Psychosom. Med., *22:*42–55.

Knapp, P. H., Bliss, C. M., and Wells, H. 1963. Addictive aspects in heavy cigarette smoking. Amer. J. Psychiat., *119:*966–972.

Knight, R. P. 1937. The psychodynamics of chronic alcoholism. J. Nerv. Ment. Dis., *86:*538–548.

Knobloch, H., Rider, R., Harper, P., and Pasamanick, B. 1956. Neuropsychiatric sequelae of prematurity. J.A.M.A., *161:*581–585.

Knopf, I. J., and Fager, R. E. 1961. Differences in gradients of stimulus generalization as a function of psychiatric disorder. *In* Sarbin, T. R. (Editor). Studies in Behavior Pathology, New York, Holt, Rinehart and Winston.

Kohn, M. L., and Carroll, E. E. 1960. Social class and the allocation of parental responsibilities. Sociometry, *23:*372–392.

Kohn, M. L., and Clausen, J. A. 1956. Parental authority behavior and schizophrenia. Amer. J. Orthopsychiat., *26:*297–313.

Kohn, M., and Clausen, J. 1955. Social isolation and schizophrenia. Amer. Sociol. Rev., *20:*265–273.

Kolb, L. 1962. Drug Addiction: A Medical Problem. Springfield, Ill., Charles C Thomas.

Kolb, L. C., and Johnson, A. M. 1955. Etiology and therapy of overt homosexuality. Psychoanal. Quart., 24:506–515.

Kolb, L. C., Masland, R. L., and Cooke, R. E. (Editors). 1962. Mental Retardation. Baltimore, The Williams & Wilkins Co. Research Publication, Assoc. Res. Nerv. Ment. Dis. Vol. 39.

Koppitz, E. 1964. The Bender-Gestalt Test for Young Children, New York, Grune & Stratton, Inc.

Koranyi, E. K., and Lehmann, H. E. 1960. On experimental sleep deprivation in psychotic patients, Arch. Gen. Psychiat., 2:534–544.

Kraepelin, E. 1907. Clinical Psychiatry. New York, The Macmillan Co.

Kraepelin, E. 1921. Manic-depressive insanity and paranoia. Edinburgh, E. and S. Livingstone, Ltd.

Kral, V. A. 1955. Postischemic dementia, J. Nerv. Ment. Dis., 122:83–88.

Kral, V. A., Berg, I., and Pivnicki, D. 1960. Carbon monoxide dementia: a case report. Compr. Psychiat., 1:164–173.

Krasner, L. 1958. Studies of the conditioning of verbal behavior. Psychol. Bull., 55:148–170.

Kreitman, N., et al. 1961. The reliability of psychiatric assessment: an analysis. J. Ment. Sci., 107:887–908.

Kreitman, N. 1961. The reliability of psychiatric diagnosis. J. Ment. Sci. 107:876–886.

Kretschmer, E. 1925. Physique and Character. (Translated by W. J. H. Sprott from Korperbau und Charakter, 2nd Ed.). New York, Harcourt, Brace and Co.

Kris, E. 1951. Ego psychology and interpretation in psychoanalytic therapy. Psychoanal. Quart. 20:15–30.

Kvaraceus, W. C. 1945. Juvenile Delinquency and the School. Yonkers-on-Hudson, World Book Co.

Lander, B. 1954. Towards an Understanding of Juvenile Delinquency. New York, Columbia University Press.

Landis, C. 1940. Sex in Development. New York, Hoeber-Harper.

Larsson, T., and Sjogren, T. 1954. A Methodological, psychiatric and statistical study of a large Swedish rural population. Acta Psychiat., Supplementum 89.

Lavin, N. I., Thorpe, J. G., Baker, J. C., Blakemore, C. B., and Conway, C. G. 1961. Behaviour therapy in a case of transvestism. J. Nerv. Ment. Dis., 133:346–353.

Lawton, J. J., Jr., and Malmquest, C. P. 1961. Gasoline addiction in children. Psychiat. Quart., 35:555–561.

Leahy, A. M. 1935. Nature-nurture and intelligence. Genet. Psychol. Monogr., 4:236–308.

Leahy, A. M. 1935. Nature-nurture and intelligence. Genet. Psychol. Monogr. 17:235–308.

Lehmann, H. E. 1963. Phenomenology and pathology of addiction. Compr. Psychiat., 4:168–180.

Lehmann, S. 1971. Community and psychology and community psychology. American Psychol. 26:554–560.

Lehrman, N. 1961. Follow-up of brief and prolonged hospitalization. Compr. Psychiat. 2:227–240.

Leighton, A. 1959. My Name is Legion. New York, Basic Books.

Leighton, A. H., Clausen, J. A., and Wilson, R. N. (Editors). 1957. Explorations in Social Psychiatry. New York, Basic Books.

Lejeune, J., Turpin, R., and Gautier, M. 1959. Quoted by Lejeune, J., and Turpin, R. 1962. Somatic chromosomes in mongolism. In Kolb, L. C., Masland, R. L., and Cooke, R. E. (Editors). Mental Retardation. Baltimore, The Williams & Wilkins Co. Research Publication, Assoc. Res. Nerv. Ment. Dis., 39:67–77.

Lennox, W. G. 1949. Psychiatry, psychology and seizures. Amer. J. Orthopsychiat., 19:432–446.

Lennox, W. G. 1953. Significance of febrile convulsions. Pediatrics, 11:341–356.

Lennox, W. G., and Jolly, D. H. 1954. Seizures, brain waves and intelligence tests of epileptic twins. In Genetics and the Inheritance of Integrated Neurological and Psychiatric Patterns. Research Publications, Assoc. Res. Nerv. Ment. Dis. 33:325–345.

LeShan, L., and LeShan, E. 1961. Psychotherapy and the patient with limited life span. Psychiatry, 24:318–323.

Levine, M. 1952. Principles of psychiatric treatment. In Alexander, F., and Ross, H. (Editors). Dynamic Psychiatry. Chicago, The University of Chicago Press.

Levine, S. 1962. The effects of infantile experience on adult behavior. In Bachrach, A. J. (Editor). Experimental Foundations of Clinical Psychology. New York, Basic Books.

Levine, S. 1960. Infantile stimulation. Sci. Amer., 202:81–86.

Levy, D. M. 1962. Early infantile deprivation. In Kolb, L. C., Masland, R. L., and Cooke, R. E. (Editors). Mental Retardation. Baltimore, The Williams & Wilkins Co. Research Publication, Assoc. Res. Nerv. Ment. Dis., 39:243–255.

Levy, D. M. 1934. Experiments on the sucking reflex and social behavior of dogs. Amer. J. Orthopsychiat. 4:203–224.

Levy, D. M. 1928. Fingersucking and accessory movements in early infancy: an etiological study. Amer. J. Psychiat. 7:881–918.

Levy, D. M. 1943. Maternal Overprotection. New York, Columbia University Press.

Levy, D. M. 1951. Psychopathic behavior in infants and children: A critical survey of the existing concepts. Amer. J. Orthopsychiat., 21:250–254.

Levy, D. M. 1938. Release therapy in young children. Psychiatry, 1:387–390.

Lewin, B. D. 1950. The Psychoanalysis of Elation. New York, W. W. Norton & Co.

Lichtenstein, M., and Brown, A. W. 1938. Intelligence and achievement of children in a delinquency area. J. Juv. Res., 22:1–25.

Liddell, H. S. 1952. Experimental induction of psychoneuroses by conditioned reflex with stress. In Milbank Memorial Fund. The Biology of Mental Health and Disease. New York, Hoeber-Harper.

Liddell, H. S. 1960. Experimental neuroses in animals. In Tanner, J. M. (Editor). Stress and Psychiatric Disorders. Oxford, Blackwell Scientific Publications.

Liddell, H. S. 1954. Sheep and goats: The psychological effects of laboratory experiences of deprivation and stress upon certain experimental animals. In Galdston, I. (Editor). Beyond the Germ Theory. New York, New York Academy of Medicine, Health Education Council.

Liddell, N. S. 1944. Conditioned reflex method and experimental neurosis. In Hunt, J. (Editor) Personality and the Behavior Disorders. New York, Ronald Press.

Lidz, R. W., and Lidz, T. 1949. The family environment of schizophrenic patients. Amer. J. Psychiat., 106:332–345.

Lidz, T. 1959. General concepts of psychosomatic medicine. In Arieti, S. (Editor). American Handbook of Psychiatry. New York, Basic Books.

Lidz, T., and Fleck, S. 1960. Schizophrenia, human integration and the role of the family. In Jackson, D. D. (Editor). The Etiology of Schizophrenia. New York, Basic Books.

Lifton, R. J. 1961. Thought Reform and the Psychology of Totalism. New York, W. W. Norton & Co.

Lilly, J. 1956. Mental Effects of Reduction of Ordinary Levels of Physical Stimuli on Intact, Healthy Persons, Washington, D.C., American Psychiatric Association, Psychiatric Research Reports, No. 5.

Lindner, R. 1944. Rebel Without A Cause. New York, Grune & Stratton, Inc.

Lindner, R. 1955. Songs my mother taught me. *In* The Fifty-Minute Hour. New York, Holt, Rinehart and Winston, Inc. Reprinted 1956. Bantam Books, H-2304.

Linton, R. 1956. Culture and Mental Disorders. Springfield, Ill., Charles C Thomas.

Lippman, H. S. 1962. Treatment of the Child in Emotional Conflict. 2nd Ed., New York, Blakiston Division, McGraw-Hill Book Co., Inc.

Liverant, S. 1959. MMPI differences between parents of disturbed and non-disturbed children. J. Consult. Psychol., *23:*256–260.

Loftus, T. A. 1960. Meaning and Method of Diagnosis in Clinical Psychiatry. Philadelphia, Lea & Febiger.

Lorr, M. 1953. Multidimensional Scale for Rating Psychiatric Patients. Hospital Form. Washington, D.C. Veterans Administration Technical Bulletin TB 10–507.

Lorr, M. 1954. Rating scales and check lists for the evaluation of psychopathology. Psychol. Bull., *51:*119–127.

Lorr, M., Klett, C., McNair, D., and Lasky, J. 1962. Inpatient Multidimensional Psychiatric Scale, Washington, D.C., Veterans Administration.

Lourie, R. S., et al. 1958. A study of the etiology of pica in young children, an early pattern of addiction. *In* Hoch, P. H., and Zubin, J. (Editors). Problems of Addiction and Habituation. New York, Grune & Stratton, Inc. pp. 74–86.

Luby, E. D., Frohman, C. E., Grisell, J. L., Lenzo, J. E., and Ax, A. 1959. Sleep deprivation, A multi-disciplinary study. *In* Gottlieb, J. S., and Tourney, G. (Editors). Scientific Papers and Discussions. Washington, D.C., American Psychiatric Association, District Branches Publication 1.

Luby, E. D., Gottlieb, J. S., Cohen, B. D., Rosenbaum, G., and Domino, E. F. 1962. Model psychoses and schizophrenia. Amer. J. Psychiat., *119:*61–67.

Lucas, C. J., Sainsburg, P., and Collins, J. G. 1962. A social and clinical study of delusions in schizophrenia. J. Ment. Sci., *108:*747–758.

Lykken, D. T. 1957. A study of anxiety in the sociopathic personality. J. Abnorm. Soc. Psychol., *55:*6–10.

McCandless, B. 1961. Children and Adolescents. New York, Holt, Rinehart and Winston.

McCarthy, R. G. 1951. Facts about Alcohol. Chicago, Science Research Associates, Guidance Series Booklet No. 120.

McClelland, D. C., and Atkinson, J. W. 1948. The projective expression of needs: I. The effect of different intensities of the hunger drive on perception. J. Psychol., *25:*205–223.

McCord, W., and McCord, J. 1956. Psychopathy and Delinquency. New York, Grune & Stratton, Inc.

McCord, W., McCord, J., and Gudeman, J. 1959. Some current theories of alcoholism: a longitudinal evaluation. Quart. J. Stud. Alcohol, *20:*727–749.

McCord, W., McCord, J., and Howard, A. 1961. Familial correlates of aggression in nondelinquent male children. J. Abnorm. Soc. Psychol., *62:*79–93.

McCurdy, H. 1961. The Personal World. New York, Harcourt, Brace and World.

McFarland, R. A. 1952. Anoxia: Its effects on the physiology and biochemistry of the brain and on behavior. *In* The Biology of Mental Health and Disease. New York, Hoeber-Harper.

McGhie, A. 1961. A comparative study of the mother-child relationship in schizophrenia. Brit. J. Med. Psychol., *34:*195–221.

McIntosh, W. J. 1949. Follow-up study of one thousand non-academic boys. J. Except. Child., *15:*166–170.

Maas, H. S., Kahn, A. J., and Sumner, D. 1955. Socio-cultural factors in psychiatric clinic services for children: a collaborative study in the New York and San Francisco metropolitan areas. Smith College Study. Soc. Work, *25:*1–90.

Macfarlane, J. W., Allen, L., and Honzik, M. P. 1954. A Developmental Study of the Behavior Problems of Normal Children Between 21 Months and 14 Years. University of California Press, Vol. 2, pp. 1–222.

MacIver, R. 1942. Social Causation. Boston, Ginn and Co.

Maclean, N., et al. 1962. A survey of sex-chromosome abnormalities among 4,514 mental defectives. Lancet, *1*(1):293–296.

Mahler, M. S., Furer, M., and Settlage, C. F. 1959. Severe emotional disturbances in childhood: psychosis. *In* Arieti, S. (Editor). American Handbook of Psychiatry. New York, Basic Books, pp. 816–839.

Mahrer, A. 1963. Psychological symptoms as a function of psychiatric hospitalization. Newsletter, Res. Psychol. *5:*15–16.

Maier, H. W. 1965. Three Theories of Child Development. New York, Harper & Row.

Maier, N. R. F. 1949. Frustration. New York, McGraw-Hill Book Co., Inc.

Malinowski, B. 1927. Sex and Repression in Savage Society. New York, Harcourt, Brace and Co.

Malzberg, B. 1959. Important statistical data about mental illness. *In* Arieti, S. (Editor). American Handbook of Psychiatry. New York, Basic Books.

Malzberg, B. 1938. Outcome of insulin treatment of one thousand patients with dementia praecox. Psychiat. Quart., *12:*528–553.

Malzberg, B. 1940. Social and Biological Aspects of Mental Disease. Utica, N.Y., State Hospital Press.

Mardones, R. J., Segovia, N. M., and Hederra, A. D. 1953. Heredity of experimental alcohol preference in rats. II. Coefficient of heredity. Quart. J. Stud. Alcohol, *14:*1–2.

Mark, J. C. 1953. The attitudes of the mothers of male schizophrenics toward child behavior. J. Abnorm. Soc. Psychol. *48:*185–189.

Marks, P. A. 1961. An Assessment of the Diagnostic Process in a Child Guidance Setting. Psychological Monographs, No. 507 (Vol. 75, No. 3).

Marmor, J., and Pumpian-Mindlin, E. 1950. Toward an integrative conception of mental disorder. J. Nerv. Ment. Dis., *3:*19–29.

Martin, I. 1960. Somatic reactivity. *In* Handbook of Abnormal Psychology, London, Pitman Medical Publishing Co.

Masland, R. L., Sarason, S. B., and Gladwin, T. 1958. Mental Subnormality: Biological, Psychological and Cultural Factors. New York, Basic Books.

Masserman, J. H. 1961. Principles of Dynamic Psychiatry. 2nd Ed. Philadelphia, W. B. Saunders Co.

Masserman, J. H., and Fechtel, C. 1956. How brain lesions affect normal and neurotic behavior. Amer. J. Psychiat., *112:*865–872.

Masserman, J. H., and Yum, K. S. 1946. An analysis of the influence of alcohol on experimental neuroses in cats. Psychosom. Med., *8:*36–52.

Matarazzo, J. D., and Saslow, G. 1960. Psychological and related characteristics of smokers and nonsmokers. Psychol. Bull., *57:*493–513.

May, Rollo (Ed.) 1969. Existential Psychology. New York, Random House.

May, R. 1950. The Meaning of Anxiety. New York, The Ronald Press Co.

Mayer-Gross, W., Slater, E., and Roth, M. 1960. Clinical Psychiatry, 2nd Ed. Baltimore, The Williams & Wilkins Co., pp. 305–543.

Mead, M. 1949. Male and Female. Reprinted 1955. New York, Mentor No. M.D. 150.

Mead, M. 1935. Sex and Temperament. Reprinted 1950. New York, Mentor No. M.D. 133.

Medearis, D. N., Jr. 1962. Cytomegalic inclusion disease as an example of a viral infection acquired in utero which may result in mental retardation. In Kolb. L. C., Masland, R. L., and Cooke. R. E. (Editors). Mental Retardation. Baltimore, The Williams & Wilkins Co. Research Publication, Assoc. Res. Nerv. Ment. Dis., 39:130–140.

Mednick, S., Garner, A. M., and Stone, H. K. 1959. A test of some behavioral hypotheses drawn from Alexander's specificity theory. Amer. J. Orthopsychiat., 29:592–598.

Meduna, L. Von. 1938. General discussion of the Cardiazol therapy. Amer. J. Psychiat., 94:40–50.

Meehl, P. E. 1962. Schizotoxia, schizotypy, schizophrenia. Amer. J. Psychol., 17:827–838.

Meier, M. J., and French, L. A. 1965. Some personality correlates of unilateral and bilateral EEG abnormalities in psychomotor epileptics. J. Clin. Psychol., 21:3–9.

Menninger, K. A. 1938. Man Against Himself. New York, Harcourt, Brace and Co.

Menninger, K., et al. 1958. The unitary concept of mental illness. Bull. Menninger Clin., 22:4–12.

Mensh, I. N. 1959. Psychiatric diagnosis in the institutionalized aged. Geriatrics, 14:511–517.

Mental Health in Corrective Institutions. 1941. New York, Proceedings of the Seventy-first Annual Congress of the American Prison Association.

Mesnikoff, A. M., Rainer, J. D., Kolb, L. C., and Carr, A. C. 1963. Intrafamilial determinants of divergent sexual behavior in twins. Amer. J. Psychiat., 119:732–738.

Meyer, A. 1948. The Commonsense Psychiatry of Dr. Adolf Meyer. New York, McGraw-Hill Book Co.

Meyer, R., Schiff, L., and Becker, A. 1967. The home treatment of psychotic patients: An analysis of 154 cases. Amer. J. Psychiat. 123:1430–1438.

Meyer, V. 1961. Psychological effects of brain damage. In Eysenck, H. J. (Editor). Handbook of Abnormal Psychology. New York, Basic Books, pp. 529–565.

Milbank Memorial Fund. 1950. Epidemiology of Mental Disorder. New York, Milbank Memorial Fund.

Milbank Memorial Fund. 1953. Interrelations Between the Social Environment and Psychiatric Disorders. New York, Milbank Memorial Fund.

Milbank Memorial Fund. 1957. The Nature and Transmission of the Genetic and Cultural Characteristics of Human Populations. New York, Milbank Memorial Fund.

Miles, W. R. 1932. Psychological effects of alcohol in man. In Emerson, H. (Editor). The Effect of Alcohol on Man in Health and Disease. New York, The Macmillan Co.

Miller, C. W. 1942. Factors affecting the prognosis of paranoid disorders. J. Nerv. Ment. Dis., 95:580–588.

Miller, C. W. 1941. The paranoid syndrome. A.M.A. Arch. Neurol. Psychiat., 45:953–963.

Miller, D. R., and Swanson, G. E. 1960. Inner Conflict and Defense. New York, Henry Holt and Co.

Miller, N. 1948. Theory and experiment relating psychoanalytic displacement to stimulus-response generalization. J. Abnorm. Soc. Psychol., 43:155–178.

Mohr, J. W., Turner, R. E., and Ball, R. B. 1962. Exhibitionism and Pedophilia. Corr. Psychiat., J. Soc. Ther., 8, No. 4.

Mohr, J. W., Turner, R. E., and Jerry, M. B. 1964. Pedophilia and Exhibitionism. Toronto, University of Toronto Press.

Money, J. 1963. Cytogenetic and psychosexual incongruities with a note on space-form blindness. Amer. J. Psychiat., 119:820–827.

Moreno, J. 1946. Psychodrama, Vol. 1. 2nd Ed. New York, Beacon House.

Morgan, C. D., and Murray, H. A. 1935. A method for investigating fantasies: the thematic apperception test. Arch. Neurol. Psychiat., 34:289–306.

Mosher, L. 1970. Madness and the Community. Attitude, 1:2–7.

Mowrer, O. H. 1950. Learning Theory and Personality Dynamics. New York, Ronald Press.

Muench, G. A. 1947. An Evaluation of Non-Directive Psychotherapy by Means of the Rorschach and Other Indices. Appl. Psychol. Monogr., No. 13.

Muench, G. A. 1944. A follow-up of mental defectives after eighteen years. J. Abnorm. Soc. Psychol., 39:407–418.

Mulder, D. W. 1959. Psychoses with brain tumors and other chronic neurologic disorders. In Arieti, S. (Editor). American Handbook of Psychiatry. New York, Basic Books, pp. 1144–1162.

Munroe, M. 1935. Reading Aptitude Tests, Primary Form. Boston, Houghton Mifflin.

Murphy, G. 1949. Historical Introduction to Modern Psychology. New York, Harcourt, Brace and Co.

Murphy, J. M. 1962. Cross-cultural studies of the prevalence of psychiatric disorders. World Ment. Health, 14:53–65.

Murray, E. J., and Cohen, C. 1959. Mental illness, milieu therapy and social organization in ward groups. J. Abnorm. Soc. Psychol., 58:48–54.

Murray, H. A. 1938. Explorations in Personality. New York, Oxford University Press.

Murray, H. A. 1943. Thematic Apperception Test. Cambridge, Harvard University Press.

Myers, J. K., and Roberts, B. H. 1959. Family and Class Dynamics in Mental Illness. New York, John Wiley & Sons, Inc.

Nabokov, V. 1955. Lolita. Reprinted 1959. Crest Giant D-338.

Nash, H. 1962. The double-bind procedure: Rationale and empirical evaluation. J. Nerv. Ment. Dis., 134:34–47.

Neel, J. V., and Schull, W. J. 1954. Human Heredity, Chicago, The University of Chicago Press.

Nelson, W. E. (Editor). 1964. Textbook of Pediatrics. 8th Ed. Philadelphia, W. B. Saunders Co.

Nemiah, J. C. 1961. Foundations of Psychopathology. New York, Oxford University Press.

Neuer, H. 1947. The relationship between behavior disorders in children and the syndrome of mental deficiency. Amer. J. Ment. Defic., 52:143–147.

Newman, H. H., Freeman, S. N., and Holzinger, K. 1937. Twins: A Study of Heredity and Environment. Chicago, The University of Chicago Press.

Norris, V. 1959. Mental Illness in London, Maudsley Monograph No. 6. London, Chapman & Hall, Ltd.

Norton, A. 1952. Incidence of neurosis related to maternal age and birth order. Brit. J. Soc. Med., 6:256.

Noyes, A. P., and Kolb, L. C. 1963. Modern Clinical Psychiatry, 6th Ed. Philadelphia, W. B. Saunders Co.

Nyswander, M. 1959. Drug addictions. In Arieti, S. (Editor). American Handbook of Psychiatry. New York, Basic Books.

O'Connor, J. et al. 1964. The effects of psychotherapy on the course of ulcerative colitis: A preliminary report. Amer. J. Psychiat., 120:738–742.

O'Connor, N. 1953. The occupational success of feeble-minded adolescents. Occup. Psychol., 27:157–163.

O'Connor, N., and Franks, C. M. 1960. Childhood upbringing and other environmental factors. *In* Eysenck, J. H. (Editor). Handbook of Abnormal Psychology. London, Pitman Medical Publishing Co., Ltd., pp. 393–416.

O'Connor, N., and Tizard, J. 1956. The Social Problem of Mental Deficiency. London, Pergamon Press.

Offer, D., and Sabshin, M. 1966. Normality. New York, Basic Books.

Olds. J. 1955. Physiological mechanisms of reward. *In* Jones, M. R. (Editor). Nebraska Symposium on Motivation, Vol. 3. Lincoln, University of Nebraska Press.

Olson, G., and Peterson, D. 1962. Intermittent chemotherapy for chronic psychiatric inpatients. J. Nerv. Ment. Dis., *134:*145–149.

O'Neal, P., and Robins, L. N. 1958. Childhood patterns predictive of adult schizophrenia: a thirty-year follow-up study. Amer. J. Psychiat., *115:*385–391.

O'Neal, P., and Robins, L. N. 1958. The relation of childhood behavior problems to adult psychiatric status: a 30-year follow-up study of 150 subjects. Amer. J. Psychiat., *114:* 961–969.

O'Neal, P., Robins, L. N., King, L. J., and Schaefer, J. 1962. Parental deviance and the genesis of sociopathic personality. Amer. J. Psychiat., *118:*1114–1124.

Opler, M. K. (Editor). 1959. Culture and Mental Health. New York, The Macmillan Co.

Opler, M. K. 1956. Culture, Psychiatry and Human Values: The Methods and Values of a Social Psychiatrist. Springfield, Ill., Charles C Thomas.

Orlinsky, N., and D'Elia, E. 1964. Rehospitalization of the schizophrenic patient. Arch. Gen. Psychiat., *10:*47–54.

Osmond, H., and Smythies, J. 1952. Schizophrenia: a new approach. J. Ment. Sci., *98:*309–315.

Parnell, R. W. 1958. Behaviour and Physique. London, Edward Arnold and Co.

Partridge, G. D. 1928. Psychopathic personalities among boys in a training school for delinquents. Amer. J. Psychiat., *8:*159–186.

Pasamanick, B. (Editor). 1959. Epidemiology of Mental Disorder. Washington, D.C., American Association for the Advancement of Science, Publication No. 60.

Pasamanick, B., and Knapp, P. H. (Editors). 1958. Social Aspects of Psychiatry. Washington, D.C., American Psychiatric Association, Psychiatric Research Reports No. 10.

Pasamanick, B., and Knobloch, H. 1961. Epidemiologic studies on the complications of pregnancy and the birth process. *In* Caplan, G. (Editor). Prevention of Mental Disorders in Children. New York, Basic Books, pp. 74–94.

Pasamanick, B., Dinitiz, S., and Lefton, M. 1959. Psychiatric orientation and its relation to diagnosis and treatment in a mental hospital. Amer. J. Psychiat., *116:*127–32.

Paterson, D. G., and Rundquist, E. A. 1933. The occupational background of feeblemindedness. Amer. J. Psychol., *45:* 118–124.

Paul, G. 1966. Insight vs. Desensitization in Psychotherapy. Stanford, Calif., Stanford University Press.

Pauly, I. B. 1963. Female Psychosexual Inversion: Transsexualism. Paper presented at the annual meeting of the American Psychiatric Association.

Pavlov, I. P. 1928. Lectures on Conditioned Reflexes. New York, International Publishers Co., Inc.

Pavlov, I. P. 1941. Lectures on Conditioned Reflexes, Vol. 2. New York, International Publishers Co., Inc.

Penrose, L. S. 1938. A Clinical and Genetic Study of 1280 Cases of Mental Defect. London, H. M. Stationery Office, Med. Research Council Special Report Series No. 229.

Penrose, L. S. 1954. The Biology of Mental Defect., Rev. Ed. London, Sidgwick and Jackson, Ltd.

Penrose, L. S. 1964. The Biology of Mental Defect, 2nd Ed. New York, Grune & Stratton, Inc.

Penrose, L. S. 1959. Outline of Human Genetics. New York, John Wiley & Sons, Inc.

Penrose, L. S. 1950. Research Methods in Human Genetics. *In* Congres International de Psychiatrie, Paris, 1950. VI. Psychiatrie Sociale. Paris, Hermann & Cie.

Pescor, M. J. 1943. A Statistical Analysis of the Clinical Records of Hospitalized Drug Addicts. Public Health Reports, Supplement No. 143.

Peterson, D. R., Becker, W. C., Hellmer, L. A., Shoemaker, D. J., and Quay, H. C. 1959. Parental attitudes and child adjustment. Child Develop., *30:*119–130.

Peterson, L., and Smith, L. L. 1960. The post-school adjustment of educable mentally retarded adults in comparison with that of adults of normal intelligence. Except. Child., *26:*404–408.

Phillips, L. 1953. Case history data and prognosis in schizophrenia. J. Nerv. Ment. Dis., *117:*515–525.

Pinneau, S. R. 1950. A critique on the articles by Margaret Ribble. Child Develop., *21:*203–228.

Pinneau, S. R. 1955. The infantile disorders of hospitalism and anaclitic depression. Psychol. Bull., *52:*429–452.

Pinneau, S. R. 1955. Reply to Dr. Spitz. Psychol. Bull., *52:*459–462.

Pittman, F., Langsley, D., Kaplan, D., Flomenhaft, K., and DeYoung, D. 1965. Family therapy as an alternative to psychiatric hospitalization. Paper presented at Regional Research Conference, American Psychiatric Association, Galveston, Texas.

Plunkett, R. J., and Gordon, J. E. 1960. Epidemiology and Mental Illness: Joint Commission on Mental Illness and Health, Monograph Series No. 6, New York, Basic Books.

Pokorny, A. D. 1960. Characteristics of 44 patients who subsequently committed suicide. A.M.A. Arch. Gen. Psychiat., *2:*314–323.

Pollard, J. C., Baker, C., Uhr, L., and Feuerfile, D. F. 1960. Controlled sensory in-put: a note on the technic of drug evaluation with a preliminary report on a comparative study of Sernyl, Psilocybin and LSD-25. Compr. Psychiat., *1:*377–380.

Pollock, H. M. 1945. Mental disease among mental defectives. Amer. J. Ment. Defic., *49:*477–480,

Popham, R. E. 1953. A critique of the genetotrophic theory of the etiology of alcoholism. Quart. J. Stud. Alcohol, *15:*228–237.

Popham, R. E. 1959. Some social and cultural aspects of alcoholism. Canad. Psychiat., Assoc. J., *4:*222–229.

Popham, R. E., and Schmidt, W. 1962. A Decade of Alcoholism Research. Brookside Monograph No. 3, Toronto, University of Toronto Press.

Porteus, S. D., and Peters, H. N. 1947. Maze test validation and psychosurgery. Genet. Psychol. Monogr., *36:*3–86.

Prichard, J. C. 1835. Treatise on Insanity. London, Sherwood, Gilbert and Piper.

Prince, M. 1906. The Dissociation of Personality (Reprinted 1920, Meridian). New York, Longmans, Green and Co.

Pritchard, M. 1962. Homosexuality and genetic sex. J. Ment. Sci., *108:*616–623.

Pritchard, M. 1967a. Prognosis of schizophrenia before and after pharmacotherapy: I. Short-term outcome. Brit. J. Psychiat., *113:*1345–1352.

Pritchard, M. 1967b. Prognosis of schizophrenia before and after pharmacotherapy: II. Three-year follow-up. Brit. J. Psychiat., *113:*1353–1359.

Querido, A. 1969. The shaping of community mental health care. Int. J. Psychiat., 7:300–311.

Rabinovitch, R. D. 1959. Reading and learning disabilities. In Arieti, S. (Editor). American Handbook of Psychiatry. New York, Basic Books, pp. 857–869.

Rado, S. 1949. An adaptational view of sexual behavior. In Hoch, P. H., and Zubin, J. (Editors). Psychosexual Development. New York, Grune & Stratton, Inc.

Rado, S. 1961. The automatic motivating system of depressive behavior. Compr. Psychiat., 2:248–260.

Rado, S. 1954. Hedonic control, action-self and the depressive spell. In Hoch, P. H., and Zubin, J. (Editors). New York, Grune & Stratton, Inc.

Rado, S. 1958. Narcotic bondage: A general theory of the dependence on narcotic drugs. In Hoch, P. H., and Zubin, J. (Editors). Problems of Addiction and Habituation. New York, Grune & Stratton, Inc.

Rado, S. 1928. The problem of melancholia. Int. J. Psychoanal., 9:420–438.

Rado, S. 1933. The psychoanalysis of pharmacothymia (drug addiction). Psychoanal. Quart., 2:1–23.

Rado, S. 1960. Theory and therapy: The theory of schizotypal organization and its application to the treatment of decompensated schizotypal behavior. In Sher, S. C., and Davis, H. R. (Editors). The Out-Patient Treatment of Schizophrenia. New York, Grune & Stratton, Inc.

Randell, J. B. 1959. Tranvestitism and trans-sexualism. Brit. Med., J., 2:1448–1452.

Rapaport, D. 1945. Diagnostic Psychological Testing (two volumes). Chicago, Year Book Publishers, Inc.

Rapaport, D., 1960. The structure of psychoanalytic theory. A systematory attempt. Psychol. Issues, 2, No. 2, New York, International Universities Press.

Raskin, N., and Ehrenberg, R. 1956. Senescence, senility and Alzheimer's disease. Amer. J. Psychiat., 113:133–136.

Rechtshaffen, A. 1959. Psychotherapy with geriatric patients: a review of the literature. J. Gerontol., 14:73–88.

Reed, E. W., and Reed, S. C. 1965. Mental Retardation: A Family Study. Philadelphia, W. B. Saunders Co.

Rees, L. 1960. Constitutional factors and abnormal behavior. In Eysenck, H. J. (Editor). Handbook of Abnormal Psychology. London, Pitman Medical Publishing Co.

Rees, L., and Eysenck, H. J. 1945. A factorial study of some morphological and psychological aspects of human constitution. J. Ment. Sci., 91:8.

Reichard, S., and Tillman, C. 1950. Patterns of parent-child relationships in schizophrenia. Psychiatry, 13:247–257.

Reid, D. D. 1960. Epidemiological Methods in the Study of Mental Disorders. Geneva, World Health Organization, Public Health Papers No. 2.

Reid, E. C. 1960. Epidemiological Methods in the Study of Mental Disorders. Geneva, World Health Organization, Public Health Papers No. 2.

Reiss, M. (Editor). 1958. Psychoendocrinology. New York, Grune & Stratton, Inc.

Rennie, P. A. C. 1942. Prognosis in manic-depressive psychoses. Amer. J. Psychiat., 98:801–814.

Report of the Commission on Obscenity and Pornography. 1970. New York, Bantam Books.

Ribble, M. 1944. Infantile experience in relation to personality development. In Hunt, J. McV. (Editor). Personality and Behavior Disorders. New York, The Ronald Press Co.

Rice, Laura. 1965. Therapist's style of participation and case outcome. J. Consult. Psychol., 29:155–160.

Rimland, B. 1964. Infantile Autism. New York, Appleton-Century-Crofts.

Ritter, C. 1954. A Woman in the Polar Night. New York, E. P. Dutton & Co.

Roach, J. L., Gurrslin, O., and Hunt, R. G. 1958. Some social psychological characteristics of a child guidance clinic caseload. J. Consult. Psychol., 22:183–186.

Roback, A. A. 1961. History of Psychology and Psychiatry. New York, Philosophical Library.

Roberts, J. A. F. 1952. The genetics of mental deficiency. Eugen. Rev., 44:71–83.

Roberts, J. A. F. 1950. The genetics of oligophrenia. In Congrès International de Psychiatrie, Paris, 1950, VI, Psychiatrie Sociale, Génétique et Eugénique. Paris, Hermann, pp. 55–117.

Roberts, J. A. F. 1959. An Introduction to Medical Genetics, 2nd Ed. New York, Oxford University Press.

Robins, E., et al., 1959. Some clinical considerations in the prevention of suicide based on a study of 134 successful suicides. Amer. J. Public Health.

Roe, A., Burks, B., and Mittelman, B. 1945. Adult Adjustment of Foster Children of Alcoholic and Psychotic Parentage and the Influence of the Foster Home. Memoria of the Section on Alcohol. New Haven, Yale University Press.

Rogers, C. 1951. Client-Centered Therapy. Boston, Houghton Mifflin Co.

Rogers, C. 1957. The necessary and sufficient conditions of therapeutic personality change. J. Consult. Psychol., 21:95–103.

Rogers, C. R. 1961. On Becoming a Person. Boston, Houghton-Mifflin.

Rohrer, J. H., and Edmonson, M. S. (Editors). 1960. Eighth Generation: Cultures and Personalities of New Orleans Negroes. New York, Harper & Row, Publishers, Inc.

Rome, H. P., and Robinson, D. B. 1959. Psychiatric conditions associated with metabolic, endocrine and nutritional disorders. In Arieti, S. (Editor). American Handbook of Psychiatry. New York, Basic Books, pp. 1260–1288.

Rosanoff, A. J., Handy, L. M., and Plesset, I. R. 1941. The Etiology of Child Behavior Difficulties, Juvenile Delinquency and Adult Criminality, with Special Reference to their Occurrence in Twins. Psychiat. Monogr. No. 1. Sacramento, Calif. Department of Institutions.

Rosanoff, A. J., Handy, L. M., and Plesset, I. R. 1937. The etiology of mental deficiency. Psychol. Monogr. 48(4):1–137.

Rosanoff, A. J., Handy, L. M., and Rosanoff, J. A. 1934. Etiology of epilepsy with special reference to its occurrence in twins. A.M.A. Arch. Neurol. Psychiat., 31:1165–1193.

Rose, A. M. (Editor). 1955. Mental Health and Mental Disorder. New York, W. W. Norton & Co.

Rosen, E. 1949. George X: the self-analysis of an avowed fascist. J. Abnorm. Soc. Psychol., 44:528–540.

Rosen, E., and Rizzo, G. 1961. Preliminary standardization of the MMPI for use in Italy: A case study of inter-cultural differences. Educ. Psychol. Measmt., 21:629–636.

Rosen, G. 1961. Cross-cultural and historical approaches. In Hoch, P. H., and Zubin, J. (Editors). Psychopathology of Aging. New York, Grune & Stratton, Inc., pp. 1–20.

Rosen, G. 1959. Social stress and mental disease from the Eighteenth Century to the present: Some origins of social psychiatry. Milbank Mem. Fund Quart. 37:5–32.

Rosenthal, D. 1962. Problems of sampling and diagnosis in the major twin studies of schizophrenia. J. Psychiat., Res. 1:116–134.

Rosenthal, D. 1961. Sex distribution and the severity of illness among samples of schizophrenic twins. J. Psychiat. Res. 1:26–36.

Rosenthal, D. 1959. Some factors associated with concordance and discordance with respect to schizophrenia in monozygotic twins. J. Nerv. Ment. Dis., 129:1–10.

Rosenthal, H. R. 1959. Psychotherapy for the aging. Amer. J. Psychother. 13(1):55–65.

Rosenzweig, S. 1949. Psychodiagnosis. New York, Grune & Stratton, Inc.

Rosenzweig, S. 1954. A transvaluation of psychotherapy: a reply to Hans Eysenck. J. Abnorm. Soc. Psychol., 49:298–304.

Rosenzweig, S., and Cass, L. K. 1954. The extension of psychodiagnosis to parents in the child guidance setting. Amer. J. Orthopsychiat., 24:715–722.

Rosenzweig, S., and Sarason, S. 1942. An experimental study of the Treadic hypotheses: reaction to frustration, ego defense, and hypnotizability. Charac. Personality, 11:1–20.

Ross, A. O. 1959. The Practice of Clinical Child Psychology. New York, Grune & Stratton, Inc.

Roth, M. 1955. The natural history of mental disorder in old age. J. Ment. Sci., 101:281–301.

Rothschild, D. 1956. Senile psychoses and psychoses with cerebral arteriosclerosis. In Kaplan, O. J. (Editor). Mental Disorders in Later Life. Stanford, Calif., Stanford University Press.

Roueché, B. 1954. Ten feet tall. In The Incurable Wound. New York, Berkley Books.

Ruch, T. C. 1961. Neurophysiology of emotion and motivation. In Ruch, T. C., and Fulton, J. F. (Editors). Medical Physiology and Biophysics, 18th Ed. Philadelphia, W. B. Saunders Co.

Ruesch, J., et al. 1946. Chronic Disease and Psychosomatic Invalidism. Psychosom. Med. Monogr., No. 9. New York, Hoeber-Harper.

Ruesch, J., and Bateson, G. 1951. Communication, The Social Matrix of Psychiatry. New York, W. W. Norton & Co.

Ruesch, J., and Bowman, K. 1946. Prolonged post-traumatic syndromes following head injury. Amer. J. Psychiat., 102:145–163.

Ruesch, J., and Kees, W. 1961. Non-verbal Communication. Berkeley, University of California Press.

Rush, B. 1794. Medical Inquiries and Observations. 2nd Ed. Philadelphia, Thomas Dobson.

Ryan, J. 1962. The therapeutic value of the closed ward. J. Nerv. Ment. Dis. 134:256–262.

Salzman, L. 1947. An evaluation of shock therapy. Amer. J. Psychiat., 103:669–679.

Sarason, S. B. 1953. Psychological Problems in Mental Deficiency, 2nd Ed. New York, Harper & Bros.

Sarbin, T. R. (Editor). 1961. Studies in Behavior Pathology. New York, Holt, Rinehart and Winston.

Sargant, W., and Slater, E. 1954. An Introduction to Physical Methods of Treatment in Psychiatry, 3rd Ed. Baltimore, The Williams & Wilkins Co.

Sarte, J. P. 1956. Being and Nothingness. (Trans. by H. Barnes), New York, Philosophical Library.

Scarpitti, F. R., Murray, E., Dinitz, S., and Reckless, W. S. 1960. The "good" boy in a high delinquency area: 4 years later. Amer. Sociol. Rev., 25:555–558.

Schilder, P. 1941. The psychogenesis of alcoholism. Quart. J. Stud. Alcohol, 2:227–292.

Schilder, P. 1939. The psychology of schizophrenia. Psychoanal. Rev., 26:380–398.

Schmidt, H. O., and Fonda, C. 1956. The reliability of psychiatric diagnosis: A new look. J. Abnorm. Soc. Psychol., 52:262–267.

Schofield, W., and Balian, L. 1959. A comparative study of the personal histories of schizophrenic and nonpsychiatric patients. J. Abnorm. Soc. Psychol., 59:216–225.

Schonbar, R. A. 1959. Some manifest characteristics of recallers and non-recallers of dreams. J. Consult. Psychol., 23:414–418.

Schuell, H., Jenkins, J. J., and Jimenez-Pabon, E. 1964. Aphasia in Adults; Diagnosis, Prognosis and Treatment. New York, Hoeber-Harper.

Schuham, A. 1967. The double-bind hypothesis a decade later. Psychol. Bull., 68:409–416.

Schulberg, H., and Baker, F. 1969. Unitization: Decentralizing the Mental Hospitalopolis. Int. J. Psychiat., 7:213–223.

Schulman, J. L. 1963. Management of the child with early infanile autism. Amer. J. Psychiat., 120:250–254.

Schwartz, P. 1957. Birth Trauma as a Cause of Mental Deficiency. Pennsylvania Department of Welfare.

Sears, P. S. 1953. Child-rearing factors related to playing of sex-typed roles. Amer. Psychol., 8:431.

Sears, R. R., Maccoby, E. E., and Levin, H. 1957. Patterns of Child-rearing. Evanston, Ill., Row, Peterson and Co.

Sears, R. R., Whiting, J. W. M., Nowles, V., and Sears, P. S. 1953. Some Child-rearing Antecedents of Aggression and Dependency in Young Children. Genet. Psychol. Monogr., No. 47.

Selling, L. S. 1943. Men Against Madness. New York, Garden City Publishing Co.

Selye, H. 1952. The general adaptation syndrome. In The Biology of Mental Health and Disease. New York, Hoeber-Harper.

Selye, H. 1956. The Stress of Life. New York, McGraw-Hill Book Co., Inc.

Shagass, C. 1957. Neurophysiological studies of anxieties and depression. In Kline, N. S. (Editor). Research in Affects. Washington, D.C., American Psychiatric Association, Psychiatric Research Reports No. 8.

Sharp, A. 1938. An experimental test of Freud's doctrine of the relation of hedonic tone to memory revival. J. Exp. Psychol., 22:395–418.

Shaw, C. 1930. The Jack-Roller. Chicago, The University of Chicago Press.

Shaw, C., and MacKay, H. D. 1942. Juvenile Delinquency and Urban Areas. Chicago, The University of Chicago Press.

Shaw, M. W. 1962. Familial mongolism. Cytogenetics, 1:141–179.

Sheldon, W. H. 1954. Atlas of Men. New York, Harper and Bros.

Sheps, J. 1959. New developments in family diagnosis in emotional disorders of old age. Geriatrics, 14:443–449.

Sherman, M., and Henry, T. R. 1933. Hollow Folk, New York, Thomas Y. Crowell Co.

Shields, J., and Slater, E. 1960. Heredity and psychological abnormality. In Eysenck, H. J. (Editor). Handbook of Abnormal Psychology. London, Pitman Medical Publishing Co.

Shinfuku, N., Matsumoto, H., Omura, M., and Sugihara, H. 1959. Long term observation of bodily changes in a cyclothymic patient. Yonago Acta Med., 3:164–172.

Shipley, W. C. 1940. Shipley-Hartford Retreat Scale: Manual of Directions and Scoring Key. Hartford, Conn., Hartford Retreat.

Silverman, D. 1943. Clinical and electroencephalographic studies of criminal psychopaths. Arch. Neurol. Psychiat., 50:18–33.

Silverman, D. 1944. The electroencephalograph and therapy of criminal psychopaths. J. Crim. Psychopathol., 5:439–466.

Simon, A., and Cahan, R. B. 1963. The acute brain syndrome in geriatric patients. In Mendel, W. M., and Epstein, L. J. (Editors). Acute Psychotic Reactions. Washington, D.C., American Psychiatric Association, Psychiat., Res. Rep. No. 16, pp. 8–21.

Singer, J. L., and Opler, M. K. 1961. Contrasting patterns of fantasy and motility in Irish and Italian schizophrenics. *In* Sarbin, T. R. (Editor). Studies in Behavior Pathology. New York, Holt, Rinehart and Winston.

Singer, J. L., and Schonbar, R. A. 1961. Correlates of day-dreaming: a dimension of self-awareness. J. Consult. Psychol., *25*:1–6.

Singer, M. T., and Wynne, L. C. 1963. Differentiating characteristics of the parents of childhood schizophrenics, childhood neurotics and young adult schizophrenics. Amer. J. Psychiat., *120*:234–243.

Skeels, H. M., and Fillmore, E. A. 1937. Mental development of children from underprivileged homes. J. Genet. Psychol., *50*:427–439.

Skinner, B. F. 1938. The Behavior of Organisms: An Experimental Approach. New York, Appleton-Century-Crofts.

Skinner, B. F. 1953. Science and Human Behavior. New York, The Macmillan Co.

Sklar, J., and O'Neill, F. J. 1961. Experiments with intensive treatment in a geriatric ward. *In* Hoch, P. H., and Zubin, J. (Editors). Psychopathology of Aging. New York, Grune & Stratton, Inc., pp. 266–273.

Slater, E. 1953. Psychotic and Neurotic Illness in Twins. London, Her Majesty's Stationery Office, Medical Research Council Special Reports Series No. 278.

Slavson, S. R. 1950. Analytic Group Psychotherapy. New York, Columbia University Press.

Sloan, W., and Birch. J. 1955. A rationale for degrees of retardation. Amer. J. Ment. Defic., *60*:258–264.

Sloane, P., and Karpinski, E. 1942. Effects of incest on the participants. Amer. J. Orthopsychiat., *12*:666–673.

Smith, A. D. M. 1960. Megaloblastic madness. Brit. Med. J., *2*(2):1840–1845.

Smith, J. O. 1962. Criminality and mental retardation. Train. Sch. Bull. *59*(3):74–80.

Smith, T., Bower, W., and Wignall, C. 1965. Influence of policy and drugs on Colorado State Hospital population. Arch. Gen. Psychiat. *12*:352–362.

Society for Psychosomatic Research. 1959. The Nature of Stress Disorder. Springfield, Ill., Charles C Thomas.

Soddy, K. 1960. Clinical Child Psychiatry. Baltimore, The Williams & Wilkins Co.

Soddy, K. (Editor). 1961. Cross-cultural Studies in Mental Health. London, Tavistock Publications.

Solomon, P., Kusmansky, P. E., Leiderman, P. H., Trumbull, R., and Wexler, D. (Editors). 1961. Sensory Deprivation. Cambridge, Harvard University Press.

Solomon, R. L., and Wynne, L. C. 1954. Traumatic avoidance learning: the principles of anxiety conservation and partial irreversibility. Psychol. Rev., *61*:353–385.

Speers, R., and Lansing, C. 1965. Group Therapy in Childhood Psychosis. Chapel Hill, N.C., University of North Carolina Press.

Spiegel, D., and Newringer, C. 1963. The role of dread in suicidal behavior. J. Abnorm. Soc. Psychol., *66*:507–511.

Spitz, H. A. 1963. Field theory in mental deficiency. *In* Ellis, N. R. (Editor). Handbook of Mental Deficiency. New York, McGraw-Hill Book Co., Inc.

Spitz, R. A. 1946. Anaclitic depression. Psychoanal. Stud. Child, *2*:313–340.

Spitz, R. A. 1945. Hospitalism: an inquiry into the genesis of psychiatric conditions in early childhood. Psychoanal. Stud. Child, *1*:53–74.

Spitz, R. A. 1955. Reply to Dr. Pinneau. Psychol. Bull., *52*:453–459.

Spitz, R. A. 1949. The role of ecological factors in emotional development in infancy. Child Develop., *20*:145–156.

Spitz, R. A. 1954. Unhappy and fatal outcomes of emotional deprivation and stress in infancy. *In* Galdston, I. (Editor).

Beyond the Germ Theory. New York, New York Academy of Sciences, Health Education Council.

Spitz, R. A., and Wolf, K. M. 1946. Anaclitic depression: an enquiry into the genesis of psychiatric conditions in early childhood, II. *In* Freud, A., et al. (Editors). The Psychoanalytic Study of the Child, Vol. II. New York, International Universities Press.

Sprenger, J., and Kraemer, H. (Henricus Institoris). Malleus Maleficarum. (Translated by Montague Summers, 1948.) London, The Pushkin Press.

Srole, L., Langner, T. S., Michael, S. C. Opler, M. K., and Rennie, P. A. C. 1962. Mental Health in the Metropolis: The Midtown Manhattan Study, Vol. 1. New York, McGraw-Hill Book Co., Inc.

Stacey, C. L., and DeMartino, M. F. (Editors). 1957. Counseling and Psychotherapy with the Mentally Retarded. Glencoe, Ill., The Free Press.

Stainbrook, E. 1953. *In* Hoch, P., and Zubin, J. (Editors). Current Problems in Psychiatric Diagnosis. New York, Grune & Stratton, Inc.

Statan, C. 1969. Community psychiatry—stretcher bearer of the social order? Int. J. Psychiat., *7*:312–321.

Stein, M. I. (Editor). 1961. Contemporary Psychotherapies. Glencoe, Ill., The Free Press.

Steinberg, A. G. 1959. Methodology in human genetics. J. Med. Educ., *34*:315–334.

Stengel, E. 1960. Classification of mental disorders. Bull. W.H.O. *21*:601–663.

Stephens, E. 1953. Defensive reactions of mentally retarded adults. Soc. Casewk., *34*:119–124.

Stern, C. 1960. Principles of Human Genetics, 2nd Ed. San Francisco, W. H. Freeman and Co.

Stern, R. L. 1947. Diary of a War Neurosis. J. Nerv. Ment. Dis., *106*:583–586.

Stevens, H. A. and Heber, R. (Editors). 1964. Mental Retardation. Chicago, University of Chicago Press.

Stevens, S. 1954. An ecological study of child guidance intake. Smith Coll. Stud. Soc. Work, *25*:73–84.

Stevenson, I. 1959. The psychiatric interview. *In* Arieti, S. (Editor). American Handbook of Psychiatry. New York, Basic Books.

Stevenson, I., and Sheppe, W. M. 1959. The psychiatric examination. *In* Arieti, S. (Editor). American Handbook of Psychiatry. New York, Basic Books.

Stewart, A. H., Weiland, I. H., Leider, A. R., Mangham, C. A., Holmes, T. H., and Ripley, H. S. 1954. Excessive infant crying (colic) in relation to parent behavior. Amer. J. Psychiat., *110*:687–694.

Stott, D. H. 1962. Abnormal mothering as a cause of mental subnormality. I.Q. critique of some classic studies of maternal deprivation in the light of possible congenital factors. J. Child Psychol. Psychiat., *3*:79–91.

Stott, D. H. 1962. Evidence for a congenital factor in maladjustment and delinquency. Amer. J. Psychiat., *118*:781–794.

Stott, D. H. 1959. Infantile illness and subsequent mental and emotional development. J. Genet. Psychol. *94*:233–251.

Strauss, A. A. 1939. Typology in mental deficiency. Proc. Amer. Assoc. Ment. Defic., *44*:85–90.

Strauss, A. A., and Kephart, N. C. 1955. Psychopathology and Education of the Brain-Injured Child. New York, Grune & Stratton, Inc.

Strauss, A. A., and Lehtinen, L. E. 1947. Psychopathology and Education of the Brain-Injured Child. New York, Grune & Stratton, Inc.

Strauss, H. 1959. Epileptic disorders. *In* Arieti, S. (Editor). American Handbook of Psychiatry. New York, Basic Books.

Strecker, E. A. 1941. Chronic alcoholism: A psychological survey. Quart. J. Stud. Alcohol, *3*:12–17.

Strömgren, E. 1950. Statistical and genetical population studies within psychiatry, methods and principal results. *In*

Congrès International de Psychiatrie, Paris, 1950. VI. Psychiatrie Sociale Génétique et Eugénique. Paris, Hermann et Cie.

Strupp, H. H. 1957. Freud and Modern Psychoanalysis. Woodbury, New York, Barron's Educational Series, Inc.

Strupp, H. H. 1960. Psychotherapists in Action: Explorations of the Therapist's Contribution to the Treatment Process. New York, Grune & Stratton, Inc.

Strupp, H. H. 1971. Psychotherapy and the Modification of Abnormal Behavior. New York, McGraw-Hill.

Strupp, H., Fox, R., and Lessler, K. 1969. Patients View Their Psychotherapy. Baltimore, Johns Hopkins Press.

Strupp, H., and Bergin, A. 1969. Some empirical and conceptual bases for coordinated research in psychotherapy: A critical review of issues, trends, and evidence. Int. J. Psychiat., 7:18–90.

Sullivan, H. S. 1947. Conceptions of Modern Psychiatry, Washington, D.C., William Alanson White Psychiatric Foundation.

Sullivan, H. S. 1953. The Interpersonal Theory of Psychiatry. New York, W. W. Norton & Co.

Suter, C. 1952. Psychological Factors in Epilepsy. Neuropsychiatry. Vol. 3, No. 3.

Suttenfield, V. 1954. School phobia: a study of five cases. Amer. J. Orthopsychiat., 24:368–380.

Taggart, S. R., Russell, S. B., and Price, E. V. 1956. Report of syphilis follow-up program among veterans after World War II. J. Chron. Dis., 4:579–588.

Takala, A. 1960. Child-rearing practices and attitudes as measured by different techniques: II. Child-rearing practices and attitudes in different social environments. Acta Acad. Paedogogical Jyvasky Iaensis, 19:77–152.

Thigpen, C. H., and Cleckley, H. M. 1957. The Three Faces of Eve. Reprinted 1961. New York, Popular Library, No. SP 117.

Thompson, G. N. 1959. Acute and chronic alcoholic conditions. In Arieti, S. (Editor). American Handbook of Psychiatry. New York, Basic Books.

Thompson, W. R. 1954. The inheritance and development of intelligence. In Hooker, D., and Hare, C. C. (Editors). Genetics and the Inheritance of Integrated Neurological and Psychiatric Patterns. Research Publication, Assoc. Res. Nerv. Ment. Dis., Vol. 33. Baltimore, The Williams & Wilkins Co.

Thorne, F. C. 1950. Principles of Personality Counseling. Brandon, Vermont, Journal of Clinical Psychology.

Tietze, T. 1959. A study of mothers of schizophrenic patients. Psychiatry, 12:55–65.

Tillich, P. 1952. The Courage to Be. New Haven, Yale University Press.

Tizard, B. 1962. The personality of epileptics: a discussion of the evidence. Psychol. Bull., 59:196–210.

Tomlinson, P. 1948. Subcoma insulin therapy: an analysis of 300 cases. Psychiat. Quart., 22:609–620.

Toverud, K. U., Stearns, G., and Macy, I. G. 1950. Maternal Nutrition and Child Health: An Interpretative Review. Washington, D.C., National Research Council, Bulletin 123.

Travis, J. H. 1933. Precipitating factors in manic depressive psychoses. Psychiat. Quart. 7:411–418.

Tredgold, A. S., and Soddy, K. 1963. A Textbook of Mental Deficiency, 10th Ed. Baltimore, The Williams & Wilkins Co.

Trouton, D., and Eysenck, H. J. 1960. The effects of drugs on behavior. In Eysenck, H. J. (Editor). Handbook of Abnormal Psychology. London, Pitman Medical Publishing Co.

Truax, C. and Carkhuff, R. 1967. Toward Effective Counseling and Psychotherapy: Training and Practice. Chicago, Aldine Press.

Truax, C., Silber, L., and Wargo, D. 1966. Effects of group psychotherapy with high accurate empathy and nonpossesive warmth upon female institutionalized delinquents. J. Abnorm. Psychol., 71:267–274.

Tryon, R. C. 1942. Individual differences. In Moss, F. A. (Editor). Comparative Psychology. New York, Prentice-Hall, Inc.

Tuckman, J., and Connor, H. 1962. Attempted suicide in adolescents. Amer. J. Psychiat., 119:228–232.

Tuckman, J., and Regan, R. 1966. Intactness of the home and behavioral problems in children. J. Child. Psychol. Psychiat. 7:225–233.

Tuckman, J., and Youngman, W. 1968. A scale for assessing suicide risk of attempted suicides. J. Clin. Psychol., 24:17–19.

Tulchin, S. H. 1939. Intelligence and Crime. Chicago, The University of Chicago Press.

Turnbull, E. P. N., and Baird, D. 1957. Maternal age and foetal oxygenation. Brit. Med. J., 2(2):1021–1024.

Tutko, T. A., and Spence, J. T. 1962. The performance of process and reactive schizophrenics and brain injured subjects on a conceptual task. J. Abnorm. Soc. Psychol. 65:387–394.

Tyler, L. E. 1956. The Psychology of Human Differences. New York, Appleton-Century-Crofts, Inc.

Uhr, L., and Miller, J. G. (Editors). 1960. Drugs and Behavior. New York, John Wiley & Sons, Inc.

Ullman, A. D. 1958. Sociocultural backgrounds of alcoholism. Ann. Amer. Acad. Polit. Soc. Sci., 315:48–54.

United States Department of Commerce. 1958. Current Population Reports. Illustrative Projections of the Population of the United States, by Age and Sex, 1960–1980. Washington, D.C., Bureau of the Census. Series P-25, No. 187.

United States Public Health Service, 1966. Minimal Brain Dysfunction in Children. Terminology and Identification. No. 1415.

Vandenberg, S. G. 1962. The hereditary abilities study: hereditary components in a psychological test battery. Amer. J. Hum. Genet. 14:220–237.

Vandenberg, S. G. 1962. Psychophysiological Reactions of Twins: Heritability, Estimates of PGR, Heart Beat and Breathing Rates. Paper presented at Annual Meeting of American Society of Human Genetics, August, 1962.

Vigotsky, L. S. 1934. Thought in schizophrenia. A.M.A. Arch. Neurol. Psychiat., 31:1063–1077.

Vogel, V. H., and Vogel, V. E. 1951. Facts About Narcotics. Chicago, Science Research Associates, Guidance Series Booklet No. 121.

Wallach, M. A., and Greenberg, C. 1960. Personality Functions of Symbolic Sexual Arousal to Music. Psychol. Monogr., No. 7, Vol. 74.

Wallerstein, R. 1968. The challenge of the community mental health movement to psychoanalysis. Amer. J. Psychiat. 124:1049–1056.

Wallin, J. E. W. 1955. Education of Mentally Handicapped Children. New York, Harper & Bros.

Wallin, J. E. W. 1956. Mental Deficiency in Relation to Problems of Genesis, Social and Occupational Consequences, Utilization, Control and Prevention. Brandon, Vermont, Journal of Clinical Psychology.

Wanklin, J. M., Buck, C. W., and Hobbs, G. E. 1956. The distribution of mental disease. Ment. Hyg. 40:275–282.

Watson, J. B., and Raynor, R. 1920. Conditioned emotional reaction. J. Exp. Psychol., 3:1–4.

Wattenberg, W. W. 1954. Factors associated with repeating among pre-adolescent delinquents. J. Genet. Psychol., 84:189–195.

Weakland, J. H. 1960. The "double bind" hypothesis of schizophrenia and three-party interaction. In Jackson, D. D. (Editor). The Etiology of Schizophrenia. New York, Basic Books.

Weakland, J. H., and Fry, W. F. 1962. Letters of mothers of schizophrenics. Amer. J. Orthopsychiat., 32:604–623.

Weaver, T. R. 1946. The incidence of maladjustment among mental defectives in military environment. Amer. J. Ment. Defic., 51:238–246.

Webb, W. B. 1969. Partial and differential sleep deprivation. In Kales, A. (Ed.) Sleep: Physiology and Pathology. Philadelphia, J. B. Lippincott.

Wechsler, I. 1963. Clinical Neurology, 9th Ed. Philadelphia, W. B. Saunders Co.

Wechsler, D. 1955. Manual for the Wechsler Adult Intelligence Scale. New York, The Psychological Corporation.

Wechsler, D. 1944. The Measurement of Adult Intelligence, 3rd Ed. Baltimore, The Williams & Wilkins Co.

Wechsler, D. 1949. Wechsler Intelligence Scale for Children (Manual). New York, The Psychological Corporation.

Weil, W. F. 1953. Clinical data and dynamic considerations in certain cases of childhood schizophrenia. Amer. J. Orthopsychiat., 23:518–527.

Weinberg, S. K. 1955. Incest Behavior. New York, Citadel Press.

Weinberg, S. K. 1952. Society and Personality Disorders. New York, Prentice-Hall, Inc.

Weiner, H., Thaler, M., Reiser, M. F., and Mirsky, I. A. 1957. Etiology of duodenal ulcer. I. Relation of specific psychological characteristics to rate of gastric secretion (serum pepsinogen). Psychosom. Med. 19:1–10.

Weinstein, E. A. 1962. Cultural Aspects of Delusion: A Psychiatric Study of the Virgin Islands. Glencoe, Ill., The Free Press.

Weiss, E., and English, O. S. 1957. Psychosomatic Medicine, 3rd Ed. Philadelphia, W. B. Saunders Co.

West, L. J. (Editor). 1962. Hallucinations. New York, Grune & Stratton, Inc.

West, L. J., and Greenblatt, M. (Editors). 1960. Explorations in the Physiology of Emotions. Washington, D.C., American Psychiatric Association, Psychiatric Research Reports No. 12.

Westwood, G. 1960. A Minority—A Report on the Life of the Male Homosexual in Great Britain. London, Longmans, Green and Co.

Weybrew, B. D., and Parker, J. W. 1960. Bibliography of Sensory Deprivation, Isolation and Confinement. New London, Connecticut, U.S. Naval Medical Research Laboratory, Memorandum Report No. 60–1.

Weyer, J. 1579. Histoires, Disputes et Discours des Illusions et Impostures des Diables, des Magiciens Infames, Sorciers et Empoisonneurs. Reprinted 1885. Paris, Aux Bureaux du Progès Médical.

Wheeler, L. R. 1942. A comparative study of the intelligence of East Tennessee mountain children. J. Educ. Psychol., 33:321–334.

Wheeler, L. R. 1932. The intelligence of East Tennessee mountain children. J. Educ. Psychol., 23:351–370.

White, W. A. 1926. The language of schizophrenia. A.M.A. Arch. Neurol. Psychiat., 16:395–413.

Whitehorn, J. C. 1956. The healthful benefits of stress. J. Chron. Dis., 4:646–647.

Whitehorn, J., and Betz, B. 1960. Further studies of the doctor as a crucial variable in the outcome of treatment with schizophrenic patients. Amer. J. Psychiat., 117:215–223.

Wildenskov, H. O. 1934. Investigations into the Causes of Mental Deficiency. Copenhagen, Munksgaard and London, Humphrey Milford.

Wilkins, L. 1962. The effects of thyroid deficiency upon the development of the brain. In Kolb, L. C., Masland, R. L., and Cooke, R. E. (Editors). Mental Retardation. Baltimore, The Williams & Wilkins Co. Research Publication, Assoc. Res. Nerv. Ment. Dis., 39:150–158.

Williams, R. J. 1956. Biochemical Individuality. New York, John Wiley & Sons, Inc.

Williams, R. J. 1947. The etiology of alcoholism: A working hypothesis involving the interplay of heredity and environmental factors. Quart. J. Stud. Alcohol, 7:567–587.

Williams, R. J., et al. 1957. Identification of blood characteristics common to alcoholic males. Science, 126:1237.

Williams, W. S., and Jaco, E. G. 1958. An evaluation of functional psychosis in old age. Amer. J. Psychiat., 114:910–916.

Williams, W. S., and Jaco, E. G. 1957. A re-examination of mental illness in old age. Dis. Nerv. Sys., 18:375–379.

Wilson, J. G. 1959. Experimental studies on congenital malformations. J. Chron. Dis., 10:111–130.

Windle, W. F. 1952. Anoxia: its effects on structure of the brain. In The Biology of Mental Health and Disease. New York, Hoeber-Harper.

Windle, W. F., et al. 1962. Structural and Functional Sequelae of Asphyxia Neonatorum in Monkeys. In Kolb, L. C., Masland, R. L., and Cooke, R. E. (Editors). Mental Retardation. Baltimore, The Williams & Wilkins Co. Research Publication, Assoc. Res. Nerv. Ment. Dis., 39:169–182.

Wing, J. 1962. Institutionalism in mental hospitals. Brit. J. Soc. Clin. Psychol. 1:38–51.

Wirt, R. D., and Briggs, P. F. 1959. Personality and Environmental Factors in the Development of Delinquency. Psychol. Monogr. Vol. 73, No. 15.

Witmer, H. L., Hertzog, E., Weinstein, E. A., and Sullivan, M. E. 1963. Independent Adoptions: A Follow-up Study. New York, Russell Sage Foundation.

Wittkower, E. D., and Cleghorn, R. A. (Editors). 1954. Recent Developments in Psychosomatic Medicine. Philadelphia, J. B. Lippincott Co.

Wittkower, E. D., and Fried, J. 1959. A cross-cultural approach to mental health problems. Amer. J. Psychiat. 116:423–428.

Wittman, P., Sheldon, W. H., and Katz, C. J. 1948. A study of the relationship between constitutional variations and fundamental psychotic behavior reactions. J. Nerv. Ment. Dis., 108:470–476.

Wolberg, L. R. 1947. Hypnotic experiments in psychosomatic medicine. Psychosom. Med., 9:337–342.

Wolberg, L. R. 1954. The Technique of Psychotherapy. New York, Grune & Stratton, Inc.

Wolf, I., Sacks, J. M., and Mason, A. S. 1959. A research treatment program for geriatric mental patients. J. Gerontol., 14:469–472.

Wolf, S., and Wolff, H. G. 1942. Evidence on the genesis of peptic ulcer in man. J.A.M.A., 120:670–675.

Wolf, S., and Wolff, H. G. 1953. Headaches: Their Nature and Treatment. Boston, Little, Brown, and Co.

Wolf, S., and Wolff, H. G. 1947. Human Gastric Function: An Experimental Study of a Man and His Stomach. New York, Oxford University Press.

Wolfenden, J. 1963. The Wolfenden Report. New York, Stein and Day.

Wolff, G. E. 1959. Geriatric mental patients and how we can help them. Geriatrics, *14*:94–98.

Wolff, G. E. 1957. Results of four years of active therapy for chronic mental patients and the value of an individual maintenance dose of ECT. Amer. J. Psychiat., *114*:453–456.

Wolfgang, M. E., Savitz, L., and Johnston, N. (Editors). 1962. The Sociology of Crime and Delinquency. New York, John Wiley & Sons, Inc.

Wolking, W. D., Quast, W., and Lawton, J. J., Jr. 1964. MMPI profiles of the parents of behaviorally disturbed and non-disturbed children. Paper presented at American Psychological Association meetings, Sept. 1964.

Wolpe, J. 1952. Experimental neurosis as learned behavior. Brit. J. Psychol., *43*:243–268.

Wolpe, J. 1958. Psychotherapy by Reciprocal Inhibition. Stanford, Calif., Stanford University Press.

Woodward, S. B. 1855. Twenty-second Annual Report. Boston, Mass.

Woodworth, R. S. 1941. Heredity and Environment. New York, Social Science Research Council, Bulletin 47.

Woollam, D. H., and Millen, J. W. 1956. Role of vitamins in embryonic development. Brit. Med. J., *1*(2):1262–1265.

World Health Organization. 1962. Deprivation of Maternal Care: A Reassessment of Its Effects. Public Health Papers No. 14. Geneva, W.H.O.

World Health Organization, 1967. Manual of the International Statistical Classification of Diseases, Inquiries, and Causes of Death: Based on Recommendations of the Eighth Conference, 1965 and Adapted by the Nineteenth World Health Assembly, Vol. 1, Geneva, W.H.O.

World Health Organization. 1959. Mental Problems of Aging and the Aged. Report of the Expert Committee on Mental Health, Geneva, W.H.O.

World Health Organization. 1954. The Mentally Subnormal Child. Technical Report Series No. 75. Geneva, W.H.O.

World Health Organization. 1950–1955. Technical Report Series Nos. 19, 21, 42, 48, 57, 76, 84, 94, 95. Geneva, W.H.O.

Wortis, J. (Editor). 1960. Recent Advances in Biological Psychiatry. New York, Grune & Stratton, Inc.

Yolles, S. 1969. Mental Health's Homeostatic State. A new territory. Int. J. Psychiat. *7*:327–332.

Zahn, T. P. 1960. Size estimation of pictures associated with success and failure as a function of manifest anxiety. J. Abnorm. Soc. Psychol., *61*:457–462.

Zeleny, L. D. 1931. A Comparative Study of the Investigations of Intelligence of Criminals: U.S., 1910–1930. Unpublished doctoral dissertation, University of Minnesota.

Zeller, A. 1951. An experimental analogue of repression: III. The effect of induced failure and success on memory measured by recall. J. Exp. Psychol., *42*:32–38.

Zigler, E., and Phillips, L. 1961. Social competence and outcome in psychiatric disorder. J. Abnorm. Soc. Psychol., *63*:264–271.

Zigler, E., and Phillips, L. 1962. Social competence and the process-reactive distinction in psychopathology. J. Abnorm. Soc. Psychol., *65*:215–222.

Zilboorg, G., and Henry, G. W. 1941. A History of Medical Psychology. New York, W. W. Norton & Co.

Zubek, J. P., et al. Canad. J. Psychol., 1963, *17*, 118.

Zubin, J. 1967. Classification of the behavior disorders. Annual Review of Psychology, *18*:373–406.

Zubin, J., Sutton, S., Salzinger, K., Salzinger, S., Burdock, E., and Peretz, D. 1961. A biometric approach to prognosis in schizophrenia. *In* Hoch, P., and Zorbin, J. (Editors). Comparative Epidemiology in the Mental Disorders. New York, Grune & Stratton, Inc.

Zuckerman, M., Oltean, M., and Monashkin, I. 1958. The parental attitudes of the mothers of schizophrenics. J. Consult. Psychol., *22*:307–310.

Zuckerman, M., Ribback, B. B., Monashkin, I., and Norton, J. A. 1958. Normative data and factor analysis on the parental attitude research instrument. J. Consult. Psychol., *22*:165–171.

Zwerling, I., and Rosenbaum, M. 1959. Alcoholic addiction and personality. *In* Arieti, S. (Editor). American Handbook of Psychiatry. New York, Basic Books.

NAME INDEX

See also Selected References on page 481.

Abraham, K., 203, 311
Ackerman, N., 456
Ackerman, N. W., 409
Adler, A., 30, 310
Aichhorn, A., 271
Alexander, F., 185, 186, 352, 443
Allen, F. H., 449, 455
Allport, G. W., 42
Alzheimer, A., 330, 331
Amark, C., 308
Anastasi, A., 369
Andry, R. G., 405
Angus, L. R., 363
Apperson, L., 295
Aretaeus, 192
Arieti, S., 130, 196, 207, 223, 234, 240, 242
Asclepiades, 21, 31
Asher, E. J., 376
Auerbach, A. H., 343
Ayd, F. J., Jr., 86, 195, 196

Babigian, H., 47
Bachrach, A., 447
Bacon, M. K., 269
Bacon, S. D., 304
Bagnara, J. T., 172
Baird, D., 371
Baker, F., 467
Baldwin, A., 121
Bales, R. F., 314
Balian, L., 236
Baller, W. R., 365, 378
Bandura, A., 264, 459
Banta, T. J., 367
Bard, M., 470
Barry, H., 117, 269
Barthell, C., 234
Bateson, G., 239
Beach, F. A., 292
Beatman, F., 456
Becker, W. C., 122, 205
Beckett, P. G., 121, 233
Beers, C., 30
Beier, E. G., 373

Bell, J. E., 409
Benda, C. E., 360
Bender, L., 295, 396, 403
Benedict, P. K., 240
Berenson, B. G., 453
Bergin, A., 458, 459
Bernard, C., 90
Bernheim, H. M., 28
Berry, J., 466
Bettelheim, B., 409
Betz, B., 459
Bexton, W. H., 114
Bieber, I., 295
Binet, A., 383
Birch, J., 356, 357
Blacker, K., 87
Blackwell, B., 86
Bleuler, E., *27*, 213, 214, 215, 216, 220
Bleuler, M., 308, 311
Blum, R., 322
Böök, J. A., 364
Bovet, L., 408
Bowen, M., 238, 395
Bowlby, J., 405
Bowman, K., 342
Boyles, P. D., 471
Bradley, C., 395
Bradway, K. P., 369
Brady, J. V., 106, 107, 186
Braid, J., 28
Brancale, R., 275
Bray, D. W., 375
Breed, N., 206
Breger, L., 68
Breuer, J., 29
Brill, H., 322
Bromberg, W., 365
Bronner, A., 365, 379
Bronson, W. C., 295
Brown, A. W., 376
Brown, F., 117, 405
Brown, F. W., 83, 84, 162
Brown, W., 204
Browne, W. A. F., 135
Bruetsch, W. L., 332, 333, 339
Bruhn, J. G., 204

Buck, C., 184
Buell, B., 139
Buhler, C., 10
Burgess, E. W., 128
Burks, B. S., 377
Burlingham, D. T., 111
Burney, C., 114
Burrows, G., 135
Burt, C., 81
Burton, R. F., 202
Busse, E. W., 343, 344, 353
Byrd, R. E., 114
Byrum, M., 405

Cabeen, C. W., 298
Cameron, D. E., 12, 443
Cameron, N., 12, 215, 245, 246
Camus, A., 64
Cannon, W. B., 90
Carkhuff, R., 453, 458
Carothers, J. C., 135
Carrier, N. A., 362
Carroll, E. E., 407
Carter, M. P., 268
Casey, J. F., 431
Castaneda, A., 362
Caveness, W. F., 344
Celsus, A. C., 26
Chapanis, A., 376
Chapman, L. F., 328
Charcot, J. M., 28
Charles, D. C., 365, 378
Chein, I., 321
Child, I. L., 116, 269
Christmas, J., 470
Christoffel, H., 278
Clausen, J. A., 206, 235, 238, 319, 320
Cleckley, H., 155, 255, 256, 257, 270
Cleland, C. C., 362
Cochran, I. L., 362
Cohen, A. K., 267
Cohen, C., 243
Cohen, G. B., 205
Colby, K. M., 452
Coleman, J. C., 298
Conger, J. J., 310
Connor, H., 206
Conrad, K., 342
Coppen, A. J., 97, 292
Cormier, B. M., 288
Cornelison, A., 238
Cowen, E. L., 379
Crawshaw, R. S., 353
Cressler, L., 471
Cronback, L. J., 417

Darling, H. F., 269
Davis, W. A., 406
Dekaban, A. S., 371
D'Elia, E., 243
Democritus, 202
de Sade, Marquis, 281
DeSanctis, S., 395
Despert, J. L., 236, 395, 396

Dewan, J. G., 335, 343
DiMichael, S. G., 379
Diogenes, 449
Diven, K., 58
Dix, D., 26, 27
Dollard, J., 105
Doorbar, R., 275
Dorcus, R. M., 153
Doust, J. W. L., 98, 232, 233
DuBois, P., 450
Dunaif, S. L., 229
Dunham, H. W., 142, 208
Dunn, W. L., Jr., 235

Eaton, J. W., 136, 207
Edmonson, M. S., 269
Edwards, A. S., 376
Ehrenberg, R., 344, 350
Eisenberg, L., 395, 396
Eisler, F., 204
Ellis, A., 270, 275
Engel, G. L., 177
English, O. S., 179
Epps, P., 205
Erikson, E. H., 32, 52, 53, 54, 55, 63
Erwin, W., 447
Estes, H. R., 393
Ewing, J., 311
Eysenck, H. J., 66, 67, 68, 162, 163, 201, 202, 459, 460

Fager, R. E., 11
Fairweather, G., 471
Falret, J. P., 192
Farber, I. E., 115
Farina, A., 238
Faris, E., 135
Faris, R. E. L., 142, 208
Fechtel, C., 327
Feffer, M. H., 235
Feldhausen, J. F., 362
Fenichel, O., 58, 149, 167, 265, 293, 311, 439
Fielding, H., 303
Fillmore, E. A., 376
Fisher, C., 90
Fleck, S., 237, 238
Fonda, C., 47
Fontana, A., 235
Ford, C. S., 292
Foucault, M., 24
Fouls, L. B., 295
Fox, R., 147, 311, 453, 460
Franck, K., 422
Frank, J. D., 455, 460
Frank, L. K., 128
Frankl, V., 64
Franks, C. M., 385
Franks, J., 185
Freedman, A. M., 381
Freeman, D., 350
Freeman, F. N., 377
Freeman, S. N., 376
Fremming, K. H., 132, 134
French, I., 443
French, L. A., 338

French, T., 185
Freud, A., 111, 454
Freud, S., 12, 28, 29, 32, 51, 52, 55, 56, 57, 58, 63, 64, 163, 164, 166, 203, 216, 234, 250, 273, 275, 276, 283, 293, 297, 310, 352, 443, 446
Freund, K., 297
Friedman, A., 194
Fromm, E., 68, 147
Fromm-Reichmann, F., 52, 147, 234
Frumkin, R., 140
Fry, W. F., 239
Fuller, J. L., 79, 84, 162
Funkenstein, D. H., 163

Galen, 21, 22, 32
Gallagher, J. J., 367
Gallinek, A., 350
Garmezy, N., 230, 235, 238
Garner, A. M., 185
Gellhorn, E., 162
Gerard, D. L., 237, 241, 315, 321
Gesell, A., 384
Gibby, R. B., 374
Gibson, R. W., 205
Gilbert, J. A., 88
Ginzberg, E., 375
Glickman, S., 236
Glueck, B. C. Jr., 275
Glueck, E., 263, 265, 365, 404, 405
Glueck, S., 263, 265, 273, 282, 288, 294, 296, 365, 404, 405
Goddard, H. H., 365, 368
Goldberg, E., 241
Goldberg, T. B., 393
Goldfarb, A. I., 344, 353
Goldfarb, W., 117, 395, 403
Goldhamer, H., 136
Goldman-Eisler, F., 116, 204
Goldstein, K., 367, 419
Goldstein, M. J., 290
Good, W. W., 431
Goodstein, L. D., 405
Gordon, H., 268, 376
Gorlow, L., 373
Gottesman, I., 79, 81, 83, 232
Grace, W. J., 175
Graham, D. T., 175
Gralnick, A., 250
Grayson, H. M., 243
Green, E., 269
Green, R., 290
Greenberg, C., 150
Greenfield, N. S., 123, 164
Greenwald, H., 258, 270
Gregory, I., 117, 149, 162, 232, 264, 265
Griesinger, W., 24, 25
Guilleband Report, 345
Gullingsrud, M. J. O., 350
Gunzberg, H. C., 379

Hall, S. B., 195
Halliday, A., 134
Halliday, J. L., 187
Halperin, S. L., 369

Hamilton, M., 183
Hammer, E. F., 275, 294
Hampson, J. L., 294
Hanvik, L. J., 405
Hare, E. H., 241
Harlow, H. F., 119, 120, 121, 234, 293, 404, 406
Harrell, R. F., 372
Hartman, A., 293
Hartmann, H., 32
Hathaway, S. R., 268
Havighurst, R. J., 407
Hazell, K., 345
Healy, W., 365, 379
Hebb, D. O., 113, 114, 356
Hederra, A. D., 309
Helfand, I., 220
Hendrick, I., 270
Henry, T. R., 140
Heron, W., 113, 114
Herskovitz, H. H., 264
Hess, E., 285
Heston, L., 232
Hetherington, E. M., 367
Higgins, J. V., 379
Hilgard, E. R., 101, 170
Hill, D., 264
Hinko, E., 435
Hippocrates, 20, 32
Hirschfeld, M., 279, 282, 283, 291
Hirsh, J., 197
Hobbs, G. E., 184
Hoch, P. H., 204, 229, 431, 433, 435
Hofmann, A., 86
Hollingshead, A. B., 13, 140, 166, 208, 241, 268, 345
Holmes, O. W., 234, 380
Holtzman, W., 431
Holway, A. R., 116
Holzinger, K., 163, 376, 377
Hood, A., 97
Horney, K., 30, 68, 129
Horton, D., 314
Horwitt, M. K., 233
Houston, L. G., 241
Howard, A., 122
Howard, M., 81
Howells, J. G., 409, 410
Hull, C. L., 66
Huntington, G., 339
Huschka, M., 118
Hutt, M. L., 374

Inouye, E., 232
Itard, J. M. G., 355

Jacks, I., 240
Jackson, C., 304
Jackson, D., 456
Jackson, J. H., 338
Jaco, E. G., 345, 349, 351
James, I., 197
Janet, P., 28, 151
Jarvik, L. F., 343
Jellinek, E. M., 304, 315
Jenkins, R., 236, 436

Jenness, A. R., 150
Jephcott, P., 268
Jervis, G. A., 371
Johnson, A. M., 116, 266, 295, 393, 405, 406
Johnson, L. C., 88
Johnson, S., 58
Johnson, Samuel, 302
Jolly, D. H., 342
Jones, D., 195
Jones, L., 376
Jones, M., 271
Juda, A., 366
Judd, L. L., 290
Jung, C. G., 30, 68, 214

Kaij, L., 308
Kalinowsky, L. B., 433, 435
Kallmann, F. J., 201, 202, 231, 291, 343, 368, 403
Kanner, L., 123, 373, 374, 380, 383, 384, 387, 395, 396, 405, 407
Kant, H. S., 290
Kaplan, J., 318, 322
Kaplan, S. D., 203
Kardiner, A., 129
Karpinski, E., 289
Karpman, B., 273
Kasanin, J., 236
Katz, S., 93, 232
Kawi, A. A., 403
Kay, D. W. K., 251
Kemp, T., 380
Kennedy, R. J. R., 379
Kennedy, W. A., 394
Kephart, N. C., 367
Kestenberg, J. S., 396
Keys, A., 87, 88
Kierkegaard, S., 64
Kiernan, I., 266
King, G. F., 230, 263
Kinsey, A. C., 277, 284, 288
Kirsner, J., 176
Klaber, M. M., 180
Klatskin, E. H., 407
Klausmeier, H. J., 362
Klein, E., 235
Klein, M., 454
Kline, N. S., 74
Knapp, P. H., 175, 318
Knight, R. P., 236, 311
Knobloch, H., 371, 381
Knopf, I. J., 11
Kohn, M. L., 206, 235, 238, 407
Kolb, L. C., 180, 198, 295
Koppitz, E., 420
Koranyi, E. K., 92
Kornetsky, C., 321
Kraemer, H., 23
Kraepelin, E., 24, 25, 26, 192, 204, 213, 221, 245
Kraines, S. H., 197
Krasner, L., 66, 448
Kretschmer, E., 92, 93, 202
Kris, E., 32
Kvaraceus, W. C., 365

Lander, B., 267
Landis, C., 164
Lansing, C., 408
Larsson, T., 132, 191, 364
Lavin, N. I., 297
Leahy, A. M., 377
Lehmann, H. E., 92
Lehmann, S., 466
Lehrman, N., 466
Lehtinen, L. E., 367
Leighton, A. H., 128, 267, 320
Lejeune, J., 369, 370
Lennox, W. G., 342, 400, 401
LeShan, E., 352
LeShan, L., 352
Lessler, K., 147, 453, 460
Levin, H., 110
Levin, S., 197
Levine, M., 264, 448
Levine, S., 121
Levy, D. M., 110, 454
Lichtenstein, M., 376
Liddell, H. S., 106, 111, 112
Liddell, N. S., 66
Lidz, R. W., 237, 238
Lidz, T., 169, 237
Liébault, A. A., 28
Lifton, R. J., 115
Lindemann, E., 117
Lindner, R., 270, 281
Lippman, H. S., 392
Lipschutz, L., 435
Liverant, S., 122, 405
Lorr, M., 417
Luby, E. D., 90, 233
Lucas, C. J., 251
Lykken, D. T., 104, 158, 266

McAdoo, W., 295
McCandless, B., 294
McCord, J., 122, 255
McCord, W., 122, 255
McCurdy, H., 113, 122
McFarland, R. A., 89, 92
McGaugh, J., 68
McGhie, A., 237
McGlashan, A., 205
McIntosh, W. J., 379
McKay, H. D., 267
Maas, H. S., 386
Maccoby, E. E., 110
Macfarlane, J. W., 386
MacIver. R., 256
Maclean, N., 370
Mahrer, A., 467
Maier, N. R. F., 109
Malinowski, B., 135, 296
Malzberg, B., 137, 435
Mardones, R. J., 309
Mark, J. C., 237
Marks, P. A., 384, 386, 405
Marmor, J., 115
Marshall, A. W., 136

Maslow, A., 10
Masserman, J. H., 59, 60, 106, 107, 108, 109, 247, 310, 327
Mawrer, H., 68
May, R., 64, 65
Mayer-Gross, W., 224, 344
Maynard, H., 471
Mednick, S., 185
Meduna, L. Von, 432
Meehl, P. E., 103, 214, 218
Meier, M. J., 338
Menninger, K. A., 311
Mensh, I. N., 349
Mesmer, F. A., 28
Mesnikoff, A. M., 295
Meth, J. M., 130
Meyer, A., 31
Meyer, R., 468
Miller, C. W., 250
Miller, D. R., 151
Miller, N., 58
Miller, N. E., 105
Mitchell, B. C., 377
Mohr, J. W., 278, 287, 447
Monachesi, E. D., 268
Money, J., 294
Morel, B., 213
Morrison, S., 241
Mosher, L., 471
Mower, O. H., 68
Muench, G. A., 379
Munroe, M., 402
Murphy, J. M., 128, 130
Murray, E. J., 243
Murray, H. A., 43
Myers, J. K., 141

Neel, J. V., 79, 80, 82, 379
Nelson, W. E., 359, 361
Nemetz, S. J., 175
Nemiah, J. C., 48, 203
Netter, F. H., 195, 196
Neuer, H., 363
Neumann, H., 47
Newman, H. H., 376
Newringer, C., 197
Nicoloy, R., 293
Norris, V., 48, 197
Norton, A., 164

O'Connor, J., 188
O'Connor, N., 379, 385
Offer, D., 10
Olds, J., 103, 322
Olinger, L. B., 243
Olson, G., 431
O'Neal, P., 262, 263, 265, 410
O'Neill, F. J., 350
Opler, M. K., 13
Orlinsky, N., 243
Osmond, H., 86

Palmai, G., 268
Parker, J., 205
Pasamanick, B., 47, 381, 403
Paster, S., 295
Paterson, D. G., 369
Patrick, G. T. W., 88
Paul, G., 459
Pavlov, I. P., 30, 66, 102, 105, 445, 446
Penrose, L. S., 97, 363, 364, 368, 369, 370
Pescor, M. J., 321
Pestalozzi, J. H., 383
Peters, H. N., 436
Peterson, D., 431
Peterson, D. R., 122
Peterson, L., 365
Peterson, L. V., 353
Phillips, L., 143, 230
Pick, A., 331
Pickering, G. W., 183
Pinel, P., 26
Pinneau, S. R., 111
Pittman, F., 468
Plato, 21
Plutarch, 21
Pokorny, A. D., 197
Polatin, P., 229
Pollock, H. M., 363
Popham, R. E., 314, 315
Porter, M., 266
Porteus, S. D., 436
Prell, D. B., 162
Prichard, J. C., 256
Prince, M., 156
Pritchard, M., 291, 430
Pumpian-Mindlin, E., 115

Querido, A., 469

Rado, S., 68, 192, 198, 203, 204, 218, 310, 322
Randell, J. B., 279
Rank, O., 68
Rapaport, D., 63
Raskin, N., 344
Rechtshaffen, A., 352
Redlich, F. C., 13, 140, 166, 208, 241, 268, 345
Reed, E. W., 367, 375
Reed, S. C., 367, 375
Rees, L., 163, 232, 241
Regan, R., 405
Reichard, S., 237
Rennie, P. A. C., 193
Ribble, M., 110
Rice, C. J., 290
Rice, L., 459
Rimland, B., 403
Ritter, C., 114
Rizzo, G., 136
Roach, J. L., 386
Robbins, S. L., 340
Roberts, J. A. F., 141, 182, 183, 368, 369
Robins, E., 197, 263

Robins, L. N., 410
Rodnick, E. H., 230, 235, 238
Roe, A., 309
Rogers, C., 10, 444
Rogers, C. R., 446
Rohrer, J. H., 269
Rorschach, H., 420
Rosanoff, A. J., 263, 342, 366
Rosen, E., 136, 245, 246, 422
Rosen, G., 131, 351
Rosenthal, D., 231
Rosenthal, H. R., 352, 353
Rosenzweig, S., 460
Roth, M., 224, 251, 349, 403
Rothschild, D., 343
Roueché, B., 202
Rowley, V. N., 405
Ruesch, J., 184, 342
Rundquist, E. A., 369
Rush, B., 26, 138
Ryan, J., 467

Sabshin, M., 10
Saenger, G., 315
Sage, p., 236
Sakel, M., 434
Salzman, L., 434
Sanddal, J. W., 269
Sanders, D., 471
Sarason, S. B., 367, 379
Sartre, J. P., 64
Scarpitti, F. R., 267
Scheerer, M., 419
Schilder, P., 234, 311
Schmidt, H. O., 47
Schmidt, W., 314
Schofield, W., 236
Schonbar, R. A., 150
Schuell, H., 329
Schuham, A., 240
Schulberg, H., 467
Schull, W. J., 79, 80, 82, 379
Schwartz, P., 371
Scot, R., 24, 25
Sears, P. S., 116, 294
Sears, R. R., 110, 294, 407
Segovia, N. M., 309
Séguin, E., 355
Seltzer, A., 285
Selye, H., 90, 91, 173
Shaffer, G. W., 153
Shagass, C., 203
Sharp, A., 58
Shaw, C., 267
Shaw, C. R., 262
Shaw, G. B., 141
Shaw, M. W., 370
Sheldon, W. H., 92, 93, 94, 95, 96, 163, 202, 232
Sheps, J., 344, 351, 353
Sherman, M., 140
Sherman, S., 456
Shields, J., 80, 83, 201, 202, 232, 263, 403
Shinfuku, N., 203
Shipley, W. C., 419
Shlien, J., 285
Siegel, J., 237

Silber, L., 270
Silverman, D., 264, 269
Singer, J. L., 13, 150
Sjögren, T., 132, 191, 364
Skeels, H. M., 376
Skinner, B. F., 66, 447
Sklar, J., 350
Slater, E., 80, 201, 202, 224, 231, 263, 403
Sloan, W., 356, 357
Sloane, P., 289
Smith, J. O., 366
Smith, L. L., 365
Smith, T., 467
Smith, W. D., 295
Smythies, J., 86
Soddy, K., 364, 366
Solomon, R. L., 109
Soranus, 21
Sowry, G. S. C., 183
Spaulding, W. B., 335, 343
Speers, R., 408
Spence, J. T., 230
Spiegel, D., 197
Spielberger, C., 205
Spitz, H. H., 367
Spitz, R. A., 111
Spivak, G., 264
Sprenger, J., 23
Srole, L., 131, 141, 142
Stacey, C. L., 373
Stein, M. I., 455
Stephens, E., 374
Sterling, M., 431
Stewart, A. H., 406
Stone, H. K., 185
Stott, D. H., 263, 403
Strauss, A. A., 367
Strauss, H., 414
Strupp, H. H., 147, 453, 458, 459, 460
Sullivan, H. S., 30, 68, 236, 461
Suttenfield, V., 393
Swanson, G. E., 151
Szurek, S. A., 116, 406

Takala, A., 407
Thigpen, C. H., 155
Thompson, C. B., 365
Thompson, G. N., 307
Thompson, W. R., 79, 81, 84, 162
Thorne, F. C., 450
Thurber, J., 62
Tillich, P., 64
Tillman, C., 237
Tizard, B., 338
Toverud, K. U., 371
Travis, J. H., 204
Tredgold, A. S., 364, 366
Truax, C., 270, 458
Tryon, R. C., 81
Tuckman, J., 206, 209, 405
Tuke, W., 26
Tulchin, S. H., 365
Turnbull, E. P. N., 371
Turner, C. D., 172
Tutko, T. A., 230
Twain, M., 304
Tyler, L. E., 377

Ullman, A. D., 314
Ullmann, L., 448

Vandenberg, S. G., 182
Vander Veer, A. H., 247
Vigotsky, L. S., 214
Vives, J. L., 24
von Fellenberg, P. E., 383
von Sacher-Masoch, L., 282

Waldrop, G. S., 471
Wallach, M. A., 150
Wallerstein, R., 470
Wallin, J. E. W., 365
Walters, R., 264
Wargo, D., 270
Wattenberg, W. W., 365
Watterson, D., 264
Weakland, J. H., 239
Weaver, T. R., 363
Webb, W. B., 90
Wechsler, D., 6, 418
Wechsler, I., 331, 360
Weil, R. J., 136
Weil, W. F., 207
Weinberg, S. K., 264, 289, 291
Weiner, H., 186
Weinstein, E. A., 251
Weiss, E., 179
Westwood, G., 295
Weyer, J., 24
Wheeler, L. R., 376
Whitehorn, J. C., 351

Whitehorn, J., 459
Wildenskov, H. O., 368
Wile, R., 315
Williams, R. J., 309
Williams, W. C., 376
Williams, W. S., 345, 349, 351
Wilson, R. N., 320
Windle, W. F., 371
Wing, J. K., 466, 467
Wittman, P., 93, 232
Wolberg, L. R., 169, 437, 439, 442
Wolf, K. M., 111
Wolf, S., 176
Wolfenden, J., 284
Wolff, G. E., 328, 350
Wolking, W. D., 405, 406
Wolpe, J., 66, 68, 109, 298, 446
Woodward, S., 135
Woodworth, R. S., 376
Wynne, L. C., 109

Yolles, S., 470
Youngman, W., 209
Yum, K. S., 310

Zahn, T. P., 150
Zeleny, L. D., 365
Zeller, A., 58
Ziboorg, G., 23
Zigler, E., 143, 230
Zimmermann, R. R., 119
Zubek, J. P., 114
Zubin, J., 46, 47, 48, 204

SUBJECT INDEX

See also Selected References on page 481.

abnormal behavior, symptoms, 36 ff.
  syndromes of, 44 ff.
abnormal psychology, definition of, 3
  historical background, 17 ff.
  in relation to other disciplines, 11 ff.
abnormality, classification of, 35 ff.
  definitions of, 5 ff.
  etiology of, 71 ff.
  expectancy of, 132, 134
  frequency of, 130 ff.
  incidence of, 131, 140
  multiple causes of, 71 ff.
  prevalence of, 132, 140
  socioeconomic status in, 140 ff.
abscess, brain, 331
abulia, 42
acceptance of child, 123
accident proneness, 258
acrocephaly, 357
acute brain syndromes, 325 ff.
acute depression, 194
acute mania, 198
acute schizophrenia, 229
addiction, in childhood, 398 ff.
  to alcohol, 303
  to drugs, 316 ff.
adjustment reactions, 387 ff.
adolescence, adjustment reactions of, 390–391
  behavior disorders of, 45
adrenalin, 171
advice in therapy, 449
affect, disordered, 39
  inappropriate, 41
    in schizophrenia, 214, 216
  labile, 40
affective disorders, 191 ff.
aggression, passive, 148
agitated depression, 196
agraphia, 329
alarm reaction, 90
alcoholic hallucinosis, 307
Alcoholics Anonymous, 316
alcoholism, 301 ff.
  nutritional deficiencies in, 306
  sex ratio in, 313
alexia, 329

Alzheimer's disease, 330
amaurotic idiocy, 361, 369
ambivalence, 40, 148
  in schizophrenia, 214, 216
amenorrhea, 178
amentia, 355 ff.
amnesia, 37
  hysterical, 155
amok, 135
amphetamines, 316
Amytal, 316
anal period in development, 53 ff.
anesthesia, hysterical, 36, 152
anhedonia, 104, 220
ano-genital activity, 275, 277
anorexia, 42
anorexia nervosa, 177, 178, 447–448
anoxia, 88, 342, 371
Antabuse, 315
antidepressive drugs, 208, 432
antisocial personality, 255 ff.
anxiety, 147, 150 ff.
apathy, 40, 221
aphasia, 329
approach-approach conflict, 43
approach-avoidance conflict, 43
arteriosclerosis, cerebral, 333
associations, loose, in schizophrenia, 214
astasia-abasia, 152
asthenic physique, 92
asthma, 174
ataractic drugs, 430
ataxia, 81
athletic physique, 92
atrophy of brain, 329
autism, early infantile, 395–396
autistic thinking, 38, 214, 227
autistic withdrawal, 216
automatism, 44
autonomic nervous system, 171 ff.
aversive conditioning, 315
aversive motivation in schizophrenia, 235
avoidance-avoidance conflict, 43
avoidance learning, 109
  in schizophrenia, 234

barbiturates, 316, 317, 319, 320
Beauchamp, Miss, 156
bed-wetting, 386
behavior disorder, 255
behavior modification, 445 ff.
behavior therapy, 67
behavioral observations, 417–418
Bender-Gestalt Test, 419
bestiality, 275–276, 288
Bibliography, 481 ff.
biological determinants, of abnormal behavior, 84 ff., 144
   of affective disorders, 92, 202, 203
   of alcoholism, 308 ff.
   of antisocial personality, 263–264
   of delinquency, 263–264
   of mental retardation, 366
   of neuroses, 163
   of organic brain syndromes, 341 ff.
   of psychophysiologic disorders, 182, 183
   of schizophrenias, 92, 232–234
   of sexual deviations, 97, 292
   of sociopathic personality, 263–264
birth, premature, 371
blackouts, alcoholic, 302
blocking, 38
brain syndromes, 325 ff.
   in childhood, 400
   organic, 45
brainwashing, 115
bufotenin, 316

caffeine, 316, 318
cardiovascular reaction, psychophysiologic, 173
castration anxiety, 293–294
catalepsy, 44
catastrophic reaction, 327
catatonia, 213
catatonic schizophrenia, 223 ff.
causation, categories of, 71 ff.
   hereditary, 77 ff.
   psychological, 101 ff.
   socio-cultural, 127 ff.
   summary of, 143–145
cerebral arteriosclerosis, 333
cerebral palsy, 360, 371
cerebrotonic temperament, 93, 96
character disorder, 255
child guidance clinics, 384
childhood, adjustment reactions of, 387–388
   behavior disorders of, 45, 383
   schizophrenia of, 229
child-rearing, 123
chlorpromazine, 430–431
chorea, 44
chromosome anomalies, 291–292, 370
chronic brain syndrome, 325 ff.
chronic undifferentiated schizophrenia, 229
clarification in therapy, 452
classification of abnormality, 25, 35 ff.
client-centered therapy, 444–445
cocaine, 316, 318
codeine, 316, 318
cognitive slippage, 218
colitis, 177
color-blindness, 78

coma, 327
combat fatigue, 107
communication, double-bind, 239, 240
   nonverbal, 116
community, therapeutic, 271
community approaches, effectiveness of, 470
community mental health, 465 ff.
community services, comprehensive, 468 ff.
compulsion, 44
concrete thinking, 38, 214
conditioning, classical, 101 ff.
conduct disorder, 255
confabulation, 38
conflict, 43
   psychological, 105, 106
   social, 127 ff.
   unconscious, 439
congenital factors, 78
consistency of diagnoses, 46 ff.
constitutional factors, 78, 91 ff.
conversion hysteria, 148
convulsive therapy, 432 ff.
cretinism, 87, 357, 361
crime, 255 ff.
cross-cultural studies, 134 ff.
cultural lag, 140
culture and personality, 129
cunnilingus, 277
cytomegalic inclusion disease, 370–371

decentralization of hospitals, 467
defense mechanisms, 56 ff.
deficiencies, vitamin, 87, 371
deficiency, mental, 355 ff.
déjà vu, 39
delinquency, 255 ff.
   group, 262
   in childhood, 398 ff.
deliriant drugs, 316
delirious mania, 199
delirium, 326
delirium tremens, 306–307
delusions, 39
   erotic, 248
   in depression, 197
   in schizophrenia, 218
   of grandeur, 227, 246
   of influence, 227, 247
   of persecution, 227, 246
   of reference, 227
   sexual, 248
dementia, 328
dementia praecox, 213
Demerol, 316, 319
demonology, 18, 22 ff.
denial, 60
dependence on drugs, 317
dependency, 148, 220, 221
depersonalization, 39, 197
depression, 39
   simple, 194
depressive stupor, 198
deprivation, biological, 87 ff.
   dream, 90
   emotional, 111
   maternal, 110

deprivation (*Continued*)
  oral, 116
  parental, 117, 264, 265
  psychological, 105, 110 ff.
  sensory, 113
  sleep, 88 ff.
  sociocultural, 127 ff.
desensitization, 297–298
  systematic, 445–447
determinants, summary of, 143–145
determinism, psychic, 441
development of personality, 51 ff.
deviant behavior, 4 ff.
deviation, sexual, 273 ff.
Dexedrine, 316, 319
diagnosis, consistency of, 46 ff.
direct discipline, 123
directive psychotherapy, 449
discipline, direct and indirect, 123
  indirect, 164
disintoxication, 315, 322
disorganization, social, 127, 142
disorientation, 37
displacement of affect, 58
dissociation, 28
disulfiram (Antabuse), 135
dizygotic twins, 79
dominance, maternal, 238, 239
Don Juan complex, 118
double-bind communication, 239, 240
double-blind study, 431
dream deprivation, 90
dream interpretation, 439
drug addiction, 316 ff.
drug therapy, 430 ff.
dynamic approach, 51 ff.
dyslexia, 78

echolalia, 219, 223
echopraxia, 44, 223
ectomorphic physique, 92 ff.
eczema, 180
ego-defenses, 56 ff.
elation, 39
Elavil, 208
electroconvulsive therapy, 208, 432 ff.
electroencephalogram, 414–415
electro-stimulation, experimental, 103
empiricism, development of, 17
encephalitis, 331
encopresis, 386
endocrine disorders, 341
endocrine reaction, psychophysiologic, 180
endomorphic physique, 92 ff.
enuresis, 118, 386
environmental manipulation, 460–462
epilepsy, grand mal, 334, 336
  idiopathic, 334
  in childhood, 401
  Jacksonian, 338
  petit mal, 334, 337
  psychomotor, 335–337
  symptomatic, 334–335
  treatment of, 347
epiloia, 369
epinephrine, 171

Equanil, 432
etiology, of abnormality, 71 ff.
  summary of, 143–145
euphoria, 39
evaluation, 413 ff.
excitement, catatonic, 223
exhibitionism, 275, 278 ff.
existential approach, 64 ff.
expectancy of abnormality, 132, 134
experimental neurosis, 30, 106
extinction of learning, 103, 104
extrapunitive behavior, 258, 259

families, multi-problem, 139
family constellations, 122
family therapy, 409, 456–458
fantasy, 62
fear, free-floating, 150
feeblemindedness, 355 ff.
fellatio, 277
fetishism, 286
fever therapy, 332, 348
first-admission rates, 131
fixation, 59
flagellation, 282–283
flight of ideas, 38
folie à deux, 249, 250
foster child studies, 79
  of schizophrenias, 232
free association, 29, 439
frequency of abnormality, 130 ff.
frigidity, 148, 180
frustration, 105, 109
frustration tolerance, low, 259
fugue, hysterical, 38, 155
functional psychoses, 45
Funkenstein test, 163

gargoylism, 357, 369
gastrointestinal disorders, psychophysiologic, 175 ff.
general adaptation syndrome, 90
general paralysis (paresis), 331, 348
genes, dominant and recessive, 78
genitourinary reaction, psychophysiologic, 178 ff.
geriatrics, 351
Glossary, 473 ff.
Goldstein-Scheerer Test, 419
gratification, vicarious, 266
grimacing, 224
group therapy, 455–456

habituation, 318
hallucination, 36, 85
  in schizophrenia, 218
hallucinogenic drugs, 85
hashish, 316
head-banging, 386
hebephilia, 287–288
hebephrenia, 213
hebephrenic schizophrenia, 222
hemiplegia, 333

hereditary determinants, of abnormal behavior, 78 ff., 143
  of affective disorders, 201, 202
  of alcoholism, 308–309
  of antisocial personality, 262–263
  of delinquency, 262–263
  of epilepsy, 82, 342
  of Huntington's chorea, 82
  of intelligence, 79 ff., 366 ff.
  of mental retardation, 366 ff.
  of neuroses, 83, 162, 163
  of organic brain syndromes, 342–343
  of psychophysiologic disorders, 83, 182
  of schizophrenias, 83, 231–232
  of sexual deviations, 291
  of sociopathic personality, 262–263
hermaphrodite, 294
heroin, 316
historical background of abnormal psychology, 17 ff.
home treatment, 468
homosexuality, 97, 283
hospitalization, partial, 468
hospitals, changes in, 466 ff.
  first admission rates, 131
humanitarianism, development of, 17
humors, 20
Huntington's chorea, 339, 341
hydrocephaly, 357, 360, 377
hyperesthesia, hysterical, 152
hypertelorism, 357, 369
hypertension, 83, 173
hyperthyroidism, 180
hyperventilation, 174
hypnoanalysis, 451
hypnosis, 28 ff., 153, 166, 417
  in therapy, 450
hypnotic drugs, 316
hypochondriasis, 161
hypoesthesia, hysterical, 152
hypoglycemia, 435
hypomania, 198
hypothalamus, 173
hypothyroidism, 87, 341
  congenital, 361
hysmenorrhea, 178
hysteria, 29

identification, 59, 165
  psychosexual, 294–296
idiot, 357
illusion, 36, 85
imbecile, 358
imipramine, 432
immigration, 138
impairment, intellectual, 37, 45, 220
impotence, 148, 178, 179
incest, 275–276, 288
incidence of abnormality, 131, 140
indirect discipline, 123
infancy, adjustment reaction of, 387
infections causing brain syndromes, 331
insight, 29
  in therapy, 442
institutionalism, 466
instrumental learning, 103 ff.
insulin coma treatment, 87, 434

intellectual impairment, 37, 45, 220
  tests of, 419
intellectual subnormality, 37
intelligence, disordered, 37
  subnormal, 355 ff.
  tests of, 418–419
interaction of causes, 143
interpretation, in therapy, 451
  therapeutic, 439
interview, 415 ff.
intoxication, alcoholic, 302
introjection, 59
inversion, psychosexual, 284
involuntary movements, 386
involutional melancholia, 200
isolation, 62
  social, 114, 119, 142, 234, 344–345, 351

jaundice, 371
Joint Commission on Mental Illness and Health, 468
juvenile paresis, 401

kernicterus, 371
kleptomania, 158, 159, 286
Klinefelter's syndrome, 291–292, 370
koro, 135
Korsakoff's syndrome, 307

lability of affect, 40
laboratory tests, 413–414
latah, 135
latent homosexuality, 251
latent period in development, 55 ff.
latent schizophrenia, 229
learning, 101 ff.
learning theory approach, 66 ff.
lesbianism, 283
leucotomy, 435–436
libido, 30
litigious behavior, paranoid, 248
lobotomy, 435–436
logorrhea, 44, 219
Lorr behavioral rating scale, 417–418
LSD, 86
lying, pathological, 260 ff.

manic-depressive illness, 193 ff.
manic episodes, 198 ff.
marijuana, 316, 318, 322
marital schism and skew, 238
marital status, 139
masochism, 275–276, 282–283
masturbation, 275, 276, 277
mechanisms of defense, 56 ff.
Mecholyl, 163
megalomania, 246
melancholia, involutional, 200
memory, impairment of, 37
meningioma, 338
meningitis, 331

menstrual disturbances, 178
mental deficiency, 37
mental health acts, 468
mental health movement, 465
mental retardation, 37, 45, 355 ff.
meprobamate, 316, 432
mescaline, 85, 316
mesmerism, 28
mesomorphic physique, 92 ff.
metabolic disorders, 341
methadone, 316
Metrazol therapy, 432
microcephaly, 357, 360, 369
migraine, 173
milieu therapy, 460–462
Miltown, 432
mind-body problem, 13
minimal brain dysfunction, 401
Minnesota Multiphasic Personality Inventory, 420
misidentification, 39
mobility, residential (horizontal), 139, 142
    social (vertical), 141, 142
modern trends in treatment, 465 ff.
mongolism, 357, 359, 370
monozygotic twins, 79
moral insanity, 256
moron, 358, 362
morphine, 316
motivation, disordered, 41
multiple causes of abnormality, 71 ff.
multiple diagnoses, 45
multiple personality (hysterical), 156
mutism, 44
myxedema, 87

nail-biting, 386
narcissism, 43
    in paranoid states, 246
    in schizophrenia, 234
narcotic drugs, 316
naturalism, development of, 17
negativism, 44, 223
Nembutal, 316, 319
neologisms, 44, 216
neoplasm of brain, 338
neurasthenia, 161
neurodermatitis, 180
neurosis(es), 45, 147 ff.
    anxiety, 150
    conversion hysteria, 151 ff.
    depressive, 160 ff.
    dissociative hysteria, 154 ff.
    experimental, 106
    in childhood, 391 ff.
    obsessive-compulsive, 158 ff.
    phobic, 157 ff.
    symptom, 148 ff.
    war, 107
neurotic personality with drug addiction, 320
nicotine, 316, 318
    non-directive psychotherapy, 449
nonverbal communication, 116
normal personality development, 51 ff.
normal probability curve, 356
normalcy, definitions of, 6 ff.
nosology, 25 ff.

noxious agents, 85 ff.
nuclear schizophrenia, 230
nutritional deficiencies in alcoholism, 306
nutritional disorders, 341
nymphomania, 273, 276

obscenity, 289, 291
observations, behavioral, 417–418
obsession, 38
Oedipal complex, 55
Oedipal relationship, 288
oligophrenia, 355 ff.
operant conditioning in therapy, 447
opium, 316
oral stage in development, 52 ff.
organ neurosis, 170
organic brain syndrome(s), 45, 325 ff.
    in childhood, 400
oro-genital activity, 275, 277
outcome of psychotherapy, 459
overgratification, 110
overinclusive thinking, 215
overindulgence, 265
overprotection, 123, 164, 236, 385

pan-anxiety in schizophrenia, 220, 229
paralogical thinking, 214, 227
paralysis, general (paresis), 331, 348
    hysterical, 152
paranoia, 245
paranoid personality, 251
paranoid schizophrenia, 227 ff.
paranoid states, 245 ff.
paraphilia, 273 ff.
parasympathetic nervous system, 171 ff.
parental behavior, inconsistent, 265
paresis, 331, 348
    juvenile, 401
paresthesia, hysterical, 152
Parnate, 208
passive aggression, 148
pederasty, 277, 288
pedophilia, 286, 287
peeping Tom, 277
pellagra, 87
penicillin, 348
Pentothal, 417
peptic ulcer, 83, 106, 175, 176
perception, disorders of, 36
perfectionism, 123, 237
peripheral schizophrenia, 230
persecution complex, 228, 248
personality, antisocial, 255 ff.
    development of, 51 ff.
    disorders of, 45
    neurotic, 148 ff., 257
    paranoid, 251
    premorbid, 230
    psychopathic, 255 ff.
    schizoid, 236
    sociopathic, 255 ff.
personality tests, 420
persuasion in therapy, 450
perversion, sexual, 273 ff.

peyote, 316
phallic period in development, 54 ff.
phenothiazine drugs, 430
phenylketonuria (PKU), 361, 369, 377
phenylthiocarbamide (PTC), 78
Phillips Scale, 230
phobia, 38
  school, 384, 392–394
physical examination, 414
physiological responses in anger and fear, 170
physique, 92
pica, 400
Pick's disease, 330, 331
placebo, 430
polygenic inheritance, 78 ff.
pornography, 289, 291
postencephalitic syndrome, 401
postmature birth, 371
postpartum depression, 193
posturing, 223, 224
premature birth, 371
premorbid personality in schizophrenia, 230
presenile dementia, 329 ff.
prevalence of abnormality, 132, 140
primary process thinking, 216
primary sociopath, 266
primary symptoms of impairment, 328
primary symptoms of schizophrenia, 214 ff.
problem families, 139
process schizophrenia, 230
projection, 59, 227, 250 ff.
projective tests, 420
promiscuity, 257, 275, 276, 277
prophecy, self-fulfilling, 246
prostitution, 276, 289
pseudo-community, paranoid, 246
pseudo-homosexuality, 283
pseudo-neurotic schizophrenia, 229
pseudo-psychopathic schizophrenia, 229
pseudo-retardation, 362, 396
psilocybin, 316
psychoanalysis, 29 ff., 51 ff., 438 ff.
  in antisocial personality, 270
  in neuroses, 167
  in psychophysiologic disorders, 188
  in schizophrenias, 242
  in sexual deviations, 297
psychodynamics, 51 ff.
psychological determinants, of abnormal behavior, 101 ff., 144
  of affective disorders, 203 ff.
  of alcoholism, 310 ff.
  of antisocial personality, 264 ff.
  of delinquency, 116, 264 ff., 406
  of drug addiction, 321
  of mental retardation, 372 ff.
  of neuroses, 163 ff.
  of paranoid states, 250 ff.
  of psychophysiologic disorders, 184 ff.
  of schizophrenias, 234 ff.
  of sexual deviations, 292 ff.
  of sociopathic personality, 264 ff.
psychological tests, 418 ff.
psychoneurosis. See *neurosis.*
psychoneurotic disorders, 147 ff.
psychopathic personality, 255 ff.
psychophysiologic disorders, 45, 169 ff.
psychoses, functional, 45
  in childhood, 394 ff.

psychosexual development, 51 ff.
psychosomatic disorders, 170
psychosurgery, 435 ff.
psychotherapeutic relationship, 448–449
psychotherapy, 437 ff.
  changes during, 453–454, 458 ff.
  effectiveness of, 458 ff.
  in affective disorders, 208
  in alcoholism, 315
  in childhood disorders, 408
  in delinquency, 270–271
  in drug addiction, 322–323
  in mental retardation, 379
  in neuroses, 166, 167
  in paranoid states, 252
  in psychophysiologic disorders, 188
  in schizophrenias, 242, 243
  in sexual deviations, 297–298
  in sociopathic personality, 270–271
  studies of, 453–454, 458 ff.
  techniques of, 449 ff.
psychotomimetic drugs, 85
public education programs, 465
punishment, 104, 105
  need for, 258, 266, 275
pyknic physique, 92
pyknolepsy, 401
pyromania, 158, 286

racial origin, 138
rape, 275–276
  statutory, 288
rationalization, 61
reaction formation, 58
reactive schizophrenia, 230
reading problems, 384, 402
reassurance in therapy, 451
reconditioning therapy, 297, 315
References, 481 ff.
reflection in therapy, 452
reflex, conditioned, 102
regression, 59, 220, 234, 293
reinforcement of learning, 103, 104
rejection, 110, 123, 236, 264, 265
  parental, 385
relationship, psychotherapeutic, 448–449
reliability of diagnoses, 46 ff.
repression, 28, 57
residence, urban vs. rural, 138
residential mobility, 139
residual schizophrenia, 229
resistance in therapy, 439
respiratory disorders, psychophysiologic, 174
restitutional symptoms, 220
retardation, mental, 37, 45, 355 ff.
retarded depression, 195
retirement, 351
Rorschach Test, 420–421
rubella, 370

sadism, 275–276, 281–282
sadomasochism, 283
satyriasis, 273, 276
schism, marital, 238
schizoid personality, 236

schizophrenia, 213
 acute, 229
 catatonic, 223 ff.
 childhood, 229, 395
 chronic undifferentiated, 229
 hebephrenic, 222
 latent, 229
 nuclear, 230
 paranoid, 227 ff.
 peripheral, 230
 premorbid personality in, 230
 primary symptoms of, 214 ff.
 process, 230
 pseudo-neurotic, 229
 pseudo-psychopathic, 229
 reactive, 230
 residual, 229
 secondary symptoms of, 218 ff.
 simple, 221
 twin studies in, 231, 232
 undifferentiated, 229
schizophrenogenic mother, 237
school phobia, 384, 392–394
sclerosis, tuberous, 369
scoptophilia, 277
Seconal, 316, 319
secondary process thinking, 216
secondary symptoms of schizophrenia, 218 ff.
sedative drugs, 316, 432
seizures, hysterical, 152
self-esteem, 147
self-fulfilling prophecy, 246
senile dementia, 329 ff.
sensation, disorders of, 36
sex-linked inheritance, 78 ff.
sex ratio in alcoholism, 313
sex-typing, 294–295
sexual deviation, 273 ff.
sexual ignorance, 164
shell shock, 107
sibling rivalry, 123
simple depression, 194
simple schizophrenia, 221
situational disturbances, 45
skew, marital, 238
skin disorders, psychophysiologic, 180, 181
sleep deprivation, 88 ff.
social isolation, 114, 119, 142, 234, 344–345, 351
socialization, 116
society, open vs. closed, 128
socioeconomic status and abnormality, 140 ff.
sociopathic personality, 255 ff.
 with alcoholism, 312, 313
 with drug addiction, 319
Sodium Amytal, 417
sodomy, 277
solitary confinement, 114
somatic therapy, 429 ff.
somatization reaction, 170
somatotonic temperament, 93, 96
somnambulism, 156
speech, disordered, 43
stammering, 43
status, ascribed vs. achieved, 128
stereotypy, 44
sterilization, compulsory, 380
stimulant drugs, 316
stimulus-generalization, 102

stress, biological, 87 ff.
 psychological, 105 ff.
 sociocultural, 127 ff.
stroke, 333
studies of psychotherapy, 453–454, 458 ff.
stupor, 44
 catatonic, 223
 organic, 327
stuttering, 43
sublimation, 58
subnormality, mental, 355 ff.
suggestibility in hysteria, 153
suggestion in therapy, 450
suicidal gestures and threats, 259
suicide, 130, 139, 197, 206
 in childhood, 395
suicide prevention, 209, 210
superego defect, 257 ff., 266
surgery, multiple, 149
sympathectomy, 187
sympathetic nervous system, 171 ff.
symptom neuroses, 148 ff.
syndromes, brain, 325 ff.
syphilis, 331–333, 348
 congenital, 370, 377

task setting in therapy, 449
Tay-Sachs disease, 361
techniques of psychotherapy, 449 ff.
technological change, 140
temperament, 93, 96
terminology, 10. See also *Glossary,* 473 ff.
tests, Bender-Gestalt, 419
 Goldstein-Scheerer, 419
 intellectual impairment, 419
 intelligence, 418–419
 laboratory, 413–414
 Minnesota Multiphasic, 420
 personality, 420
 projective, 420
 psychological, 418 ff.
 Rorschach, 420–421
 Shipley-Hartford, 419
 Thematic Apperception, 421
 vocational, 422
 Wassermann, 332
 Wechsler-Bellevue, 418
Thematic Apperception Test, 421
therapeutic community, 271, 461
therapy, 429 ff.
 behavior modification, 445
 client-centered, 444–445
 electroconvulsive, 432 ff.
 in affective disorders, 208
 in alcoholism, 315–316
 in antisocial personality, 269–271
 in childhood disorders, 407
 in delinquency, 269–271
 in drug addiction, 322–323
 in mental retardation, 377 ff.
 in neuroses, 166, 167
 in organic brain syndromes, 346 ff.
 in paranoid states, 252
 in psychophysiologic disorders, 187, 188
 in schizophrenias, 241 ff.
 in sexual deviations, 296–298

therapy (*Continued*)
  in sociopathic personality, 269–271
  with children, 454
·thinking, autistic, 38
  concrete, 38
  disordered, 37
three wishes (projective test), 228
thumb-sucking, 386
thyroid disorders, 341
tic, 44, 386
  hysterical, 152
Tofranil, 208, 432
tolerance, alcohol, 303
  for drugs, 317
toxoplasmosis, 370–371
tranquilizing drugs, 316, 430
transference, 439, 441
transient situational disturbances, 45
trans-sexualism, 279, 281
transvestism, 275, 279 ff.
treatment, 429 ff.
  in affective disorders, 208 ff.
  in alcoholism, 315–316
  in antisocial personality, 269–271
  in delinquency, 269–271
  in disorders of childhood, 407
  in drug addiction, 322–323
  in mental retardation, 377
  in neuroses, 166, 167
  in organic brain syndromes, 346 ff.
  in paranoid states, 252
  in psychophysiologic disorders, 187, 188
  in schizophrenias, 241 ff.
  in sexual deviations, 296–298
  in sociopathic personality, 269–271
tremor, 44
  hysterical, 152
trephining, 18
"truth serum," 417
tuberous sclerosis, 369
tumor of brain, 338
Turner's syndrome, 291–292, 370
twin studies, 79 ff.
  in affective disorders, 201–202
  in alcoholism, 308–309
  in epilepsy, 342
  in schizophrenia, 231, 232
  in senile psychoses, 343

ulcer, peptic, 83, 106, 175, 176
ulcerative colitis, 177
uncertainty, 105, 106
unconscious, 29
underachievement, 221, 236
undifferentiated schizophrenia, 229
undoing, 62
unemployment, 127, 138, 139
unsocialized aggressive reaction, 388
urinary disturbances, 178

vicarious gratification, 266
victim of sexual offenses, 291
vigilance, 105, 106
Vineland Social Maturity Scale, 378
viscerotonic temperament, 93, 96
vitamin deficiencies, 87, 371
  in alcoholism, 306
vocational tests, 422
voodoo death, 135
voyeurism, 275, 277 ff.

war, 127, 138
war neuroses, 107
Wassermann test, 332
waxy flexibility, 44, 223
Wechsler-Bellevue Test, 418
Wernicke's syndrome, 307
witchcraft, 19, 22 ff., 135
withdrawal drug, psychoses in, 317
  seizures, 317
  symptoms, 317
witigo, 135
working through, therapeutic, 443

zoophilia, 288
zygosity, determination of, 79

INDEX CASE -
CO-TWIN -
ETIOLOGY - the causes of disease
ATROPHY -
CONCORDANCE - both dev. symptoms under study.

TUNNEL VISION -
VICERAL -
multiple sclerosis
FREE FLOATING -

193 - post-partum ?
P 230 - poor + good premorbid
P184

BIC PENS - (no)
TOILET PAPER
WORM (TEQUILLA)

l reappraisal
J Clin Exp Psychop.
1954, 1 15 219 -33

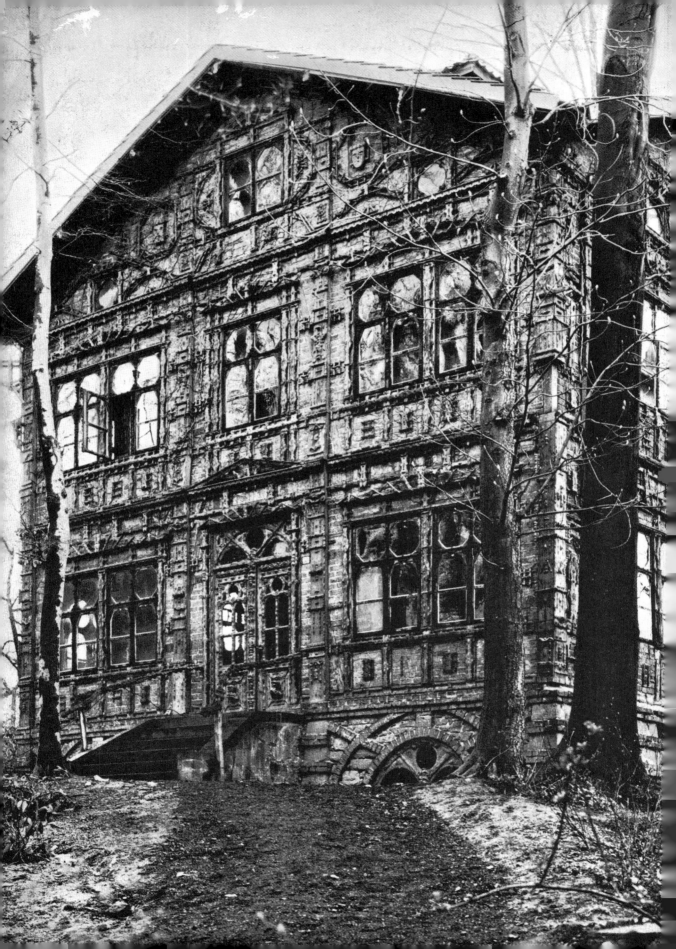